Causes, Diagnosis and Treatment of Arthritis

Causes, Diagnosis and Treatment of Arthritis

Edited by Mary Kellar

hayle medical
New York

Hayle Medical,
750 Third Avenue, 9th Floor,
New York, NY 10017, USA

Visit us on the World Wide Web at:
www.haylemedical.com

ISBN: 978-1-63241-446-5

The publisher's policy is to use permanent paper from mills that operate a sustainable forestry policy. Furthermore, the publisher ensures that the text paper and cover boards used have met acceptable environmental accreditation standards.

Printed in China.

Cataloging-in-Publication Data

Causes, diagnosis and treatment of arthritis / edited by Mary Kellar.
p. cm.
Includes bibliographical references and index.
ISBN 978-1-63241-446-5
1. Arthritis. 2. Rheumatoid arthritis. 3. Arthritis--Diagnosis. 4. Arthritis--Treatment. I. Kellar, Mary.

RC933 .C38 2017
616.722--dc23

Table of Contents

Preface

Over the recent decade, advancements and applications have progressed exponentially. This has led to the increased interest in this field and projects are being conducted to enhance knowledge. The main objective of this book is to present some of the critical challenges and provide insights into possible solutions. This book will answer the varied questions that arise in the field and also provide an increased scope for furthering studies.

Arthritis is a disorder that affects the joints of the human body. This book on arthritis deals with the causes and symptoms of this medical condition. A common treatment for arthritis patients includes pain management as well as various physical therapy techniques. This field consists of interventional and surgical techniques that can treat those who suffer from arthritis. This book on arthritis is a collective contribution of a renowned group of international experts. It aims to equip students and experts with the advanced topics and upcoming concepts in this area. This book is a compilation of chapters that discuss the most vital concepts and emerging trends in the field of arthritis. It is a resource guide for experts as well as students.

I hope that this book, with its visionary approach, will be a valuable addition and will promote interest among readers. Each of the authors has provided their extraordinary competence in their specific fields by providing different perspectives as they come from diverse nations and regions. I thank them for their contributions.

Editor

A Systematic Critical Appraisal of Non-Pharmacological Management of Rheumatoid Arthritis with Appraisal of Guidelines for Research and Evaluation II

Lucie Brosseau[1]*, Prinon Rahman[2], Stéphane Poitras[1], Karine Toupin-April[3], Gail Paterson[5], Christine Smith[1], Judy King[1], Lynn Casimiro[1,4], Gino De Angelis[1], Laurianne Loew[1], Sabrina Cavallo[7], Jessica Mc Ewan[6]

1 School of Rehabilitation Sciences, Faculty of Health Sciences, University of Ottawa, Ottawa, Ontario, Canada, **2** Department of Community Health and Epidemiology, Dalhousie University, Halifax, Nova Scotia, Canada, **3** Centre for Global Health, Institute of Population Health, Ottawa, Ontario, Canada, **4** Department of Academic Affairs, Montfort Hospital, Ottawa, Ontario, Canada, **5** The Arthritis Society, Ottawa, Ontario, Canada, **6** University of Ottawa Library, Ottawa, Ontario, Canada, **7** École de Santé Publique, Université de Montréal, Montréal, Quebec, Canada

Abstract

Clinical practice guidelines (CPGs) have been developed to summarize evidence about the management of rheumatoid arthritis (RA) and facilitate the uptake of evidence-based knowledge by consumers, health professionals, health administrators and policy makers. The objectives of this review was to assess the quality of CPGS on non-pharmacological management of RA with a standardized and validated instrument - the Appraisal of Guidelines for Research and Evaluation (AGREE II) tool and summarize the key recommendations from these CPGs. Scientific literature databases from 2001 to 2013 were systematically searched and a total of 13 CPGs for RA was identified. Only a minority of AGREE II domains were effectively addressed by the CPGS. Scope and purpose was effectively addressed in 10 out of 13 CPGs, stakeholder involvement in 11 CPGs, rigor of development in 6 CPGs, clarity/presentation in 9 CPGs, editorial independence in 1 CPGs, and applicability in none of the CPGs. The overall quality of the included CPGs according to the 7-point AGREE II scoring system was 4.8 ± 1.04. Patient education/self-management, aerobic, dynamic and stretching exercises were the commonly recommended for the non-pharmacological management of RA by the high-quality CPGs. The general clinical management recommendations tended to be similar among high-quality CPGs. Non-pharmacological management interventions were superficially addressed in more than half of the selected CPGs. CPGs creators should use the AGREE II criteria when developing guidelines. Innovative and effective methods of CPGs implementation to users are needed to ultimately enhance the quality of life of arthritic individuals. In addition, it was difficult to establish between strongly recommended, recommended and weakly recommended, as there is no consensus between the strength of the recommendations between the appraised CPGs.

Editor: Adrian V. Hernandez, Universidad Peruana de Ciencias Aplicadas (UPC), Peru

Funding: The authors are thankful for the financial support of the Canadian Institutes of Health Research's (CIHR) Community Outreach Program for Non-Governmental Organizations. This project was funded by the CIHR Institute of Musculoskeletal Health and Arthritis Community Outreach Grant: #ICS-123828. The funders had no role in study design, data collection and analysis, decision to publish, or preparation of the manuscript.

Competing Interests: LB was involved in the development of the series of Ottawa Panel CPGs, but did not review the quality of her own CPGs to avoid possible competing interests. Also, other authors (LC, GD, LL, SP, JK, JM) were involved in the Ottawa panel CPGs, but not in the evaluation of the quality of CPGs in the actual review. To ensure objectivity of the discussion, the remaining authors were not involved in any of the CPGs and were involved in the discussion of results and the review of the manuscript prior to submission (PR, GP, CS & SC). There are no patents, products in development or marketed products to declare. This does not alter the authors' adherence to all the PLOS ONE policies on sharing data and materials.

* E-mail: Lucie.Brosseau@uottawa.ca

Introduction

Rheumatoid arthritis (RA) is an autoimmune pathology characterised by inflammation at the joints and in tissues surrounding other organs, which is usually accompanied by severe pain [1]. The prevalence of RA in the US in 2007 was about 1.5 million adults [2], and women were affected three times more than men [3]. The incidence is highly variable between nations, but is typically around 40 cases per 100,000 [4]. RA carries a great economic impact due to higher incidence in adults during their peak productivity years and the fact that long term treatment is required [5]. The estimated medical expenses for arthritis and rheumatism (excluding cost of time lost from paid or unpaid work) were estimated to be between $1.7 billion and $2.5 billion [6].

Evidence-based practice (EBP) is defined as the application and integration of the best available research evidence with clinical expertise and patient values by health care professionals delivering health care services [7]. There is a need for health professionals to include the best evidence-based practice (EBP) in order to provide optimal care to their patients [8]. EBP can include the use of clinical practice guidelines (CPGs) which are "systematically developed statements to guide the daily practice of health professionals about optimal health care for specific clinical circumstances" [9].

Health professionals working in rheumatology should appraise CPGs in their daily practice [10] in order to make the best informed decision about the optimal intervention for patient care. The Appraisal of Guidelines for Research and Evaluation II (AGREE II) (www.agreetrust.org) is an updated validated instrument that assesses the methodological quality of CPGs to ensure their high quality [11–13].

Numerous CPGs exist in the scientific literature, especially in the field of rheumatology. The CPG content can vary from a broad spectrum of recommendations including diagnosis, pharmacological and non-pharmacological management, surgery, multidisciplinary care, service delivery, or management of co-morbid conditions [14]. In the past, only one critical appraisal using AGREE I instrument has been conducted on CPGs available for the non-pharmacological management of RA [15]. Although the AGREE II instrument has been used to assess the quality of some CPGs for the management of osteoarthritis [10,16–17], the quality of non-pharmacological CPGs for the management of RA have not been assessed with this updated instrument. Therefore, there is a need to appraise non-pharmacological CPGs for RA – so that health care providers can identify which CPGs in RA are high-quality and reliable to use in their practice. To our knowledge, no publications have used AGREE II to appraise CPGs for RA before this paper. The objectives of this critical appraisal review were: 1) to systematically identify CPGs for the non-pharmacological management of RA found in the scientific literature for use by multidisciplinary healthcare providers; 2) assess the quality of the selected CPGs using the AGREE II instrument and 3) identify and compare the non-pharmacological recommendations from the selected CPGs.

Methodology

The PRISMA statement [18] was used to report this systematic review (Checklist S1) and the Cochrane methodology (www.cochrane.org) [19] was used to identify, select and analyze the data.

Systematic Search and Selection of CPGs

A librarian (JM) used specific key words to complete a systematic literature search (Appendix S1) in the following databases: AMED, CINHAL, Medline, and Embase (Figure S1). A hand search was also performed with existing guideline inventories such as PEDro (http://www.pedro.fhs.usyd.edu.au/index.html) [20], the National Guideline Clearinghouse (http://www.guideline.gov/) [21], Guideline International Network (http://www.g-i-n.net/) [22], Turning Research into Practice (TRIP) (http://www.tripdatabase.com/) [23] and by searching the reference lists of the selected CPGs. Two trained research assistants followed the selection criteria described in appendix S2, to identify and select CPGs that considered non-pharmacological management of RA for quality appraisal. CPGs which contained at least one recommendation related to the non-pharmacological management of RA, used a systematic review to identify and grading systems to evaluate the evidence were included. In addition, CPGs that were published before 2001 and written in a language other than English were not considered. Ethics approval was not required as this is a systematic literature review.

Evaluation of the CPG Quality

The AGREE II instrument is a CPG appraisal instrument consisting of 23 items across six domains: 1) scope and purpose; 2) stakeholder involvement; 3) rigour of development; 4) clarity and presentation; 5) applicability; and 6) editorial independence. Each item is scored with a 7-point scoring system. If a CPG fulfilled none of the criteria for an item, it is graded with a 1, but if all the criteria are met and presented in good quality a grade of 7 is assigned. The purpose of this instrument is to provide a framework to: 1) assess the quality of guidelines; 2) provide a methodological strategy for the development of guidelines; and 3) provide what information should be reported in the guidelines (http://agree.machealth.ca/players/open/index.html) [24].

Three evaluators were trained over two months with the AGREE II instrument using the tutorial found on its website (http://agree.machealth.ca/players/open/index.html) [24]. A senior research assistant with experience with AGREE II, one of the instrument's developers, and the director of the Cochrane Effective Practice and Organization of Care and Cochrane Collaboration group were available to provide assistance with evaluating the CPGs when necessary.

Two pairs of experienced evaluators independently assessed the selected CPGs with the AGREE II instrument and to prevent a potential information bias a third experienced evaluator was involved when a co-author of the present review was also a co-creator of an included CPG. A standardised electronic form found on the AGREE II website was used to compile the data (www.agreetrust.org) [11]. A score between one and seven was assigned depending on whether the items met the criteria or considerations, and the completeness and quality of reporting. Some of the AGREE II items were not relevant to the guidelines assessed and because AGREE II does not include a 'not applicable' response item in the scale these items was given a score of one. After completing the appraisal of all 23 items, each appraiser provided an overall quality assessment score out of 7 on the CPG and stated whether they 1) recommend the CPG for practice 2) recommend the CPG for practice but with modifications or 3) do not recommend the CPG for practice (p. 10 http://www.agreetrust.org/wp-content/uploads/2013/06/AGREE_II_Users_Manual_and_23-item_Instrument_ENGLISH.pdf). According to the AGREE II user manual (www.agreetrust.org), the overall quality assessment requires the user to make a judgment about the quality of the CPG, taking into account that the potential bias of the guidelines has been adequately addressed and the recommendations are both internally and externally valid and feasible for practice [12–13].

Non-pharmacological Interventions of RA

In addition to assessing the methodological quality, all the non-pharmacological interventions assessed in the included CPGs were compiled with the strength of the recommendations (Table S1). Standardised categories were created for equal comparison of the strength of recommendations across CPGs. They were: 1) strongly recommended; 2) recommended; 3) weak evidence; and 4) insufficient evidence (Table S1). The categories took into consideration that CPGs had different scoring systems such that any recommendation was put in an equivalent category than it had in the original CPG. A "strongly recommended" grade was assigned to the highest CPG grading that would include one or more high-quality randomised controlled trials (RCT). A "recommended" grade was assigned when a grading had one or more controlled clinical trials (CCTs) or a lower quality RCT; this grade signifies that the intervention is still reliable to guide practice most of the time. Strong clinical or expert opinions founded on current practice are graded as "weak evidence" and should be applied with caution. If scientific evidence is lacking or there are conflicting results that have not been supported by clinical or expert opinion, it was given a grade of "insufficient evidence".

Data Analysis

The AGREE II instrument was used for the broad appraisal of the quality of CPGs. The quality score of each CPG was calculated for each of the AGREE II domains. Domain scores were calculated by summing up all the scores of the individual items and calculating the total as a percentage of the maximum possible score for that domain.

The scaled domain score:

(Obtained score- Minimum possible score)/(Maximum possible score).

Maximum possible score = 7 (strongly agree) × 3 (items) × 2 (appraisers).

Minimum possible score = 1 (strongly disagree) × 3 (items) × 2 (appraisers).

The scaled domain score were obtained by calculating the mean of the 2 evaluators' scores as shown in the AGREE II user manual (www.agreetrust.org) [11]. The two evaluators used the concordance calculator developed by McMaster University (http://fhswedge.csu.mcmaster.ca/cepftp/qasite/AGREEIIRaterConcordanceCalculator.html) [25] to obtain accurate quality ratings for each domain of the AGREE II criteria Items scores were discussed by the two reviewers when large scoring discrepancies (≤3 points difference in the score assigned by the appraisers to the same item) or if the individual item scores of the two reviewers are greater than or equal 1.5SD from the mean for each of the domain. The purpose of the discussion was to resolve the discrepancies in scoring by consensus between the two raters.

Identifying High Quality Guidelines

The AGREE II consortium has not set a minimum or maximum range for the domain quality and this makes it difficult to distinguish between high and low CPGs. Therefore the criteria of previous critical appraisals using the AGREE I [10,15,26–28] were used with the updated AGREE II instrument to identify and recommend high quality guidelines. Domain scores ≥60% is considered effectively addressed. A guideline is considered high quality and recommended if it effectively targets at least 3 out of the 6 domains including rigour of development (domain 3).

Inter-rater Reliability Study

To ensure a high inter-rater reliability between the two appraisers who had equal training, an intra-class coefficient (ICC) based on ANOVA was calculated in SPSS (Version 20) [28]. The sub-total for the item scores in each domain obtained by one evaluator were compared with those rated by the second evaluator. This statistical procedure was performed after the consensus process explained above.

Descriptive Analysis

A scatterplot was conducted on excel 2013 plotting the overall quality assessment scores of each included CPG and the year it was published. This additional analysis was conducted to ascertain if the quality of CPGs improved over time.

Results

Of the 1136 citations systematically searched, duplicates were eliminated leaving 827 residual citations for title and abstract review (Figure S1). Based on the title and abstract, 811 citations were subsequently excluded because they did not address a CPG related to non-pharmacological management of RA and twelve CPGs were included (Figure S1). One additional CPG was identified and included after consulting the reference list of the included publications (Figure S1).

Based on the selection criteria (Appendix S2) a total of thirteen CPGs on the non-pharmacological management of RA [30–44] were retrieved by the two trained evaluators (Figure S1).

Six CPGs were developed for the early stage RA (first two years from the onset) [30–31,33,35,43,44] and the residual CPGs (n = 7) were more general in terms of the evolution of RA [31,33,35–39]. Three separate guidelines and an accompanying online guideline aid [41] were developed by the Ottawa Panel, but as the guideline development process was identical for all three guidelines they were evaluated as one. The 13 CPGs can be divided into two categories: general management [30–35,37,41–42] and non-pharmacological management of RA [34–36,38–42] (see Table 1).

Evaluation of Selected CPGs

The quality assessments of the CPGs based on the AGREE II scores are presented in Table 2 and Appendix S3 presents the individual item scores for each domain graded by the two evaluators for the six domains. Based on the quality scores from the AGREE II, 6 [34,36,38–42] out of the 13 CPGs are considered high quality CPGs. All six CPGs adequately addressed (≥60%) domain 3: rigour of development and 2 or more additional domains. The overall quality for these six CPGs ranged from 5 to 6.5 out of 7 (see table 2). The majority of the CPGs effectively addressed domain 1, 2 and 4 with a mean quality score of 70% ±42%, 71% ±26% and 64.0% ±28% respectively. Conversely, domain 3, 5 and 6 were poorly addressed by the majority of the guidelines. All three domains had a low mean quality score (<60%) of 52.4%±23%, 18.5%±35% and 38.3%±23%.

According to the number of domains effectively addressed (Table 2) and overall assessment (Appendix S3), 6 CPGs [34,36,38–42,36] are recommended, 6 CPGs [30–32,35,37,44] are recommended but with modifications and 1 CPG [33] is not recommended for practice by the evaluators.

Non-pharmacological Recommendations for the Management of RA

Table S1 presents specific non-pharmacological recommendations cited in the selected CPGs for the management of RA. The strength of the recommendations for each intervention was provided by the developers of the included CPGs [30–44] including the People Getting a Grip on Arthritis Program (PGRIP) [42] based on the Ottawa Panel CPGs [39–41] is also provided. The recommendations formulated by these CPGs were categorized by alphabetical order: 1) electrotherapy; 2) other intervention; 3) team approaches; 4) therapeutic exercises; and 5) weight management. Generally speaking, the strength of the recommendations varied largely amongst the 13 CPGs (Table S1). All CPGs failed to mention whether these non-pharmacological recommendations were contraindicated or represented harms in the management of RA.

Electrotherapy. CPGs which considered electrotherapy for RA focus on electrical stimulation of muscle, TENS, Low Intensity Laser Therapy (LILT) and therapeutic ultrasound. Large discrepancies on the strength of recommendations existed for TENS, LILT and therapeutic ultrasound. For these particular electrotherapeutic modalities, the recommendations ranged from insufficient evidence to a strong recommended. Amongst the thirteen CPGs, four CPGs [36,38–42] found insufficient evidence to recommend electrical stimulation of muscle. Both high and low frequency TENS were recommended by the NICE guidelines and strongly recommended by the Ottawa Panel Guidelines [37,41]. The Ottawa Panel guideline was the only non-pharmacological CPGs which strongly recommended TENS, Low Level Laser

Table 1. Guidelines that considered pharmacological and non-pharmacological interventions.

Guidelines that considered pharmacological+non-pharmacological interventions	Guidelines that only considered non-pharmacological interventions.
ACR [30]	Forrestier et al. [34]
BSR [31]	Gossec et al. [35]
BSR [32]	Hurkman et al. [36]
EULAR [33]	Ottawa Panel [38–42]
NICE [37]	
RACGP [43]	
SIGN [44]	

ACR: American College of Rheumatology, BSR: British society of rheumatology; EULAR: The European League against rheumatism; NICE: National Institute for health and Clinical Excellence; SIGN: Scottish Intercollegiate Guidelines Network.

Therapy and therapeutic ultrasound. The Remaining nine CPGs either found insufficient evidence to recommend any of the four modalities in electrotherapy or these modalities were not applicable to the CPG.

Other therapies. A larger variety of other interventions were also assessed. These non-pharmacological interventions included acupuncture, assistive devices, balneotherapy, complementary and alternative therapies, energy conservation, foot orthoses and insoles, heat therapy, cryotherapy, hydrotherapy, joint protection, paraffin wax application combined with or without exercises, patient education and splinting.

The 13 CPGs [30–44] recognised that acupuncture, assistive devices, heat therapy/cryotherapy provided either insufficient evidence or was weakly recommended. Balneotherapy [33], complementary and alternative therapies [43], energy conservation [30], hydrotherapy [33], and paraffin wax application alone [37], Paraffin wax application combined with or without exercises is either recommended or strongly recommended by 1 CPG [41].

Six out of the thirteen CPGs either recommended or strongly recommended "joint protection and splinting" [30,32,36–43] and foot orthoses and insoles were recommended by four CPGs [31,35,40,44]. Joint protection was recommended or strongly recommended by seven CPGs [30,32,40,43]. Patient education/self-management was strongly recommended or recommended by 10 CPGs [30–34,36–42] and the remaining 3 CPGs [35,43–44] found weak to insufficient evidence. Splinting was recommended or strongly recommended by two CPGs [39,45].

Team approach. All CPGs [30–34,37,44] that assessed Multidisciplinary Team Approach in the management of RA unanimously recommended its use. These CPGs alternatively either weakly recommended or recommended the representation of several professions to be part of the team (i.e. Nutrition, Medicine, Nursing, Occupational Therapy, Podiatry/Chiropodiatry, Pharmacy, Physiotherapy, Psychology, Social Work).

Therapeutic exercises. Aerobic exercises was either recommended or strongly recommended by 12 of the 13 CPGs [30–42,44] and dynamic exercises were strongly recommended or recommended by all 13 [30–44] CPGs. Strengthening exercises and whole body exercises were recommended by 12 [30–42,44]. Stretching was cited and recommended by only one CPG [37]. Two CPGs [38,44,] strongly recommended specific low intensity exercises in the management of RA.

Weight management. There was a large variation regarding the strength of recommendations for weight management in RA for the 6 CPGs that assessed this intervention [33–35,37,43–44]. One CPG [43] either strongly recommended or recommended diet, diet supplement and diet combined with physical activity, diet supplement and diet alone for the management of RA. Another CPG [44] found evidence to recommend control of weight and diet for weight management.

Inter-rater Reliability Study

The AGREE II scores exhibited an overall very good inter-rater reliability with an ICCs values ranging from 0.91 to 0.95 (high reliability) depending on the domain assessed (Table 3). The high ICC scores confirm that the results obtained between the two evaluators are highly reliable (Table 3).

Descriptive Analysis

Based on the overall quality scores out of 7 (figure S2) there is an improvement from the earliest published CPG ACR [30] to the CPGs published 11 years later such as Hurkman et al. 2011 [36], Ottawa Panel 2011 [40] and SIGN 2011 [44]. However the results from figure S2 illustrates that the quality of CPGs does not improve overtime, Eular (2007) [33] and NICE (2009) [37] received lower quality scores compared to Ottawa Panel [2004] guidelines which was published earlier in 2004.

Discussion

This systematic review identified a total of 13 CPGs, of which 7 were more general and comprised a larger proportion of pharmacological compared to non-pharmacological recommendations [30–33,37,43–44]. Only 6 CPGs were entirely devoted to non-pharmacological interventions for RA [34–36,38–43]. Based on the AGREE II quality scoring instrument 6 CPGs [34,36,38–43] were considered high quality CPGs (adequately addressed rigor of development >60% in addition to addressing two or more domains effectively) and recommended for the non-pharmacological management of RA and the remaining CPGs were recommended for practice but with modifications. The majority of the 13 CPGs [30–44] recommended that non-pharmacological interventions be combined with pharmacological interventions in the global management of RA. Only two CPGs distinguish specific recommendations for the management of RA during the first two years since onset [31,34] and after the two first years [32]. Foot orthosis/insoles, joint protection, patient education/self-management, multidisciplinary team approach, aerobic, dynamic, stretching, strengthening and whole body exercises were the common non-pharmacological interventions recommended by majority of the selected CPGs.

Table 2. Quality Scores using AGREE II Instruments for included CPGs on RA.

Agree II domains	ACR	BSR	BSR & BHP	Eular	Forestier et al.	Gossec et al.	Hurkman et al.	NICE	Ottawa Panel	RACGP	SIGN	(mn ±SD)
	[30]	[31]	[32]	[33]	[34]	[35]	[36]	[37]	[38–42]	[43]	[44]	
Domain 1	17%	83%	89%	17%	86%	89%	47%	75%	97%	97%	81%	70.4%±42%
Domain 2	25%	75%	75%	36%	67%	64%	86%	89%	72%	86%	94%	70.6%±26%
Domain 3	11%	34%	32%	44%	71%	58%	69%	52%	65%	84%	55%	52.4%±23%
Domain 4	11%	83%	67%	14%	100%	39%	94%	39%	61%	100%	97%	64.0%±28%
Domain 5	17%	50%	8%	0%	46%	0%	4%	17%	10%	17%	35%	18.5%±35%
Domain 6	38%	38%	46%	0%	50%	21%	8%	92%	42%	33%	54%	38.3%±23%
Quality of CPGs (mn±SD)	3.5±0.5	4.5±0.71	4.5±0.71	4±1.41	5.5±0.5	5±0	5±0	4±0	5.5±0.71	6.5±0.71	5±1.41	4.8±0.61
Assessed by	PR & LB	PR &LB	PR & LB	PR & LB	PR & LB	PR & LB	PR & LB	PR & LB	PR & KTA	PR & LB	PR & LB	PR & LB

ACR: American College of Rheumatology, BSR: British society of rheumatology; EULAR: The European League against rheumatism; NICE: National Institute for health and Clinical Excellence; SIGN: Scottish Intercollegiate Guidelines Network; $\bar{x}$: mean; SD: standard deviation.

Table 3. Inter rater reliability study results for included CPGs [a].

Agree II Domain	P(G)MS[b]	RMS	EMS	*n*	K	ICC (Random)	Lower 95% CI	Upper 95% CI	P value
Domain 1	54.382	.045	.545	12	2	.990 (high)	.963	.997	.000
Domain 2	34.778	3.200	1.422	12	2	.959 (high)	.835	.990	.000
Domain 3	165.756	16.200	.494	12	2	.987(high)	.947	.997	.000
Domain 4	58.482	3.682	5.082	12	2	.913(high)	.677	.977	.000
Domain 5	35.64	.182	.482	12	2	.986(high)	.950	.996	.000
Domain 6	21.467	.200	.533	12	2	.975(high)	.900	.994	.000

[a]CP Gs= clinical practice guidelines; P(G)MS=Patients' (Guideline's) Mean Square; RMS= Rater's Mean Square; EMS= Error Mean Square; n= sample size; K= number of measurements; ICC= intraclass correlation coefficient; CI= confidence interval.
[b]Temporary PMS, RMS, and EMS value.

Quality Scores of CPGs

None of the CPGs were found to adequately address all six of the domains when using the AGREE II appraisal instrument. The majority of the included CPGs obtained a high AGREE II quality score for domain 1 (scope and purpose), domain 2 (stakeholder involvement) and domain 4 (clarity of presentation). The scope and purpose were well addressed in 10 [31–32,34–35,37–44] out of the 13 CPGs and the 3 [30,33,36] CPGs that were not able to effectively target this domain lacked information on the target population [36] and the clinical question addressed by the CPG [30,33,36]. Eleven [31–32,34–44] out of the 13 CPGs effectively addressed stakeholder involvement. However, 2 CPGs [30,33] received a score <60% due to insufficient information on how the views and preferences of the target population were sought and the target users of the CPGs. While all the CPGs considered the views and preferences of patient and patient representatives, most CPGs lacked information on the methods by which the views and preferences were sought and how these outcomes impacted the development and formation of the recommendation. Generally most of the CPGs received high scores for clarity of presentation (domain 4), however 4 CPGs [30,33,35,37] were not able to effectively target this domain, because the recommendations presented were unclear especially regarding the duration and dosage for non-pharmacological interventions.

Domain 3 (rigour of development) obtained a relatively low mean AGREE II score for the 13 CPGS and 6 CPGs effectively targeted (≥60%) this domain [34,36,38–43]. Special attention should be given to the rigor of development when examining the quality of the results [26], as CPGs were considered high quality if the rigor of development was effectively targeted (>60%) in addition to targeting 2 or more other domains. Receiving a high score for this domain indicated minimum bias and evidence based design in the development of the CPGs. All 13 CPGs [30–44] reported the relevant data bases used and explicit link between the recommendations and supporting evidence. The majority of the CPGs were unsuccessful in targeting this domain due to insufficient information on the inclusion and exclusion criteria used [30–31,34,36,43], the methods for formulating the recommendations [30–32,35,37,44] and an explicit statement about when and what method will be used to update the guideline [30–33,35]. Although most CPGs provided the benefits when considering non-pharmacological recommendations, insufficient information about the risks and side effects for a weak evidence recommendation was provided. This might be due to the fact that RCTs on non-pharmacological interventions rarely reported side effects (i.e harm) and risks. "Harm" is difficult to assess when developing a CPG, as it is based on the RCT which studies the effectiveness. As a result some CPGs [30–32,35] received low scores for this domain because the information was not available to the evaluators. It is unrealistic to expect busy clinicians to search for required or supplementary information; therefore CPGs should be reported in sufficient details with the additional information included and easily accessible.

Domain 5 (Applicability) obtained the lowest mean AGREE II ratings for all 13 CPGs and none were able to effectively address this domain. A rational for such low scores can be attributed to the criteria for this domain. In order for CPGs to receive high ratings, it should report the tools for application, the barriers and cost in applying the recommendations, and monitoring and auditing criteria. It might be premature to use these criteria to assess the applicability of the CPGs, because the developers usually focus on planning the dissemination and implementation of the CPGs [24]. The inclusion of the "applicability" domain is controversial, as the development of a CPG takes considerable time with extensive human and financial resources. Applicability requires well conducted RCTs and cluster RCTs in order to be properly implemented [45] and should ideally include an economic evaluation. The Knowledge-To-Action Cycle [46] should be taken into account when conducting an implementation study. These missing items and the prematurely assessed domain could directly affect the evaluation of the overall quality of the CPGs included in this synthesis paper. AGREE II should be applied in two phases: 1) the development phase and 2) the implementation phase.

Domain 6 (editorial independence) also received a low mean quality score for the 13 CPGs [30–44] and only one CPG [37] effectively targeted this domain. The scores for this domain was low, because several CPGs failed to mention the information related to conflict of interest [31–32] in their publication and whether the views of the funding body have influenced the content of the guideline [30–32,34–35].

The quality scores for the CPGs in the review are important to consider and are useful when making decisions as to recommend a specific CPG. The criteria from previous critical appraisals with AGREE I are used with the AGREE II instrument to identify high quality guidelines in this systematic reviews. While the new AGREE II instrument does not provide a threshold to identify "high" quality CPGs from "low" CPGs, the domain scores are helpful for comparing guidelines [26]. CPG developers should use the AGREE II criteria (www.agreetrust.org) [11] when developing their CPG in order to publish higher quality CPGs [10,15].

The results of this review can be partially compared to the only known systematic review done for the quality appraisal done of CPGs on the use of physiotherapy in RA with AGREE I [15]. Although the same CPGs were considered in both reviews, the present review used the updated AGREE tool (AGREE II) to assess the CPG quality. The findings of this review agree with the results of Hurkman et al [15], where none of the CPGs for both reviews effectively targeted all six of the domains. Both reviews found that rigor of development and applicability were not well addressed by most of the CPGs and finally for both reviews the domain scores ranged from >70% for domain 1 (scope and purpose) to <50% for domain 5 (applicability).

Strength of Non-pharmacological Recommendations

Surprisingly the strength of the recommendations differed among the CPGs. Part of the reason for this discrepancy could be attributed to the difference in the years of the CPGs developed. However, recently published CPGs based on the same available literature also differed in strength for the recommendations. A reason for this might be due to the method of analysis in order to ensure consensus about the strength of the recommendations for each non-pharmacological intervention.

The strength of recommendations may also vary according to the stages of RA [31–32]. Furthermore, non-pharmacological management of RA depends on the stage and progression of the disease, the patient's personality, environment, objectives as well as clinical assessment, and must be regularly adjusted [34,49,50]. Some CPGs [36] provided a disclaimer for certain non-pharmacological recommendations, such as heat therapy which was not recommended for inflamed joints. Clinical algorithms may facilitate clinical decision making [30–32,34,44].

Often, physiotherapy and occupational therapy are classified as interventions, but in fact they are professions. Physiotherapists and occupational therapists provide a large spectrum of non-pharmacological interventions to patients with RA. Consequently more precision needs to be provided, especially regarding therapeutic interventions. The adoption of a PICOT [7] format to report the recommendation would be an asset for clinicians. P indicates the characteristics of the population for which the intervention is effective (e.g. stage of disease, disease duration etc...); I represents the characteristics of the intervention (e.g. dosage etc...); C is the comparator (placebo, control etc.); O indicates outcomes for which the intervention is effective; T is the time (short vs. long term effects) to apply the intervention in order to improve effectiveness or to learn the retention effect after stopping the intervention). Luqmani et al. [30] discussed the need for reporting the lasting impact of the effective intervention. The Ottawa Panel CPG [38–42] is the only one that used the PICOT format to frame its recommendations.

Almost all CPGs recommended or strongly recommended patient education, aerobic exercise, dynamic exercise and strengthening exercises. Further, majority of the CPGs recommended joint protection, splinting, multidisciplinary team approach and whole body exercises. Although therapeutic exercises to maintain joint range of motion and mobility were generally recommended by all the CPGs. However, there is a need for a more specific scientific basis of the benefits and potential harms related to types of exercises [44]. Exercise dose-response in relation to disease activity, joint symptoms, level of fatigue and quality of life need to be determined for the optimal management of RA [15,47].

More precisions on dosage are also needed on the use of splints (e.g. static vs. dynamic/working exercise) [31,41], patient education (e.g. group vs. individual; self-management) [31,41] and thermotherapy (e.g. heat application vs. cryotherapy) [31] and needs to be categorized or more detailed in some CPGs. Operational definitions also need to be provided (e.g. hydrotherapy vs. balneotherapy vs. aquatics).

Most CPGs recognized that the management of RA must include pharmacological and non-pharmacological interventions [30–35,37,42–44]. Additionally, non-pharmacological approaches should also explore the consideration of combined interventions to be more representative of the clinical context. Primary RCTs that were used to build the CPG, examined the specific effect of monotherapy, whereas combined interventions are current practice in rehabilitation. These need to be explored to reflect current practices, as many interventions may be effective or more effective when used in combination, such as paraffin wax alone versus paraffin wax combined with exercise.

Descriptive Analysis

The sample size of the included CPGs was too small to perform any additional analysis such as a student t test or ANOVA test and test for statistical significance of the improvement of CPGs over time. Based on figure S2 the overall quality of the CPG does not improve over time, many of the CPGs published earlier [39–40] were considered to be of higher quality CPGs compared to those published more recently. A rationale for why some of the earlier published CPGs had a much higher quality than the more recently published CPGs could be attributed to the methodology each guideline used. The Ottawa panel guidelines follows the Cochrane methodology when developing their guidelines and this rigorous evidence based method resulted in higher quality CPGs compared to the CPGs published more recently using another method of development.

Limitations

The AGREE II instrument is updated versions of the initial AGREE I instrument [12–13]. AGREE II was available in 2009 with validation studies conducted in 2010 [12–13,52]. Despite this fact, more recent CPGs published after this date [33,38,45] did not receive a high overall quality score and did not effectively address all the domains, especially for items in domain 5 (applicability) and domain 6 (editorial independence). Another limitation of the AGREE II is it evaluates only the quality of the reporting versus the quality of the development [48,51]. As only the published and available documents were evaluated, the ratings for rigor of development were lower than they might have been if we had contacted the developers for the required documentation. We considered the scoring system (e.g. discrimination between a score of 4 or 5) and the subjectivity of interpreting the domain criteria as a limit to the AGREE II instrument. The 7-point scale used in AGREE II is based on the idea that if all the elements of a particular item are fully addressed, then it is given a score of seven for that particular item. Conversely, if none of the elements were present then it was given a score of one. An initial score of one (absence of information) can be considered a systematic error, because AGREE II does not consider "not applicable" a response according to its scoring system. Finally, there is a potential publication bias that may limit generalizability of our results as only CPGs published in English were selected.

Conclusion

In summary, the literature search yielded 13 CPGs that targeted non-pharmacological interventions for RA. Six CPGs were found to be of high quality based on the AGREE II instrument and the non-pharmacological interventions that were recommended were: patient education/self-management, aerobic, dynamic and stretching exercises. The authors found that the recommendations presented in the CPGs provided insufficient information on the mode of delivery, dosage, intensity, frequency and duration. Future CPG developers should focus more on addressing all six AGREE II domains, in particular rigor of development and applicability to ensure the recommendations presented can easily be implemented in daily health care practice.

Supporting Information

Figure S1 Prisma flow diagram of included CPGs.

Figure S2 CPG Quality Over Time.

Table S1 Recommendations for the Management of Rheumatoid Arthritis. ACR: American College of Rheumatology, BSR: British society of rheumatology; EULAR: The European League against rheumatism; NICE: National Institute for health and Clinical Excellence; PGrip: People Getting A Grip on Arthritis (www.arthritis.ca/PeopleGettingaGrip); SIGN: Scottish Intercollegiate Guidelines network Scottish Intercollegiate Guidelines network; NA: Not Assessed; TENS: Transcutaneous Electric Nerve Stimulation.

Appendix S1 Literature Search Strategy.

Appendix S2 Selection criteria for clinical practice guidelines.

Appendix S3 Raw data of the AGREE II items.

Checklist S1 Prisma 2009 Checklist.

Acknowledgments

The authors of this paper would like to acknowledge and thank the support of Ms. Jennifer Burt, President, the Arthritis Health Professions Association (AHPA) and Ms. Carol Miller, Director, Practice and Research, the Canadian Physiotherapy Association.

Author Contributions

Conceived and designed the experiments: LB PR KTA JK LC GDA LL SC JM. Analyzed the data: PR KTA GP CS SP SC. Wrote the paper: LB PR KTA GP CS JK LC GDA LL SP SC.

References

1. Choy EH, Panayi GS (2001) Cytokine pathways and joint inflammation in rheumatoid arthritis. N Engl J Med 344(12): 907–16.
2. Myasoedova E, Davis JM 3rd, Crowson CS, Gabriel SE (2010) Epidemiology of rheumatoid arthritis: Rheumatoid arthritis and mortality. Curr Rheumatol Rep 12(5): 379–85.
3. Jawaheer D, Lum RF, Gregersen PK, Criswell LA (2006) Influence of male sex on disease phenotype in familial rheumatoid arthritis. Arthritis Rheum 54(10): 3087–94.
4. Symmons DP (2002) Epidemiology of rheumatoid arthritis: Determinants of onset, persistence and outcome. Best Pract Res Clin Rheumatol 16(5): 707–22.
5. Simons WR, Rosenblatt LC, Trivedi DN (2012) The economic consequences of rheumatoid arthritis: Analysis of medical expenditure panel survey 2004, 2005, and 2006 data. J Occup Environ Med 54(1): 48–55.
6. Maetzel A, Li LC, Pencharz J, Tomlinson G, Bombardier C, et al. (2004) The economic burden associated with osteoarthritis, rheumatoid arthritis, and hypertension: A comparative study. Ann Rheum Dis 63(4): 395–401.
7. Sackett DL, Rosenberg WM, Gray JA, Haynes RB, Richardson WS (2007) Evidence based medicine: what it is and what it isn't. 1996. Clin Orthop Relat Res 455: 3–5.
8. Akobeng AK (2005) Evidence in practice. Arch Dis Child 90(8): 837–40.
9. Grossman JH, Field MJ (1990) Clinical practice guidelines: Directions for a new program, Washington: National Academy Press. 38 (161p).
10. Poitras S, Avouac J, Rossignol M, Avouac B, Cedraschi C, et al. (2007) A critical appraisal of guidelines for the management of knee osteoarthritis using Appraisal of Guidelines Research and Evaluation Criteria. Arthritis Res Ther 9(6): 1–12.
11. Appraisal of Guidelines for Research and Evaluation [www.agreetrust.org]
12. Brouwers MC, Kho ME, Browman GP, Burgers JS, Cluzeau F, et al. (2010) AGREE next steps consortium. Development of the AGREE II, part 1: Performance, usefulness and areas for improvement. CMAJ 182(10): 1045–52.
13. Brouwers MC, Kho ME, Browman GP, Burgers JS, Cluzeau F, et al. (2010) AGREE next steps consortium. Development of the AGREE II, part 2: Assessment of validity of items and tools to support application. CMAJ 2010, 182(10): E472–8.
14. Ward MM (2009) Guidelines for the management of RA: Breadth versus depth. Nat Rev Rheumatol 5(6): 302–303.
15. Hurkmans EJ, van der Giesen FJ, Bloo H, Boonman DC, van der Esch M, et al. (2011) Physiotherapy in rheumatoid arthritis: Development of a practice guideline. Acta Reumatol Port 36(2): 146–158.
16. Toupin KA, Benkhalti MJ, Paterson G, Ueffing E, Rader T, et al. (2013) Clinical practice guidelines for osteoarthritis. In: Martel-Pelletier J, Pelletier JP, editors. Addressing unmet needs in osteoarthritis. London: Future Medicine Ltd. 122–138.
17. Pencharz JN, Grigoriadis E, Jansz GF, Bombardier C (2002) A critical appraisal of clinical practice guidelines for the treatment of lower-limb osteoarthritis. Arthritis Res 4: 36–44.
18. Moher D (2009) Preferred reporting items for systematic reviews and meta-analyses: The PRISMA statement. Annals of Internal Medicine, 151(4): 264. doi: 10.7326/0003-4819-151-4-200908180-00135.
19. Cochrane Collaboration methodology. Available: www.cochrane.org.
20. Physiotherapy Evidence Database (PEDro) Available: http://www.pedro.fhs.usyd.edu.au/index.html. Accessed 2013 May 23.
21. National Guideline Clearinghouse Available: http://www.guideline.gov/. Accessed 2013 May 23.
22. Guidelines International Network (GIN). Available: http://www.g-i-n.net/. Accessed 2013 May 23.
23. Trip Database Available: http://www.tripdatabase.com/. Accessed 2013 October 11.
24. Appraisal of Guidelines Research and Evaluation II Overview Tutorial. Available: http://agree.machealth.ca/players/open/index.html.
25. McMaster AGREE II score calculator Excel spreadsheet. Available: http://fhswedge.csu.mcmaster.ca/cepftp/qasite/CriticalAppraisal.html.
26. Brooks D, Solway S, MacDermid J, Switzer-McIntyre S, Brosseau L, et al. (2005) Quality of clinical practise guidelines in physical therapy. Physiother Can 57: 123–4.
27. Hurdowar A, Graham ID, Bayley M, Harrison M, Wood-Dauphinee S, et al. (2007) Quality of stroke rehabilitation clinical practice guidelines. J Eval Clin Pract 13(4): 657–64.
28. Brosseau L, Graham I, Casimiro L, MacLeay L, Cleaver S, et al. (2004) What is the quality of clinical practice guidelines accessible on the world wide web for the treatment of musculoskeletal conditions in physiotherapy? Physiother Theory Pract 20: 91–105.
29. McGraw KO, Wong SP (1996) Forming inferences about some intraclass correlation coefficients. Psychological Methods 1(1): 30–46.
30. American College of Rheumatology (2002) Guidelines for the management of rheumatoid arthritis. Arthritis Rheum 46(2): 328–346.
31. Luqmani R, Hennel S, Estrach C, Birrell F, Bosworth A, et al. (2006) British Society for Rheumatology and British Health Professionals in Rheumatology guideline for the management of rheumatoid arthritis (the first 2 years). Rheumatology 45(9): 1167–1169.
32. Luqmani R, Hennel S, Estrach C, Birrell F, Bosworth A, et al. (2009) British Society for Rheumatology and British Health Professionals in Rheumatology Guideline for the management of Rheumatoid Arthritis (after the first 2 years). Rheumatology 48(4): 436–439.
33. Combe B, Landewe R, Lukas C, Bolosiu HD, Breedveld F, et al. (2007) EULAR recommendations for the management of early arthritis: Report of a task force of the European standing committee for international clinical studies including therapeutics (ESCISIT). Ann Rheum Dis 66(1): 34–45.
34. Forestier R, Andre-Vert J, Guillez P, Coudeyre E, Lefevre-Colau M, et al. (2009) Non-drug treatment (excluding surgery) in rheumatoid arthritis: Clinical practice guidelines. Joint Bone Spine 76(6): 691–698.
35. Gossec L, Pavy S, Pham T, Constantin A, Poiraudeau S, et al. (2006) Nonpharmacological treatments in early rheumatoid arthritis: Clinical practice guidelines based on published evidence and expert opinion. Joint Bone Spine 73(4): 396–402.
36. Hurkmans EJ, van der Giesen FJ, Bloo H, Boonman DC, van der Esch M, et al. (2011). Physiotherapy in rheumatoid arthritis: Development of a practice guideline. Acta Reumatologica Portuguesa 36(2): 146–158.
37. The National Institute for Health and Clinical Excellence (NICE) (2009). Rheumatoid Arthritis: National Clinical Guideline for Management and Treatment in Adults. (NICE Clinical guidelines, No. 79) London: Royal College of Physicians.
38. Brosseau L, Wells G, Tugwell P, Egan M, Dubouloz CJ, et al. (2004) Ottawa Panel evidence clinical practice guidelines for therapeutic exercises and manual therapy in the treatment of rheumatoid arthritis. Physical Therapy 84: 934–981.
39. Brosseau L, Wells G, Tugwell P, Egan M, Dubouloz CJ, et al. (2004) Ottawa Panel evidence clinical practice guidelines for electrotherapy and thermotherapy interventions in the treatment of rheumatoid arthritis. Physical Therapy 84: 1016–1043.
40. Brosseau L, Wells G, Tugwell P, Egan M, Dubouloz CJ, et al. (2011) Ottawa Panel evidence-based clinical practice guidelines for patient education programs in the management of rheumatoid arthritis (RA). Health Educ J 71(4): 397–451.
41. People Getting a Grip on Arthritis Program (PGRIP). Available: www.arthritis.ca/peoplegettingagrip.
42. Brosseau L, Lineker S, Bell M, Wells G, Casimiro L, et al. (2012) People getting a grip on arthritis: A knowledge transfer strategy to empower patients with rheumatoid arthritis and osteoarthritis. Health Education Journal 71(3): 255–267.
43. The Royal Australian College of General Practitioners (2009) Clinical guideline for diagnosis and management of early rheumatoid arthritis. Melbourne.
44. Scottish Intercollegiate Guidelines Network (SIGN) (2011) The management of early rheumatoid arthritis. Edinburgh.
45. Davis DA, Taylor-Vaisey A (1997) Translating guidelines into practice. A systematic review of theoretic concepts, practical experience and research evidence in adoption of clinical practice guidelines. CMAJ 157(4): 408–16.
46. Straus SE, Tetroe J, Graham ID (2013) Knowledge translation in health care: Moving from evidence to practice. Chichester: Wiley-Blackwell/BMJ.
47. Regnaux JP, Trinquart L, Boutron I, Nguyen C, Brosseau L, et al (2012) High-intensity versus low-intensity physical activity or exercise in patients with hip or knee osteoarthritis. Cochrane Database of Systematic Reviews 2012, Issue 11.
48. Jadad AR, Moore RA, Carroll D, Jenkinson C, Reynolds DJM, et al. (1996) Assessing the quality of reports of randomized clinical trials: Is blinding necessary? Control Clin Trials 17: 1–12.
49. Macedo LG, Elkins MR, Maher CG, Moseley AM, Herbert RD, et al. (2010) There was evidence of convergent and construct validity of Physiotherapy Evidence Database quality scale for physiotherapy trials. J Clin Epidemiol 63(8): 920–5.
50. Olivo SA, Macedo LG, Gadotti IC, Fuentes J, Stanton T, et al. (2008) Scales to assess the quality of randomized controlled trials: A systematic review. Phys Ther 88: 156–175.
51. Shea BJ, Grimshaw JM, Wells GA, Boers M, Andersson N, et al. (2007) Development of AMSTAR: a measurement tool to assess the methodological quality of systematic reviews. BMC Med Res Methodol 7: 1–10.
52. Shekelle PG, Ortiz E, Rhodes S, Morton CS, Eccles PM, et al. (2001) Validity of the Agency for Healthcare Research and Quality clinical practice guidelines: How quickly do guidelines become outdated? JAMA 286(12): 1461–1467.

Increase of Hemoglobin Levels by Anti-IL-6 Receptor Antibody (Tocilizumab) in Rheumatoid Arthritis

Motomu Hashimoto[1]*, Takao Fujii[1,2], Masahide Hamaguchi[3], Moritoshi Furu[1], Hiromu Ito[1,4], Chikashi Terao[5], Keiichi Yamamoto[6], Wataru Yamamoto[1,7], Takashi Matsuo[2], Masato Mori[2], Koichiro Ohmura[2], Hiroshi Kawabata[8], Tsuneyo Mimori[2]

1 Department of the Control for Rheumatic Diseases, Graduate School of Medicine, Kyoto University, Kyoto, Japan, 2 Department of Rheumatology and Clinical Immunology, Graduate School of Medicine, Kyoto University, Kyoto, Japan, 3 Department of Experimental Immunology, Immunology Frontier Research Center, Osaka University, Osaka, Japan, 4 Department of Orthopedic Surgery, Graduate School of Medicine, Kyoto University, Kyoto, Japan, 5 Center for Genomic Medicine, Graduate School of Medicine, Kyoto University, Kyoto, Japan, 6 Division of Clinical and Epidemiological Database, Department of Information Governance, National Cerebral and Cardiovascular Center, Osaka, Japan, 7 Department of Health Information Management, Kurashiki Sweet Hospital, Kurashiki, Japan, 8 Department of Hematology and Oncology, Graduate School of Medicine, Kyoto University, Kyoto, Japan

Abstract

Objective: To compare the effect of tocilizumab (TCZ) with other biologic therapies in improving anemia of rheumatoid arthritis (RA) patients.

Methods: We compared the change of hemoglobin (Hb) levels in a cohort of 147 consecutive RA patients who were treated with biologics for more than 12 weeks. Twenty eight patients were treated with TCZ, and 119 patients were treated with biologics other than TCZ (87 with TNF inhibitors and 32 with abatacept). The change of Hb levels from baseline to week 12 was compared between the TCZ and the non-TCZ groups. We performed univariate and multivariate analyses with adjustment of potential confounders such as baseline characteristics, concomitant treatment, and the clinical response to treatment.

Results: Hb levels generally increased after biologic therapies both in the TCZ and the non-TCZ groups. The increase of Hb levels was greater in the TCZ group than in the non-TCZ groups (1.1 g/dL in the TCZ group vs 0.3 g/dL in the non-TCZ group, $p = 0.009$). Univariate analysis revealed that increase of Hb levels was also significantly associated with lower Hb, higher Low Hemoglobin Density, and higher CRP levels at baseline and greater reduction in the clinical disease activity index. TCZ therapy was significantly associated with the increase of Hb levels even after adjustment for these factors by multivariate analysis ($p<0.001$, effect size 0.08–0.12).

Conclusion: TCZ therapy is an independent factor associated with the increase of Hb level after biologic therapies in RA patients. It will help in selecting appropriate biologics for RA patients with anemia.

Editor: Ivan Cruz Moura, Institut national de la santé et de la recherche médicale (INSERM), France

Funding: The authors have no support or funding to report.

Competing Interests: The authors have read the journal's policy and have the following conflicts: M. Hashimoto, T.F., M.F., H.I., and T. Mimori are affiliated with a department that is supported financially by five pharmaceutical companies (Mitsubishi Tanabe Pharma Co., Bristol-Myers K.K., Chugai Pharmaceutical Co., Ltd., AbbVie GK., Eisai Co., Ltd.). M.H. and M.F. has received grant and research support from Astellas Pharma Inc. and Pfizer Japan Inc. H.I. has received grant and research support from Astellas Pharma Inc., Pfizer Japan Inc., NTT communications, and Takeda Pharmaceutical Co., Ltd. T.F. has received grant and research support from Takeda Pharmaceutical Co., Santen Pharmaceutical Co., Ltd., Astellas Pharma Inc., Asahi Kasei Pharma Corporation, and Daiichi Sankyo Co., Ltd. T.M. has received grant and research support from Asahi Kasei Pharma Corporation, Astellas Pharma Inc., Bristol-Myers Squibb K.K., Chugai Pharmaceutical Co., Ltd., Eisai Co., Ltd., Mitsubishi Tanabe Pharma Corporation, Pfizer Japan Inc., Santen Pharmaceutical Co., Ltd., and Takeda Pharmaceutical Co., Ltd., and speakers bureau from AbbVie GK., Bristol-Myers Squibb K.K., Chugai Pharmaceutical Co., Ltd., Eisai Co., Ltd., Mitsubishi Tanabe Pharma Corporation, Pfizer Japan Inc., and Takeda Pharmaceutical Co., Ltd. K.O. has received grant and research support from AbbVie GK., Astellas Pharma Inc., Bristol-Myers Squibb K.K., Chugai Pharmaceutical Co., Ltd., Eisai Co., Ltd., Mitsubishi Tanabe Pharma Corporation, and speakers bureau from AbbVie GK., Astellas Pharma, Bristol-Myers Squibb K.K., Chugai Pharmaceutical Co., Ltd., Eisai Co., Ltd., Mitsubishi Tanabe Pharma Corporation, Pfizer Japan Inc., and Takeda Pharmaceutical Co., Ltd. The sponsors were not involved in the study design; in the collection, analysis, interpretation of data; in the writing of this manuscript; or in the decision to submit the article for publication. The authors, their immediate families, and any research foundations with which they are affiliated have not received any financial payments or other benefits from any commercial entity related to the subject of this article. The authors declare that although they are affiliated with a department that is supported financially by pharmaceutical companies, the authors received no current funding for this study and this does not alter their adherence to all the PLOS ONE policies on sharing data and materials.

* E-mail: mohashim@kuhp.kyoto-u.ac.jp

Introduction

Anemia is an important complication in rheumatoid arthritis (RA) which is associated with physical disability and increased mortality [1] [2]. Anemia of chronic disease (ACD), also known as anemia of chronic inflammation, is the major reason for developing anemia in RA patients. Recent studies suggest that

ACD develops via multiple mechanisms including pathogenic iron homeostasis, impaired erythropoiesis, and the blunted erythropoietin response [1]. Inflammatory cytokines such as IL-6 and tumor necrosis factor α (TNFα) are critically involved in its process. For example, IL-6 induces hepcidin, a critical regulator of iron metabolism in ACD [3] [4], while TNFα and IL-1 impair erythropoiesis and induce the blunted erythropoietin response [5]. Among various mechanisms, recent studies suggest the central role of hepcidin and IL-6 for the pathophysiology of ACD [3].

Recently, the treatment of RA has significantly advanced over past decade by the introduction of biologic therapies (biologics) [6]. Today, several biologics that target different molecules are used in RA clinical practice with comparable efficacy and side effects [6]. These include TNF inhibitors (infliximab, etanercept, adalimumab, golimumab, and certolizumab); an IL-6 receptor antagonist, tocilizumab (TCZ); a T cell co-stimulatory blocker, abatacept; and a B cell specific depletor, rituximab, and so on. Because IL-6 and other cytokines are critically involved in the pathogenesis of ACD, biologic therapies such as TCZ and TNF inhibitors could potentially increase hemoglobin (Hb) levels after treatment. Indeed, increase of Hb levels after biologic therapies has been demonstrated in RA and in other inflammatory diseases [5] [7] [8] [9] [10] [11] [12].

Given the central role of IL-6 in ACD, it is possible that TCZ therapy would improve anemia more effectively than other biologics. However, it should be determined carefully because the etiology of anemia in RA is multifactorial and ACD is not the only cause of anemia in RA. The Hb levels after treatment may be influenced by various factors such as baseline characteristics, concomitant treatment, or clinical response to treatment. For example, age, sex, renal function, or initial levels of Hb and inflammatory markers would apparently affect the change in Hb levels [13] [14]. Methotrexate treatment frequently causes folate deficiency and macrocytic anemia, while the use of non-steroidal anti-inflammatory drugs (NSAIDs) or glucocorticoids might cause gastrointestinal bleeding that may lead to iron deficiency and microcytic anemia. The change in Hb levels may correlate with the clinical response to treatment or the reduction of inflammatory markers. Therefore, clinical research is necessary to determine which biologics are optimal in improving anemia of RA. Because anemia is associated with not only the patient's subjective symptoms such as fatigue [2], but also with the radiological progression of RA [15], such studies will be beneficial for clinicians aiming at remission of RA.

The aim of this study is to determine whether TCZ therapy is more effective at increasing Hb levels in RA than other non-TCZ biologics even after taking into account many confounding factors. For this aim, we conducted a cohort study by enrolling the consecutive RA patients treated by biologics in our cohort, and analyzed the effect of TCZ therapy with potential confounders for the increase of Hb levels.

Patients and Methods

Study design and population

The study population was enrolled from Kyoto University Rheumatoid Arthritis Management Alliance (KURAMA) cohort and followed up prospectively [16]. Briefly, the KURAMA cohort was established on 1st May 2011 in the Center for Rheumatic Diseases in Kyoto University Hospital aiming at the tight control of RA following recent advances in RA treatment and to utilize their sequential clinical and laboratory data for clinical investigations [6] [17]. Annually, around 400 patients are consecutively registered in the KURAMA cohort. The median age of the patients is 64.5 years old, 87.6% female, median disease duration is 13.0 years [17]. In this cohort, around 30% of the patients are on the treatment with biologics which are initiated not only for patients with high disease activity but also for patients with low to moderate disease activity to suppress the residual joint swelling [17].

In the current study, we enrolled all the patients consecutively from 1st May 2011 to 1st November 2012. Inclusion criteria were as follows: patients with written informed consent, over 18 years of age, fulfilling the American College of Rheumatology / European League Against Rheumatism classification criteria for RA in 2010 [18], and newly introduced for biologics in our institute during the study period and remained on the drug for more than 12 weeks. Patients receiving hemodialysis or erythropoietin therapy and patients who had an active gastrointestinal bleeding event during the study period were excluded. The study was designed in accordance with the declaration of Helsinki and was approved by the ethics committee of Kyoto University Graduate School and Faculty of Medicine. We followed up all the included patients for 12 weeks, and analyzed the change of Hb levels and disease conditions. Biologics used in this study were TCZ, infliximab, etanercept, adalimumab, golimumab, and abatacept. Rituximab and certollizumab were not included because they were not approved for RA patients in Japan at the time of this study.

Data collection

Clinical data included age, sex, body-mass index, disease duration of RA, swollen joint count, tender joint count, patient's global assessment of disease activity, and physician's global assessment of disease activity. Serological data and blood cell count included Hb, red blood cell count (RBC), mean corpuscular volume (MCV), mean corpuscular hemoglobin (MCH), mean corpuscular hemoglobin concentration (MCHC), and C-reactive protein (CRP). Anemia was defined as Hb level <12.0 in women and <13.0 in men. Iron status in the presence of inflammation was assessed by Low Hemoglobin Density (LHD%) transformed from MCHC, because LHD%>5.5 is a reliable marker for detecting the functional iron deficiency in ACD patients [19] [20]. Renal function was assessed by estimated glomerular filtration rate calculated by creatinine value, sex and age. RA disease activity was evaluated by clinical disease activity index (CDAI) and CRP separately, because IL-6 inhibition has a prominent effect on the production of hepatic acute phase proteins such as CRP and it is preferred to use CDAI which does not comprise CRP for the assessment of the clinical response to TCZ [21]. Physical function was assessed by modified health assessment questionnaire-disability index (mHAQ). Clinical response to biologic therapies was assessed by the reduction of CDAI, CRP or mHAQ from baseline to week 12 (ΔCDAI = CDAI at baseline - CDAI at week 12, ΔCRP = CRP at baseline - CRP at week 12, ΔmHAQ = mHAQ at baseline – mHAQ at week 12). Data for the concomitant use of methotrexate, glucocorticoids, NSAIDs, iron drugs, and folic acid were also recorded. Clinical and laboratory data were compared at baseline and week 12 after the initiation of biologic therapies.

Statistical analysis

The SPSS statistical package, version 11.0.1 J (SPSS, Inc., Chicago, IL) was used for all the statistical analyses and P value less than 0.05 was considered statistically significant. Continuous variables in two groups were assessed by Mann-Whitney u-test and frequencies were assessed by Chi square test. Univariate regression analysis was performed to analyze associations between the increase of Hb and potential confounders. The relationship

Table 1. Characteristics of the study population and increase of Hb levels after biologic therapies.

	TCZ group	non-TCZ group	P
	N = 28	N = 119	
Basic characteristics			
Age, year	62 (34–)	60 (19–86)	0.58
Female, % (n)	78.6% (22)	88.2% (105)	0.22
Duration of RA, month	127 (9–464)	77 (3–759)	0.22
BMI, kg/m^2	23.0 (16.6–32.5)	22.2 (0.2–32.5)	0.48
eGFR	78.6 (35.9–122.4)	80.7 (28.8–153.4)	0.50
Hb, g/dl	12.3 (6.3–15.9)	12.1 (8.3–16.7)	0.99
RBC, 10^6/ml	4.0 (2.6–5.3)	4.1 (2.7–5.4)	0.32
MCV	94.0 (77.2–104.9)	92.3 (69.6–105.1)	0.44
MCH, pg	30.4 (23.2–35.6)	29.9 (20.0–35.6)	0.34
LHD%	12.0 (1.5–82.0)	11.5 (1.2–94.7)	0.89
LHD%>5.5, % (n)	78.6% (22)	81.5% (97)	0.79
CDAI	17.4 (0.9–62.4)	12.2 (1.2–49.6)	0.12
CRP, mg/dl	0.4 (0–11.9)	0.5 (0–9.2)	0.67
mHAQ	0.8 (0–2.5)	0.4 (0–2.6)	0.052
Anti-CCP positivity, % (n)	91.7% (22)	91.3% (73)	1.00
Concomitant treatments			
Methotrexate, % (n)	64.3% (18)	73.9% (88)	0.35
Glucocorticoids, % (n)	75.0% (21)	42.9% (51)	0.003
NSAIDs, % (n)	71.4% (20)	54.6% (65)	0.14
Iron drugs, % (n)	10.7% (3)	5.9% (7)	0.40
Folic acid, % (n)	57.1% (16)	70.6% (84)	0.18
Previous biologics, % (n)	71.4% (20)	31.1% (37)	<0.001
Clinical response			
ΔCDAI	7.2 (−2.2–44.3)	6.2 (−10.0–33.5)	0.52
ΔCRP (mg/dl)	0.2 (−0.6–10.2)	0.2 (−6.7–6.7)	0.24
ΔmHAQ	0.125 (−1–1.3)	0.125 (−2.6–1.5)	0.33
Increase of Hb levels, g/dl			
	1.1 (−1.2–4.7)	0.3 (−1.7–2.4)	0.009

Continuous variables were compared by Mann-Whitney u-test and were expressed as median (min-max). Categorical variables were compared by Chi square test and were expressed as % (number) unless otherwise mentioned. Clinical response to biologic therapies was assessed by the reduction in CDAI, CRP or mHAQ from baseline to week 12. Increase of Hb levels (g/dl) was compared between the TCZ and the non-TCZ group and was expressed as median (Min-Max). TCZ, tocilizumab; RA, rheumatoid arthritis; BMI, body mass index; eGFR estimated glomerular filtration rate; Hb, hemoglobin; RBC, red blood cell count; MCV, mean corpuscular volume; MCH, mean corpuscular hemoglobin; LHD%, low hemoglobin density; CDAI, clinical disease activity index; CRP, C-reactive protein; mHAQ modified health assessment questionnaire-disability index; CCP, citrullinated protein/peptide; NSAIDs, non-steroidal anti-inflammatory drugs.

between the increase of Hb and potential confounders were evaluated using Spearman's Rank correlation coefficient. Multivariate analysis of covariance was used to analyze the effect size TCZ therapy and other confounding factors displaying significant associations in the univariate analyses for the increase of Hb levels. Because the effect of biologic therapies on the increase of Hb levels was unknown, a formal sample size estimate was not made a priori. Data were expressed as median (min to max) for continuous variables and percentages (numbers) for categorical variables unless otherwise mentioned.

Results

Study population

During the study period, 750 patients were registered in the KURAMA cohort and 151 patients were newly introduced for biologic therapies and remained on the drugs for more than 12 weeks. Three patients receiving hemodialysis and one patient who had gastrointestinal bleeding complication before week 12 were excluded from the study. Among the 147 study population, 28 (19.0%) patients were treated with TCZ and 119 (81.0%) patients with non-TCZ biologic therapies; 87 (59.2%) patients were treated with TNF inhibitors including 23 (15.6%) patients with etanercept, 27 (18.4%) patients with infliximab, 9 (6.1%) patients with adalimumab, 28 (19.0%) patients with golimumab, while 32 (21.8%) patients were treated by abatacept. The study population (n = 147) were divided into the TCZ group (n = 28) and the non-TCZ group (n = 119) including TNF inhibitors(infliximab, etanercept, adalimumab, golimumab, n = 87) and abatacept (n = 32) and used for the analysis.

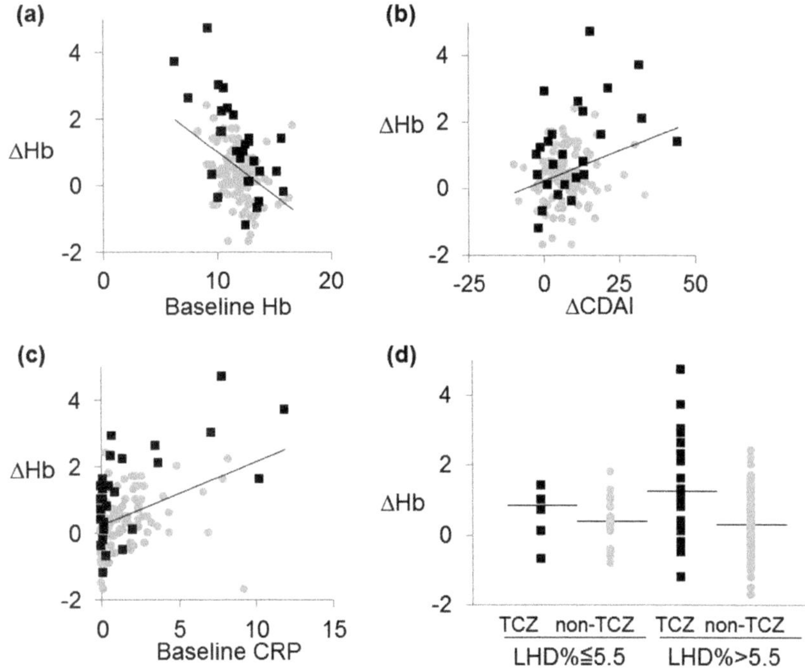

Figure 1. Correlation between the increase of hemoglobin levels and baseline hemoglobin (a), CRP (b), reduction in the clinical disease activity index (c), and baseline LHD% (d). Dot plot suggests the correlation between (a) baseline hemoglobin (Hb) and ΔHb (N = 147), (b) baseline CRP and ΔHb (N = 147), and (c) reduction in the clinical disease activity index (ΔCDAI) and ΔHb (N = 122) in rheumatoid arthritis patients treated by TCZ (black closed square) or non-TCZ biologics (gray closed circle). The straight line corresponds to the best-fit linear regression line for all samples. (d) ΔHb levels in patients treated with TCZ (black closed square) or non-TCZ biologics (gray closed circle) are expressed in two groups divided by the baseline LHD% value 5.5. The straight lines represent the median levels of ΔHb for indicated groups. (ΔHb = Hb at week 12 - Hb at baseline, ΔCDAI = CDAI at baseline – CDAI at week 12; LHD% = low hemoglobin density.)

Baseline characteristics and clinical response

The baseline characteristics including Hb, MCV, MCH, LHD%, or CRP levels and CDAI were not different between the TCZ and the non-TCZ groups (**Table1**). Anemia was present in 53.6% of the TCZ group and 47.9% of the non-TCZ group. The median levels of MCV in anemic patients were normal (91.3), but the minimum and maximum levels of MCV varied widely (69.6–105.1) suggesting that the causes of anemia in this study population are multifactorial. LHD% levels exceeded the cut off value 5.5 in 81.0% of the patients suggesting the presence of functional iron deficiency in the majority of patients. Baseline mHAQ tended to be higher in the TCZ group than in the non-TCZ group, but this tendency was not found to be statistically significant. The frequency of concomitant use of methotrexate or NSAIDs was not different between the two groups, while that of the use of glucocorticoids and iron drugs was higher in the TCZ group than in the non-TCZ group. Additionally, previous use of biologics was more frequent in the TCZ group than in the non-TCZ group (**Table 1**). The clinical responses to treatment assessed by ΔCDAI, ΔCRP, and ΔmHAQ were not different between the TCZ and the non-TCZ group (**Table 1**).

Increase of Hb levels after TCZ therapy

In the current study, we aimed to compare the effects of biologic therapies on anemia of RA. The increase of Hb levels was greater in the TCZ group than in the non-TCZ group (1.1 vs 0.3 g/dL, respectively, $p = 0.009$) (**Table 1**), while no significant difference was observed within the non-TCZ group between TNF inhibitors (infliximab, etanercept, adalimumab, golimumab) and abatacept (0.4 vs 0.2 g/dL, respectively, $p = 0.64$).

Next, we performed univariate regression analysis to determine if there were any confounding factors associated with the increase of Hb levels after biologic therapies. Increase in Hb levels was significantly correlated with lower Hb levels, higher LHD%, and higher CRP levels at baseline, and with better clinical response assessed by ΔCDAI or ΔCRP, but not ΔmHAQ (**Table 2**) (**Figure 1**). Increase of Hb levels was not associated with other continuous variables such as age, body mass index, MCV, or renal function assessed by estimated glomerular filtration index. Furthermore, categorical variables such as concomitant use of methotrexate, glucocorticoids, NSAIDs, iron drugs, folic acid, or previous use of biologics did not affect the increase in Hb levels (**Table 2**).

Thus, we selected baseline Hb levels, baseline LHD%, baseline disease activity, and clinical response to treatment as potential confounders for the multivariate analysis (**Table 3**). Because LHD%>5.5 was a reliable marker for detecting functional iron deficiency, the dichotomous variable with a cut off value LHD%> 5.5 was used in the multivariate analysis. Baseline disease activity and clinical response was assessed by CDAI and ΔCDAI in model 1, CRP and ΔCRP in model 2, respectively. In both models, TCZ remained as an independent factor associated with the increase of Hb level even after adjustment for baseline Hb levels, baseline LHD%>5.5, baseline disease activity and the clinical response to treatment. The effect size of TCZ for the increase of Hb level was 0.08 to 0.12 (**Table 3**). Baseline Hb levels, baseline LHD%>5.5, disease activity and clinical response to treatment also remained as a significant factor for the increase of Hb, suggesting that not only TCZ use but also baseline anemic state, functional iron deficiency,

Table 2. Factors associated with increase of Hb levels after biologic therapies.

	ρ	P
Basic characteristics		
Age, year	0.00	0.97
Sex (female)	−0.06	0.49
Duration of RA, month	−0.06	0.54
Body mass index, kg/m^2	0.05	0.58
Estimated glomerular filtration index	0.10	0.29
Hb, g/dl	−0.37	<0.001
RBC, 10^6/ml	−0.34	<0.001
MCV, fL	−0.02	0.80
MCH, pg	−0.10	0.29
LHD%	0.21	0.01
CDAI	0.03	0.77
CRP, mg/dl	0.32	<0.001
mHAQ	−0.07	0.51
Concomitant treatments		
Methotrexate	0.02	0.79
Glucocorticoids	0.04	0.68
NSAIDs	−0.14	0.09
Iron drugs	0.10	0.25
Folic acid	0.09	0.27
Previous biologics	−0.14	0.10
Clinical response		
ΔCDAI	0.23	0.01
ΔCRP, mg/dl	0.34	<0.001
ΔmHAQ	0.18	0.09

Association between the increase of Hb levels and characteristics of the patients were assessed by Spearman's rank test. Clinical response to biologic therapies was assessed by the reduction of CDAI, CRP, or mHAQ from baseline to week 12, (ΔCDAI = CDAI at baseline - CDAI at week 12, ΔCRP = CRP at baseline - CRP at week 12, and ΔmHAQ = mHAQ at baseline - mHAQ at week 12, respectively). ρ represents Spearman's rank correlation coefficient; RA, rheumatoid arthritis; BMI, body mass index; eGFR, estimated glomerular filtration index; Hb; hemoglobin, RBC; red blood cell count; MCV, mean corpuscular volume; MCH, mean corpuscular hemoglobin; LHD%, low hemoglobin density, CDAI, clinical disease activity index; CRP, C-reactive protein; mHAQ, modified health assessment questionnaire-disability index; NSAIDs, non-steroidal anti-inflammatory drugs.

and the state of inflammation collectively determine the change of Hb levels after biologic therapies (**Table 3**).

To exclude the possible impact of iron supplementation in our cohort, we also analyzed the data by excluding the patients who received iron drugs from the study population (excluding 3 patients in TCZ group and 7 patients in the non-TCZ group, N = 137). The increase of Hb levels was also significantly higher in the TCZ group than in the non-TCZ group (1.2 vs 0.3 g/dl,

Table 3. Effect of TCZ therapy and other confounding factors for the increase of Hb levels.

	Model 1		Model 2	
	Effect size	**P**	**Effect size**	**P**
TCZ therapy	0.12	<0.001	0.08	<0.001
Hb level at baseline	0.23	<0.001	0.13	0.001
LHD%>5.5 at baseline	0.06	0.009	0.03	0.028
Disease activity at baseline	0.08	0.002	0.01	0.40
Clinical response	0.12	<0.001	0.08	<0.001

The effect size of TCZ therapy and other confounding factors for the increase of Hb levels after treatment was analyzed by the multivariate analysis of covariance. Disease activity and clinical response was assessed by CDAI and ΔCDAI in model 1, and CRP and ΔCRP in model 2, respectively. (ΔCDAI = CDAI at baseline - CDAI at week 12, ΔCRP = CRP at baseline - CRP at week 12). TCZ, tocilizumab; Hb, hemoglobin; LHD%, low hemoglobin density; CDAI, clinical disease activity index; CRP, C-reactive protein; mHAQ, modified health assessment questionnaire-disability index.

respectively, p = 0.0003), and the multivariate analysis revealed that TCZ therapy was an independent factor associated with the increase of Hb levels (effect size 0.12–0.15).

Discussion

In this study, we have shown that Hb levels increase more after TCZ therapy than other biologic therapies. Even after adjusting for baseline characteristics, baseline disease activity, and clinical response to treatment, TCZ therapy was an independent factor that was associated with the increase of Hb levels after biologic therapies. Improvement of anemia after biologic therapies such as TCZ or TNF inhibitors has been reported previously in RA [5] [8] [11], and other inflammatory diseases such as Castleman's disease [9] [10]. However, few studies have compared the effect of different biologic therapies with possible confounding factors for the increase of Hb levels. We have recently reported the pronounced increase of Hb levels by TCZ than TNF inhibitors in RA patients in a different cohort [22]. However, in that cohort, baseline CRP levels and clinical responses were higher in the TCZ group than the TNF inhibitor's group and the effect of these confounding factors were not fully investigated [22]. Our study suggests that TCZ therapy would be beneficial for treating anemia of RA patients, in particular with severe anemia and high disease activity.

Our results are consistent with the recent studies suggesting the central role of IL-6-hepcidin axis in ACD [3] [23]. Hepcidin, a peptide hormone produced mainly by hepatocytes, reduces intestinal iron absorption and blocks iron release from macrophages to induce hypoferremia and pathogenic iron homeostasis to cause ACD [3] [4] [24]. IL-6 was the necessary and sufficient cytokine for the induction of hepcidin during inflammation because IL-6 or hepcidin knockout mice do not develop anemia upon inflammation [23] [25]. IL-6 level was the only factor other than disease stage that independently predicted Hb levels in cancer associated ACD [26]. IL-6 inhibition by TCZ was effective in correcting anemia in Castleman's disease which is characterized by the overproduction of IL-6 from lymph nodes [9]. Therefore, IL-6-hepcidin axis is central to ACD both *in vivo* and *in vitro*.

Although we have shown that TCZ therapy was an independent factor associated with the increase of Hb levels after biologic therapies by consecutively enrolling all the RA patients treated by biologics in the KURAMA cohort, our study has several limitations. First, since the study population was small, the result may not be valid for all RA patients. Second, several baseline characteristics such as concomitant use of glucocorticoids and iron drugs were different between the TCZ and the non-TCZ group in our study population, although these factors did not affect the increase of Hb levels in the univariate analysis and the result of the multivariate analysis was not affected when these factors were included as covariates. Third, due to the lack of data on markers of iron status (serum iron, ferritin, and transferrin), hepcidin, or erythropoietin, we could not assess the mechanisms of anemia in our study population. Although we postulate that ACD is the major mechanism involved because IL-6 inhibition by TCZ was effective in increasing Hb levels, we cannot rule out other possibilities; for example, IL-6 inhibition may have acted directly on erythropoiesis or the erythropoietin response [27]. Further studies will be necessary to fully determine the role of IL-6 in anemia of RA.

In conclusion, this study has shown that Hb level significantly increases after TCZ therapy compared with non-TCZ biologic therapies even after adjustment for baseline characteristics, baseline disease activity, and clinical response to treatment. It implies the central role of IL-6 in anemia of RA patients and suggests that TCZ would be a good option for RA patients with anemia.

Author Contributions

Conceived and designed the experiments: M. Hashimoto TF T. Mimori. Performed the experiments: M. Hashimoto TF MF HI KO. Analyzed the data: M. Hashimoto M. Hamaguchi CT. Contributed reagents/materials/analysis tools: KY WY T. Matsuo MM. Wrote the paper: M. Hashimoto M. Hamaguchi HK.

References

1. Weiss G, Goodnough LT (2005) Anemia of chronic disease. N Engl J Med 352: 1011–1023.
2. Han C, Rahman MU, Doyle MK, Bathon JM, Smolen J, et al. (2007) Association of anemia and physical disability among patients with rheumatoid arthritis. J Rheumatol 34: 2177–2182.
3. Raj DSC (2009) Role of interleukin-6 in the anemia of chronic disease. Semin Arthritis Rheum 38: 382–388.
4. Ganz T (2003) Hepcidin, a key regulator of iron metabolism and mediator of anemia of inflammation. Blood 102: 783–788.
5. Papadaki HA, Kritikos HD, Valatas V, Boumpas DT, Eliopoulos GD (2002) Anemia of chronic disease in rheumatoid arthritis is associated with increased apoptosis of bone marrow erythroid cells: improvement following anti-tumor necrosis factor-alpha antibody therapy. Blood 100: 474–482.
6. Smolen JS, Landewé R, Breedveld FC, Dougados M, Emery P, et al. (2010) EULAR recommendations for the management of rheumatoid arthritis with synthetic and biological disease-modifying antirheumatic drugs. Ann Rheum Dis 69: 964–975.
7. Doyle MK, Rahman MU, Han C, Han J, Giles J, et al. (2009) Treatment with infliximab plus methotrexate improves anemia in patients with rheumatoid arthritis independent of improvement in other clinical outcome measures-a pooled analysis from three large, multicenter, double-blind, randomized clinical trials. Semin Arthritis Rheum 39: 123–131.
8. Demirag MD, Haznedaroglu S, Sancak B, Konca C, Gulbahar O, et al. (2009) Circulating hepcidin in the crossroads of anemia and inflammation associated with rheumatoid arthritis. Intern Med 48: 421–426.
9. Song S-NJ, Tomosugi N, Kawabata H, Ishikawa T, Nishikawa T, et al. (2010) Down-regulation of hepcidin resulting from long-term treatment with an anti-IL-6 receptor antibody (tocilizumab) improves anemia of inflammation in multicentric Castleman disease. Blood 116: 3627–3634.
10. Furst DE, Kay J, Wasko MC, Keystone E, Kavanaugh A, et al. (2013) The effect of golimumab on haemoglobin levels in patients with rheumatoid arthritis, psoriatic arthritis or ankylosing spondylitis. Rheumatology (Oxford) 52: 1845–1855.
11. Doyle MK, Rahman MU, Frederick B, Birbara CA, de Vries D, et al. (2013) Effects of subcutaneous and intravenous golimumab on inflammatory biomarkers in patients with rheumatoid arthritis: results of a phase 1, randomized, open-label trial. Rheumatology (Oxford) 52: 1214–9.
12. Matsuyama M, Suzuki T, Tsuboi H, Ito S, Mamura M, et al. (2007) Anti-interleukin-6 receptor antibody (tocilizumab) treatment of multicentric Castleman's disease. Intern Med 46: 771–774.
13. Ferrucci L, Semba RD, Guralnik JM, Ershler WB, Bandinelli S, et al. (2010) Proinflammatory state, hepcidin, and anemia in older persons. Blood 115: 3810–3816.
14. Wolfe F, Michaud K (2006) Anemia and renal function in patients with rheumatoid arthritis. J Rheumatol 33: 1516–1522.
15. Möller B, Scherer A, Förger F, Villiger PM, Finckh A (2013) Anaemia may add information to standardised disease activity assessment to predict radiographic damage in rheumatoid arthritis: a prospective cohort study. Ann Rheum Dis 73: 691–6.
16. Terao C, Hashimoto M, Yamamoto K, Murakami K, Ohmura K, et al. (2013) Three Groups in the 28 Joints for Rheumatoid Arthritis Synovitis - Analysis Using More than 17,000 Assessments in the KURAMA Database. PLoS One 8: e59341.
17. Furu M, Hashimoto M, Ito H, Fujii T, Terao C, et al. (2014) Discordance and accordance between patient's and physician's assessments in rheumatoid arthritis. Scand J Rheumatol. In press.
18. Aletaha D, Neogi T, Silman AJ, Funovits J, Felson DT, et al. (2010) 2010 Rheumatoid arthritis classification criteria: an American College of Rheumatology/European League Against Rheumatism collaborative initiative. Arthritis Rheum 62: 2569–2581.
19. Thomas DW, Hinchliffe RF, Briggs C, Macdougall IC, Littlewood T, et al. (2013) Guideline for the laboratory diagnosis of functional iron deficiency. Br J Haematol 161: 639–648.

20. Urrechaga E, Unceta M, Borque L, Escanero JF (2012) Low hemoglobin density potential marker of iron availability. Int J Lab Hematol 34: 47–51.
21. Smolen JS, Schoels MM, Nishimoto N, Breedveld FC, Burmester GR, et al. (2013) Consensus statement on blocking the effects of interleukin-6 and in particular by interleukin-6 receptor inhibition in rheumatoid arthritis and other inflammatory conditions. Ann Rheum Dis 72: 482–492.
22. Song S-NJ, Iwahashi M, Tomosugi N, Uno K, Yamana J, et al. (2013) Comparative evaluation of the effects of treatment with tocilizumab and TNF-α inhibitors on serum hepcidin, anemia response and disease activity in rheumatoid arthritis patients. Arthritis Res Ther 15: R141.
23. Nemeth E, Rivera S, Gabayan V, Keller C, Taudorf S, et al. (2004) IL-6 mediates hypoferremia of inflammation by inducing the synthesis of the iron regulatory hormone hepcidin. J Clin Invest 113: 1271–1276.
24. Nemeth E, Valore EV, Territo M, Schiller G, Lichtenstein A, et al. (2003) Hepcidin, a putative mediator of anemia of inflammation, is a type II acute-phase protein. Blood 101: 2461–2463.
25. Laftah AH, Ramesh B, Simpson RJ, Solanky N, Bahram S, et al. (2004) Effect of hepcidin on intestinal iron absorption in mice. Blood 103: 3940–3944.
26. Macciò A, Madeddu C, Massa D, Mudu MC, Lusso MR, et al. (2005) Hemoglobin levels correlate with interleukin-6 levels in patients with advanced untreated epithelial ovarian cancer: role of inflammation in cancer-related anemia. Blood 106: 362–367.
27. Nikolaisen C, Figenschau Y, Nossent JC (2008) Anemia in early rheumatoid arthritis is associated with interleukin 6-mediated bone marrow suppression, but has no effect on disease course or mortality. J Rheumatol 35: 380–386.

3

Toll-Like Receptor 4 Mediates Endothelial Cell Activation Through NF-κB but Is Not Associated with Endothelial Dysfunction in Patients with Rheumatoid Arthritis

Rossella Menghini[1], Umberto Campia[2*], Manfredi Tesauro[1], Arianna Marino[1], Valentina Rovella[1], Giuseppe Rodia[1], Francesca Schinzari[3], Barbara Tolusso[4], Nicola di Daniele[1], Massimo Federici[1,5], Angelo Zoli[4], Gianfranco Ferraccioli[4], Carmine Cardillo[3]

1 Department of System Medicine, University of Tor Vergata, Rome, Italy, **2** Division of Cardiology, MedStar Heart Institute, Washington, DC, United States of America, **3** Department of Internal Medicine, Catholic University Medical School, Rome, Italy, **4** Department of Rheumatology, Catholic University Medical School, Rome, Italy, **5** Center for Atherosclerosis, Policlinico Tor Vergata, Rome, Italy

Abstract

Objective: To investigate the effects of TLR4 antagonism on human endothelial cells activation and cytokine expression, and whether the Asp299Gly TLR4 polymorphism is associated with better endothelial function in patients with rheumatoid arthritis (RA).

Methods: Human aortic endothelial cells (HAECs) were treated with lipopolysaccharide (LPS), OxPAPC, and free fatty acids (FFA) at baseline and after incubation with the TLR4 antagonist eritoran (E5564). Cytokine expression was assessed by quantitative real-time PCR. In vivo endothelial function was assessed as brachial artery flow-mediated dilation (FMD) in RA patients with the wild type gene (aa) and with the Asp299Gly TLR4 polymorphic variant (ag).

Results: In HAEC, TLR4 antagonism with eritoran inhibited LPS-induced mRNA expression of IL-6, IL-8, TNFα, CCL-2, VCAM and ICAM ($P<0.05$ for all) and inhibited Ox-PAPC-induced mRNA expression of IL-8 ($P<0.05$) and IL-6, albeit not to a statistically significant level ($p=0.07$). In contrast, eritoran did not affect FFA-induced mRNA expression of IL-6 ($P>0.05$). In 30 patients with RA (15 with the ag allele) undergoing measurement of FMD, no differences in FMD and plasma levels of IL-6, IL-8, VCAM, and ICAM were found between the aa and the ag phenotype ($P>0.05$ for all).

Conclusions: TLR4 signaling in endothelial cells may be triggered by LPS and oxidized phospholipids, leading to endothelial activation and inflammation, which are inhibited by eritoran. Our in vivo investigation, however, does not support an association between the Asp299Gly TLR4 polymorphism and improved endothelium-dependent vasodilator function in patients with RA. Further study is needed to better understand the potential role of TLR4 on endothelial dysfunction in this and other patient populations.

Editor: Angelo Scuteri, INRCA, Italy

Funding: This work as supported by an intramural grant of Tor Vergata University to Dr. Menghini. The funders had no role in study design, data collection and analysis, decision to publish, or preparation of the manuscript.

Competing Interests: The authors have declared that no competing interests exist.

* E-mail: umberto.campia@medstar.net

Introduction

Chronic inflammation represents a pivotal mechanism in the pathogenesis of atherosclerosis [1]. Interestingly, recent evidence suggests that innate immunity may also contribute to the development of vascular damage by interacting with inflammatory pathways [2]. In particular, toll-like receptors (TLRs) are increasingly being recognized as a link between the innate immune system, inflammation, and atherogenesis. This family of innate immune receptors is expressed by endothelial cells, in which they trigger various signaling pathways and lead to cell activation, increased expression of inflammatory cytokines and adhesion molecules, and endothelial dysfunction [3,4]. While initially identified as sensors of microbial invasion, TLRs are now known to be activated also by endogenous ligands produced in inflamed tissues, potentially leading to further inflammation and perpetuating an inflammatory milieu [3]. Among them, TLR4, a receptor for lipopolysaccharide (LPS) from Gram negative bacterial cell walls, also exhibits affinity for fatty acids [5], extracellular matrix components, fibrinogen, and various heat shock proteins [6]. Of note, TRL4 signaling leads to activation of NF-κB [4], a pathway associated with andothelial injury [7], and TRL4 expression is increased in human atherosclerotic plaques [8]. Additionally, lack of TLR4 reduces atherosclerosis and alters plaque phenotype in apoE-deficient mice fed a high-cholesterol diet [9]. In agreement with these data, clinical evidence indicates that the Asp299Gly TLR4 polymorphism, a functional variant in the TLR4 gene (896A→G) that attenuates receptor signaling and diminishes the inflammatory response to LPS [10], is associated with decreased atherosclerotic risk [11]. However, whether antagonism of TLR4 prevents TLR4-induced expression of inflammatory cytokines and adhesion molecules in human macrovascular endothelial cells has not been investigated in detail.

Rheumatoid arthritis (RA) is one of the most prevalent systemic autoimmune diseases [12] and is associated with endothelial dysfunction [13] and increased cardiovascular risk [14]. This risk is attributed to the presence of both traditional and non-traditional risk factors, including inflammation and immunologic abnormalities [15]. A growing body of knowledge indicates that TLR4 may play a relevant role of in the pathogenesis of autoimmune damage in RA [3]. In line with this evidence, the Asp299Gly TLR4 polymorphism is associated with decreased RA disease susceptibility and lower baseline disease activity [16]. However, whether the presence of the Asp299Gly TLR4 polymorphism is associated with better endothelial function compared with the wild type genotype in patients with RA has not been studied.

The current investigations were therefore designed to test the following hypotheses: 1) antagonism of TLR4 with eritoran (E5564) inhibits the expression of inflammatory cytokines and adhesion molecules in human endothelial cells; and 2) the presence of the Asp299Gly TLR4 polymorphism is associated with better endothelium-dependent vasodilation compared with the wild type genotype in patients with RA.

Materials and Methods

In-Vitro Experiments: Cell Culture and Treatment

Human aortic endothelial cells (HAECs) were purchased from Lonza (Basel, Switzerland) and cultured according to the manufacturer's instructions. All experiments were performed using HAECs between the 2th and the 5th passage. HAECs were treated with: LPS (Sigma Aldrich, St. Louis, MO) at a concentration of 100 ng/mL for 6 hours; ox-PAPC (oxidation products of 1-palmitoyl-2-arachidonoyl-sn-glycerol-3-phosphatidylcholine, Hycult Biotech, Uden, The Netherlands), an antigenic epitope of oxidized LDL, at a concentration of 100 µg/mL for 6 hours; or long chain free fatty acids (FFA, oleic acid 500 µM+palmitic acid 500 µM) for 24 hours. Cells were incubated with 10 nM eritoran for 30 minutes prior to treatments where indicated. Eritoran (Eisai Inc., Woodcliff Lake, NJ) is a synthetic analog of lipid A and a potent and specific antagonist of LPS action, which inhibits lipid A binding to MD2 and terminates MD2/TLR4-mediated signaling [17]. At the end of treatments, HAECs where collected and used for molecular analysis.

In-Vitro Experiments: Gene Expression Analysis

Total RNA was isolated from HAECs using Trizol reagents (Invitrogen Corp, Eugene, OR). A total of 2 µg of RNA was reverse-transcribed into complementary DNA (cDNA) using the High Capacity cDNA Archive kit (Applied Biosystems, Foster City, CA). Fifty nanograms of cDNA was amplified by real-time polymerase chain reaction (RT-PCR) using an ABI PRISM 7500 System and TaqMan reagents (Applied Biosystems) and normalized to 18S ribosomal RNA as an endogenous control. Each reaction was performed in triplicate, and the relative gene copy number was calculated as $2^{-\Delta\Delta Ct}$ as previously described [18].

In-Vitro Experiments: Western Blots

Total protein was isolated from HAECs and western blots were performed as previously described [19]. The following antibodies were used: anti-P65, anti-phosphoSer^{536} P65, anti-IκBα, and anti-phosphoSer$^{32/36}$ IκBα, (Cell Signaling Technology Inc., Danvers, MA).

Clinical Study: Study Population

Nonsmoker patients with a diagnosis of RA according to the ACR revised criteria [20] and age- and sex-matched healthy controls were enrolled in the study. None of the patients had history or presence of hypertension, diabetes, hypercholesterolemia, cardiovascular disease, vasculitis, or any other systemic condition. All RA patients were on chronic treatment with either disease modifying antirheumatic drugs (DMARDs), monoclonal antibodies, or their combination. When used, aspirin, coxibs or other nonsteroidal anti-inflammatory drugs were withdrawn at least one week before the study; patients were allowed to use acetaminophen (paracetamol) or tramadol as needed. The Disease Activity Score 44 (DAS 44) was calculated for each patient. This score assesses disease activity by including tender and swollen joint count and the erythrocyte sedimentation rate. The level of disease activity can be interpreted as low (DAS≤2.4), moderate (2.4< DAS≤3.7), or high (DAS>3.7) [21]. A DAS<1.6 corresponds with being in remission according to the American Rheumatism Association (ARA) criteria [22]. The study protocol was conducted according to the principles expressed in the Declaration of Helsinki, was approved by the institutional Ethics Committee of Tor Vergata University, and all participants gave written informed consent.

Clinical Study: Laboratory Methods

EDTA-collected blood samples were drawn on the study day after an overnight fast, immediately centrifuged for 15 min at 1000×g and stored at −80°C until analysis.

Detection of autoantibodies. Rheumatoid factor (RF)-IgM and RF-IgA (Orgentec Diagnostika GmbH, Mainz, Germany) and anti-CCP antibodies (Axis Shield Diagnostics, Dundee, UK) were measured using commercially available ELISA kits Equal volumes for each sample were loaded according to each specific kit's instructions. The suggested cut-off levels were 20 U/mL for RF-IgM and RF-IgA and 5 U/mL for anti-CCP antibodies. *Soluble biomarkers:* plasma levels of IL-6, IL-8, ICAM, VCAM and MCP-1 were measured using commercially available ELISA kits (R&D Systems, Minneapolis, MN, USA). Equal volumes for each sample were loaded according to each specific kit's instructions. Quantitative levels of cytokines were determined by comparison with standard curves and reported as picograms or nanograms per mL (pg/mL or ng/mL). The sensitivity of the test was of 0.7 pg/mL for IL-6, 1.5 pg/mL for IL-8, 0.1 ng/mL for ICAM, 0.6 ng/mL for VCAM and 5.0 pg/mL for MCP-1. Genomic DNA for TLR4 genotyping was prepared from frozen whole blood with the use of a blood DNA isolation kit (Genomic Prep, Amersham Pharmacia Biotech, Piscataway, NJ). Subsequent allele-specific PCR amplification for the TLR4 allele Asp299Gly was performed according to a previously described protocol [23].

Clinical Study: Endothelial Function Testing

Assessment of endothelial function was conducted in the fasting state using a standardized ultrasound procedure [24]. Brachial artery reactivity, a test of endothelium-dependent vasodilation, was assessed as previously reported [25]. Briefly, participants lay supine on a bed and were allowed to rest for at least 10 minutes. During the rest period, participants were connected to a continuous ECG monitor and a pressure cuff was applied around the upper forearm. The left brachial artery was then visualized on the anterior aspect of the arm, 2–15 cm proximal to the antecubital fossa, using a Logiq E ultrasound machine (GE

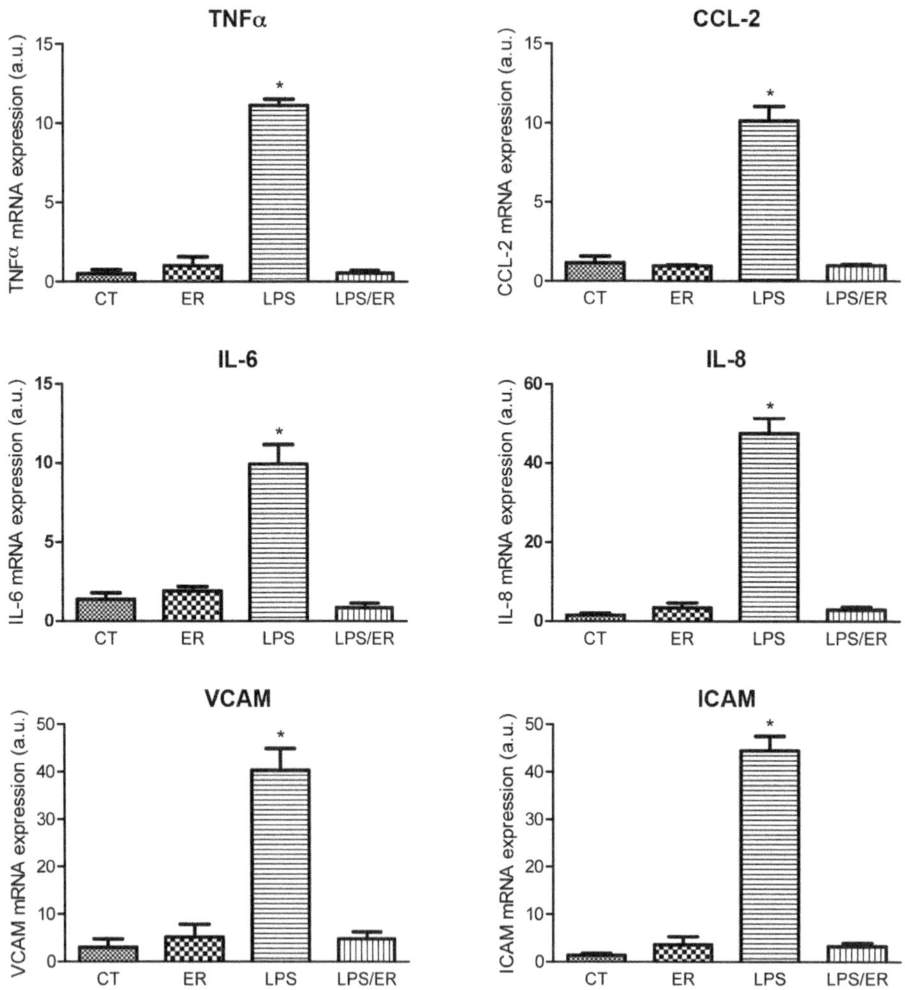

Figure 1. Effects of eritoran on LPS-induced mRNA expression (arbitrary units) of TNFα (top left panel), CCL-2 (top right panel), IL-6 (middle left panel), IL-8 (middle right panel), VCAM (bottom left panel), and ICAM (bottom right panel). Values reported as mean±SD (n = 5 per group). CT: control; ER: eritoran; LPS: lipopolysaccharide; ER/LPS: eritoran/lipopolysaccharide. *p<0.05 vs CT, ER, and LPS/ER.

Healthcare Italia, Milan, Italy) with a high-resolution probe (12-MHz linear array transducer). After baseline images and flow measurements were obtained, the pressure cuff applied on the forearm was inflated at 250 mmHg for 5 minutes. Blood flow was measured during the first 15 seconds after cuff deflation, and arterial image acquisition for diameter measurements was performed between 60 and 90 seconds after cuff deflation. Arterial diameter was measured from the anterior to the posterior interface between the lumen and the endothelium at end diastole, incident with the R wave on the ECG. Images were analyzed by an investigator, different from the sonographer, blinded to image sequence and clinical data of study participants.

Statistical Analysis

For the clinical study, sample size calculation was based on differences between the values of FMD in the three groups. Using a 2-sided paired t test, a sample of 12 subjects in each group was calculated to be necessary to detect a 2% difference in FMD with 80% power and $\alpha < 0.05$. With anticipation of up to 3 (i.e. 20%) technically inadequate vascular studies, 15 participants per group were enrolled to yield 12 evaluable participants in each group. All group data are reported as mean ± SD. Group differences were analyzed by one way ANOVA, Fisher exact test, and unpaired Student t test, as appropriate. All calculated p values are two-tailed, and a value of $p < 0.05$ was considered to indicate statistical significance. Statistical analyses were performed using commercially available software.

Results

In-Vitro Experiments: Eritoran Inhibits LPS-Induced mRNA Expression of Inflammatory Cytokines in HAECs

To determine the effects of TLR4 receptor antagonism on LPS-induced expression of inflammatory cytokines in HAECs, we assessed mRNA levels of IL-6, IL-8, TNFα, and CCL-2 mRNA after treatment with LPS, alone and following pretreatment with eritoran for 30 minutes. Incubation with eritoran did not lead to significant changes in mRNA levels of these cytokines compared to control. Treatment with LPS alone for 6 hours induced a significant increase in cytokine expression. In contrast, when HAECs were treated with LPS following pretreatment with eritoran, cytokine mRNA levels were similar to control (figure 1, top and middle panels).

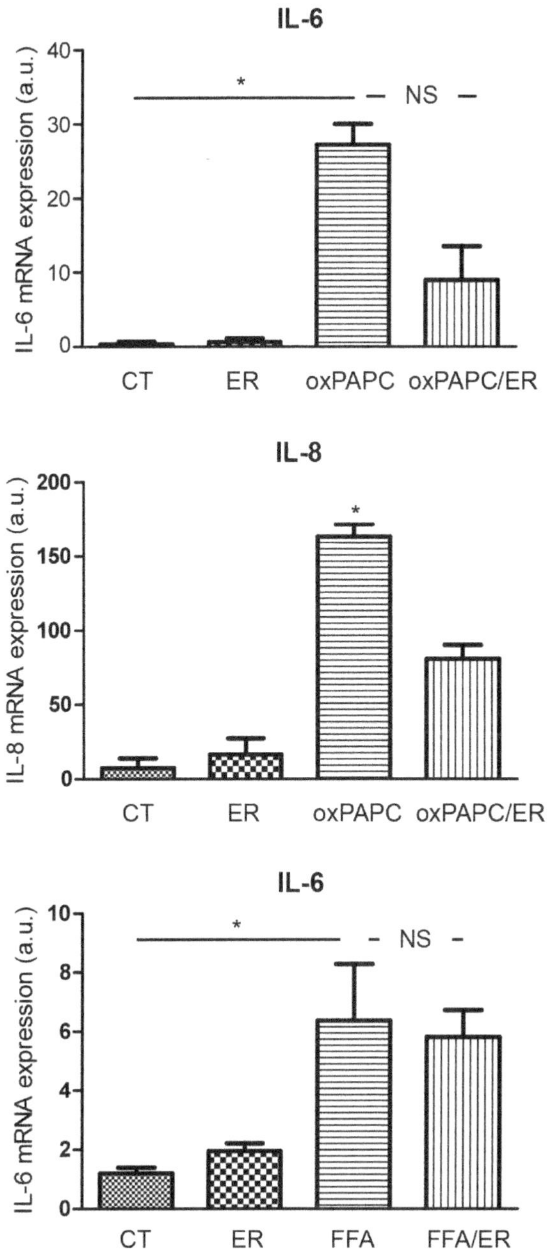

Figure 2. Effects of eritoran on OxPAPC-induced mRNA expression (arbitrary units) of IL-6 (top panel) and IL-8 (middle panel) and on FFA-induced mRNA expression (arbitrary units) of IL-6 (bottom panel). Values reported as mean±SD (n = 5 per group). CT: control; ER: eritoran; OxPAPC: oxidation products of 1-palmitoyl-2-arachidonoyl-sn-glycerol-3-phosphatidylcholine; FFA: free fatty acids; OxPAPC/ER: oxidation products of 1-palmitoyl-2-arachidonoyl-sn-glycerol-3-phosphatidylcholine/eritoran. Top panel: *$p<0.05$ vs CT and ER; NS: $p = 0.07$ vs OxPAPC/ER. Middle panel: *$p<0.05$ vs CT, ER, and OxPAPC/ER. Bottom panel: *$p<0.05$ vs CT and ER; NS: $p>0.05$ vs FFA/ER.

In-Vitro Experiments: Eritoran Inhibits LPS-Induced mRNA Expression of Adhesion Molecules in HAECs

To assess whether TLR4 receptor antagonism impacts LPS-induced expression of adhesion molecules in HAECs, we measured mRNA levels of VCAM and ICAM after treatment with LPS, alone and following pretreatment with eritoran for 30 minutes. compared with control, eritoran alone did not lead to significant changes in VCAM and ICAM mRNA levels. Treatment with LPS alone for 6 hours caused a significant increase in mRNA levels of the adhesion molecules. In contrast, when HAEC were treated with LPS following pretreatment with eritoran, mRNA levels of VCAM and ICAM were similar to control (figure 1, bottom panels).

In-Vitro Experiments: Eritoran Inhibits ox-PAPC-Induced mRNA Expression of IL-8 in HAECs

To explore the effects of TLR4 receptor antagonism on ox-PAPC-induced expression of inflammatory cytokines in HAECs, we assessed the effects of ox-PAPC treatment on mRNA levels of IL-6 and IL-8, alone and following pretreatment with eritoran for 30 minutes. Eritoran did not affect cytokine mRNA levels compared with control. ox-PAPC alone for 6 hours significantly increased cytokine mRNA levels. In contrast, when ox-PAPC treatment followed pretreatment with eritoran, mRNA levels of IL-8 were significantly reduced when compared with ox-PAPC alone (figure 2, top panel). Similarly, mRNA levels of IL-6 were reduced; however, they failed to reach statistical significance ($p = 0.07$) (figure 2, middle panel).

In-Vitro Experiments: Eritoran Does Not Affect FFA-Induced mRNA Expression of IL-6 in HAECs

To confirm that eritoran's effects on inflammatory cytokines are mediated by TLR4, we assessed the effects of FFA treatment on mRNA levels of IL-6, alone and after incubation with eritoran for 30 minutes. As in the previous experiments, eritoran did not affect IL-6 mRNA levels compared with control. FFA alone for 6 hours led to significantly increased IL-6 mRNA levels. Consistent with our hypothesis that eritoran's effects on inflammatory cytokines are mediated by TLR4, pre-treatment with eritoran did not affect FFA-induced inflammatory cytokine expression (figure 2, bottom panel).

In-Vitro Experiments: Eritoran Reduces LPS-Induced Phosphorylation of NF-κB p65 Subunit and IκB-α in HAECs

To confirm that the effects of TLR4 antagonism on the expression of inflammatory cytokines are mediated by a modulation of the NF-κB pathways, we assessed phosphorylation of NF-κB p65 subunit and of IκB-α by western blotting (figure 3, top panel). Compared with control, treatment with eritoran for 30 minutes did not induce phosphorylation of NF-κB p65 subunit and of IκB-α. In contrast, treatment of HAECs with LPS for 6 hours caused an increase in the phosphorylation of NF-κB p65 subunit and IκB-α. Pretreatment with eritoran prevented the LPS-induced phosphorylation of NF-κB p65 subunit (figure 3, bottom left panel) and IκB-α (figure 3, bottom right panel).

Clinical Study: Study Population

Thirty patients and 15 age- and sex-matched healthy controls took part in the study. Their baseline clinical characteristics are reported in Table 1. The mean DAS 44 score of all the patients was 2.2 (range: 0.5–3.9). The majority of the patients were treated with a disease-modifying anti-rheumatic drug (27/30) and/or a biologic agent (19/30). No significant differences were observed in these parameters, disease activity, and drug treatment between the two patient groups (all $P>0.05$).

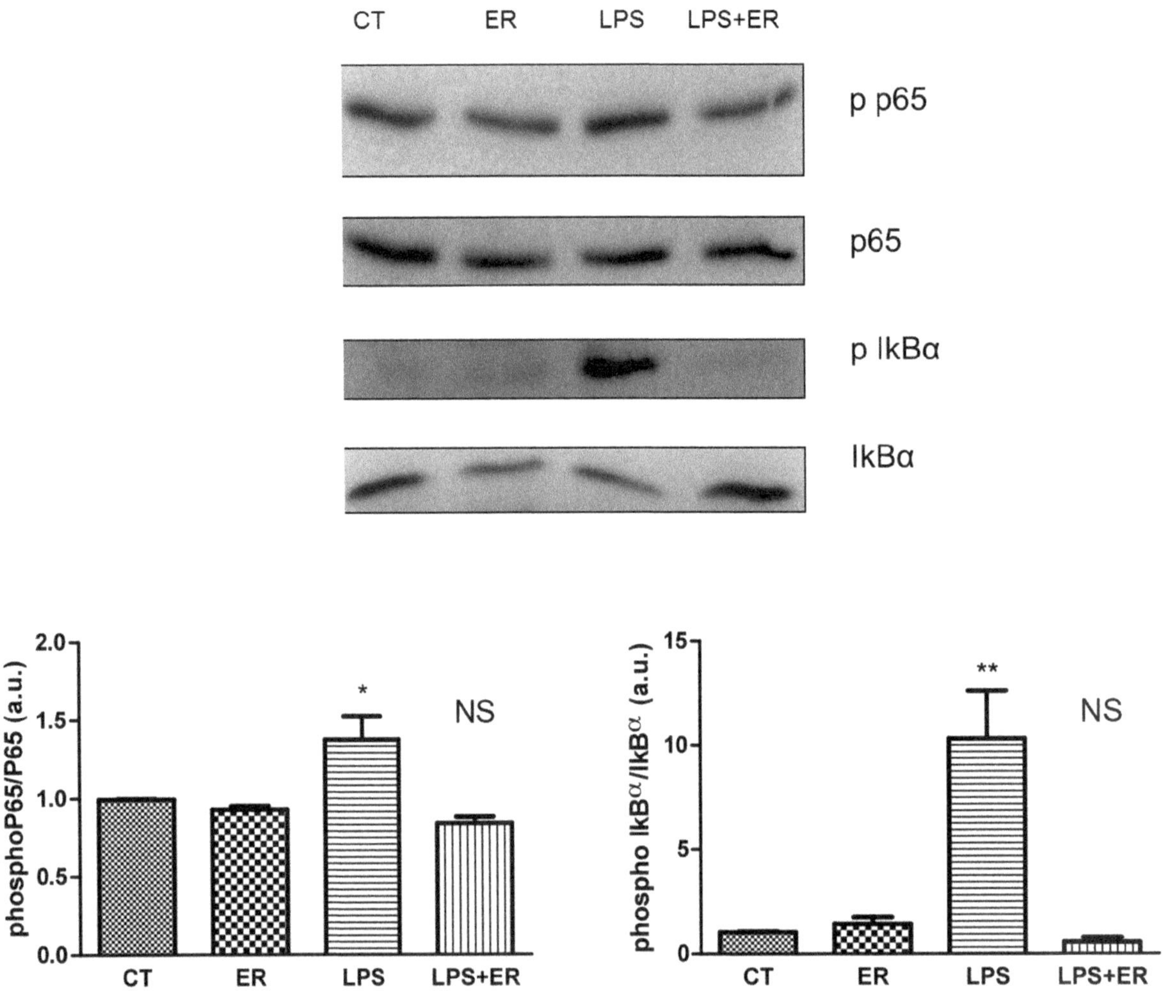

Figure 3. Representative Western blots (top panel) and bar graphs showing the effect of eritoran on LPS-induced phosphorylation of NF-κB p65 subunit (bottom left panel) and IκB-α (bottom right panel) (n = 5 per group). Bottom left panel: *$p<0.05$ vs CT; NS: $p>0.05$ vs LPS/ER. Bottom right panel: **$p<0.005$ vs CT; NS: $p>0.05$ vs LPS/ER.

Clinical Study: Brachial Artery Reactivity

Baseline brachial artery diameter was similar in the three groups (3.7±0.6 mm, 3.3±0.5 mm, and 3.4±0.7 mm in the control, aa, and ag group, respectively, p = 0.18). Flow-mediated dilation was significantly higher in the controls compared to the RA groups (p = 0.014). However, no significant differences in FMD were observed between the two patient groups (p>0.05) (figure 4 and figure 5, top left panel).

Clinical Study: Plasma Cytokines and Adhesion Molecules in RA Patients

Plasma levels of IL-6 and IL-8, of MCP-1, and of VCAM and ICAM were similar between the aa and ag groups (figure 5).

Discussion

The main results of our in-vitro investigations are that, in HAEC, TLR4 antagonism with eritoran: 1) inhibits LPS-induced mRNA expression of the inflammatory cytokines IL-6, IL-8, TNFα, and CCL-2, and of the adhesion molecules VCAM and ICAM; 2) inhibits ox-PAPC-induced mRNA expression of IL-8 and of IL-6, albeit to a borderline significant level; and 3) reduces LPS-induced phosphorylation of NF-κB p65 subunit and IκB-α. These findings indicate that TLR4 induces activation of human macrovascular endothelial cells through NF-κB-dependent pathways, leading to the expression of genes regulating the production of inflammatory mediators and adhesion molecules. Importantly, TLR4-dependent activation of these pathways is not restricted to exogenous ligands such as LPS, as mRNA expression of IL-6 and IL-8 was also triggered by Ox-PAPC. These phospholipid oxidation products are present in sites of chronic inflammation, in apoptotic cell membranes, and in oxidized LDL [26], suggesting a potential pathophysiologic role of Ox-PAPC-dependent LTR4 activation in atherosclerosis. Finally, as FFA-induced IL-6 expression was not affected by eritoran, our data suggest that TLR4 activation in macrovascular endothelial cells is possibly restricted to specific lipid ligands such as Ox-PAPC.

Our results are in agreement with the recent findings from Lu and colleagues. These authors reported that, in HAEC and in dermal microvascular endothelial cells, LPS induced an increase in mRNA expression and synthesis of IL-6, as well as a more robust gene expression of IL-8 and other inflammatory cytokines, ICAM, VCAM, chemokines, growth factors, and adhesion molecules [27]. Our study shows that also Ox-PAPC, an endogenous byproduct of phospholipid peroxidation, triggers TLR4-dependent expression

Table 1. Baseline Characteristics of Study Participants.

Parameter	TLR4 Alleles			P
	Control	AA (Wild type)	AG (Asp299Gly)	
Participants per group (number)	15	15	15	
Sex (women/men)	10/5	12/3	10/5	0.71*
Age (years)	54±4	47±12	50±14	0.22#
BMI (kg/m²)	25.0±4.3	26.3±4.8	27.0±2.7	0.40#
Fasting blood glucose (mg/mL)	94±10	94±36	105±28	0.44#
Disease duration (Years)	N/A	8.0±7.8	6.1±9.4	0.56
Disease Activity Score (DAS 44)	N/A	2.08±0.93	1.84±0.74	0.43
DMARD (yes/no)	N/A	13/2	14/1	0.54
Anti-CCP antibodies level (U/mL)	N/A	93.0±192.8	42.1±41.0	0.33
Rheumatoid Factor – IgM level (IU/mL)	N/A	69.7±130.0	59.6±67.0	0.79
Rheumatoid Factor – IgA level (IU/mL)	N/A	26.6±49.4	30.9±41.5	0.80
ESR (mm/h)	N/A	19±17	40±76	0.31
hsCRP (mg/L)	N/A	4.7±4.1	3.8±2.8	0.51

DMARD: disease-modifying anti-rheumatic drug; anti-CCP: anti-cyclic citrullinated peptide antibodies; ESR: erythrocyte sedimentation rate. hsCRP: high sensitivity C-reactive protein; BMI: body mass index.
*p value calculated using Fisher exact test and #p value calculated using one way ANOVA; all other p values calculated using unpaired t test.
Values are reported as mean ± SD unless specified otherwise.

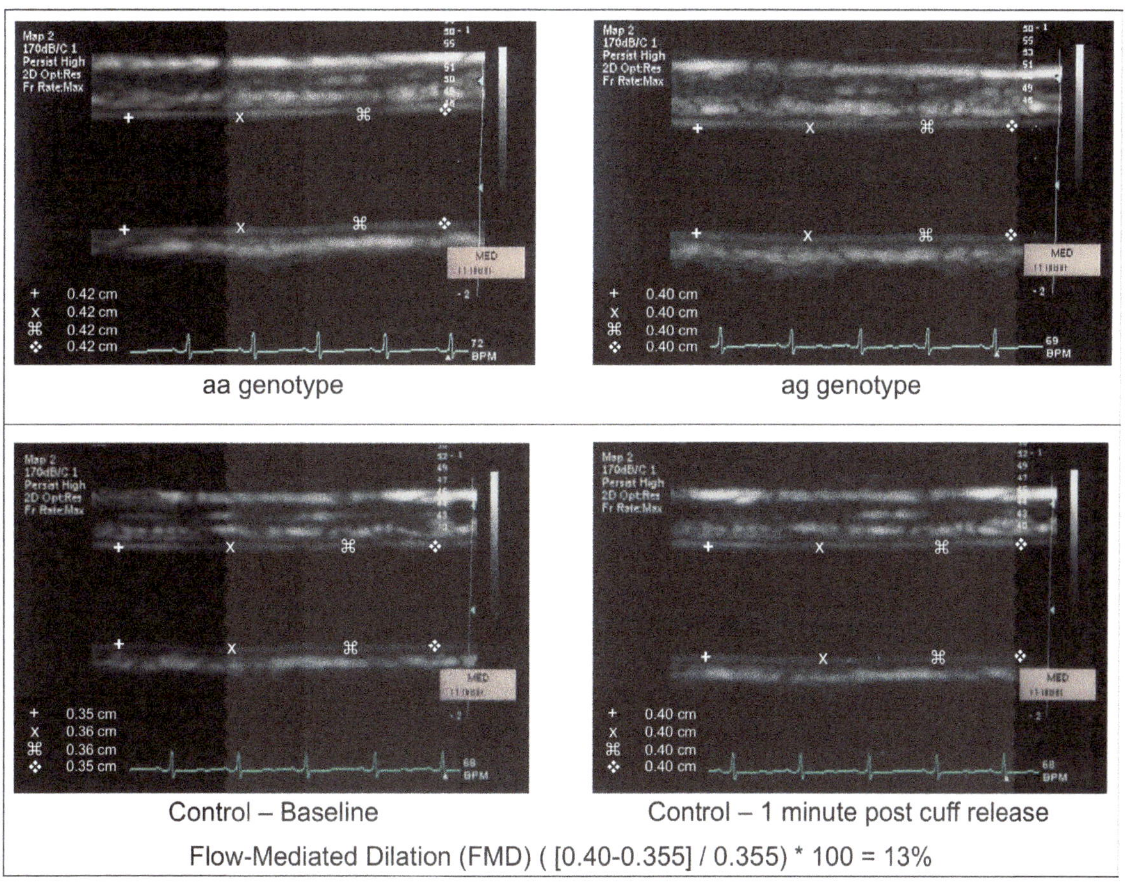

Figure 4. Representative images of the baseline brachial ultrasound of a participant with the aa genotype (top left picture), of a participant with the ag genotype (top right picture), and of the baseline and post-hyperemic ultrasound of a healthy control (bottom pictures). The calculation of flow-mediated dilation (FMD) using the values collected in the healthy control is also reported.

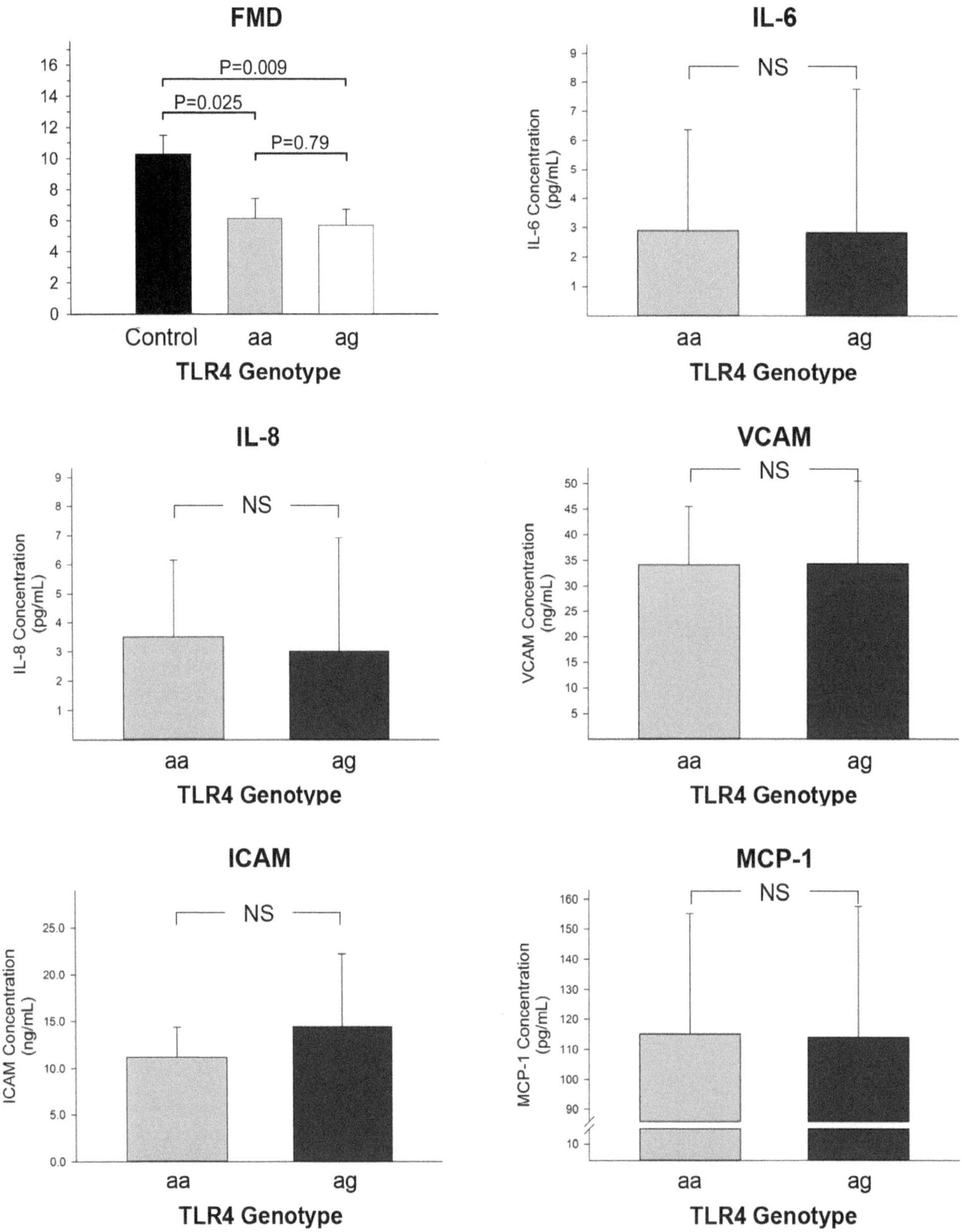

Figure 5. Flow-mediated dilation (top left panel) and plasma levels of IL-6 (top right panel), IL-8 (middle left panel), VCAM (middle right panel), ICAM (bottom left panel), and MCP-1 (bottom right panel) according to TLR4 genotype in study participants. Values reported as mean±SD.

of inflammatory mediators, confirming and further expanding previous observations [28]. In addition, we also confirm previous evidence that the synthesis of inflammatory mediators induced by TLR4 signaling is mediated by activation of NF-κB [4], which has been associated with endothelial injury [7]. Our in vitro findings complement the current understanding of the role of TLR4 signaling in the pathogenesis of endothelial dysfunction proposed by Liang and colleagues. [29] In a series of elegant ex-vivo experiments using vessels from type 2 diabetic mice with mutated TLR4 (TLR4$^{-/-}$), these investigators demonstrated that TLR4 activation leads to the transcription of NADPH oxidase 1 and 4 and increased reactive oxidative species (ROS) generation. In turn, the higher concentration of ROS impairs eNOS coupling, thereby reducing nitric oxide (NO) production; blunts endothelium-derived hyperpolarizing factor-mediated vasodilation; and increases the synthesis of vasoconstrictor prostanoids by cyclooxygenase 1. Thus, activation of TLR4 in macrovascular endothelial cells appears to trigger an inflammatory and proatherosclerotic phenotype, with enhanced expression of cytokines and adhesion molecules, increased ROS production, and abnormal synthesis of vasoactive factors. Conversely, in our study, TRL4 blockade by eritoran significantly inhibited LPS-stimulated expression of inflammatory and adhesion molecules in macrovascular endothelial cell cultures. In the same setting, TRL4 signaling inhibition was also effective in blunting IL-8 responses to Ox-PAPC treatment. These findings are in keeping with previous observations of mitigated inflammatory responses to LPS in endothelial cells pretreated by TRL4-blocking antibodies [27]. Even more importantly, our results are consistent with the recent evidence that TLR4 antagonism may inhibit vascular inflammation and atherogenesis in diabetic ApoE$^{-/-}$ mice, supporting the concept that TLR4 pathway is a potential therapeutic target [30].

The principal findings of our clinical study are that well-treated RA patients, despite low disease activity, have impaired brachial artery FMD and that the presence of the Asp299Gly TLR4 polymorphism is not associated with better endothelial function or lower plasma levels of inflammatory cytokines, adhesion molecules, and MCP-1. Of note, MCP-1 and its associated protein MCPIP are increased in experimental models of RA and exert detrimental effects on endothelial function by decreasing NO bioavailability [31]. Therefore, our investigation does not confirm the hypothesis that the Asp299Gly polymorphism, which has been reported to decrease TLR4 signaling activity [10], is associated with better vasodilator function compared to the wild type in this population. These results are apparently at odds with our and other groups' laboratory data that suggest LTR4-mediated endothelial activation and dysfunction, and are not consistent with the evidence that the Asp299Gly TLR4 polymorphism is associated with a decreased risk of atherosclerosis [11]. A number of factors may account for our negative results. The impact of the Asp299Gly variant on the endothelium may be modest and minor differences in endothelial function may have been missed due to small sample size and high variability of FMD. Alternatively, it is possible that the effects of this polymorphism on endothelial function are negligible in patients with RA, in whom other inflammatory stimuli may represent the main players in the pathogenesis of endothelial damage and atherosclerosis [32]. In this regard, it must be considered that patients with RA recruited for our study were receiving optimal medical treatment and had normal DAS 44 scores and low levels of inflammatory markers. It might be postulated, therefore, that it was difficult under those conditions to detect possible differences in endothelial activation and vasodilator function related to polymorphisms of the TRL4 gene. However, our results are in line with other studies that did not find a significant association between TLR4 Asp299Gly polymorphism and risk for development and progression of atherosclerosis, including a recently published meta-analysis [33–34].

In conclusion, the results of our in vitro study indicate that TLR4 signaling in endothelial cells may be triggered by both LPS and endogenous ligands, such as oxidized phospholipids, leading to endothelial cell activation and a proinflammatory phenotype. Importantly, TLR4 activation by endogenous ligands is likely to occur in the presence of a proatherosclerotic milieu, where it can contribute to maintain and amplify endothelial activation and vessel wall inflammation. Further investigations are needed to better understand the potential impact of TLR4 polymorphisms on endothelial function in this and other populations at onset of the disease and while on high disease activity. Certainly the findings of our in vivo investigation do not suggest that the Asp299Gly TLR4 polymorphism is associated with improved endothelial function in patients with RA, while treated and in low disease activity.

Acknowledgments

Eritoran (E5564) was kindly provided by EISAI Inc., Woodcliff Lake, NJ.

Author Contributions

Conceived and designed the experiments: RM MT VR MF AZ GF CC NDD. Performed the experiments: RM AM VR GR FS BT. Analyzed the data: RM UC MF CC. Wrote the paper: RM UC MT GF CC.

References

1. Ross R (1999) Atherosclerosis–an inflammatory disease. The New England journal of medicine 340: 115–126.
2. Michelsen KS, Doherty TM, Shah PK, Arditi M (2004) TLR signaling: an emerging bridge from innate immunity to atherogenesis. Journal of immunology 173: 5901–5907.
3. O'Neill LA (2008) Primer: Toll-like receptor signaling pathways–what do rheumatologists need to know? Nature clinical practice Rheumatology 4: 319–327.
4. Dauphinee SM, Karsan A (2006) Lipopolysaccharide signaling in endothelial cells. Laboratory investigation; a journal of technical methods and pathology 86: 9–22.
5. Shi H, Kokoeva MV, Inouye K, Tzameli I, Yin H, et al. (2006) TLR4 links innate immunity and fatty acid-induced insulin resistance. The Journal of clinical investigation 116: 3015–3025.
6. Vabulas RM, Ahmad-Nejad P, da Costa C, Miethke T, Kirschning CJ, et al. (2001) Endocytosed HSP60s use toll-like receptor 2 (TLR2) and TLR4 to activate the toll/interleukin-1 receptor signaling pathway in innate immune cells. The Journal of biological chemistry 276: 31332–31339.
7. Sun R, Zhu Z, Su Q, Li T, Song Q (2012) Toll-like receptor 4 is involved in bacterial endotoxin-induced endothelial cell injury and SOC-mediated calcium regulation. Cell biology international 36: 475–481.
8. Xu XH, Shah PK, Faure E, Equils O, Thomas L, et al. (2001) Toll-like receptor-4 is expressed by macrophages in murine and human lipid-rich atherosclerotic plaques and upregulated by oxidized LDL. Circulation 104: 3103–3108.
9. Michelsen KS, Wong MH, Shah PK, Zhang W, Yano J, et al. (2004) Lack of Toll-like receptor 4 or myeloid differentiation factor 88 reduces atherosclerosis and alters plaque phenotype in mice deficient in apolipoprotein E. Proceedings of the National Academy of Sciences of the United States of America 101: 10679–10684.
10. Arbour NC, Lorenz E, Schutte BC, Zabner J, Kline JN, et al. (2000) TLR4 mutations are associated with endotoxin hyporesponsiveness in humans. Nature genetics 25: 187–191.
11. Kiechl S, Lorenz E, Reindl M, Wiedermann CJ, Oberhollenzer F, et al. (2002) Toll-like receptor 4 polymorphisms and atherogenesis. The New England journal of medicine 347: 185–192.
12. Scott DL, Wolfe F, Huizinga TW (2010) Rheumatoid arthritis. Lancet 376: 1094–1108.

13. Murdaca G, Colombo BM, Cagnati P, Gulli R, Spano F, et al. (2012) Endothelial dysfunction in rheumatic autoimmune diseases. Atherosclerosis 224: 309–317.
14. Maradit-Kremers H, Crowson CS, Nicola PJ, Ballman KV, Roger VL, et al. (2005) Increased unrecognized coronary heart disease and sudden deaths in rheumatoid arthritis: a population-based cohort study. Arthritis and rheumatism 52: 402–411.
15. Hollan I, Meroni PL, Ahearn JM, Cohen Tervaert JW, Curran S, et al. (2013) Cardiovascular disease in autoimmune rheumatic diseases. Autoimmunity reviews.
16. Radstake TR, Franke B, Hanssen S, Netea MG, Welsing P, et al. (2004) The Toll-like receptor 4 Asp299Gly functional variant is associated with decreased rheumatoid arthritis disease susceptibility but does not influence disease severity and/or outcome. Arthritis and rheumatism 50: 999–1001.
17. Barochia A, Solomon S, Cui X, Natanson C, Eichacker PQ (2011) Eritoran tetrasodium (E5564) treatment for sepsis: review of preclinical and clinical studies. Expert Opin Drug Metab Toxicol 7: 479–494.
18. Menghini R, Menini S, Amoruso R, Fiorentino L, Casagrande V, et al. (2009) Tissue inhibitor of metalloproteinase 3 deficiency causes hepatic steatosis and adipose tissue inflammation in mice. Gastroenterology 136: 663–672 e664.
19. Casagrande V, Menghini R, Menini S, Marino A, Marchetti V, et al. (2012) Overexpression of tissue inhibitor of metalloproteinase 3 in macrophages reduces atherosclerosis in low-density lipoprotein receptor knockout mice. Arterioscler Thromb Vasc Biol 32: 74–81.
20. Aletaha D, Neogi T, Silman AJ, Funovits J, Felson DT, et al. (2010) 2010 Rheumatoid arthritis classification criteria: an American College of Rheumatology/European League Against Rheumatism collaborative initiative. Arthritis and rheumatism 62: 2569–2581.
21. van Gestel AM, Prevoo ML, van 't Hof MA, van Rijswijk MH, van de Putte LB, et al. (1996) Development and validation of the European League Against Rheumatism response criteria for rheumatoid arthritis. Comparison with the preliminary American College of Rheumatology and the World Health Organization/International League Against Rheumatism Criteria. Arthritis and rheumatism 39: 34–40.
22. Prevoo ML, van Gestel AM, van THMA, van Rijswijk MH, van de Putte LB, et al. (1996) Remission in a prospective study of patients with rheumatoid arthritis. American Rheumatism Association preliminary remission criteria in relation to the disease activity score. British journal of rheumatology 35: 1101–1105.
23. Lorenz E, Frees KL, Schwartz DA (2001) Determination of the TLR4 genotype using allele-specific PCR. BioTechniques 31: 22–24.
24. Corretti MC, Anderson TJ, Benjamin EJ, Celermajer D, Charbonneau F, et al. (2002) Guidelines for the ultrasound assessment of endothelial-dependent flow-mediated vasodilation of the brachial artery: a report of the International Brachial Artery Reactivity Task Force. J Am Coll Cardiol 39: 257–265.
25. Rizza S, Cardellini M, Porzio O, Pecchioli C, Savo A, et al. (2011) Pioglitazone improves endothelial and adipose tissue dysfunction in pre-diabetic CAD subjects. Atherosclerosis 215: 180–183.
26. Chen L, Liang B, Froese DE, Liu S, Wong JT, et al. (1997) Oxidative modification of low density lipoprotein in normal and hyperlipidemic patients: effect of lysophosphatidylcholine composition on vascular relaxation. Journal of lipid research 38: 546–553.
27. Lu Z, Li Y, Jin J, Zhang X, Lopes-Virella MF, et al. (2012) Toll-like receptor 4 activation in microvascular endothelial cells triggers a robust inflammatory response and cross talk with mononuclear cells via interleukin-6. Arterioscler Thromb Vasc Biol 32: 1696–1706.
28. Dvoracek LA, Kreisberg JI, McKinney J, Schmid G, Francis AD, et al. (2010) Lovastatin inhibits oxidized L-A-phosphatidylcholine B-arachidonoyl-gamma-palmitoyl (ox-PAPC)-stimulated interleukin-8 mRNA and protein synthesis in human aortic endothelial cells by depleting stores of geranylgeranyl pyrophosphate. Atherosclerosis 208: 50–55.
29. Liang CF, Liu JT, Wang Y, Xu A, Vanhoutte PM (2013) Toll-like receptor 4 mutation protects obese mice against endothelial dysfunction by decreasing NADPH oxidase isoforms 1 and 4. Arterioscler Thromb Vasc Biol 33: 777–784.
30. Lu Z, Zhang X, Li Y, Jin J, Huang Y (2013) TLR4 antagonist reduces early-stage atherosclerosis in diabetic apolipoprotein E-deficient mice. J Endocrinol 216: 61–71.
31. He M, Liang X, He L, Wen W, Zhao S, et al. (2013) Endothelial dysfunction in rheumatoid arthritis: the role of monocyte chemotactic protein-1-induced protein. Arterioscler Thromb Vasc Biol 33: 1384–1391.
32. Protogerou AD, Zampeli E, Fragiadaki K, Stamatelopoulos K, Papamichael C, et al. (2011) A pilot study of endothelial dysfunction and aortic stiffness after interleukin-6 receptor inhibition in rheumatoid arthritis. Atherosclerosis 219: 734–736.
33. Netea MG, Hijmans A, van Wissen S, Smilde TJ, Trip MD, et al. (2004) Toll-like receptor-4 Asp299Gly polymorphism does not influence progression of atherosclerosis in patients with familial hypercholesterolaemia. Eur J Clin Invest 34: 94–99.
34. Zhang K, Zhang L, Zhou B, Wang Y, Song Y, et al. (2012) Lack of association between TLR4 Asp299Gly polymorphism and atherosclerosis: evidence from meta-analysis. Thrombosis research 130: e203–208.

4

Multi-Dimensional Health Assessment Questionnaire in China: Reliability, Validity and Clinical Value in Patients with Rheumatoid Arthritis

Yang Song[1], Li-an Zhu[2]*, Su-li Wang[1], Lin Leng[2], Richard Bucala[2], Liang-Jing Lu[1]*

1 Department of Rheumatology, Ren Ji Hospital, School of Medicine, Shanghai Jiao Tong University, Shanghai, China, **2** Department of Medicine, Section of Rheumatology, Yale University School of Medicine, New Haven, Connecticut, United States of America

Abstract

Objective: To evaluate the psychometric properties and clinical utility of Chinese Multidimensional Health Assessment Questionnaire (MDHAQ-C) in patients with rheumatoid arthritis (RA) in China.

Methods: 162 RA patients were recruited in the evaluation process. The reliability of the questionnaire was tested by internal consistency and item analysis. Convergent validity was assessed by correlations of MDHAQ-C with Health Assessment Questionnaire (HAQ), the 36-item Short-Form Health Survey (SF-36) and the Hospital anxiety and depression scales (HAD). Discriminant validity was tested in groups of patients with varied disease activities and functional classes. To evaluate the clinical values, correlations were calculated between MDHAQ-C and indices of clinical relevance and disease activity. Agreement with the Disease Activity Score (DAS28) and Clinical Disease Activity Index (CDAI) was estimated.

Results: The Cronbach's alpha was 0.944 in the Function scale (FN) and 0.768 in the scale of psychological status (PS). The item analysis indicated all the items of FN and PS are correlated at an acceptable level. MDHAQ-C correlated with the questionnaires significantly in most scales and scores of scales differed significantly in groups of different disease activity and functional status. MDHAQ-C has moderate to high correlation with most clinical indices and high correlation with a spearman coefficient of 0.701 for DAS 28 and 0.843 for CDAI. The overall agreement of categories was satisfying.

Conclusion: MDHAQ-C is a reliable, valid instrument for functional measurement and a feasible, informative quantitative index for busy clinical settings in Chinese RA patients.

Editor: Arvind Chopra, Center for Rheumatic Diseases, India

Funding: This work was supported by grants from National Natural Sciences Foundation of China (No. 81373209; No. 30671946; No. 81072469) and Shanghai Natural Sciences Foundation (No. 09ZR1417600). The funders had no role in study design, data collection and analysis, decision to publish, or preparation of the manuscript.

Competing Interests: The authors have declared that no competing interests exist.

* E-mail: lu_liangjing@medmail.com.cn (LJL); lianzhu20032003@hotmail.com (LAZ)

Introduction

Rheumatoid arthritis (RA) is one of the few diseases where subjective patient and physician measures are the best known predictors of treatment response and future health outcomes [1]. The treatment of RA has been improved greatly by current regimens of disease modifying drugs and biologic agents. From the patients' perspective, however, many deleterious disease consequences still exist, including persistent pain, functional disability, fatigue, and depression that may be affected by health beliefs and underlying psychological problems [2]. Quantitative measurement of such information is therefore critical. Patient self-report questionnaires have been reported to be the most cost-effective in the documentation of the effectiveness of rheumatology care [3,4], and standardized patient questionnaire measures, rather than laboratory tests or radiographs, are the most significant quantitative predictors of severe outcomes of rheumatoid arthritis (RA), including work disability [5–7] and mortality [8,9].

The heath assessment questionnaire (HAQ) is widely used throughout the world to assess functional status in rheumatoid arthritis and a wide variety of rheumatic diseases. Developed in 1978, the HAQ remains the gold standard for measuring functional status in RA [10]. However, its length and relatively complex scoring could make clinical use difficult. Accordingly, several revisions have been made over past several years. The multidimensional health assessment questionnaire (MDHAQ) is the latest version of such revisions with decreased patient and provider time requirement [1]. Meanwhile, it has a broader perspective and better coverage of the scales in the International Classification of Functioning, Disability and Health (ICF) [11,12] The MDHAQ also includes the routine assessment of patient index data 3 (RAPID3), an index that includes three of the patient-reported American College of Rheumatology (ACR) core data set measures for RA: physical function, pain, and patient global estimate of status [13]. RAPID3 has been reported to give similar data as DAS28 and CDAI for distinguishing active versus placebo treatments in clinical trials [14] and is calculated much more easily and quickly than HAQ, DAS28 and CDAI [15].

In this study,the original English version of MDHAQ was translated into Chinese with an cross-cultural adaptation process, and an assessment of psychometric properties and values was performed in Chinese patients with RA.

Patients and Methods

Ethics Statement

This study was approved by the institutional review board of Shanghai Jiao Tong University and Ethics Committee of Renji hospital. They specifically approved that written informed consent was not required because data were going to be analysed anonymously. Following feedback from participants in the pretest procedure, all participants granted oral consent to participate after receiving comprehensive information about the study. Oral consent was documented by interviewers at the beginning of the interview.

Patients

One hundred and sixty-two consecutive RA patients were recruited into the study between March 2013 and November 2013 from Ren Ji Hospital, School of Medicine, Shanghai Jiao Tong University. Each patient had to fulfill the following criteria: (a) met the ACR 1987 revised criteria for the classification of RA [16] (b) was at least 18 years of age. The patients were excluded if they had chronic disabling disease other than RA or cognitive impairment. Demographic characteristics were recorded including age, sex, marital status, education, and disease duration.

MDHAQ

The MDHAQ is a 2-page version questionnaire which comprises 10 questions regarding physical function(FN), psychological status(PS), pain(PN), Rheumatoid Arthritis Disease Activity Index (RADAI) self report joint count (JTCT),global health status(PTGL), fatigue(FT), symptom checklist review of systems (ROS),morning stiffness(AM), exercise habits(EX), and change in status over the last week(CHG) as well as a recent medical history [17,18]. The FN includes 10 items, numbered Question1.a–j, on activities of daily living scaled in a Likert format (from 0 = without any difficulty to 3 = unable to do, total score ranges from 0 to 10). The sum of the raw score is divided by three to give a score between 0 and 10.Three items, numbered Question1, k–m, constitute the psychological status section scored 0–9.9(scored 0 = "without any difficulty", 1.1 = "with some difficulty", 2.2 = "with much difficulty", and 3.3 = "unable to do"). PN, PTGL, and FT were assessed by three VASs presented as 21 circles, with an arithmetic scale of 0–10 in 0.5 unit increments in Question 2, Question 4 and Question 9. The JTCT (Question 3) includes 8 joints or joint groups, scored 0, 1, 2 or 3 by the patient. ROS (Question 5) is a quantitative review of symptoms the patient experienced over the last month, scoring of which is the number of checked boxes. AM (Question 6) is scored in minutes with maximum 300 minutes. CHG, as the 7th question, is scored 1–5(1 = Much better, 2 = Better, 3 = Same, 4 = Worse,5 = Much worse). EX (question 8) cares about the frequency of aerobical exercises for at least 30 minutes, with a scoring instrument of 3 = 3 or more times a week, 2 = 1–2 times per week,1 = 1–2 times per month, 0 = Do not exercise regularly,9 = cannot exercise due to disability/handicap. And recent medical history (Question 10) is the only one that does not scored quantitatively in the whole questionnaire. RAPID3, on a 0–30 scoring scale, can be divided into four categories: high severity >12, moderate severity = 6.1–12, low severity = 3.1–6, and remission < =3.

Translation and cross-cultural adaptation

The procedure of translation and cross-cultural adaptation was performed following the guidelines by Guillemin et al. [3,19] The original MDHAQ was first translated into Chinese independently by 2 translators who were aware of the objectives of the questionnaire. The translated versions were then back translated into English by another two translators blinded to the intent and the concepts of the questionnaire. A multidisciplinary consensus committee was held to produce a synthesized version based on the translations and back-translations. This version was applied to 10 randomly selected outpatients with RA in the following pre-test. On the basis of the feedback and a discussion within the commitment, several wording revisions were introduced to suit the Chinese culture. "Walk two miles or three kilometers" was modified to "Walk six Li or three kilometers?"because most Chinese people use" Li", rather than" mile" as a commonly used unit of length in everyday life." How much of a problem has unusual fatigue or tiredness been for you" was changed to "How much unusual fatigue or tiredness have you had?" All the modifications were conceptual equivalence of the source by the commitment. An additional 10 outpatients completed this modified version and no further suggestions were feed backed. This modified instrument, referred to as the MDHAQ-China (MDHAQ-C), was administered to recruited RA patients in this study.

Evaluation methods

Patients who completed MDHAQ-C were also asked to complete the Chinese HAQ [20], the Chinese version of the 36-item Short-Form Health Survey (SF-36) [21], and the Chinese version of the Hospital anxiety and depression scales(HAD) [22] at the same time. Disease Characteristics were estimated by three different methods: laboratory tests, clinical estimates by physicians, and patient self-estimate scales. The laboratory tests included erythrocyte sedimentation rate (ESR), C reactive protein (CRP) and rheumatoid factors (RF). A physician clinically evaluated the patient by assessments of swollen joint counts (STC) and tender joint counts (TJC) and by the physician overall assessment using a visual analog scale (VAS) and ACR functional classification [23]. Patient self-estimate scales were two VASs in a 100 mm line to assess of pain and global status completed by patients independently. Reliability was tested by internal consistency with a following item analysis procedure. Convergent validity was tested by examining the correlation of MDHAQ with HAQ, SF-36 and HAD using spearman's method. The correlations between MDHAQ and the SF-36 were hypothesized to be negative and those with HAQ and HAD were expected to be positive, with all of these correlations significant. Highly strong correlation was set as the spearman's coefficient >0.70, strong as 0.5–0.7, moderate as 0.30–0.5, and weak as <0.3. Discriminant validity was estimated in patients distributed into two different groups: patients that were active versus inactive (remission) in disease activity groups by the cutoff value of 2.6 according to DAS28, and patients with disability versus without disability groups by the cutoff value of 1 in functional class. Clinical values were assessed by comparing RAPID3 and the components with disease characteristics and agreement of RAPID3 with Disease Activity core-28(DAS28) [24] and with Clinical Disease Activity Index(CDAI) [25] Categories for disease activities were also assessed according to the statistic methods by Pincus T [13] which will be shown in detail in the following statistical analyses.

Statistical Analyses

Test-retest was evaluated by intraclass correlation coefficient (ICC) or kappa statistics. Internal consistency was assessed using Cronbach's coefficient alpha. Item analysis was performed by item-total correlations and corrected item-total correlations. Comparisons between different groups were calculated by non-parametric test (Mann-Whitney). Spearman's rank-order correlation coefficient was used to evaluate correlation of RAPID3 and components with disease characteristics. Agreement of RAPID3 with DAS28 and CDAI was evaluated respectively by correlations using spearman's method. Cross-tabulations were computed to compare the number and proportion of patients classified in the four DAS28 and CDAI categories of high disease activity (DAS28 >5.1, CDAI >22), moderate disease activity (DAS28 = 3.21–5.1, CDAI = 10.1–22), low disease activity (DAS28 = 2.61–3.20, CDAI = 2.81–10), and remission (DAS28≤2.6, CDAI = 0–2.8) with the four proposed RAPID3 categories. The level of agreement of categories by the different scales was evaluated using kappa statistics. Statistics were considered to be significant when p value>0.05.

Results

156 of the 162 recruited RA patients completed the questionnaires, indicating a response rate of 96.3%. All the patients were Chinese. The mean (SD) age of the patients was 46.79(12.80), ranging from 19 to 75; 87.2% of them were female and 94.2% had been married. The mean (SD) years of education was 9.32(5.62), ranging from 0 to 31 years. The mean (SD) disease duration was 6.46(7.37) years. The mean (SD) of ESR, CRP, DAS28 and CDAI was 29.6(26.5), 11.6(26.5), 4.64(6.36), and 15.08(15.61) respectively. With respect to work status, 46.8% (73) of RA patients were engaged at work, while the other 73 patients were unemployed, with 16 disabled, 39 homemakers, and 28 retired. The detailed demographic and clinical characteristics were shown in Table 1

Reliability

The internal consistency value was 0.944 in FN and the removal of each item didn't lead to a significant change in Cronbach's alpha, ranging from 0.934 to 0.943. For the PS scale, the Cronbach's alpha was .0.768 and the Cronbach's alpha rose to 0.900 when the item k was deleted while the value fell to 0.577 and 0.548 separately for item l and m (Table 2)

Item analysis

The results of item analysis were displayed in Table 2. The associations between items and the scale were satisfactorily high. The item-total correlation analysis showed that all the items were correlated with FN significantly (0.549–0.808 for FN and0.756–0.801 for PS, p<0.001).The corrected item-total correlation analysis showed that the value ranged from 0.648 to o.838 for FN and 0.411 to 0.733 for PS.

Validity

To assess the convergent validity of the MDHAQ-C, the scales of MDHAQ-C were compared to HAQ, SF-36 and HAD. As shown in Table 3, the FN had a highly strong correlation with HAQ with a coefficient of 0.859 (p<0.001) and moderate to highly strong correlation with all the scales of SF-36, ranging from 0.528 to 0.854 (p<0.001). When comparing the rest of the scales of MDHAQ-C with these criterions, most of the results were satisfying significant. Except for EX (which showed a relatively weak correlation), the remaining scales all showed moderate to strong correlation with the criterions (p<0.001) with HAQ. The results of the comparison with SF-36 was similar, with a moderate correlation (levels of significance ranging from p<0.01 to p< 0.001). The MDHAQ-C also showed a significant correlation with HAD but at a relatively lower level(r = 0.379–0.564) for most scales. EX showed a significant correlation with SF (p<0.01) and VT (p<0.05), but were not significant for the other scales of SF-36 (Table 3).

Results of assessing of discriminant validity performed on the total10 scales of the MDHAQ-C are detailed in Table 4. Mean scores on the MDHAQ-C differed significantly between patients who were active in disease status and those who were in remission based on DAS28 scores in all scales except for CHG and EX. Similarly, all scales could differentiate subjects without functional disability from those with that situation judged by functional class in all scales except EX.

Clinical value

RAPID3 and the components were compared with results of the three different methods used in the assessment of disease characteristics which has been described in detail in the evaluation methods. As shown in Table 5, RAPID3 score had strong correlation with TJC, pain, global status and physician overall assessment (p<0.001), and had moderate correlation with ESR, CRP and SJC (p<0.001). The three components of RAPID3 showed similar results: strong correlation was seen between FN and physician overall assessment, PN and TJC, PN and physician overall assessment, PN and patient self-estimating pain and global status, and between PTGL and patient self-estimating pain and global status (p<0.001). For RF, the correlation was not significant for both RAPID3 and the components. The rest of the variables showed moderate correlation with each other.

When comparing RAPID3 with DAS28 and CDAI, Spearman's rank-order correlation coefficients were evaluated respectively. RAPID3 and DAS28 had high correlation with a coefficient of 0.701(p<0.001) (Figure 1). The kappa value was 0.467(p< 0.001). Among the 156 patients, 70.6% of them who met DAS28 high activity criteria met corresponding RAPID3 criteria. The percentage was 64.8%, 33.3% and 65.8% respectively for moderate, low, and remission groups according to the category of DAS28 (Table 6). The comparison with CDAI turned out to be similar. As was shown in Figure 2, the Spearman's rank-order correlation coefficient was 0.843(p<0.001). The kappa value was 0.491(p<0.001). The percentage of patients who met high, moderate, low and remission activity criteria of RAPID3 in those who met corresponding CDAI criteria were 74.3%,52.6%,42.9% and 96.3% respectively(Table 6).

Discussion

RA is characterized by chronic destructive inflammatory polyarthropathy with a major impact on physical and psychological health. The prevalence rates range from 0.2 to 0.93% in China [26], and as Chinese people make up almost one-quarter of the world's population, the number of RA patients is quite large in China. MDHAQ is a new instrument derived from HAQ and used in the evaluation of functional status and many other aspects regarding the quality of life of RA patients. It unifies 3 important features of a rheumatologic assessment instrument: the physical and mental aspects of the patient's functioning [27], a patient oriented perspective [28], and a brief, patient friendly format [29]. The original English version has been well validated [30] but there has not been a cross-cultural version for the substantial RA patients in China. This is the first attempt to translate the MDHAQ into Chinese and evaluate its utility in assessing the

Table 1. Demographic and clinical characteristics of the RA patients.

Variables	Measures
Age, years, mean(SD)	46.8 (12.8)
Sex,male/female(%)	20 (12.8)/136 (87.2)
Education,years,mean(SD)	9.3(5.6)
Marriage status, yes/no (%)	147 (94.2)/9 (5.8)
Disease duration,years,mean(SD)	6.46(7.37)
RF, positive,n(%)	104(66.7)
ESR, mm/h, mean(SD), median(IQR)	29.6(26.5), 20(11, 39)
CRP, mg/L, mean (SD), median(IQR)	11.6(26.5), 3.3(1, 12.2)
TJC, mean (SD), median(IQR)	5.6(7.3), 2(1, 7)
SJC, mean (SD), median(IQR)	2.9(4.8), 1(0, 3)
DAS28, mean(SD), median(IQR)	4.64 (6.36), 3.5(2.56, 4.73)
CDAI, mean(SD), median(IQR)	15.1(15.6), 9.5(4, 21)
HAQ, mean(SD), median(IQR)	0.51(1.39), 0.13(0, 0.5)
HAD, mean(SD), median(IQR)	8.02(6.19), 7(3, 11.8)
RAPID3, mean(SD), median(IQR)	7.94(6.52), 6.9(2.3, 12.0)
Work Status, n (%)	
Full-time	52 (33.33)
Part-time	6 (3.85)
Disabled	16(10.26)
Homemaker	39 (25)
Self-Employed	15 (9.62)
Retired	28 (17.95)

health status of Chinese RA patients. In addition, this is the first time when assessment of clinical utility was added to the evaluation process of a cross-cultural adapted questionnaire.

There are many dialects that are quite different from one another such as Shanghai-ese, Cantonese and Mandarin in China although the written language is the same. Mandarin was used throughout the process and all the bilingual interpreters spoke Mandarin fluently, because Mandarin is the common language in China and almost every Chinese could communicate with each other in Mandarin no matter what his or her native dialect is.

Table 2. Internal consistency and item analysis of FN and PS.

Items	Corrected Cronbach's alpha	Item-total	Corrected item-total
a.	0.936	0.670	0.800
b.	0.936	0.662	0.828
c.	0.940	0.600	0.745
d.	0.937	0.700	0.776
e.	0.935	0.725	0.815
f.	0.935	0.636	0.818
g.	0.943	0.549	0.648
h.	0.934	0.696	0.838
i.	0.940	0.738	0.743
j.	0.939	0.808	0.782
k.	0.900	0.756	0.411
l.	0.577	0.785	0.698
m.	0.548	0.801	0.733

Corrected Cronbach's alpha: the consistency coefficient of the remaining items when one item was deleted; Item-total: correlation between the item and the corresponding domains; Corrected item-total: correlation between the remaining items and the sales after one item was deleted. Statistics were significant at the level of $p<0.001$.

Table 3. Convergent validity of MDHAQ-C.

		FN	PS	PN	JCTC	PTGL	FT	EX
HAQ		0.859***	0.423***	0.676***	0.622***	0.592***	0.436***	0.195*
HAD		0.397***	0.564***	0.416***	0.426***	0.379***	0.461***	0.116
SF-36	PF	−0.854***	−0.477***	−0.519***	−0.487***	−0.520***	−0.531***	−0.198
	RP	−0.705***	−0.350***	−0.515***	0.361**	−0.467***	−0.511***	−0.189
	RE	−0.546***	−0.247**	−0.485***	0.418***	−0.523***	−0.355**	−0.037
	SF	−0.537***	−0.501***	−0.472***	0.453***	−0.451***	−0.477***	−0.346**
	BP	−0.563***	−0.305**	−0.626***	0.512***	−0.541***	−0.381***	−0.115
	GH	−0.528***	−0.373***	−0.548***	0.413***	−0.525***	−0.390***	−0.171
	VT	−0.645***	−0.509***	−0.574***	0.460***	−0.511***	−0.640***	−0.256*
	MH	−0.554***	−0.523***	−0.464***	0.495***	−0.508***	−0.543***	−0.242*

PF: physical functioning, RP and RE: physical and emotional roles, SF: social functioning, BP: bodily pain, GH: general health, VT: vitality, MH: mental health. All the above belongs to the scales of SF-36.
*: $p<0.05$, **: $p<0.01$, ***: $p<0.001$.

These efforts were made to ensure optimal cultural adaptation for the whole country.

The patients recruited were all with a consecutive diagnosis of RA. The Inclusion criteria were set to ensure all the patients included were adults. Since co-existing conditions are known to affect self-reported disabilities in the general population [31], careful selection and exclusion criteria are essential to exclude the confounding factor. The chronic disabling conditions excluded were those determined to be not from the disease itself, but could have an influence on daily activities, such as heart failure and diseases of respiratory system like COPD. The co-morbidity that was associated closely with RA such as interstitial lung disease was not included in the exclusion criteria to ensure the generalizability of the results. However, more work is needed in studying the excluded population of RA patients with these co-morbidities. Most patients were middle aged women who have been married and the female to male ratio was 6.8:1, which was similar with the epidemiological characteristics of RA in China [26]. As our clinical site is a major tertiary referral center for rheumatology in China, the recruited patients are geographically diverse and broadly representative of Chinese RA patients. These RA patients also represent a wide spectrum of disease and encompass a wide range of of age, education, and disease duration.

The internal consistency was good in FN and PS. However, when this assessment was conducted item by item, the results varied among the items. Item l and item m played an important role in the consistency as when the two items were deleted, the value of Cronbach's alpha decreased dramatically. Item k appeared to have a negative effect on the consistency. This result was also found in Finish [32] and Swedish studies [33]. The item-total correlations were satisfying while the corrected item- total correlation was 0.411, a value lower than the other two items, which also was consistent with the previous study. Arkela-Kautiainen believes the removal of the k item and altering the format of the item from the Likert scale to a VAS would be helpful [32]. However, when assessing if the item should be removed from an scale, the cutoff value for the criterion for corrected item-total was >0.4 according to Power [34] and Chiou [35]. The research by Ekback *et al* set the acceptable level to >0.3 [36]. In addition, the internal consistency of PS was at satisfyingly good level of 0.768 rather than a moderate consistency with a Cronbach's alpha of 0.66 in the Finish version. Thus, the removal of k item might be not appropriate in our MDHAQ-C version and the items of PS should be maintained as the original version according to our results.

The results from the analyses of convergent validity were consistent with the predicted hypotheses for most scales. Since ROS, AM and CHG were not relevant in the content with those questionnaires, this test was conducted in the remaining seven scales. The FN had strong correlation with HAQ and PF of SF-36, and a moderate to strong correlation between PS and HAD and MH of SF-36,between PTGL and GH of SF-36, and between FT and VT of SF-36, supporting good convergent validity. The other scales also correlated with HAD and SF-36 significantly except EX, which was only significantly correlated with SF, MH, and VT of SF-36. The possible reason for this effect could be that exercise is influenced by many factors such as motivation and belief [37], and a substantial of patients with RA were physically inactive [38]. This could lead to the insensitivity to change and could probably explain for the deficiency of discriminant validity of this scale in patients with different disease activities and functional status. Modifications and reformulation could be expected in our future researches. The CHG could distinguish patients without functional disability from those with disability while the mean score didn't

Table 4. Discriminant validity of MDHAQ-C,with functional class and disease activity being the external anchor.

	functional class		p value	DAS28		p value
	1	>1		≤2.6	>2.6	
FN	0.33(0.64)	2.63(2.19)	0.000	0.48(1.42)	1.47(0.18)	0.000
PS	0.93(1.21)	2.58(2.26)	0.000	1.04(1.45)	1.73(1.94)	0.033
PN	1.76(1.91)	5.80(2.59)	0.000	0.92(1.20)	4.16(2.94)	0.000
JCTC	3.60(5.23)	15.43(11.69)	0.000	1.90(4.79)	10.40(10.64)	0.000
PTGL	2.23(2.06)	5.28(2.15)	0.000	1.63(1.78)	4.06(2.51)	0.000
ROS	4.16(3.40)	7.98(5.42)	0.000	3.72(2.99)	6.27(4.98)	0.002
AM	19.74(55.54)	57.30(82.35)	0.000	19.87(62.80)	38.46(69.70)	0.005
CHG	2.62(0.75)	2.96(0.53)	0.047	2.73(1.56)	3.25(3.61)	0.328
FT	2.67(2.22)	5.12(2.74)	0.000	2.18(2.16)	4.01(2.73)	0.000
EX	1.62(2.16)	3.59(4.07)	0.063	1.51(1.75)	2.68(3.49)	0.466

differ significantly in active versus inactive (remission) group. As functional status was assessed by ACR functional class, of which the content was related closely with the daily activities, disability could be more easily perceived by patients than DAS 28 which contains objective results of laboratory tests. Since CHG depended totally on patients subjective feelings, that might be a possible explanation for that inconsistency. Overall, the MDHAQ-C had good discriminant validity in patients with varied disease activities and functional status.

Quantitative clinical assessment has advanced more effective treatment of RA and is associated with better outcomes than usual non-quantitative care of RA [5,39]. A formal quantitative swollen and tender joint count and indices that include the count, such as the DAS28 and CDAI, are the most specific measures of RA activity [40]. However, these are time consuming and therefore not available at most visits of patients with a rheumatologist, particularly in busy clinical settings. RAPID3 is an index without formal joint counts that can be completed in less than 10 minutes, which is less than 10% of the time of a CDAI or DAS28 [41,42], indicating considerable value for usual RA care in busy clinical settings.

Several different methods or indices are used commonly in clinical practice and research, including laboratory testing, and physician- or patient-based clinical assessments. As RAPID3 is a comprehensive instrument composed of three domains of MDHAQ, we compared RAPID3 and its components with methods or indices of assessing clinical relevance. This is the first time that both the RAPID3 and its components were assessed by comparison with the existed instruments, including simple ones such as TJC, SJC and others shown in Table 5, and comprehensive ones like DAS28 and CDAI. Moderate to strong correlations were seen between RAPID3 and almost all the disease characteristics, so were the three components. The correlations with RF were not significant. That was understandable because changes in titers of RF generally occurred slowly and often lagged behind other markers of RA activity, and it often occurred that RF values did not decrease along with clinical improvement in RA patients in clinical practice. RAPID3 scores correlated strongly with DAS28 and CDAI with a high coefficient of 0.701 and 0.843 respectively as shown in Figure 1 and Figure 2.When assessing the agreement of the categories of disease activity, the kappa values were acceptable at a fair to good level with 0.467 for DAS28, 0.491 for CDAI. Those results were consistent with the original research [13]. Thus, RAPID3 was as informative as other indices for disease status and provides a feasible, informative quantitative index for busy clinical settings, indicating substantial clinical utility.

Limitations and Further Research

The patients enrolled were chosen randomly following the inclusion and exclusion criteria. Thus, the number of patients with

Table 5. Correlations of RAPID3 and components with disease characteristics.

		FN	PN	PTGL	RAPID3
Lab	ESR	0.488***	0.408***	0.415***	0.461***
	CRP	0.447***	0.444***	0.389***	0.470***
	RF	−0.045	−0.007	0.011	0.011
Physician	SJC	0.557***	0.642***	0.521***	0.628***
	TJC	0.621***	0.738***	0.648***	0.731***
	VAS of overall assessment	0.717***	0.781***	0.686***	0.808***
Patient	VAS of Pain	0.673***	0.923***	0.773***	0.885***
	VAS of Global status	0.697***	0.720***	0.865***	0.837***

Lab: laboratory tests, Physician: clinical estimates by physicians, Patient: patient self-estimate scales.
***: p<0.001.

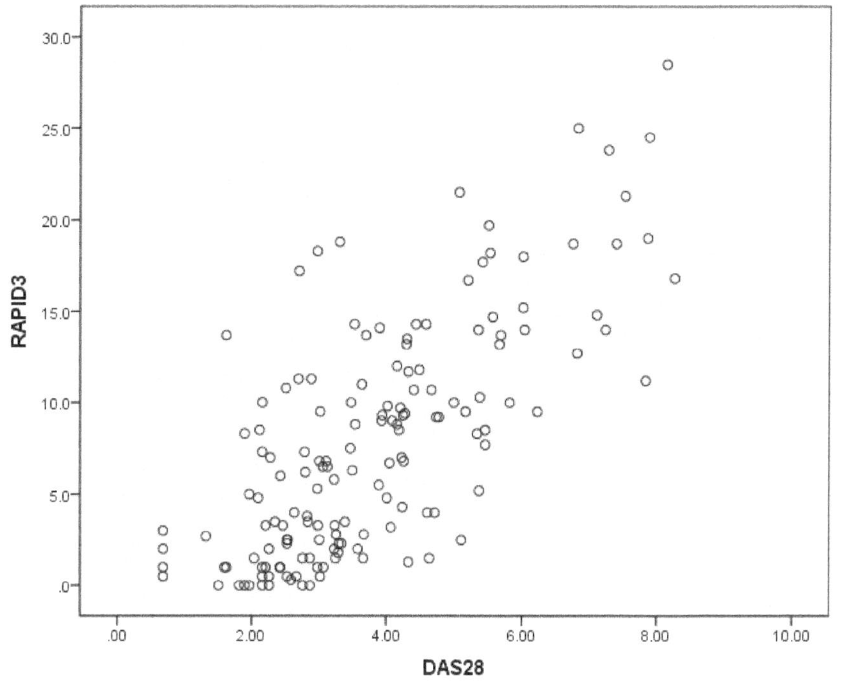

Figure 1. Scatter plots of correlation between RAPID3 and DAS28 in 156 patients with Rheumatoid Arthritis (spearman's method).

different disease activities and functional status might not be equal with one another, which is a limitation of our research. Other limitations include sensitivity to change of MDHAQ and the modification of EX domain and further researches are needed. Also, further research could be done regarding the RAPID3 and other disease variables. Our research was performed in the setting of tertiary referral center, one of the most reputable centers for rheumatology in China. Thus our patients are from around the country and geographically diverse to make certain the results were representative for all the RA patients. However, it still remains open to question whether a community setting would make a difference for MFHAQ-C, as the lack of proof regarding scorer reliability of MDHAQ. This could be figured out in further researches.

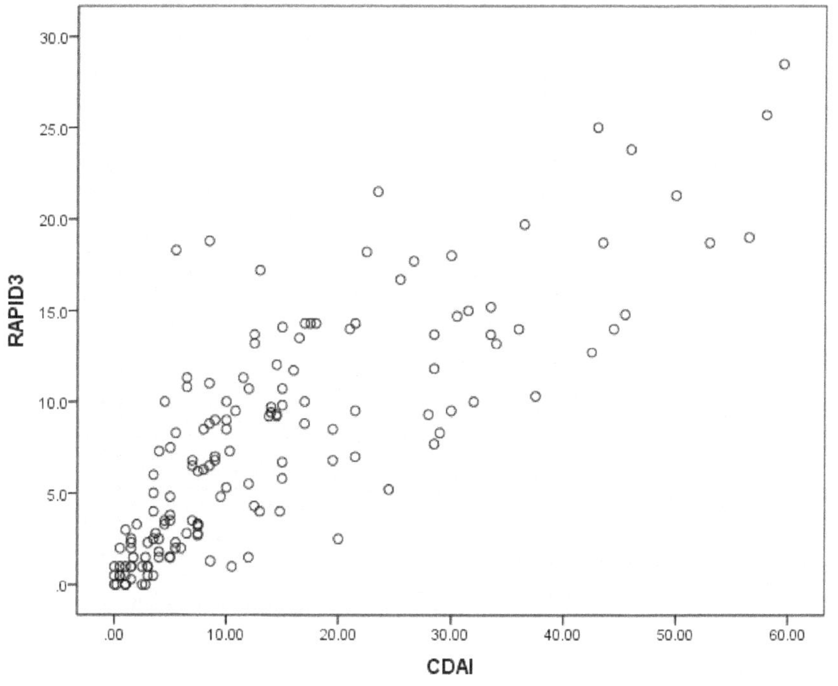

Figure 2. Scatter plots of correlation between RAPID3 and CDAI in 156 patients with Rheumatoid Arthritis (spearman's method).

Table 6. The cross-tabulation of RAPID3 scores compared with DAS28 and CDAI in four categories.

	Group	RAPID3				Total
		H	M	L	R	
DAS28	H	24(70.6%)	8(23.5%)	1(2.9%)	1(2.9%)	34(21.8%)
	M	9(16.7%)	35(64.8%)	9(16.7%)	1(1.9%)	54(34.6%)
	L	2(6.7%)	9(30.0%)	10(33.3%)	9(30.0%)	30(19.2%)
	R	1(2.6%)	6(15.8%)	6(15.8%)	25(65.8%)	38(24.4%)
Total		36(23.1%)	58(37.2%)	26(16.7%)	36(23.1%)	156(100%)
CDAI	H	26(74.3%)	8(22.9%)	1(2.9%)	0	35(22.4%)
	M	10(26.3%)	20(52.6%)	5(13.2%)	3(7.9%)	38(24.4%)
	L	2(3.6%)	20(35.7%)	24(42.9%)	10(17.9%)	56(35.9%)
	R	0	0	1(3.7%)	26(96.3%)	27(17.3%)
Total		38(24.4%)	48(30.8%)	31(19.9%)	39(25.0%)	156(100%)

All percentages are row percentages, except total in rightmost column (column percentages).The kappa value was 0.467 for DAS28 and 0.491 for CDAI ($p<0.001$).H: high activity; M: moderate activity; L: low activity; R: remission.

Conclusion

The MDHAQ-C has good reliability, validity and substantial clinical utility in Chinese RA patients. Further work should be carried out and more evidences are needed for the modification of the EX scale.

Acknowledgments

We gratefully acknowledge Prof. Ted Pincus for providing us the English version of MDHAQ and for encouraging our research in this area.

Author Contributions

Conceived and designed the experiments: YS LJL LAZ. Performed the experiments: YS LAZ LJL LL RB SLW. Analyzed the data: YS LAZ SLW LJL. Contributed reagents/materials/analysis tools: LAZ LL RB. Wrote the paper: YS LAZ LJL RB.

References

1. Maska L, Anderson J, Michaud K (2011) Measures of functional status and quality of life in rheumatoid arthritis: Health Assessment Questionnaire Disability Index (HAQ), Modified Health Assessment Questionnaire (MHAQ), Multidimensional Health Assessment Questionnaire (MDHAQ), Health Assessment Questionnaire II (HAQ-II), Improved Health Assessment Questionnaire (Improved HAQ), and Rheumatoid Arthritis Quality of Life (RAQoL). Arthritis Care Res (Hoboken) 63 Suppl 11: S4–13.
2. Pollard L, Choy EH, Scott DL (2005) The consequences of rheumatoid arthritis: quality of life measures in the individual patient. Clin Exp Rheumatol 23: S43–52.
3. Beaton DE, Bombardier C, Guillemin F, Ferraz MB (2000) Guidelines for the process of cross-cultural adaptation of self-report measures. Spine (Phila Pa 1976) 25: 3186–3191.
4. Felson DT, Anderson JJ, Boers M, Bombardier C, Chernoff M, et al. (1993) The American College of Rheumatology preliminary core set of disease activity measures for rheumatoid arthritis clinical trials. The Committee on Outcome Measures in Rheumatoid Arthritis Clinical Trials. Arthritis Rheum 36: 729–740.
5. Yelin E, Meenan R, Nevitt M, Epstein W (1980) Work disability in rheumatoid arthritis: effects of disease, social, and work factors. Ann Intern Med 93: 551–556.
6. Sokka T, Pincus T (2001) Markers for work disability in rheumatoid arthritis. J Rheumatol 28: 1718–1722.
7. Chung CP, Sokka T, Arbogast PG, Pincus T (2006) Work disability in early rheumatoid arthritis: higher rates but better clinical status in Finland compared with the US. Ann Rheum Dis 65: 1653–1657.
8. Pincus T, Callahan LF, Sale WG, Brooks AL, Payne LE, et al. (1984) Severe functional declines, work disability, and increased mortality in seventy-five rheumatoid arthritis patients studied over nine years. Arthritis Rheum 27: 864–872.
9. Sokka T, Abelson B, Pincus T (2008) Mortality in rheumatoid arthritis: 2008 update. Clin Exp Rheumatol 26: S35–61.
10. Fries JF, Spitz P, Kraines RG, Holman HR (1980) Measurement of patient outcome in arthritis. Arthritis Rheum 23: 137–145.
11. Pincus T, Sokka T (2003) Quantitative measures for assessing rheumatoid arthritis in clinical trials and clinical care. Best Pract Res Clin Rheumatol 17: 753–781.
12. Lillegraven S, Kvien TK (2007) Measuring disability and quality of life in established rheumatoid arthritis. Best Pract Res Clin Rheumatol 21: 827–840.
13. Pincus T, Swearingen CJ, Bergman M, Yazici Y (2008) RAPID3 (Routine Assessment of Patient Index Data 3), a rheumatoid arthritis index without formal joint counts for routine care: proposed severity categories compared to disease activity score and clinical disease activity index categories. J Rheumatol 35: 2136–2147.
14. Pincus T, Bergman MJ, Yazici Y, Hines P, Raghupathi K, et al. (2008) An index of only patient-reported outcome measures, routine assessment of patient index data 3 (RAPID3), in two abatacept clinical trials: similar results to disease activity score (DAS28) and other RAPID indices that include physician-reported measures. Rheumatology (Oxford) 47: 345–349.
15. Pincus T, Swearingen C, Bergman M, Colglazier C, Kaell A, et al. (2010) RAPID3 on an MDHAQ is correlated significantly with activity levels of DAS28 and CDAI, but scored in 5 versus more than 90 seconds. Arthritis Care Res 62: 181–189.
16. Arnett FC, Edworthy SM, Bloch DA, McShane DJ, Fries JF, et al. (1988) The American Rheumatism Association 1987 revised criteria for the classification of rheumatoid arthritis. Arthritis Rheum 31: 315–324.
17. Pincus T, Yazici Y, Castrejon I (2012) Pragmatic and scientific advantages of MDHAQ/RAPID3 completion by all patients at all visits in routine clinical care. Bull NYU Hosp Jt Dis 70 Suppl 1: 30–36.
18. Pincus T (2007) A multidimensional health assessment questionnaire (MDHAQ) for all patients with rheumatic diseases to complete at all visits in standard clinical care. Bull NYU Hosp Jt Dis 65: 150–160.
19. Guillemin F, Bombardier C, Beaton D (1993) Cross-cultural adaptation of health-related quality of life measures: literature review and proposed guidelines. J Clin Epidemiol 46: 1417–1432.
20. Wu B, Wilson A, Wang FF, Wang SL, Wallace DJ, et al. (2012) Cost effectiveness of different treatment strategies in the treatment of patients with moderate to severe rheumatoid arthritis in china. PLoS One 7: e47373.
21. Li L, Wang H, Shen Y (2002) Development and psychometric tests of a Chinese version of the SF-36 Health Survey Scales. Zhonghua Yu Fang Yi Xue Za Zhi 36: 109–113.

22. Leung CM, Ho S, Kan CS, Hung CH, Chen CN (1993) Evaluation of the Chinese version of the Hospital Anxiety and Depression Scale. A cross-cultural perspective. Int J Psychosom 40: 29–34.
23. Hochberg MC, Chang RW, Dwosh I, Lindsey S, Pincus T, et al. (1992) The American College of Rheumatology 1991 revised criteria for the classification of global functional status in rheumatoid arthritis. Arthritis Rheum 35: 498–502.
24. Prevoo ML, van 't Hof MA, Kuper HH, van Leeuwen MA, van de Putte LB, et al. (1995) Modified disease activity scores that include twenty-eight-joint counts. Development and validation in a prospective longitudinal study of patients with rheumatoid arthritis. Arthritis Rheum 38: 44–48.
25. Wagner E, Ammer K, Kolarz G, Krajnc I, Palkonyai E, et al. (2007) Predicting factors for severity of rheumatoid arthritis: a prospective multicenter cohort study of 172 patients over 3 years. Rheumatol Int 27: 1041–1048.
26. Li R, Sun J, Ren LM, Wang HY, Liu WH, et al. (2012) Epidemiology of eight common rheumatic diseases in China: a large-scale cross-sectional survey in Beijing. Rheumatology (Oxford) 51: 721–729.
27. Pioro MH, Kwoh CK (1996) Update on measurement of relevant outcomes in rheumatology. Curr Opin Rheumatol 8: 101–105.
28. Kwoh CK, Ibrahim SA (2001) Rheumatology patient and physician concordance with respect to important health and symptom status outcomes. Arthritis Rheum 45: 372–377.
29. Katz JN, Larson MG, Phillips CB, Fossel AH, Liang MH (1992) Comparative measurement sensitivity of short and longer health status instruments. Med Care 30: 917–925.
30. Pincus T, Sokka T, Kautiainen H (2005) Further development of a physical function scale on a MDHAQ [corrected] for standard care of patients with rheumatic diseases. J Rheumatol 32: 1432–1439.
31. Krishnan E, Hakkinen A, Sokka T, Hannonen P (2005) Impact of age and comorbidities on the criteria for remission and response in rheumatoid arthritis. Ann Rheum Dis 64: 1350–1352.
32. Arkela-Kautiainen M, Kautiainen H, Uutela T, Laiho K, Blafield H, et al. (2005) Evaluation of the MDHAQ in Finnish patients with RA [corrected]. J Rheumatol 32: 1426–1431.
33. Josefsson KA, Ekdahl C, Jakobsson U, Gard G (2013) Swedish version of the multi dimensional health assessment questionnaire — translation and psychometric evaluation. BMC Musculoskelet Disord 14: 178.
34. Power M, Quinn K, Schmidt S (2005) Development of the WHOQOL-old module. Qual Life Res 14: 2197–2214.
35. Chiou CF, Sherbourne CD, Ofman J, Lee M, Lubeck DP, et al. (2004) Development and validation of Cedars-Sinai Health-Related Quality of Life in Rheumatoid Arthritis (CSHQ-RA) short form instrument. Arthritis Rheum 51: 358–364.
36. Ekback M, Benzein E, Lindberg M, Arestedt K (2013) The Swedish version of the multidimensional scale of perceived social support (MSPSS) - a psychometric evaluation study in women with hirsutism and nursing students. Health Qual Life Outcomes 11: 168.
37. Ehrlich-Jones L, Lee J, Semanik P, Cox C, Dunlop D, et al. (2011) Relationship between beliefs, motivation, and worries about physical activity and physical activity participation in persons with rheumatoid arthritis. Arthritis Care Res (Hoboken) 63: 1700–1705.
38. Lee J, Dunlop D, Ehrlich-Jones L, Semanik P, Song J, et al. (2012) Public health impact of risk factors for physical inactivity in adults with rheumatoid arthritis. Arthritis Care Res (Hoboken) 64: 488–493.
39. Pincus T, Callahan LF (1993) What is the natural history of rheumatoid arthritis? Rheum Dis Clin North Am 19: 123–151.
40. Pincus T (2006) The DAS is the most specific measure, but a patient questionnaire is the most informative measure to assess rheumatoid arthritis. J Rheumatol 33: 834–837.
41. Yazici Y, Bergman M, Pincus T (2008) Time to score quantitative rheumatoid arthritis measures: 28-Joint Count, Disease Activity Score, Health Assessment Questionnaire (HAQ), Multidimensional HAQ (MDHAQ), and Routine Assessment of Patient Index Data (RAPID) scores. J Rheumatol 35: 603–609.
42. Pincus T, Swearingen CJ, Bergman MJ, Colglazier CL, Kaell AT, et al. (2010) RAPID3 (Routine Assessment of Patient Index Data) on an MDHAQ (Multidimensional Health Assessment Questionnaire): agreement with DAS28 (Disease Activity Score) and CDAI (Clinical Disease Activity Index) activity categories, scored in five versus more than ninety seconds. Arthritis Care Res (Hoboken) 62: 181–189.

5

Toll-Like Receptors Expressed by Synovial Fibroblasts Perpetuate Th1 and Th17 Cell Responses in Rheumatoid Arthritis

Fanlei Hu[¶], Yingni Li[¶], Li Zheng, Lianjie Shi, Hongjiang Liu, Xuewu Zhang, Huaqun Zhu, Sumei Tang, Lei Zhu, Liling Xu, Yuqin Yang, Zhanguo Li*

Department of Rheumatology and Immunology, Peking University People's Hospital, Beijing, China

Abstract

Rheumatoid arthritis (RA) is a chronic inflammatory disease characterized by synovial fibroblast hyperplasia and bone and cartilage erosion. Synovial fibroblast- and T cell-mediated inflammation plays crucial roles in the pathogenesis of RA. However how this inflammation is initiated, propagated, and maintained remains controversial. Here, we systemically examined the contribution of toll-like receptors (TLRs) to the inflammatory mediator production as well as Th1 and Th17 cell hyperactivity in RA. Our results show that rheumatoid arthritis synovial fibroblasts (RASF) express a series of TLRs, including TLR2, TLR3, TLR4, and TLR9, with the predominant expression of TLR3. Moreover, the expression levels of these TLRs were higher than those in osteoarthritis synovial fibroblasts (OASF). Ligation of TLR3, as well as TLR2 and TLR4, resulted in vigorous production of inflammatory cytokines, matrix metalloproteinases (MMPs), and vascular endothelial growth factor (VEGF) in RASF, with activation of the NF-κB, MAPK, and IRF3 pathways. More important, activation of these TLRs expressed by RASF exacerbated inflammatory Th1 and Th17 cell expansion both in cell-cell contact-dependent and inflammatory cytokine-dependent manners, which induced more IFN-γ and IL-17 accumulation. Targeting TLRs may modulate the inflammation in RA and provide new therapeutic strategies for overcoming this persistent disease.

Editor: Bruno Lourenco Diaz, Universidade Federal do Rio de Janeiro, Brazil

Funding: This work was supported by grants from the Natural Science Foundation of China (81302554 and 81030057) and the 973 program of China (2010CB529100), as well as by Peking University People's Hospital Research and Development Funds (RDB2012-04 and RDB2013-04). The funders had no role in study design, data collection and analysis, decision to publish, or preparation of the manuscript.

Competing Interests: The authors have declared that no competing interests exist.

* E-mail: li99@bjmu.edu.cn

¶ These authors contributed equally to this work.

Introduction

Rheumatoid arthritis (RA) is a chronic autoimmune inflammatory disease that causes deformity of the joints and physical disability. It affects approximately 1% of the population, and up to 30% of RA patients become permanently work disabled within 3 years of diagnosis if they do not receive medical treatment [1,2].

One of the hallmarks of RA is a dysregulated activation of the inflammatory responses, particularly the Th1 and Th17 responses. Elevated levels of proinflammatory cytokines were demonstrated in RA patient sera and synovial fluids, such as IL-6, IL-8, TNF-α, IL-17, and IL-33 [3,4,5]. TNF-α monoclonal antibodies have long been proved to be able to dramatically decrease signs and symptoms of RA. Therapeutic strategies targeting IL-6 also benefited many RA patients [6,7]. However, how the inflammation in RA is initiated and perpetuated remains controversial.

Recent evidence suggested that rheumatoid arthritis synovial fibroblasts (RASF) are one of the most important cells contributing to RA pathogenesis. They are potent participants in all aspects of the initiation, progression, and perpetuation of the disease. The hyperproliferated RASF in the synovium are aggressive to attack cartilage by secreting matrix metalloproteinases (MMPs), which would eventually lead to bone erosion and destruction [8]. More important, RASF could act as effectors of innate immunity to secrete a broad array of inflammatory mediators: cytokines (such as IL-6, IL-8, and TNF-α), chemokines (such as MCP-1, MIP-1α, and IP-10), and several other proinflammatory molecules like prostaglandins and leukotrienes. And RASF in the intimal lining were reported to be the primary source of IL-6 in RA [3,9]. In addition, RASF could interact with T cells through cell-cell contact and/or inflammatory cytokines, which induces inflammatory T cell expansion, thus exacerbating the inflammation in RA. It is of significance to understand how RASF and T cells become actived to perpetuate the inflammation in RA patients.

Exposure of cytokines and ligation of integrins by matrix molecules account for RASF and T cell activation partly. Additionally, our group as well as other groups revealed that hypoxia and hypoxia-inducible factor-1α (HIF-1α) potentiated the production of inflammatory cytokines, MMPs, and vascular endothelial growth factor (VEGF) by RASF. Moreover, HIF-1α overexpression promoted RASF-mediated inflammatory T cell expansion [5,10,11,12]. Recently, the role of toll-like receptors (TLRs) in RA has also been recognized gradually [13,14,15,16,17,18]. TLRs are a class of proteins that play a fundamental role in the innate immune system. They recognize "pathogen-associated molecular patterns (PAMP)" which are structurally conserved molecules derived from microbes and are distinguishable from host molecules, and activate the innate immune responses. Till now, more than 13 members of the TLR family have been identified in mammals [19,20]. To define the expression profile of TLRs and their pathogenic roles will improve our understanding of RA.

In this study, we systemically detected the expression of TLRs in RA, and revealed their roles in perpetuating the persistent inflammation.

Materials and Methods

Patients, Tissue Specimens, and Ethics Statement

Synovial tissue specimens used for culturing RASF (n = 5) and osteoarthritis synovial fibroblasts (OASF, n = 5) were obtained from patients during total knee replacement surgery or arthroscopy. All patients fulfilled the American College of Rheumatology 2009 criteria for RA and 1995 criteria for OA, and provided their written consents to participate in this study. The study protocols, consent forms, and consent procedure were approved by the Institutional Medical Ethics Review Board of Peking University People's Hospital.

Cell Culture and Stimulation

RASF and OASF were cultured as previously described [5], and were used at passages 4–6. For TLR stimulation, 5×10^4 RASF per well in 6-well plates were incubated with different TLR ligands for 4 h and 24 h, respectively, as follows: TLR2 ligand peptidoglycan (PGN, 10 μg/ml), TLR3 ligand polyinosinic:polycytidylic acid (ploy(I:C), 25 μg/ml), TLR4 ligand lipopolysaccharide (LPS, 100 ng/mL) from Sigma; TLR9 ligand Type B CpG (10 μg/ml) from Invitrogen (Carlsbad, CA, USA). The cells were harvested for RT-PCR and realtime PCR while the supernatants were collected for ELISA.

RASF/T cell Co-culture Assay

5×10^4 RASF per well in 6-well plates were stimulated with or without 25 μg/ml ploy(I:C) or 100 ng/ml LPS for 24 h. Then the cells were washed with serum-free RPMI 1640 and co-cultured with 2.5×10^5 allogeneic flow cytometry-sorted $CD4^+$ RA patient T cells (>99% purity) at the ratio of 1:5 in the presence of anti-CD3 and anti-CD28 (3 μg/ml each), with or without a 0.4-μm-pore-size membrane. Sometimes, the co-culture was performed under Th17 polarization conditions: 3 μg/ml anti-CD3, 3 μg/ml anti-CD28, 1 μg/ml anti-IFN-γ, 2.5 μg/ml anti-IL-4, 2.25 ng/ml TGF-β1, 30 ng/ml IL-6, 20 ng/ml IL-1β, and 30 ng/ml IL-23. 5 days later, the T cells were harvested for flow cytometry while the cell culture supernatants were collected for ELISA.

RT-PCR and Realtime PCR

Total RNA was extracted from cells using TRIzol reagent (Invitrogen) and was treated with TURBO DNase (Ambion, Austin, TX, USA) to eliminate genomic DNA contamination. Reverse transcription was performed with the RevertAid First Strand cDNA synthesis kit (Fermentas, Glen Burnie, MD, USA) according to the manufacturer's instructions. The resulting cDNA was subjected to PCR and realtime PCR analyses.

PCR was performed to analyze the expression of TLRs and inflammatory mediators in RASF. The primers used for amplification of TLR2 and TLR4 were as follows: TLR2 sense primer: 5′-ACCAAGTGAAGGTACCTGTGGGGC-3′, antisense primer: 5′-GCACCAGAGCCTGGAGGTTCAC-3′; TLR4 sense primer: 5′-CCCCGACAACCTCCCCTTCTCA-3′, antisense primer: 5′-TCCAGAAAAGGCT CCCAGGGCT-3′. The primers for TLR3, TLR9, IL-6, IL-8, TNF-α, and MMP-1 were the same as those used in our previous studies [12,21]. The PCR products were separated by gel electrophoresis on 1% agarose.

Two-step realtime PCR was also performed using SYBR Green Master Mix (Applied Biosystems, Foster City, CA, USA) according to the manufacturer's instructions. The primers for TLR2, TLR4, and TLR9 were the same as those used for PCR. The primers for TLR3, thrombospondin 1 (TSP-1), stromal cell-derived factor 1 (SDF-1), and IL-15 were as follows: TLR3 sense primer: AGGAAAGGCTAGCAGT CATCC, antisense primer: AG-CAACTTCATGGCTAACAGTG; TSP-1 sense primer: 5′-CCTATGCTGGTGGTAGACTA-3′, antisense primer: 5′-ACGTTCTAGGAGTCC ACACT-3′; SDF-1 sense primer: 5′-ACACTCCAAACTGTGCCCTTCA-3′, antisense primer: 5′-CCACGTCTTTGCCCTTTCATC-3′; IL-15 sense primer: 5′-TTCACTTG AGTCCGGAGATGC-3′, antisense primer: 5′-GCATCCAGATTCTGTTACATTCC C-3′. The other primers were as previously reported [12]. Gene expression was quantified relative to the expression of the housekeeping gene GAPDH, and normalized to control by standard $2^{-\Delta\Delta CT}$ calculation.

Western Blot Analysis

RASF were stimulated with 25 μg/ml TLR3 ligand ploy(I:C) for 0, 5, 15, and 30 min, respectively. Then the cells were collected for western blot analysis as described previously [5]. The antibodies used were as follows: anti-phospho-IκBα mAb, anti-phospho-ERK mAb, anti-phospho-p38 mAb, anti-phospho-IRF3 mAb, anti-IκBα mAb, anti-ERK mAb, anti-p38 mAb, and anti-IRF3 mAb from Cell Signalling Technology (Danvers, MA, USA); anti-actin mAb from Tianjin Sungene Biotech Co., Ltd (Tianjin, China).

Flow Cytometry Analysis

RA patient T cells were co-cultured with RASF for 5 days as described above. At the end of co-culture, the cells were stimulated with PMA (50 ng/ml) plus ionomycin (1000 ng/ml) for 5 h in the presence of Brefeldin A (10 μg/ml). Then, the cells were stained with PerCP-CY5.5–conjugated anti-CD4, fixed and permeabilized, followed by intracellular staining using FITC-conjugated anti-IFN-γ, and Alexa Fluor 647-conjugated anti-IL-17 (eBioscience, San Diego, CA, USA). Percentage of positive cells was analyzed on a FACS Arial II flow cytometer (Becton Dickinson, San Diego, CA, USA).

ELISA Assay

Commercially available ELISA kits used for measuring inflammatory cytokines and MMPs were as follows: IL-6, IL-8, and IFN-γ ELISA kits from Neobioscience Technology Co, Ltd (Beijing, China); IL-17 ELISA kit from QuantoBio Biotechnology Co, Ltd (Beijing, China); TNF-α ELISA kit from eBioscience; and MMP-3 ELISA kit from R & D Systems (Minneapolis, Minnesota, USA).

Statistical Analysis

SPSS 17.0 (SPSS, Chicago, Illinois, USA) was used for statistical analysis. Differences between various groups were evaluated by Wilcoxon signed-rank test, and were considered statistically significant when P was <0.05.

Results

Excessive Expression of Functional TLRs in RASF

We first detected the expression of TLRs in RASF by RT-PCR. As shown in Figure 1A, different TLRs, including TLR2, TLR3, TLR4, and TLR9 were present in RASF, with the highest expression levels of TLR3 and the lowest expression levels of TLR9. Realtime PCR further demonstrated that the expression levels of these TLRs were higher in RASF than in OASF (Figure 1B, a–d). To confirm these TLRs were functionally active, we stimulated RASF with TLR3 ligand ploy(I:C), and then examined the downstream signalling pathway responses, particularly the activation of the three most important pathways, NF-κB pathway, MAPK pathway, and IRF3 pathway. Our results demonstrated that after ploy(I:C) stimulation, the NF-κB pathway (Figure 1C), the MAPK pathway, including the ERK pathway (Figure 1D) and p38 pathway (Figure 1E), as well as the IRF3 pathway (Figure 1F) became activated, which could be seen from 5 minutes until 30 minutes after stimulation.

TLR Ligation Potentiated Inflammatory Cytokine Production in RASF

To reveal the contribution of TLRs to the inflammation in RA, we stimulated RASF with different TLR ligands, and then detected the corresponding inflammatory cytokine production. Ligation of TLR2 with PGN, TLR3 with ploy(I:C), and TLR4 with LPS resulted in robust inflammatory cytokine production, including IL-6 (Figure 2A), IL-8 (Figure 2B), and TNF-α (Figure 2C), as demonstrated by RT-PCR (a), realtime PCR (b), and ELISA (c) analyses. Nonetheless, ligation of TLR9 with CpG merely induced weak production of these inflammatory cytokines (Figure 2A–C), which may be attributed to the relatively low expression levels of TLR9 in RASF.

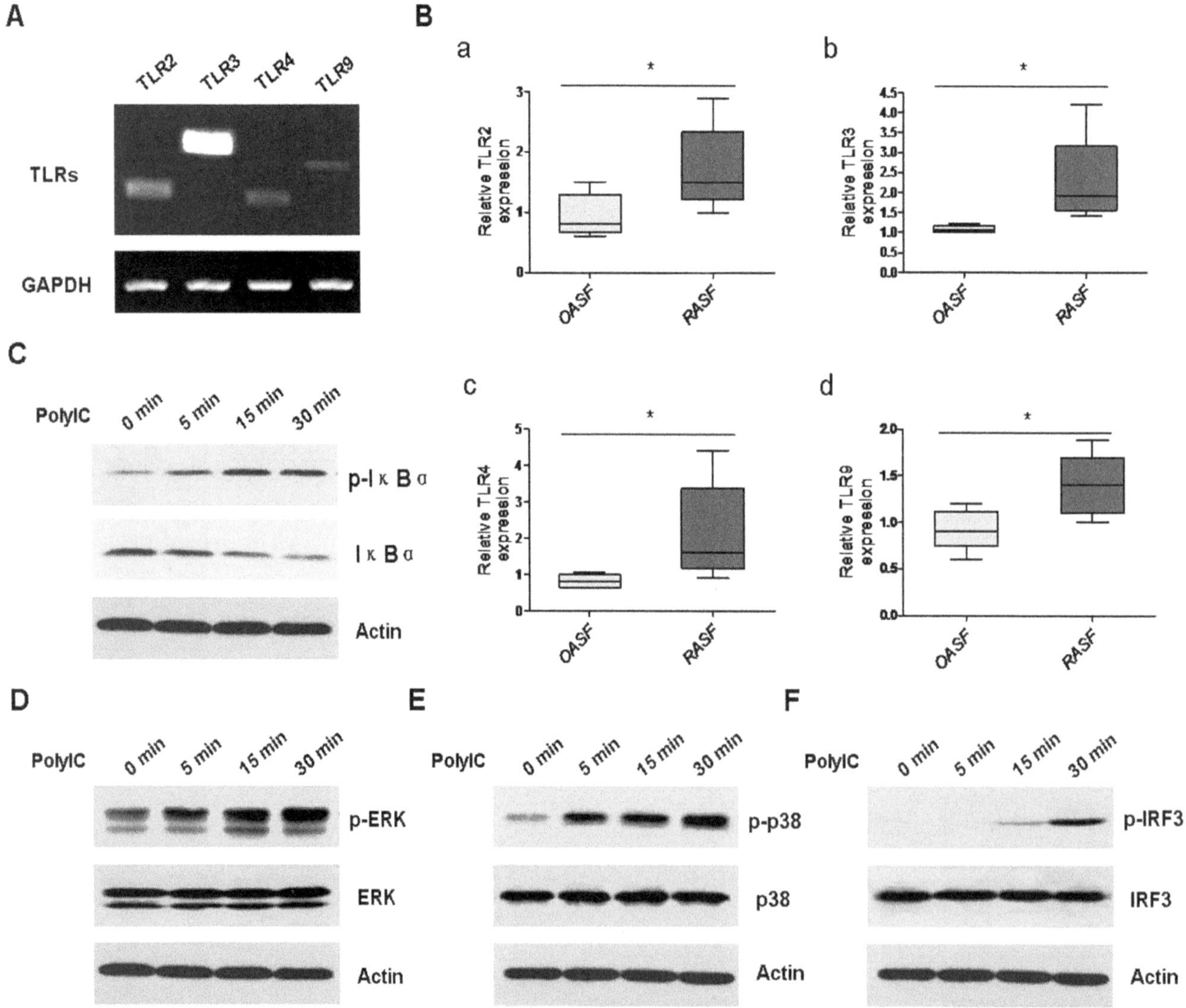

Figure 1. Functional TLRs were excessively expressed in RASF. A, The expression of TLRs, including TLR2, TLR3, TLR4, and TLR9 in RASF was detected by RT-PCR analysis. GAPDH was used as the loading control. B, The expression of TLR2, TLR3, TLR4, and TLR9 in RASF (n = 5) and OASF (n = 5) was determined by realtime PCR (Wilcoxon signed-rank test, *$P<0.05$). RASF were stimulated with 25 μg/ml ploy(I:C) for 5 min, 15 min, and 30 min, respectively. Then the cells were harvested and lysised for western blot analysis of p-IκBα (C), p-ERK (D), p-p38 (E), and p-IRF3 (F). β-actin was used as the loading control. The results were representative of at least three experiments.

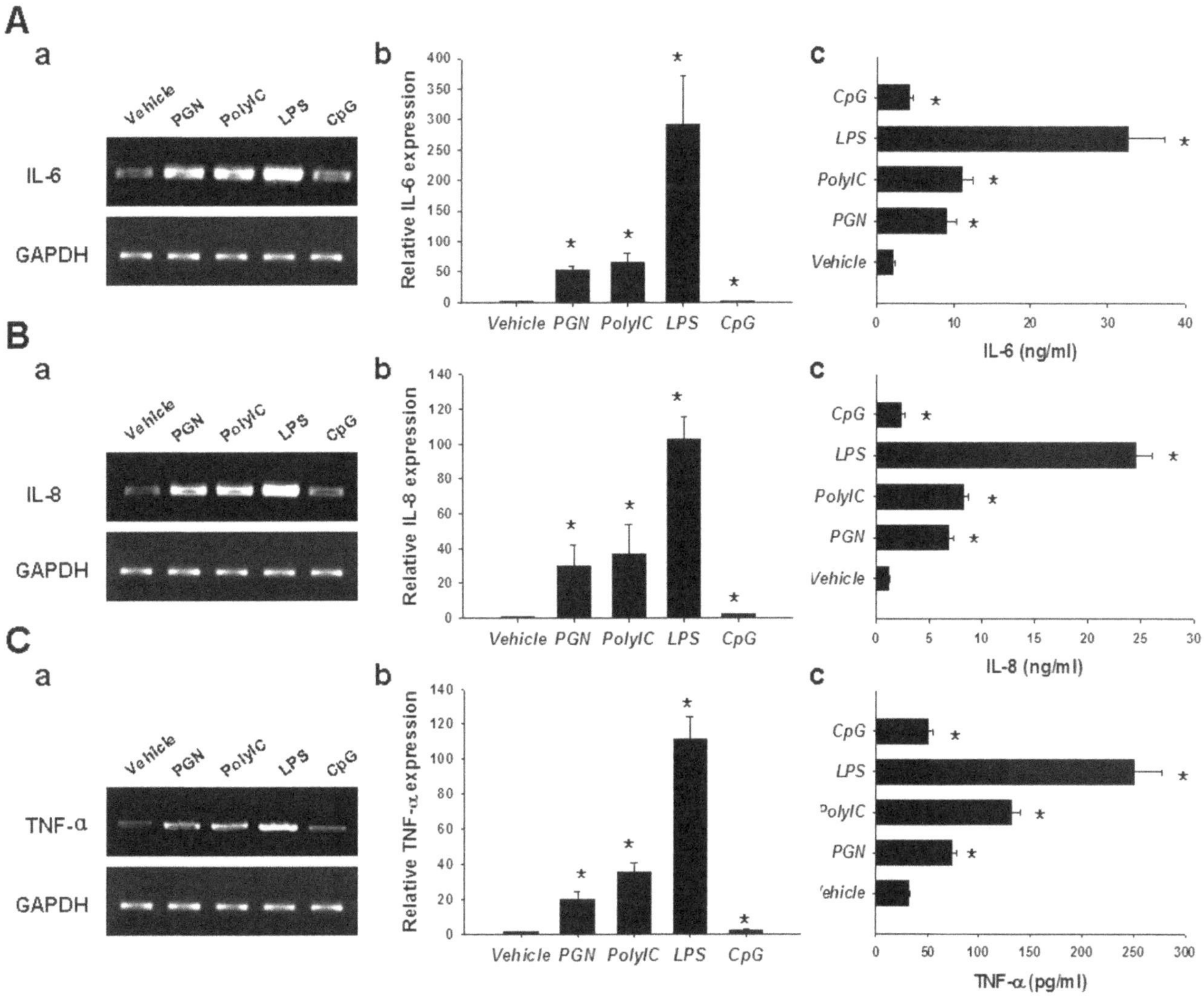

Figure 2. TLR agonists promoted RASF to produce inflammatory cytokines. RASF were stimulated with TLR2 agonist PGN (10 μg/ml), TLR3 agonist ploy(I:C) (25 μg/ml), TLR4 agonist LPS (100 ng/mL), or TLR9 agonist CpG (10 μg/ml). 4 h later, the cells were harvested for RT-PCR (A–C, a) and realtime PCR (A–C, b) analyses of IL-6, IL-8, and TNF-α; 24 h later, the cell culture supernatants were collected for ELISA analyses of IL-6, IL-8, and TNF-α (A–C, c). The results were presented as mean+SEM of five independent experiments (Wilcoxon signed-rank test, *$P<0.05$ *vs.* vehicle control).

TLR Ligands Stimulated RASF to Produce MMPs and VEGF

Cartilage destruction, bone erosion, and angiogenesis are also important phenotypes of RASF which are characterized by producing large amounts of MMPs and VEGF. So, we further determined the effects of TLR ligation on RASF-mediated MMP and VEGF production. RT-PCR showed that TLR ligands, particularly PGN, ploy(I:C), and LPS could stimulate RASF to produce MMP-1 (Figure 3A), which was further confirmed by realtime PCR analysis (Figure 3B). Similar results were also seen for MMP-3 (Figure 3C, D), MMP-9 (Figure 3E), and VEGF (Figure 3F) production as revealed by realtime PCR and ELISA analyses. All these results suggest that RASF could express functionally active TLRs.

TLR Activation Exacerbated RASF-mediated Inflammatory Th1 and Th17 Cell Expansion

RASF could inhibit the apoptosis of T cells through cell–cell interaction and/or the elaboration of soluble factors, which elicits spontaneous proliferation of inflammatory T cells. The increased inflammatory T cells then in turn induce more robust RASF activation, thus forming a RASF/T-cell regulatory circuit that perpetuates the inflammation in RA [22]. So we next determined the impact of TLR activation on RASF-mediated inflammatory T cell expansion. After stimulation with ploy(I:C) or LPS for 24 h, the molecules mediating RASF-T interactions, including TSP-1, SDF-1, and IL-15, were upregulated in RASF (Figure 4A). When co-cultured with RA patient T cells for 5 days, these RASF induced more inflammatory Th1 and Th17 cells than the unstimulated ones, as shown by flow cytometry analysis (Figure 4B). Accordingly, higher levels of IFN-γ and IL-17 were seen in the cell culture supernatants (Figure 4C). More interestingly, this effect could also be seen when the cells were co-cultured under Th17 polarization conditions (Figure 4D). Cell-cell contact and inflammatory cytokines were both involved in this inflammation exacerbation. As shown in Figure 4C, comparable proportional increase of IFN-γ and IL-17 in ploy(I:C)- or LPS-stimulated cultures was seen in the direct contact and transwell systems. The

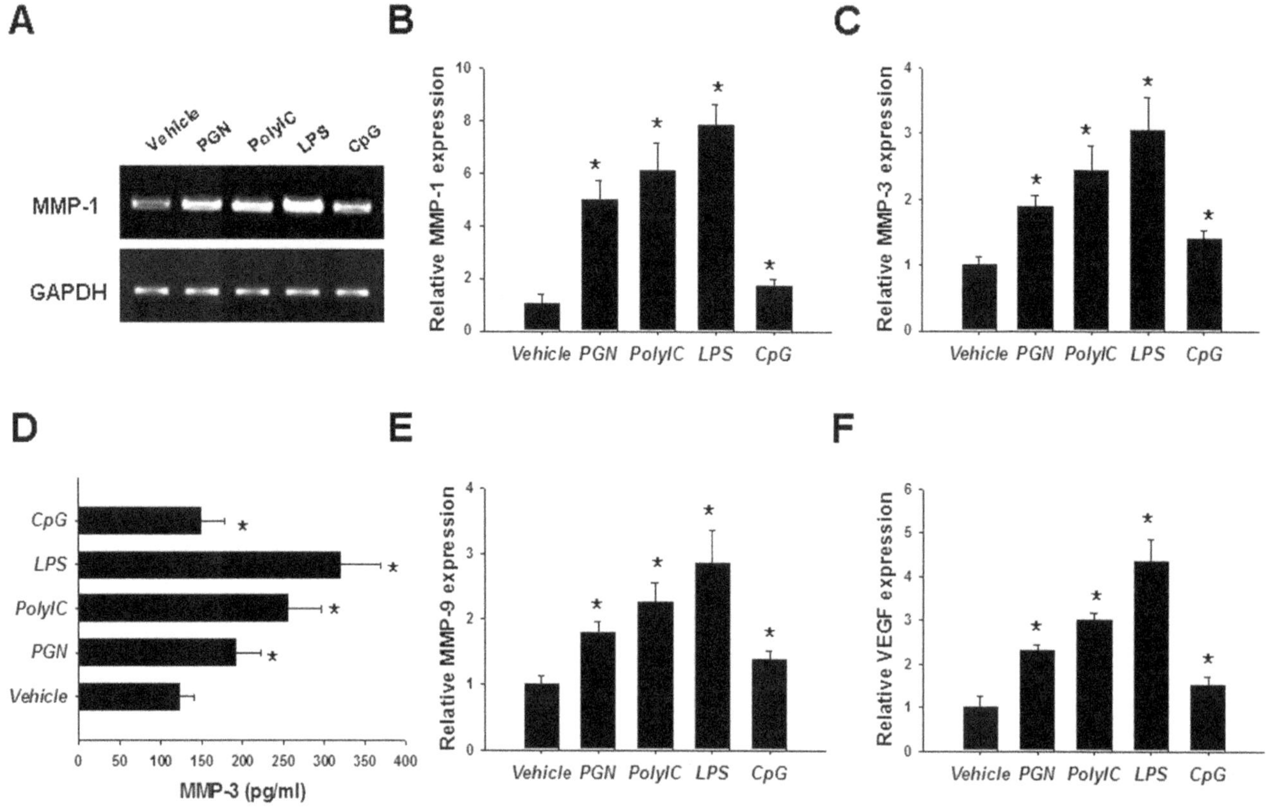

Figure 3. vLigation of TLRs stimulated MMPs and VEGF production in RASF. RASF were stimulated with 10 µg/ml PGN, 25 µg/ml ploy(I:C), 100 ng/mL LPS, or 10 µg/ml CpG for 4 h. Then the cells were harvested for RT-PCR analysis of MMP-1 (A); realtime PCR analyses of MMP-1 (B), MMP-3 (C), MMP-9 (E), and VEGF (F). And also, after stimulation for 24 h, the cell culture supernatants were collected for MMP-3 ELISA (D). The results were presented as mean+SEM of five independent experiments (Wilcoxon signed-rank test, *$P<0.05$ *vs.* vehicle control).

absolute concentration differences may be attributed to the allogenic responses of RASF and T cells. However, no or little production of IL-10 and IL-4 which are potent anti-inflammatory cytokines in RA was detected after RASF/T co-culture (data not shown). Taken together, all these suggest that TLR activation could enhance RASF-mediated expansion of inflammatory T cells.

Discussion

In this study, we revealed the distinct expression pattern of TLRs in RA. These receptors, particularly TLR2, TLR3, and TLR4 played crucial roles in the production of inflammatory cytokines, MMPs, and VEGF by RASF. More important, ligation of these TLRs expressed by RASF promoted inflammatory Th1 and Th17 responses. Thus TLRs contribute not only to the initiation but also to the perpetuation of the inflammation in RA which would be served as new therapeutic targets for the disease.

One of the most significant characteristics of RA is the intensive inflammation that is out of control. Managing to control the inflammation could prevent the disease progression, which would be the optimal strategy for RA therapy. One direct strategy is targeting the pathogenic inflammatory cytokines. Indeed, inhibitors of TNF-α have greatly advanced the management of RA, dramatically decreasing signs and symptoms of the diseases. At present, at least three agents are available which differ in pharmacokinetics and ability to bind lymphotoxin, crosslink membrane-bound TNF and induce apoptosis [6,23]. Recently, IL-6 has also been proved to be a therapeutic target for RA. IL-6R monoclonal antibody tocilizumab showed promising perspective in treating RA patients [7]. Biological reagents targeting other inflammatory cytokines would appear in the following studies. However, RA is a complicated disease involving many inflammatory cytokines. So, targeting the upstream sources of the inflammation would demonstrate better efficacy for RA therapy.

Nonetheless, how the inflammation in RA is initiated, propagated, and maintained remains controversial. Infection has long been speculated to be an underlying factor contributing to RA pathogenesis. Indeed, peptidoglycan, bacterial and viral DNA as well as viral RNA were proved to be present in RA patient inflamed joints [24,25]. These PAMPs would activate the corresponding TLRs, inducing robust inflammatory mediator production. In addition, endogenous heat shock protein, fibrinogen, hyaluronan, and double stranded RNA from apoptotic cells also exist in RA joints [13,25]. These "danger-associated molecular patterns (DAMP)" could also provoke TLRs to induce inflammation. In this study, we proved that peptidoglycan (PGN), ploy(I:C) (a synthetic mimic of double stranded RNA from virus or apoptotic cells), LPS, and CpG (a synthetic mimic of DNA from bacteria or apoptotic cells) could activate RASF to induce vigorous inflammatory mediator production. This suggests that TLRs serve as an important contributor to the initiation and propagation of the inflammatory responses in RASF, which would eventually exacerbate the inflammation in RA.

In addition, in the current study, we showed for the first time that TLR activation exacerbated RASF-mediated inflammatory Th1 and Th17 responses. Th1 cells are considered to be the

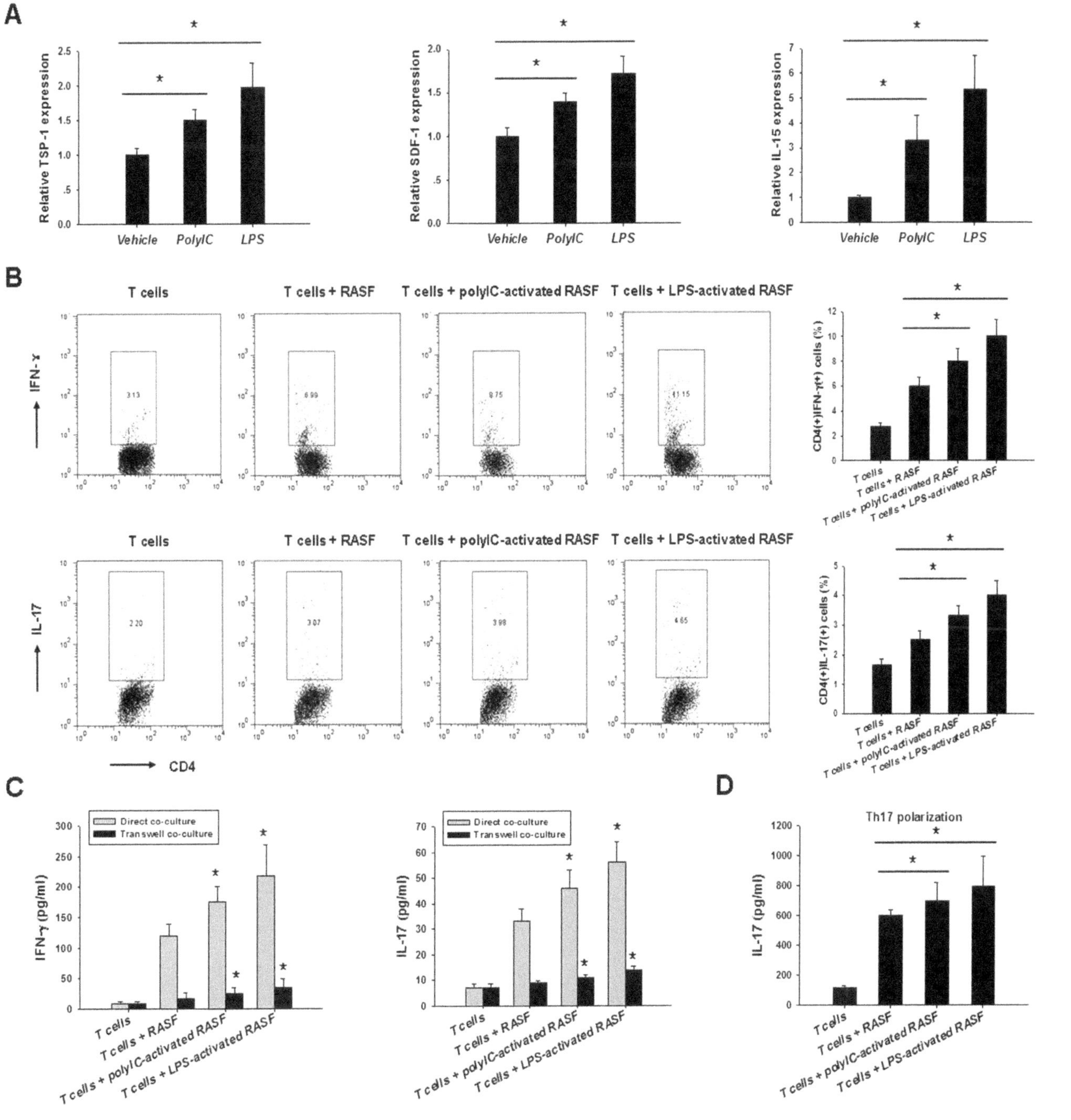

Figure 4. TLR activation enhanced RASF-mediated inflammatory Th1 and Th17 responses. A, RASF were stimulated with 25 µg/ml ploy(I:C) or 100 ng/ml LPS for 24 h, then the expression levels of TSP-1, SDF-1, and IL-15 were determined by realtime PCR analyses (Wilcoxon signed-rank test, **P*<0.05). B, After activation with 25 µg/ml ploy(I:C) or 100 ng/ml LPS for 24 h, RASF were co-cultured with allogeneic $CD4^+$ RA patient T cells in the direct contact or the transwell systems for 5 days. Then the T cells were harvested for flow cytometry analysis of the percentage of Th1 and Th17 cells (Wilcoxon signed-rank test, **P*<0.05). Accordingly, the cell culture supernatants were collected for ELISA analyses of IFN-γ and IL-17 (C) levels (Wilcoxon signed-rank test, **P*<0.05 *vs.* unstimulated control). D, RASF/T cell co-culture was performed as described above under Th17 polarization conditions. 5 days later, the cell culture supernatants were collected for IL-17 ELISA (Wilcoxon signed-rank test, **P*<0.05). The data were shown as mean+SEM of four separate assays.

conventional pathogenic cells in RA, because RA is thought to be a Th1-biased disease with Th1/Th2 imbalance. Recently, attention has increasingly focused on the role of Th17 cells, a subset that produces IL-17A, 17F, 21, and 22 and TNF-α [26]. IL 17A, which synergizes with TNF-α to promote activation of fibroblasts and chondrocytes, is currently being targeted in clinical trials [27]. In RA, synovial fibroblasts and T cells form a co-stimulatory circuit to perpetuate the inflammation. RASF could inhibit the apoptotic process of T cells and elicit their spontaneous proliferation; the increased inflammatory T cells then in turn induce more robust RASF activation. Cell-cell contact and soluble factors, such as inflammatory cytokines, contribute to this interaction. As demonstrated in our study, after TLR ligation, RASF could secrete more inflammatory mediators and express higher levels of surface TSP-1, SDF-1, and IL-15. These factors together with other unknown elements may eventually lead to the amplification of Th1 and Th17 cells. Thus TLRs also contribute to the maintenance and perpetuation of the inflammation in RA.

Given the integral roles of TLRs in the initiation, propagation, and perpetuation of the inflammation in RASF as well as T cells, targeting TLRs would be a preferred therapeutic strategy. In fact, several groups have been testing the feasibility of this hypothesis by both animal and human studies. In a serum-transfer model, disease duration was shortened in TLR4 null mice [28]. In the pristane-induced arthritis rat model, TLR3 expression was significantly upregulated during early disease stages. TLR3 agonist stimulation augmented the disease severity, and small interfering RNA (siRNA) targeting TLR3 in vivo reduced disease severity [29]. The recombinant analogue of chaperonin 10, XToll, targeting TLR4 developed by Cbio Ltd, is now being tested in a phase II clinical trial for RA treatment given by subcutaneous injection. Antibodies targeting TLR2, OPN-305 and OPN-301, have been proved to be able to abrogate spontaneous cytokine release by RASF [14]. DNA-based TLR7/9 antagonist, IMO-3100, has been tested in phase I clinical trials and showed promising results for RA. All these prove that targeting TLRs or their activation represents an attractive therapeutic option for RA.

However, we should notice that there are different types of TLRs in RA as demonstrated in our study. They might interact or work cooperatively with each other during the disease. Targeting one specific TLR might not suffice for RA amelioration. More indepth studies should be taken to further elucidate the pathogenic roles of TLRs in RA and the potential of targeting them for overcoming the chronic and persistent disease.

Author Contributions

Conceived and designed the experiments: FH ZL. Performed the experiments: FH YL. Analyzed the data: FH ZL. Contributed reagents/materials/analysis tools: LiZ LS HL XZ HZ ST LZ LX YY. Wrote the paper: FH ZL.

References

1. Gabriel SE, Michaud K (2009) Epidemiological studies in incidence, prevalence, mortality, and comorbidity of the rheumatic diseases. Arthritis Res Ther 11: 229.
2. Sokka T (2003) Work disability in early rheumatoid arthritis. Clin Exp Rheumatol 21: S71–74.
3. Brennan FM, McInnes IB (2008) Evidence that cytokines play a role in rheumatoid arthritis. J Clin Invest 118: 3537–3545.
4. Chiang EY, Kolumam GA, Yu X, Francesco M, Ivelja S, et al. (2009) Targeted depletion of lymphotoxin-alpha-expressing TH1 and TH17 cells inhibits autoimmune disease. Nat Med 15: 766–773.
5. Hu F, Shi L, Mu R, Zhu J, Li Y, et al. (2013) Hypoxia-inducible factor-1alpha and interleukin 33 form a regulatory circuit to perpetuate the inflammation in rheumatoid arthritis. PLoS One 8: e72650.
6. van Oosterhout M, Levarht EW, Sont JK, Huizinga TW, Toes RE, et al. (2005) Clinical efficacy of infliximab plus methotrexate in DMARD naive and DMARD refractory rheumatoid arthritis is associated with decreased synovial expression of TNF alpha and IL18 but not CXCL12. Ann Rheum Dis 64: 537–543.
7. Samson M, Audia S, Janikashvili N, Ciudad M, Trad M, et al. (2012) Inhibition of IL-6 function corrects Th17/Treg imbalance in rheumatoid arthritis patients. Arthritis Rheum.
8. Han Z, Boyle DL, Chang L, Bennett B, Karin M, et al. (2001) c-Jun N-terminal kinase is required for metalloproteinase expression and joint destruction in inflammatory arthritis. J Clin Invest 108: 73–81.
9. Patel DD, Haynes BF (2001) Leukocyte homing to synovium. Curr Dir Autoimmun 3: 133–167.
10. Ahn JK, Koh EM, Cha HS, Lee YS, Kim J, et al. (2008) Role of hypoxia-inducible factor-1alpha in hypoxia-induced expressions of IL-8, MMP-1 and MMP-3 in rheumatoid fibroblast-like synoviocytes. Rheumatology (Oxford) 47: 834–839.
11. Ng CT, Biniecka M, Kennedy A, McCormick J, Fitzgerald O, et al. (2010) Synovial tissue hypoxia and inflammation in vivo. Ann Rheum Dis 69: 1389–1395.
12. Hu F, Mu R, Zhu J, Shi L, Li Y, et al. (2013) Hypoxia and hypoxia-inducible factor-1alpha provoke toll-like receptor signalling-induced inflammation in rheumatoid arthritis. Ann Rheum Dis.
13. Brentano F, Schorr O, Gay RE, Gay S, Kyburz D (2005) RNA released from necrotic synovial fluid cells activates rheumatoid arthritis synovial fibroblasts via Toll-like receptor 3. Arthritis Rheum 52: 2656–2665.
14. Ultaigh SN, Saber TP, McCormick J, Connolly M, Dellacasagrande J, et al. (2011) Blockade of Toll-like receptor 2 prevents spontaneous cytokine release from rheumatoid arthritis ex vivo synovial explant cultures. Arthritis Res Ther 13: R33.
15. Brentano F, Kyburz D, Schorr O, Gay R, Gay S (2005) The role of Toll-like receptor signalling in the pathogenesis of arthritis. Cell Immunol 233: 90–96.
16. Ospelt C, Brentano F, Rengel Y, Stanczyk J, Kolling C, et al. (2008) Overexpression of toll-like receptors 3 and 4 in synovial tissue from patients with early rheumatoid arthritis: toll-like receptor expression in early and longstanding arthritis. Arthritis Rheum 58: 3684–3692.
17. Carrion M, Juarranz Y, Perez-Garcia S, Jimeno R, Pablos JL, et al. (2011) RNA sensors in human osteoarthritis and rheumatoid arthritis synovial fibroblasts: immune regulation by vasoactive intestinal peptide. Arthritis Rheum 63: 1626–1636.
18. Karpus ON, Heutinck KM, Wijnker PJ, Tak PP, Hamann J (2012) Triggering of the dsRNA sensors TLR3, MDA5, and RIG-I induces CD55 expression in synovial fibroblasts. PLoS One 7: e35606.
19. Akira S, Hemmi H (2003) Recognition of pathogen-associated molecular patterns by TLR family. Immunol Lett 85: 85–95.
20. Trinchieri G, Sher A (2007) Cooperation of Toll-like receptor signals in innate immune defence. Nat Rev Immunol 7: 179–190.
21. Hu F, Zhang L, Zheng J, Zhao L, Huang J, et al. (2012) Spontaneous production of immunoglobulin M in human epithelial cancer cells. PLoS One 7: e51423.
22. Bartok B, Firestein GS (2010) Fibroblast-like synoviocytes: key effector cells in rheumatoid arthritis. Immunol Rev 233: 233–255.
23. Taylor PC (2010) Pharmacology of TNF blockade in rheumatoid arthritis and other chronic inflammatory diseases. Curr Opin Pharmacol 10: 308–315.
24. Stahl HD, Hubner B, Seidl B, Liebert UG, van der Heijden IM, et al. (2000) Detection of multiple viral DNA species in synovial tissue and fluid of patients with early arthritis. Ann Rheum Dis 59: 342–346.
25. van der Heijden IM, Wilbrink B, Tchetverikov I, Schrijver IA, Schouls LM, et al. (2000) Presence of bacterial DNA and bacterial peptidoglycans in joints of patients with rheumatoid arthritis and other arthritides. Arthritis Rheum 43: 593–598.
26. Miossec P, Korn T, Kuchroo VK (2009) Interleukin-17 and type 17 helper T cells. N Engl J Med 361: 888–898.
27. Genovese MC, Van den Bosch F, Roberson SA, Bojin S, Biagini IM, et al. (2010) LY2439821, a humanized anti-interleukin-17 monoclonal antibody, in the treatment of patients with rheumatoid arthritis: A phase I randomized, double-blind, placebo-controlled, proof-of-concept study. Arthritis Rheum 62: 929–939.
28. Choe JY, Crain B, Wu SR, Corr M (2003) Interleukin 1 receptor dependence of serum transferred arthritis can be circumvented by toll-like receptor 4 signaling. J Exp Med 197: 537–542.
29. Meng L, Zhu W, Jiang C, He X, Hou W, et al. (2010) Toll-like receptor 3 upregulation in macrophages participates in the initiation and maintenance of pristane-induced arthritis in rats. Arthritis Res Ther 12: R103.

6

Protective Effect of the *HLA-DRB1*13:02* Allele in Japanese Rheumatoid Arthritis Patients

Shomi Oka[1], Hiroshi Furukawa[1*], Aya Kawasaki[2], Kota Shimada[3,4], Shoji Sugii[4], Atsushi Hashimoto[3], Akiko Komiya[1], Naoshi Fukui[1], Satoshi Ito[5], Tadashi Nakamura[6], Koichiro Saisho[7], Masao Katayama[8], Shinichiro Tsunoda[9], Hajime Sano[9], Kiyoshi Migita[10], Akiko Suda[11,12], Shouhei Nagaoka[11], Naoyuki Tsuchiya[2¶], Shigeto Tohma[1¶]

1 Clinical Research Center for Allergy and Rheumatology, Sagamihara Hospital, National Hospital Organization, Sagamihara, Japan, **2** Molecular and Genetic Epidemiology Laboratory, Faculty of Medicine, University of Tsukuba, Tsukuba, Japan, **3** Department of Rheumatology, Sagamihara Hospital, National Hospital Organization, Sagamihara, Japan, **4** Department of Rheumatology, Tokyo Metropolitan Tama Medical Center, Fuchu, Japan, **5** Department of Rheumatology, Niigata Rheumatic Center, Shibata, Japan, **6** Department of Rheumatology, Kumamoto Shinto General Hospital, Kumamoto, Japan, **7** Department of Orthopedics/Rheumatology, Miyakonojo Hospital, National Hospital Organization, Miyakonojo, Japan, **8** Department of Internal Medicine, Nagoya Medical Center, National Hospital Organization, Nagoya, Japan, **9** Division of Rheumatology, Department of Internal Medicine, Hyogo College of Medicine, Nishinomiya, Japan, **10** Clinical Research Center, Nagasaki Medical Center, National Hospital Organization, Omura, Japan, **11** Department of Rheumatology, Yokohama Minami Kyosai Hospital, Yokohama, Japan, **12** Center for Rheumatic Diseases, Yokohama City University Medical Center, Yokohama, Japan

Abstract

Rheumatoid arthritis (RA) is a chronic systemic inflammatory disease. Certain *HLA-DRB1* "shared-epitope" alleles are reported to be positively associated with increased RA susceptibility, whereas some of the other alleles may be negatively associated. However, studies on the latter are rare. Here, we focus on the protective effects of *DRB1* alleles in Japanese RA patients in an association study. Relative predispositional effects (RPE) were analyzed by sequential elimination of carriers of each allele with the strongest association. The protective effects of *DRB1* alleles were investigated in patients stratified according to whether they possessed anti-citrullinated peptide antibodies (ACPA). The *DRB1*13:02* allele was found to be negatively associated with RA ($P = 4.59 \times 10^{-10}$, corrected P (Pc) $= 1.42 \times 10^{-8}$, odds ratio [OR] 0.42, 95% CI 0.32–0.55, P [RPE] $= 1.27 \times 10^{-6}$); the genotypes *DRB1*04:05/*13:02* and **09:01/*13:02* were also negatively associated with RA. The protective effect of **13:02* was also present in ACPA-positive patients ($P = 3.95 \times 10^{-8}$, $Pc = 1.22 \times 10^{-6}$, OR 0.42, 95%CI 0.31–0.58) whereas **15:02* was negatively associated only with ACPA-negative RA ($P = 8.87 \times 10^{-5}$, $Pc = 0.0026$, OR 0.26, 95%CI 0.12–0.56). Thus, this study identified a negative association of *DRB1*13:02* with Japanese RA; our findings support the protective role of *DRB1*13:02* in the pathogenesis of ACPA-positive RA.

Editor: Masataka Kuwana, Keio University School of Medicine, Japan

Funding: This work was supported by Grants-in-Aid for Scientific Research (B, C) (22390199, 22591090), for Exploratory Research (25670458) and for Young Scientists (B) (24791018) from the Japan Society for the Promotion of Science, Health and Labour Science Research Grants from the Ministry of Health, Labour and Welfare of Japan, Grants-in-Aid for Clinical Research from National Hospital Organization, Research Grants from Daiwa Securities Health Foundation, Research Grants from Japan Research Foundation for Clinical Pharmacology, Research Grants from The Nakatomi Foundation, Research Grants from Takeda Science Foundation, Research Grants from Mitsui Sumitomo Insurance Welfare Foundation, Research Grants from SENSHIN Medical Research Foundation and research grants from pharmaceutical companies: Abbott Japan Co., Ltd., Astellas Pharma Inc., Chugai Pharmaceutical Co., Ltd., Eisai Co., Ltd., Mitsubishi Tanabe Pharma Corporation, Merck Sharp and Dohme Inc., Pfizer Japan Inc., Takeda Pharmaceutical Company Limited, Teijin Pharma Limited. The funders had no role in study design, data collection and analysis, decision to publish or preparing the manuscript.

Competing Interests: HF has the following conflicts: The following funders are supported in whole or in part by the indicated pharmaceutical companies. The Japan Research Foundation for Clinical Pharmacology is run by Daiichi Sankyo, the Takeda Science Foundation is supported by an endowment from Takeda Pharmaceutical Company and the Nakatomi Foundation was established by Hisamitsu Pharmaceutical Co., Inc. The Daiwa Securities Health Foundation was established by Daiwa Securities Group Inc. and Mitsui Sumitomo Insurance Welfare Foundation was established by Mitsui Sumitomo Insurance Co., Ltd. AH was supported by research grants from Mitsubishi Tanabe Pharma Corporation. NT is supported by SENSHIN Medical Research Foundation, which is supported by an endowment from Mitsubishi Tanabe Pharma Corporation. ST was supported by research grants from 9 pharmaceutical companies: Abbott Japan Co., Ltd., Astellas Pharma Inc., Chugai Pharmaceutical Co., Ltd., Eisai Co., Ltd., Mitsubishi Tanabe Pharma Corporation, Merck Sharp and Dohme Inc., Pfizer Japan Inc., Takeda Pharmaceutical Company Limited, Teijin Pharma Limited. The other authors declare no financial or commercial conflict of interest. This does not alter the authors' adherence to PLOS ONE policies on sharing data and materials.

* E-mail: h-furukawa@sagamihara-hosp.gr.jp

¶ These authors contributed equally to this work.

Introduction

Rheumatoid arthritis (RA) is a chronic systemic inflammatory disease that affects about 1% of the population. Its pathogenesis is multifactorial and disease susceptibility is associated with genetic and environmental factors [1,2,3]. Human Leukocyte Antigen (HLA) alleles are associated with RA in most ethnic groups and represent the strongest genetic risk factors for the disease. Most reports are of *HLA-DRB1* alleles positively associated with RA susceptibility. A conserved amino acid sequence at position 70–74

(QKRAA, RRRAA, or QRRAA) in the HLA-DRβ chain is shared between the RA susceptibility-associated *DRB1* alleles; this was designated the "shared epitope" (SE) [4]. A gene dosage effect was noted in the associations of *HLA-DRB1* alleles with susceptibility to RA in that homozygosity for susceptibility alleles does confer higher disease risk than heterozygosity for these alleles.

The presence of anti-citrullinated peptide antibodies (ACPA) is associated with RA with higher specificity than rheumatoid factor; thus, ACPA is thought to play some role in the pathogenesis of RA, especially as SE alleles are strongly associated with ACPA-positive RA but only relatively weakly with ACPA-negative RA [5]. Several studies have found that *DRB1*04:01* and **04:05*, both SE alleles, were mainly associated with RA in European and East Asian populations, respectively.

As well as associations with disease susceptibility, some *DRB1* alleles are reported to be negatively associated with RA. An amino acid sequence (DERAA) at position 70–74 [6], isoleucine at position 67 (I67) [7], aspartic acid at position 70 (D70) [8], or a conserved amino acid sequence at position 71–74 (S1; ARAA or ERAA) [9,10] in the HLA-DRβ chain seem to be protective in European populations. It was also reported that *DRB1*13* alleles are negatively associated with ACPA-positive and -negative RA in European populations [11]. A meta-analysis concluded that *DRB1*13:01* was protective against ACPA-positive RA in European populations [12]. However, there are very few studies on the protective effects of *DRB1* alleles in Japanese patients, although reduced frequencies of some *DRB1* alleles have been reported in Asian RA [13,14,15,16,17]. In this study, we focus on the protective effects of *HLA-DRB1* alleles in Japanese RA patients with or without ACPA.

Materials and Methods

Patients and controls

RA patients (n = 1480) were recruited at Sagamihara Hospital, Tama Medical Center, Nagoya Medical Center, Nagasaki Medical Center, Yokohama Minami Kyosai Hospital, Kumamoto Center for Arthritis and Rheumatology, Miyakonojo Hospital, Niigata Rheumatic Center, and Hyogo College of Medicine. Of these 1480 RA patients, 919 were ACPA-positive and 110 were ACPA-negative. ACPA data were not available for the remaining 451 patients. Healthy controls (n = 800; mean age ± SD, 36.7±10.7 years, 238 male [30.1%]) were recruited at Sagamihara Hospital and University of Tokyo, or by the Pharma SNP Consortium (Tokyo, Japan) [18]. All patients and healthy individuals were native Japanese living in Japan. All patients with RA fulfilled the 1987 American College of Rheumatology criteria for RA [19]. Rheumatoid factor and ACPA were detected using the N-latex RF kit (Siemens Healthcare Diagnostics, München, Germany) and the Mesacup-2 test CCP (Medical & Biological Laboratories, Nagoya, Japan), respectively. This study was reviewed and approved by the Research Ethics Committees of each participating institute: Nagasaki Medical Center Research Ethics Committee, Yokohama Minami Kyosai Hospital Research Ethics Committee, Tama Medical Center Research Ethics Committee, University of Tsukuba Research Ethics Committee, Miyakonojo Hospital Research Ethics Committee, Kumamoto Center for Arthritis and Rheumatology Research Ethics Committee, Niigata Rheumatic Center Research Ethics Committee, Hyogo College of Medicine Research Ethics Committee, and the University of Tokyo Research Ethics Committee. Written informed consent was obtained from all study participants. This study was conducted in accordance with the principles expressed in the Declaration of Helsinki.

Genotyping

Genotyping of *HLA-DRB1* was performed by a polymerase chain reaction technique using sequence-specific oligonucleotide probes (WAKFlow HLA typing kits, Wakunaga, Hiroshima, Japan), using a Bio-Plex 200 system (Bio-Rad, Hercules, CA), or using MPH-2 High Resolution HLA typing kits (Wakunaga) for four-digit allele typing. The following *DRB1* alleles contain the SE [4]: **01:01, *04:01, *04:04, *04:05, *04:10, *10:01, *14:02*, and **14:06*. *DRB1* allele groups, D70, I67, S1, and DERAA, were reported to be protective in European populations [6,7,8,9,10]; the protective effects of these allele groups in Japanese were validated in this study. *DRB1* alleles containing D70 [8] are **07:01, *08:02, *08:03, *08:09, *08:23, *11:01, *11:06, *12:01, *12:02, *12:05, *13:01, *13:02, *13:07, *14:03, *14:12*, and **16:02*. *DRB1* alleles containing I67 [7] are **07:01, *08:03, *08:23, *12:01, *12:05, *13:01, *13:02, *14:45, *15:01, *15:02*, and **15:11*. *DRB1* alleles containing DERAA [6] are the same as *DRB1*13* (i.e. **13:01*, and **13:02*). Finally, *DRB1* alleles containing S1 [20] are **13:01, *13:02, *15:01*, and **15:02*. Results of *DRB1* genotyping for some of the healthy controls were reported previously [14]. Some of the RA patients were also included in another study which reported on susceptibility effects for interstitial lung disease or positivity for autoantibodies [21,22,23]. *HLA-DRB1* genotype of each subject was not deposited in publicly available resources.

Statistical analysis

The exact tests for deviation from Hardy-Weinberg equilibrium were conducted by the Markov chain method under the condition

Table 1. Characteristics of the RA patients studied.

	RA	ACPA(+) RA	ACPA(−) RA	*P*
Number	1480	919	110	
Mean age, years (SD)	63.9 (12.2)	63.7 (12.2)	63.4 (12.3)	0.8582*
Male, n (%)	272 (19.0)	171 (18.7)	21 (19.3)	0.8969
Age at onset, years (SD)	49.3 (14.4)	49.2 (14.2)	50.1 (16.7)	0.6092*
Steinbrocker stage III and IV, n (%)	560 (37.8)	521 (56.7)	45 (40.9)	0.0703
Rheumatoid factor positive, n (%)	1002 (67.7)	826 (89.9)	40 (36.4)	9.39×10^{-37}

RA: rheumatoid arthritis, ACPA: anti-citrullinated peptide antibody, ACPA(+): ACPA-positive, ACPA(−): ACPA-negative. Association was tested by Fisher's exact test using 2×2 contingency tables or Student's t-test. *Student's t-test was employed.

Table 2. *HLA-DRB1* allele carrier frequency in RA patients and controls.

	RA (n = 1480)	Control (n = 800)	*P*	OR	*Pc*	95%CI	*P* (RPE)
*DRB1*04*	901 (60.9)	315 (39.4)	1.00×10^{-22}	2.40		(2.01–2.86)	
*DRB1*08*	188 (12.7)	181 (22.6)	2.02×10^{-9}	0.50		(0.40–0.62)	
*DRB1*12*	143 (9.7)	87 (10.9)	0.3820	0.88		(0.66–1.16)	
*DRB1*13*	112 (7.6)	134 (16.8)	4.69×10^{-11}	0.41		(0.31–0.53)	
*DRB1*14*	180 (12.2)	143 (17.9)	0.0003	0.64		(0.50–0.81)	
*DRB1*15*	405 (27.4)	262 (32.8)	0.0080	0.77		(0.64–0.93)	
SE	1035 (69.9)	315 (39.4)	2.35×10^{-45}	3.58		(2.99–4.29)	
D70	503 (34.0)	434 (54.3)	1.15×10^{-20}	0.43		(0.36–0.52)	
I67	691 (46.7)	501 (62.6)	3.67×10^{-13}	0.52		(0.44–0.62)	
S1	504 (34.1)	375 (46.9)	2.51×10^{-9}	0.59		(0.49–0.70)	
*DRB1*01:01*	210 (14.2)	83 (10.4)	0.0104	1.43	0.3239	(1.09–1.87)	3.75×10^{-5}
*DRB1*03:01*	2 (0.1)	0 (0.0)	0.5443	2.71	NS	(0.13–56.46)	
*DRB1*04:01*	84 (5.7)	17 (2.1)	4.30×10^{-5}	2.77	0.0013	(1.63–4.70)	0.0002
*DRB1*04:03*	38 (2.6)	42 (5.3)	0.0012	0.48	0.0374	(0.30–0.74)	
*DRB1*04:04*	5 (0.3)	4 (0.5)	0.7280	0.67	NS	(0.18–2.52)	
*DRB1*04:05*	738 (49.9)	185 (23.1)	1.41×10^{-36}	3.31	4.37×10^{-35}	(2.73–4.01)	1.41×10^{-36}
*DRB1*04:06*	58 (3.9)	59 (7.4)	0.0005	0.51	0.0148	(0.35–0.74)	
*DRB1*04:07*	4 (0.3)	15 (1.9)	0.0001	0.14	0.0035	(0.05–0.43)	
*DRB1*04:10*	70 (4.7)	21 (2.6)	0.0136	1.84	0.4224	(1.12–3.02)	0.0109
*DRB1*07:01*	10 (0.7)	7 (0.9)	0.6155	0.77	NS	(0.29–2.03)	
*DRB1*08:02*	56 (3.8)	61 (7.6)	0.0001	0.48	0.0042	(0.33–0.69)	
*DRB1*08:03*	135 (9.1)	124 (15.5)	8.60×10^{-6}	0.55	0.0003	(0.42–0.71)	
*DRB1*08:09*	1 (0.1)	2 (0.3)	0.2829	0.27	NS	(0.02–2.98)	
*DRB1*08:23*	1 (0.1)	0 (0.0)	1.0000	1.62	NS	(0.07–39.89)	
*DRB1*09:01*	423 (28.6)	213 (26.6)	0.3282	1.10	NS	(0.91–1.34)	7.32×10^{-5}
*DRB1*10:01*	25 (1.7)	2 (0.3)	0.0017	6.86	0.0536	(1.62–29.02)	0.0128
*DRB1*11:01*	40 (2.7)	33 (4.1)	0.0803	0.65	NS	(0.40–1.03)	0.0236
*DRB1*12:01*	95 (6.4)	58 (7.3)	0.4830	0.88	NS	(0.63–1.23)	
*DRB1*12:02*	50 (3.4)	29 (3.6)	0.8105	0.93	NS	(0.58–1.48)	
*DRB1*13:01*	5 (0.3)	8 (1.0)	0.0752	0.34	NS	(0.11–1.03)	
*DRB1*13:02*	107 (7.2)	126 (15.8)	4.59×10^{-10}	0.42	1.42×10^{-8}	(0.32–0.55)	1.27×10^{-6}
*DRB1*14:02*	2 (0.1)	0 (0.0)	0.5443	2.71	NS	(0.13–56.46)	
*DRB1*14:03*	32 (2.2)	38 (4.8)	0.0009	0.44	0.0271	(0.27–0.72)	
*DRB1*14:04*	0 (0.0)	3 (0.4)	0.0431	0.08	NS	(0.00–1.49)	
*DRB1*14:05*	28 (1.9)	35 (4.4)	0.0011	0.42	0.0348	(0.25–0.70)	

Table 2. Cont.

	RA (n = 1480)	Control (n = 800)	*P*	OR	*Pc*	95%CI	*P* (RPE)
*DRB1*14:06*	45 (3.0)	22 (2.8)	0.7952	1.11	NS	(0.66–1.86)	0.0041
*DRB1*14:07*	2 (0.1)	2 (0.3)	0.6159	0.54	NS	(0.08–3.84)	
*DRB1*14:54*	76 (5.1)	45 (5.6)	0.6254	0.91	NS	(0.62–1.33)	
*DRB1*15:01*	178 (12.0)	107 (13.4)	0.3537	0.89	NS	(0.68–1.14)	
*DRB1*15:02*	233 (15.7)	168 (21.0)	0.0019	0.70	0.0574	(0.56–0.88)	
*DRB1*16:02*	17 (1.1)	15 (1.9)	0.1912	0.61	NS	(0.30–1.22)	

RA: rheumatoid arthritis, OR: odds ratio, CI: confidence interval, *Pc*: corrected *P* value, NS: not significant, RPE: relative predispositional effects. Allele carrier frequencies are shown in parenthesis (%). Association was tested by Fisher's exact test using 2×2 contingency tables. RPE were tested by sequential elimination of carriers of each of the alleles *DRB1*04:05, *13:02, *04:01, *09:01, *01:01, *14:06, *10:01, *04:10,* and **11:01*. Allele groups SE, D70, I67, and S1 were as defined in the Materials and Methods section. *DRB1* alleles encoding the DERAA were the same as *DRB1*13* (i.e. **13:01* and **13:02*).

of 10000 each of dememorization, batches, and iterations per batch (Genepop on the web; http://genepop.curtin.edu.au/) [24]. Differences of allele carrier frequencies, genotype frequencies or amino acid residue carrier frequencies were analyzed by Fisher's exact test using 2×2 contingency tables. In order to estimate the protective effects of alleles in multi-allelic locus on individuals for RA, differences of allele carrier frequencies, or amino acid residue carrier frequencies were analyzed under the dominant model. Adjustment for multiple comparisons was performed using the Bonferroni method. *Pc* values were calculated by multiplying the *P* value by the number of alleles or amino acid residues tested.

Alleles with low carrier frequencies in RA patients may not be detectably protective because predisposing SE alleles with higher carrier frequencies could obscure their influence. To investigate the protective effects of HLA alleles, relative predispositional effects (RPE) were analyzed by sequential elimination of carriers of each allele with the strongest association [25]. In order to obtain an accurate estimate of the effects of alleles other than SE, analyses of these alleles in RA patients were also stratified in the following manner: For SE-negative subjects, the effect in "*A/A*" and "*A*/other than SE or *A*" genotype groups was investigated using "other than SE or *A*/other than SE or *A*" genotype group as the reference. For SE-positive subjects, the effect of "SE/*A*" genotype group was analyzed using "SE/other than *A*" genotype group as the reference. The protective effects of the **13:02* allele were confirmed in the presence of predisposing allele "*B*". The effect in "*B*/**13:02*" genotype group was investigated using the "*B*/other than **13:02*" genotype group as the reference. The protective effects of the **15:02* allele were confirmed in the analysis of "*B*/**15:02*" using the "*B*/other than **15:02*" genotype group as the reference in the same manner.

Results

Characteristics of RA patients

Characteristics of ACPA-positive [ACPA(+)] and ACPA-negative [ACPA(−)] RA patients are given in Table 1. The proportion of rheumatoid factor-positive patients in the ACPA(+) group was higher than in ACPA(−) RA. There were no significant differences in terms of mean age, percentage of males, age at onset, or Steinbrocker stage [26] between ACPA(+) and ACPA(-) patients.

Reduced *HLA-DRB1*13:02* allele carrier frequency in Japanese RA

HLA-DRB1 genotyping was performed in 1480 RA patients and 800 healthy controls to compare HLA allele carrier frequencies (Table 2). No deviation from Hardy-Weinberg equilibrium was observed in the controls ($P = 0.6329$), though a deviation was detected in the RA patients ($P < 0.0001$). A strong positive association between the frequency of *DRB1*04* and RA ($P = 1.00\times10^{-22}$, Corrected *P* [Pc] $= 1.31\times10^{-21}$, odds ratio [OR] 2.40, 95% confidence interval [CI] 2.01–2.86, Table 2) was confirmed. Additionally, *DRB1*13* (i.e. the DERAA allele group) was found to be negatively associated with RA ($P = 4.69\times10^{-11}$, $Pc = 6.10\times10^{-10}$, OR 0.41, 95% CI 0.31–0.53). The D70, I67, and S1 allele groups were also negatively associated with RA (D70: $P = 1.15\times10^{-20}$, OR 0.43, 95% CI 0.36–0.52; I67: $P = 3.67\times10^{-13}$, OR 0.52, 95% CI 0.44–0.62; S1: $P = 2.51\times10^{-9}$, OR 0.59, 95% CI 0.49–0.70). Finally, a predisposing association was confirmed between SE and RA ($P = 2.35\times10^{-45}$, OR 3.58, 95% CI 2.99–4.29).

We further explored associations between these *DRB1* alleles and RA by high-resolution typing, using RPE testing [25] (Table 2). RPE were analyzed by sequential elimination of carriers

Table 3. *HLA-DRB1* allele carrier frequency in RA patients and controls in subjects stratified for the presence of SE.

		RA (n = 1480)	Control (n = 800)	*P*	OR	95%CI
**03*	SE negative	1 (0.2)	0 (0.0)	0.4785	3.28	(0.13–80.65)
	SE positive	1 (0.1)	0 (0.0)	1.0000	0.91	(0.04–22.52)
**04* other than SE	SE negative	46 (10.3)	81 (16.7)	0.0055	0.58	(0.39–0.85)
	SE positive	54 (5.2)	34 (10.8)	0.0010	0.45	(0.29–0.71)
**07*	SE negative	5 (1.1)	5 (1.0)	1.0000	1.09	(0.31–3.79)
	SE positive	5 (0.5)	2 (0.6)	0.6680	0.76	(0.15–3.93)
**08*	SE negative	114 (25.6)	140 (28.9)	0.2703	0.85	(0.64–1.13)
	SE positive	74 (7.1)	41 (13.0)	0.0018	0.51	(0.34–0.77)
**09*	SE negative	230 (51.7)	161 (33.2)	1.44×10^{-8}	2.15	(1.65–2.81)
	SE positive	193 (18.6)	52 (16.5)	0.4051	1.16	(0.83–1.62)
**11*	SE negative	17 (3.8)	29 (6.0)	0.1336	0.62	(0.34–1.15)
	SE positive	23 (2.2)	4 (1.3)	0.3635	1.77	(0.61–5.15)
**12*	SE negative	63 (14.2)	66 (13.6)	0.8496	1.05	(0.72–1.52)
	SE positive	80 (7.7)	21 (6.7)	0.6248	1.17	(0.71–1.93)
**13*	SE negative	48 (10.8)	102 (21.0)	2.43×10^{-5}	0.45	(0.31–0.66)
	SE positive	64 (6.2)	32 (10.2)	0.0235	0.58	(0.37–0.91)
**14* other than SE	SE negative	63 (14.2)	89 (18.4)	0.0918	0.73	(0.52–1.04)
	SE positive	72 (7.0)	33 (10.5)	0.0537	0.64	(0.41–0.98)
**15*	SE negative	182 (40.9)	207 (42.7)	0.5950	0.93	(0.72–1.21)
	SE positive	223 (21.5)	55 (17.5)	0.1305	1.30	(0.94–1.80)
**16*	SE negative	10 (2.2)	9 (1.9)	0.8174	1.22	(0.49–3.02)
	SE positive	7 (0.7)	6 (1.9)	0.0900	0.35	(0.12–1.05)
**13:01*	SE negative	1 (0.2)	7 (1.4)	0.0712	0.15	(0.02–1.26)
	SE positive	4 (0.4)	1 (0.3)	1.0000	1.22	(0.14–10.94)
**13:02*	SE negative	47 (10.6)	95 (19.6)	0.0001	0.48	(0.33–0.71)
	SE positive	60 (5.8)	31 (9.8)	0.0148	0.56	(0.36–0.89)
D70	SE negative	242 (54.4)	320 (66.0)	0.0004	0.61	(0.47–0.80)
	SE positive	261 (25.2)	114 (36.2)	0.0002	0.59	(0.45–0.78)
I67	SE negative	301 (67.6)	371 (76.5)	0.0027	0.64	(0.48–0.86)
	SE positive	390 (37.7)	130 (41.3)	0.2614	0.86	(0.67–1.11)
S1	SE negative	217 (48.8)	288 (59.4)	0.0012	0.65	(0.50–0.84)
	SE positive	287 (27.7)	87 (27.6)	1.0000	1.01	(0.76–1.33)
D70 other than **13:02*	SE negative	212 (47.6)	253 (52.2)	0.1892	0.83	(0.64–1.08)
	SE positive	201 (19.4)	83 (26.3)	0.0092	0.67	(0.50–0.90)
I67 other than **13:02*	SE negative	280 (62.9)	310 (63.9)	0.7852	0.96	(0.73–1.25)
	SE positive	330 (31.9)	99 (31.4)	0.8904	1.02	(0.78–1.34)
S1 other than **13:02*	SE negative	182 (40.9)	213 (43.9)	0.3536	0.88	(0.68–1.15)
	SE positive	227 (21.9)	56 (17.8)	0.1147	1.30	(0.94–1.80)

RA: rheumatoid arthritis, SE: Shared epitope, OR: odds ratio, CI: confidence interval, Allele carrier frequencies are shown in parenthesis (%). Association was tested by Fisher's exact test using 2×2 contingency tables. SE negative: "*A*/*A*" or "*A*/other than SE or *A*" vs. "other than SE or *A*/other than SE or *A*". SE positive: "SE/*A*" vs. "SE/other than *A*". Allele groups SE, D70, I67, and S1 were as defined in the Materials and Methods section.

of each allele with the strongest association (Table 2, right column). The prime strongest association was between *DRB1*04:05* and RA ($P = 1.41 \times 10^{-36}$, $Pc = 4.37 \times 10^{-35}$, OR 3.31, 95% CI 2.73–4.01). Thus, a second round of comparisons was conducted after the elimination of *DRB1*04:05* carriers, revealing the next strongest association to be between *DRB1*13:02* and RA ($P = 1.27 \times 10^{-6}$, $Pc = 3.68 \times 10^{-5}$). A third round after the elimination of both *DRB1*04:05* or **13:02* carriers now showed the strongest association of RA with *DRB1*04:01* ($P = 0.0002$, $Pc = 0.0065$). Further rounds after elimination of *DRB1*04:05*, **13:02* and **04:01* carriers revealed associations between the remaining *DRB1* alleles and RA, particularly for *DRB1*09:01* ($P = 7.32 \times 10^{-5}$, $Pc = 0.0020$), **01:01* ($P = 3.75 \times 10^{-5}$, $Pc = 0.0010$), **14:06* ($P = 0.0041$, $Pc = 0.0995$), **10:01* ($P = 0.0128$, $Pc = 0.2936$), **04:10* ($P = 0.0109$, $Pc = 0.2399$), and **11:01* ($P = 0.0236$, $Pc = 0.4948$). The results from association

Table 4. *HLA-DRB1* genotype frequency in RA patients and controls.

	RA (n = 1480)	Control (n = 800)	*P*	OR	95%CI
**04:05/*13:02*	45 (6.1)	21 (11.4)	0.0168	0.51	(0.29–0.87)
**04:01/*13:02*	6 (7.1)	2 (11.8)	0.6190	0.58	(0.11–3.14)
**09:01/*13:02*	12 (2.8)	21 (9.9)	0.0004	0.27	(0.13–0.55)
**01:01/*13:02*	5 (2.4)	3 (3.6)	0.6917	0.65	(0.15–2.79)

RA: rheumatoid arthritis, OR: odds ratio, CI: confidence interval, Allele carrier frequencies are shown in parenthesis (%). Association was tested by Fisher's exact test using 2×2 contingency tables. Comparison: "*B/*13:02*" vs. *B*/other than **13:02*".

studies under the recessive and the allele models were represented in Table S1 and S2, respectively. Similar tendencies were observed in these analyses. We therefore focused on the *DRB1* allele with the most significantly reduced allele carrier frequency, namely *DRB1*13:02*.

Protective effects of the **13:02* allele against RA in both SE-positive and -negative subjects

In order to obtain an accurate estimate of the effects of alleles other than SE, associations were estimated in subjects stratified into those with or without SE (Table 3). Although *DRB1*09* ($P = 1.44 \times 10^{-8}$, OR 2.15, 95% CI 1.65–2.81) predisposes to RA in SE-negative people, **04* other than SE (**04:03, *04:06, *04:07*: SE negative, $P = 0.0055$, OR 0.58, 95% CI 0.39–0.85; SE positive, $P = 0.0010$, OR 0.45, 95% CI 0.29–0.71), **13* (**13:01, *13:02*: SE negative, $P = 2.43 \times 10^{-5}$, OR 0.45, 95% CI 0.31–0.66; SE positive, $P = 0.0235$, OR 0.58, 95% CI 0.37–0.91), and D70 (SE negative, $P = 0.0004$, OR 0.61, 95% CI 0.47–0.80; SE positive, $P = 0.0002$, OR 0.59, 95% CI 0.45–0.78) were negatively associated with RA in both SE-positive and -negative individuals. *DRB1*08* ($P = 0.0018$, OR 0.51, 95% CI 0.34–0.77) alleles were negatively associated with RA in SE-positive people. I67 ($P = 0.0027$, OR 0.64, 95% CI 0.48–0.86) and S1 ($P = 0.0012$, OR 0.65, 95% CI 0.50–0.84) alleles were negatively associated with RA in SE-negative subjects. However, D70 alleles other than **13:02* were negatively associated with RA in SE-positive ($P = 0.0092$, OR 0.67, 95% CI 0.50–0.90) but not in SE-negative individuals. I67 alleles other than **13:02* and S1 alleles other than **13:02* did not have any negative associations. These data suggest that the negative associations of D70, I67 and S1 alleles with RA in SE-negative subjects were mainly mediated by **13:02*, although the negative association of D70 in SE-positive people was due to **08* alleles. Thus, **13:02* was negatively associated with RA in SE-negative people and relatively weakly also in SE-positive subjects.

The protective effects of the **13:02* allele were analyzed in the presence of predisposing alleles (Table 4). Although **04:05* and **09:01* are positively associated with RA in Japanese, the risk of disease in people carrying these alleles was decreased in heterozygotes also carrying **13:02* (**04:05*: $P = 0.0168$, OR = 0.51, 95% CI 0.29–0.87; **09:01*: $P = 0.0004$, OR = 0.27, 95% CI 0.13–0.55).

Although the age at RA onset in **04:05* allele carriers was lower than in non-carriers (mean age ± standard deviation [SD] [years], carriers vs. non-carriers, 48.2±13.8 vs. 50.5±14.9, $P = 0.0070$) the age at onset in people with **13:02* or **01:01* was higher than in non-carriers (53.8±14.0 vs. 48.9±14.4, $P = 0.0027$, and 52.9±13.3 vs. 48.7±14.5, $P = 0.0021$, respectively) (Table S3).

Protective effects of **13:02* against ACPA(+) RA and **15:02* against ACPA(−) RA

Predisposing effects of the **04:05* allele were confirmed in ACPA(+) RA (Table 5, $P = 3.64 \times 10^{-35}$, $Pc = 1.13 \times 10^{-33}$, OR 3.59, 95% CI 2.91–4.42), whereas *DRB1*13:02* was negatively associated with ACPA(+) RA ($P = 3.95 \times 10^{-8}$, $Pc = 1.22 \times 10^{-6}$, OR 0.42, 95% CI 0.31–0.58). The DERAA allele group was still negatively associated with RA even when only ACPA(+) patients were considered ($P = 2.05 \times 10^{-9}$, OR 0.40, 95% CI 0.29–0.54). D70, I67, and S1 were also negatively associated with ACPA(+) RA (D70: $P = 5.78 \times 10^{-21}$, OR 0.39, 95% CI 0.32–0.48; I67: $P = 3.66 \times 10^{-12}$, OR 0.50, 95% CI 0.42–0.61; S1: $P = 2.31 \times 10^{-8}$, OR 0.57, 95% CI 0.47–0.70), and the predisposing association was confirmed between SE and ACPA(+) RA ($P = 1.16 \times 10^{-48}$, OR 4.41, 95% CI 3.59–5.41).

The predisposing association was also confirmed between SE and ACPA(−) RA ($P = 0.0229$, OR 1.60, 95% CI 1.07–2.38), albeit weakly. A tendency towards a positive association of **04:05* and **14:54* with ACPA(−) RA was observed (**04:05*: $P = 0.0126$, $Pc = 0.3667$, OR 1.75, 95% CI 1.15–2.69;**14:54*: $P = 0.0202$, OR 2.25, $Pc = 0.5861$, 95% CI 1.17–4.32). On the other hand, *DRB1*15:02* was negatively associated with ACPA(−) RA ($P = 8.87 \times 10^{-5}$, $Pc = 0.0026$, OR 0.26, 95% CI 0.12–0.56).

We next examined associations of alleles other than SE with ACPA(+) and ACPA(−) RA stratified by the presence or absence of SE (Table 6). This analysis showed that *DRB1*13:02* and D70 were negatively associated with ACPA(+) RA in both SE-positive and -negative subjects (SE-negative: $P = 0.0212$, OR 0.59, 95% CI 0.38–0.92; SE-positive: $P = 0.0144$, OR 0.53, 95% CI 0.32–0.87 and SE-negative: $P = 0.0011$, OR 0.59, 95% CI 0.43–0.81: SE-positive, $P = 0.0001$, OR 0.56, 95% CI 0.42–0.75, respectively). D70 alleles other than **13:02* were protectively associated with ACPA(+) RA in SE-positive ($P = 0.0076$, OR 0.65, 95% CI 0.47–0.89), but not in SE-negative subjects. These data suggest that the negative association of D70 alleles with ACPA(+) RA in SE-negative patients is mainly mediated by **13:02*. Thus, the negative association of **13:02* with ACPA(+) RA was confirmed in SE-negative and -positive subjects.

The *DRB1*15:02* allele was negatively associated with ACPA(−) RA in SE-negative people ($P = 0.0008$, OR 0.22, 95% CI 0.08–0.61). I67 and S1 alleles were negatively associated with ACPA(−) RA in SE-negative subjects ($P = 0.0080$, OR 0.45, 95% CI 0.25–0.80 and $P = 0.0008$, OR 0.37, 95% CI 0.21–0.67, respectively). However, I67 alleles other than **15:02* or S1 alleles other than **15:02* were not associated with ACPA(−) RA. These data suggest that the negative associations of I67 and S1 with ACPA(−) RA in SE-negative subjects are mainly mediated by **15:02*. Thus, the negative association of **15:02* with ACPA(−) RA was detected in SE-negative people.

Table 5. *HLA-DRB1* allele carrier frequency in ACPA(+) and ACPA(−) RA patients and controls.

	ACPA(+) RA	ACPA(−) RA	Control	ACPA(+) RA				ACPA(−) RA			
	(n = 919)	(n = 110)	(n = 800)	*P*	OR	*Pc*	95%CI	*P*	OR	*Pc*	95%CI
*DRB1*01:01*	146 (15.9)	10 (9.1)	83 (10.4)	0.0008	1.63	0.0251	(1.22–2.18)	0.8664	0.86	NS	(0.43–1.72)
*DRB1*03:01*	1 (0.1)	1 (0.9)	0 (0.0)	1.0000	2.61	NS	(0.11–64.28)	0.1209	21.93	NS	(0.89–541.76)
*DRB1*04:01*	65 (7.1)	4 (3.6)	17 (2.1)	1.12×10^{-6}	3.51	3.48×10^{-5}	(2.04–6.03)	0.3069	1.74	NS	(0.57–5.26)
*DRB1*04:03*	22 (2.4)	1 (0.9)	42 (5.3)	0.0020	0.44	0.0632	(0.26–0.75)	0.0512	0.17	NS	(0.02–1.22)
*DRB1*04:04*	4 (0.4)	0 (0.0)	4 (0.5)	1.0000	0.87	NS	(0.22–3.49)	1.0000	0.80	NS	(0.04–14.98)
*DRB1*04:05*	477 (51.9)	38 (34.5)	185 (23.1)	3.64×10^{-35}	3.59	1.13×10^{-33}	(2.91–4.42)	0.0126	1.75	0.3667	(1.15–2.69)
*DRB1*04:06*	32 (3.5)	9 (8.2)	59 (7.4)	0.0003	0.45	0.0106	(0.29–0.70)	0.7014	1.12	NS	(0.54–2.33)
*DRB1*04:07*	3 (0.3)	0 (0.0)	15 (1.9)	0.0017	0.17	0.0514	(0.05–0.59)	0.2387	0.23	NS	(0.01–3.86)
*DRB1*04:10*	46 (5.0)	3 (2.7)	21 (2.6)	0.0122	1.95	0.3768	(1.16–3.30)	1.0000	1.04	NS	(0.31–3.55)
*DRB1*07:01*	7 (0.8)	0 (0.0)	7 (0.9)	0.7956	0.87	NS	(0.30–2.49)	1.0000	0.48	NS	(0.03–8.44)
*DRB1*08:02*	27 (2.9)	10 (9.1)	61 (7.6)	1.39×10^{-5}	0.37	0.0004	(0.23–0.58)	0.5703	1.21	NS	(0.60–2.44)
*DRB1*08:03*	80 (8.7)	13 (11.8)	124 (15.5)	1.83×10^{-5}	0.52	0.0006	(0.39–0.70)	0.3931	0.73	NS	(0.40–1.34)
*DRB1*08:09*	0 (0.0)	0 (0.0)	2 (0.3)	0.2164	0.17	NS	(0.01–3.62)	1.0000	1.45	NS	(0.07–30.30)
*DRB1*08:23*	1 (0.1)	0 (0.0)	0 (0.0)	1.0000	2.61	NS	(0.11–64.28)				
*DRB1*09:01*	252 (27.4)	30 (27.3)	213 (26.6)	0.7440	1.04	NS	(0.84–1.29)	0.9086	1.03	NS	(0.66–1.62)
*DRB1*10:01*	15 (1.6)	0 (0.0)	2 (0.3)	0.0054	6.62	0.1669	(1.51–29.04)	1.0000	1.45	NS	(0.07–30.30)
*DRB1*11:01*	26 (2.8)	4 (3.6)	33 (4.1)	0.1463	0.68	NS	(0.40–1.14)	1.0000	0.88	NS	(0.30–2.52)
*DRB1*12:01*	53 (5.8)	14 (12.7)	58 (7.3)	0.2379	0.78	NS	(0.53–1.15)	0.0579	1.87	NS	(1.00–3.47)
*DRB1*12:02*	27 (2.9)	5 (4.5)	29 (3.6)	0.4963	0.80	NS	(0.47–1.37)	0.5922	1.27	NS	(0.48–3.34)
*DRB1*13:01*	1 (0.1)	1 (0.9)	8 (1.0)	0.0149	0.11	0.4632	(0.01–0.86)	1.0000	0.91	NS	(0.11–7.33)
*DRB1*13:02*	67 (7.3)	14 (12.7)	126 (15.8)	3.95×10^{-8}	0.42	1.22×10^{-6}	(0.31–0.58)	0.4819	0.78	NS	(0.43–1.41)
*DRB1*14:02*	1 (0.1)	0 (0.0)	0 (0.0)	1.0000	2.61	NS	(0.11–64.28)				
*DRB1*14:03*	17 (1.8)	4 (3.6)	38 (4.8)	0.0008	0.38	0.0257	(0.21–0.67)	0.8088	0.76	NS	(0.26–2.16)
*DRB1*14:04*	0 (0.0)	0 (0.0)	3 (0.4)	0.1006	0.12	NS	(0.01–2.40)	1.0000	1.03	NS	(0.05–20.09)
*DRB1*14:05*	18 (2.0)	6 (5.5)	35 (4.4)	0.0048	0.44	0.1482	(0.25–0.78)	0.6219	1.26	NS	(0.52–3.07)
*DRB1*14:06*	32 (3.5)	3 (2.7)	22 (2.8)	0.4086	1.28	NS	(0.74–2.21)	1.0000	0.99	NS	(0.29–3.37)
*DRB1*14:07*	1 (0.1)	0 (0.0)	2 (0.3)	0.6007	0.43	NS	(0.04–4.80)	1.0000	1.45	NS	(0.07–30.30)
*DRB1*14:54*	43 (4.7)	13 (11.8)	45 (5.6)	0.3824	0.82	NS	(0.54–1.26)	0.0202	2.25	0.5861	(1.17–4.32)
*DRB1*15:01*	106 (11.5)	15 (13.6)	107 (13.4)	0.2711	0.84	NS	(0.63–1.13)	0.8824	1.02	NS	(0.57–1.83)
*DRB1*15:02*	145 (15.8)	7 (6.4)	168 (21.0)	0.0058	0.70	0.1797	(0.55–0.90)	8.87×10^{-5}	0.26	0.0026	(0.12–0.56)
*DRB1*16:02*	10 (1.1)	2 (1.8)	15 (1.9)	0.2255	0.58	NS	(0.26–1.29)	1.0000	0.97	NS	(0.22–4.30)
SE	681 (74.1)	56 (50.9)	315 (39.4)	1.16×10^{-48}	4.41		(3.59–5.41)	0.0229	1.60		(1.07–2.38)
D70	292 (31.8)	55 (50.0)	434 (54.3)	5.78×10^{-21}	0.39		(0.32–0.48)	0.4160	0.84		(0.57–1.26)
I67	421 (45.8)	57 (51.8)	501 (62.6)	3.66×10^{-12}	0.50		(0.42–0.61)	0.0364	0.64		(0.43–0.96)

Table 5. Cont.

	ACPA(+) RA	ACPA(−) RA	Control	ACPA(+) RA				ACPA(−) RA			
	(n = 919)	(n = 110)	(n = 800)	*P*	OR	*Pc*	95%CI	*P*	OR	*Pc*	95%CI
S1	309 (33.6)	35 (31.8)	375 (46.9)	2.31×10^{-8}	0.57		(0.47–0.70)	0.0030	0.53		(0.35–0.81)
DERAA	68 (7.4)	15 (13.6)	134 (16.8)	2.05×10^{-9}	0.40		(0.29–0.54)	0.4922	0.78		(0.44–1.40)

ACPA: anti-citrullinated peptide antibody, ACPA(+): ACPA-positive, ACPA(−): ACPA-negative, RA: rheumatoid arthritis, OR: odds ratio, CI: confidence interval, *Pc*: corrected *P* value, NS: not significant. Allele carrier frequencies are shown in parenthesis (%). Association was tested by Fisher's exact test using 2×2 contingency tables. Allele groups SE, D70, I67, S1, and DERAA were as defined in the Materials and Methods section.

Then we examined the protective effects of **13:02* against ACPA(+) RA in the presence of predisposing alleles for ACPA(+) RA, *DRB1*04:05* and **09:01* (Table 5). As shown in Table 7, the risk for RA was decreased when these alleles were present together with **13:02* (**04:05*: $P = 0.0202$, OR = 0.49, 95% CI 0.27–0.88; **09:01*: $P = 0.0035$, OR = 0.30, 95% CI 0.13–0.69).

The protective effects of the **15:02* allele against ACPA(−) RA were also analyzed in the presence of predisposing alleles (Table 7). *DRB1*04:05* and **14:54* are potentially risk alleles for ACPA(−) RA (Table 5). The risk for ACPA(−) RA showed tendency towards decrease when these alleles were present together with **15:02* (**04:05*: $P = 0.2665$, OR = 0.39; **14:54*: $P = 0.6686$, OR = 0.45), but these differences were not statistically significant.

Certain amino acid residues in the HLA-DRβ chain are associated with RA

Finally, we analyzed the association with RA with respect to each amino acid residue in the HLA-DRβ chain. Tyrosine at position 10 (10Y, $P = 1.34\times10^{-20}$, OR = 0.44, $Pc = 4.59\times10^{-19}$, 95% CI 0.37–0.52), serine at position 11 (11S, $P = 1.35\times10^{-20}$, OR = 0.44, $Pc = 4.59\times10^{-19}$, 95% CI 0.37–0.52), threonine at position 12 (12T, $P = 1.35\times10^{-20}$, OR = 0.44, $Pc = 4.59\times10^{-19}$, 95% CI 0.37–0.52), and aspartic acid at position 70 (70D, $P = 1.15\times10^{-20}$, OR = 0.43, $Pc = 3.91\times10^{-19}$, 95% CI 0.36–0.52) in the DRβ chain showed strong protective associations with RA (Figure 1A, open circles). Similar associations were observed with ACPA(+) RA (Figure 1B), whereas aspartic acid at position 57 (57D, $P = 0.0006$, OR = 0.46, $Pc = 0.0191$, 95% CI 0.30–0.71) in the DRβ chain showed a slight protective association with ACPA(−) RA (Figure 1C). Thus, association analysis suggested roles for specific amino acid residues in the HLA-DRβ chain.

Discussion

Many groups have investigated associations between *HLA-DRB1* alleles and RA disease susceptibility. However, few studies have focused on protective effects of *DRB1* alleles against RA [11,12]. In the present study, we determined that the *DRB1*13:02* allele plays a protective role in Japanese RA, especially in ACPA(+) RA, using RPE analysis (Table 2). A lower frequency of **13:02* alleles in Asian patients with RA has been reported before [13,14,15,16,17]. In the genotype analysis, lower frequencies of the "*HLA-DRB1*04:05/*13:02*", or "**09:01/*13:02*" genotypes in RA were observed (Table 4). Thus, the protective effects of **13:02* seem to overcome the predisposing effects of **04:05* or **09:01*. Several studies have shown that certain *DRB1* alleles are negatively associated with RA and also some negatively associated allele groups defined by amino acid sequences, such as D70, I67, S1 and DERAA (Table 3) [6,7,8,9,10]. Our results indicated that the protective effects of these allele groups were mainly attributable to **13:02* in Japanese RA, whereas they are attributable to **13:01* in European RA [12]. The age at onset of **13:02* allele carriers was higher than non-carriers (Table S3), suggesting that the allele carriers of **13:02* may be associated with RA subsets with higher age at onset, and/or the age at onset may be delayed in the presence of the **13:02* allele.

*DRB1*13:02* commonly belongs to the haplotype *DRB1*13:02-DQB1*06:04-DPB1*04:01*, which shows evidence for positive selection in Japanese in recent history [27]. The *DRB1*13:02* allele is also a protective allele for cervical cancer [28], autoimmune hepatitis [29], and *DPB1*04:01* is protective for hepatitis B infection [30]. Certain genes of this haplotype could be protective for these diseases, in addition to RA.

Table 6. *HLA-DRB1* allele carrier frequency in ACPA(+) and ACPA(−) RA patients and controls stratified for the presence of SE.

		ACPA(+) RA	ACPA(−) RA	Control	ACPA(+) RA			ACPA(−) RA		
		(n = 919)	(n = 110)	(n = 800)	*P*	OR	95%CI	*P*	OR	95%CI
**03*	SE negative	0 (0.0)	1 (1.9)	0 (0.0)	1.0000	2.04	(0.04–102.91)	0.1002	27.22	(1.10–676.68)
	SE positive	1 (0.1)	0 (0.0)	0 (0.0)	1.0000	1.39	(0.06–34.24)	1.0000	5.58	(0.11–284.33)
**04* other than SE	SE negative	24 (10.1)	5 (9.3)	81 (16.7)	0.0183	0.56	(0.34–0.91)	0.1755	0.51	(0.20–1.32)
	SE positive	33 (4.8)	5 (8.9)	34 (10.8)	0.0009	0.42	(0.26–0.69)	0.8156	0.81	(0.30–2.17)
**07*	SE negative	4 (1.7)	0 (0.0)	5 (1.0)	0.4862	1.64	(0.44–6.17)	1.0000	0.80	(0.04–14.69)
	SE positive	3 (0.4)	0 (0.0)	2 (0.6)	0.6540	0.69	(0.12–4.17)	1.0000	1.11	(0.05–23.42)
**08*	SE negative	57 (23.9)	17 (31.5)	140 (28.9)	0.1826	0.78	(0.54–1.11)	0.7523	1.13	(0.62–2.08)
	SE positive	50 (7.3)	4 (7.1)	41 (13.0)	0.0062	0.53	(0.34–0.82)	0.2704	0.51	(0.18–1.50)
**09*	SE negative	129 (54.2)	20 (37.0)	161 (33.2)	8.63×10^{-8}	2.38	(1.73–3.27)	0.6488	1.18	(0.66–2.12)
	SE positive	123 (18.1)	10 (17.9)	52 (16.5)	0.5916	1.11	(0.78–1.59)	0.8459	1.10	(0.52–2.32)
**11*	SE negative	11 (4.6)	3 (5.6)	29 (6.0)	0.4942	0.76	(0.37–1.55)	1.0000	0.92	(0.27–3.14)
	SE positive	15 (2.2)	1 (1.8)	4 (1.3)	0.4558	1.75	(0.58–5.32)	0.5609	1.41	(0.16–12.89)
**12*	SE negative	30 (12.6)	11 (20.4)	66 (13.6)	0.8157	0.92	(0.58–1.45)	0.2158	1.62	(0.80–3.31)
	SE positive	50 (7.3)	6 (10.7)	21 (6.7)	0.7915	1.11	(0.65–1.88)	0.2699	1.68	(0.65–4.37)
**13*	SE negative	30 (12.6)	8 (14.8)	102 (21.0)	0.0056	0.54	(0.35–0.84)	0.3732	0.65	(0.30–1.43)
	SE positive	38 (5.6)	7 (12.5)	32 (10.2)	0.0110	0.52	(0.32–0.85)	0.6357	1.26	(0.53–3.02)
**14* other than SE	SE negative	28 (11.8)	15 (27.8)	89 (18.4)	0.0242	0.59	(0.38–0.94)	0.1031	1.71	(0.90–3.24)
	SE positive	51 (7.5)	6 (10.7)	33 (10.5)	0.1406	0.69	(0.44–1.10)	1.0000	1.03	(0.41–2.57)
**15*	SE negative	100 (42.0)	13 (24.1)	207 (42.7)	0.8732	0.97	(0.71–1.33)	0.0085	0.43	(0.22–0.82)
	SE positive	148 (21.7)	9 (16.1)	55 (17.5)	0.1283	1.31	(0.93–1.85)	1.0000	0.91	(0.42–1.96)
**16*	SE negative	6 (2.5)	0 (0.0)	9 (1.9)	0.5838	1.37	(0.48–3.89)	0.6090	0.46	(0.03–8.02)
	SE positive	4 (0.6)	2 (3.6)	6 (1.9)	0.0813	0.30	(0.09–1.09)	0.3460	1.91	(0.38–9.70)
**13:01*	SE negative	0 (0.0)	0 (0.0)	7 (1.4)	0.1024	0.13	(0.01–2.35)	1.0000	0.59	(0.03–10.39)
	SE positive	1 (0.1)	1 (1.8)	1 (0.3)	0.5327	0.46	(0.03–7.41)	0.2794	5.71	(0.35–92.64)
**13:02*	SE negative	30 (12.6)	8 (14.8)	95 (19.6)	0.0212	0.59	(0.38–0.92)	0.4690	0.71	(0.33–1.56)
	SE positive	37 (5.4)	6 (10.7)	31 (9.8)	0.0144	0.53	(0.32–0.87)	0.8102	1.10	(0.44–2.77)
**15:01*	SE negative	41 (17.2)	9 (16.7)	89 (18.4)	0.7578	0.93	(0.62–1.39)	0.8542	0.89	(0.42–1.89)
	SE positive	65 (9.5)	6 (10.7)	18 (5.7)	0.0481	1.74	(1.01–2.99)	0.2315	1.98	(0.75–5.23)
**15:02*	SE negative	62 (26.1)	4 (7.4)	131 (27.0)	0.8580	0.95	(0.67–1.35)	0.0008	0.22	(0.08–0.61)
	SE positive	83 (12.2)	3 (5.4)	37 (11.7)	0.9167	1.04	(0.69–1.58)	0.2395	0.43	(0.13–1.43)
D70	SE negative	127 (53.4)	35 (64.8)	320 (66.0)	0.0011	0.59	(0.43–0.81)	0.8804	0.95	(0.53–1.71)
	SE positive	165 (24.2)	20 (35.7)	114 (36.2)	0.0001	0.56	(0.42–0.75)	1.0000	0.98	(0.54–1.77)
I67	SE negative	168 (70.6)	32 (59.3)	371 (76.5)	0.1018	0.74	(0.52–1.05)	0.0080	0.45	(0.25–0.80)
	SE positive	253 (37.2)	25 (44.6)	130 (41.3)	0.2338	0.84	(0.64–1.11)	0.6610	1.15	(0.65–2.03)

Table 6. Cont.

		ACPA(+) RA	ACPA(−) RA	Control	ACPA(+) RA			ACPA(−) RA		
		(n = 919)	(n = 110)	(n = 800)	*P*	OR	95%CI	*P*	OR	95%CI
S1	SE negative	123 (51.7)	19 (35.2)	288 (59.4)	0.0552	0.73	(0.54–1.00)	0.0008	0.37	(0.21–0.67)
	SE positive	186 (27.3)	16 (28.6)	87 (27.6)	0.9392	0.98	(0.73–1.33)	0.8724	1.05	(0.56–1.97)
D70 other than **13:02*	SE negative	110 (46.2)	29 (53.7)	253 (52.2)	0.1542	0.79	(0.58–1.08)	0.8863	1.06	(0.61–1.87)
	SE positive	128 (18.8)	14 (25.0)	83 (26.3)	0.0076	0.65	(0.47–0.89)	1.0000	0.93	(0.48–1.79)
I67 other than **13:02*	SE negative	156 (65.5)	27 (50.0)	310 (63.9)	0.6802	1.07	(0.78–1.49)	0.0538	0.56	(0.32–0.99)
	SE positive	216 (31.7)	19 (33.9)	99 (31.4)	0.9417	1.01	(0.76–1.35)	0.7560	1.12	(0.61–2.05)
S1 other than **13:02*	SE negative	100 (42.0)	13 (24.1)	213 (43.9)	0.6329	0.93	(0.68–1.27)	0.0055	0.40	(0.21–0.77)
	SE positive	149 (21.9)	10 (17.9)	56 (17.8)	0.1520	1.30	(0.92–1.82)	1.0000	1.01	(0.48–2.11)
I67 other than **15:02*	SE negative	123 (51.7)	30 (55.6)	290 (59.8)	0.0455	0.72	(0.53–0.98)	0.5617	0.84	(0.48–1.48)
	SE positive	170 (25.0)	22 (39.3)	93 (29.5)	0.1420	0.79	(0.59–1.07)	0.1594	1.54	(0.86–2.78)
S1 other than **15:02*	SE negative	67 (28.2)	17 (31.5)	180 (37.1)	0.0194	0.66	(0.47–0.93)	0.4590	0.78	(0.43–1.42)
	SE positive	103 (15.1)	13 (23.2)	50 (15.9)	0.7771	0.94	(0.65–1.36)	0.1799	1.60	(0.80–3.19)

ACPA: anti-citrullinated peptide antibody, ACPA(+): ACPA-positive, ACPA(−): ACPA-negative, RA: rheumatoid arthritis, SE: Shared epitope, OR: odds ratio, CI: confidence interval, Allele carrier frequencies are shown in parenthesis (%). Association was tested by Fisher's exact test using 2×2 contingency tables. SE negative: "*A/A*" or "*A*/other than SE or *A*" vs. "other than SE or *A*/other than SE or *A*". SE positive: "SE/*A*" vs. "SE/other than *A*". Allele groups SE, I67, D70, and S1 were as defined in the Materials and Methods section.

Table 7. *HLA-DRB1* genotype frequency in ACPA(+) and ACPA(−) RA patients and controls.

	ACPA(+) RA (n = 919)	Control (n = 800)	*P*	OR	95%CI
**04:05/*13:02*	28 (5.9)	21 (11.4)	0.0202	0.49	(0.27–0.88)
**09:01/*13:02*	8 (3.2)	21 (9.9)	0.0035	0.30	(0.13–0.69)
**04:01/*13:02*	3 (4.6)	2 (11.8)	0.2755	0.36	(0.06–2.37)
**01:01/*13:02*	4 (2.7)	3 (3.6)	0.7061	0.75	(0.16–3.44)
**14:54/*13:02*	0 (0.0)	6 (13.3)	0.0263	0.07	(0.00–1.28)
	ACPA(−) RA (n = 110)	Control (n = 800)	*P*	OR	95%CI
**04:05/*15:02*	2 (5.3)	23 (12.4)	0.2665	0.39	(0.09–1.74)
**09:01/*15:02*	1 (3.3)	28 (13.1)	0.2228	0.23	(0.03–1.74)
**04:01/*15:02*	1 (25.0)	1 (5.9)	0.3524	5.33	(0.26–110.80)
**01:01/*15:02*	0 (0.0)	5 (6.0)	1.0000	0.68	(0.04–13.19)
**14:54/*15:02*	1 (7.7)	7 (15.6)	0.6686	0.45	(0.05–4.06)

ACPA: anti-citrullinated peptide antibody, ACPA(+): ACPA-positive, ACPA(−): ACPA-negative, RA: rheumatoid arthritis, SE: Shared epitope, OR: odds ratio, CI: confidence interval, Allele carrier frequencies are shown in parenthesis (%). Association was tested by Fisher's exact test using 2×2 contingency tables. Upper row: "*B/*13:02*" vs. "*B/* other than **13:02*". Lower row: "*B/*15:02*" vs. "*B/*other than **15:02*".

It was reported that SE alleles are strongly associated with ACPA(+) RA, but weakly with ACPA(−) RA [1], and this was confirmed in the present study. We documented protective effects of *DRB1*13:02* against ACPA(+) RA and *DRB1*15:02* against ACPA(−) RA in Japanese. Although the sample size of ACPA(−) RA is not large enough, the protective effect of **15:02* against ACPA(−) RA was also reported in another study [31], supporting the results. These findings could be explained by differences in the pathogenesis of ACPA(+) and ACPA(−) RA. Although the genotype of *DRB1*03/*13* was reported to be associated with ACPA(−) RA in a European population [11], such an association was not found in the current study.

Amino acid residues 10Y, 11S, 12T, and 70D of the HLA-DRβ chain were negatively associated with RA (Figure 1A). Amino acid residues 11 and 70 form the HLA-DR peptide-binding groove [32]. These data suggest the involvement of peptide antigens bound to specific HLA molecules in controlling the development of RA. Associations of amino acid residues 10, 11, 12, 13, 33, 37, 47, 67, 70, 96 and 98 of the HLA-DRβ chain were reported in European ACPA(+) RA [33], showing slightly different association pattern from the results of this study (Figure 1B). However, associated amino acid residues 10, 11, 12, 13, 33, 57, 70, 96 and 98 of HLA-DRβ chain in Korean ACPA(+) RA [33] were more similar to the results (Figure 1B), reflecting the difference of DRB1 allele frequencies between European and Asian populations.

The negative association with the *DRB1*13:02* allele needs to be confirmed in future independent studies. Because the distribution of *HLA* alleles in other ethnic populations is different from the Japanese, the protective role of some *DRB1* alleles in RA in other populations should be determined.

Thus, the present study identified a negative association of *DRB1*13:02* with Japanese RA; our findings support the protective role of *DRB1*13:02* alleles in the pathogenesis of ACPA(+) RA.

Supporting Information

Table S1 ***HLA-DRB1*** **homozygous frequency in the RA patients and controls.**

Table S2 ***HLA-DRB1*** **allele frequency in the RA patients and controls.**

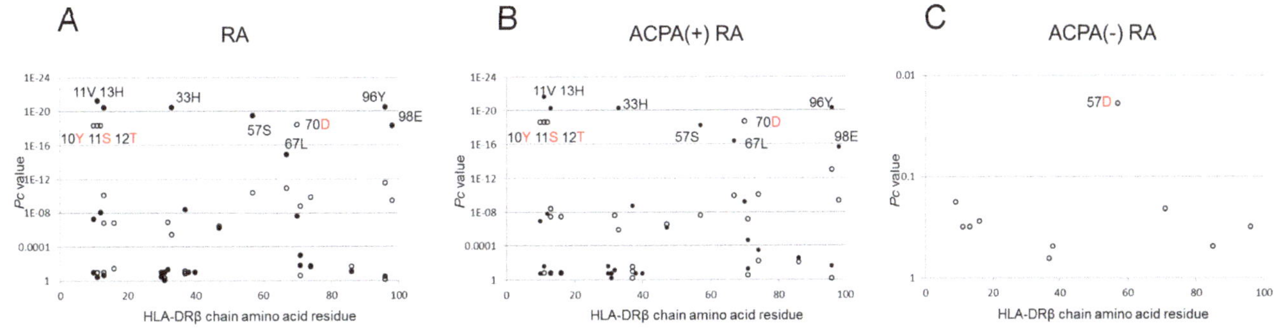

Figure 1. Associations of amino acid residues in the DRβ chain with RA (A), ACPA-positive [ACPA(+)] RA (B), and ACPA-negative [ACPA(−)] RA (C). Corrected *P* (*Pc*) values were calculated by multiplying the *P* value by the number of amino acid residues tested. Associations were established by Fisher's exact test using 2×2 contingency tables. Positive associations are indicated by filled circles and negative associations by open circles.

Table S3 Age at onset of *HLA-DRB1* allele carrier or non-carrier in the RA patients.

Acknowledgments

We thank Ms. Mayumi Yokoyama (Sagamihara Hospital) for secretarial assistance.

Author Contributions

Conceived and designed the experiments: HF NT S. Tohma. Performed the experiments: SO HF A. Kawasaki. Contributed reagents/materials/analysis tools: HF K. Shimada SS AH A. Komiya NF SI TN K. Saisho MK S. Tsunoda HS KM AS SN NT S. Tohma. Contributed to the writing of the manuscript: SO HF NT S. Tohma.

References

1. Perricone C, Ceccarelli F, Valesini G (2011) An overview on the genetic of rheumatoid arthritis: a never-ending story. Autoimmun Rev 10: 599–608.
2. Scott IC, Steer S, Lewis CM, Cope AP (2011) Precipitating and perpetuating factors of rheumatoid arthritis immunopathology: linking the triad of genetic predisposition, environmental risk factors and autoimmunity to disease pathogenesis. Best Pract Res Clin Rheumatol 25: 447–468.
3. Lewis SN, Nsoesie E, Weeks C, Qiao D, Zhang L (2011) Prediction of disease and phenotype associations from genome-wide association studies. PLoS ONE 6: e27175.
4. Reveille JD (1998) The genetic contribution to the pathogenesis of rheumatoid arthritis. Curr Opin Rheumatol 10: 187–200.
5. Holoshitz J (2010) The rheumatoid arthritis HLA-DRB1 shared epitope. Curr Opin Rheumatol 22: 293–298.
6. van der Horst-Bruinsma IE, Visser H, Hazes JM, Breedveld FC, Verduyn W, et al. (1999) HLA-DQ-associated predisposition to and dominant HLA-DR-associated protection against rheumatoid arthritis. Hum Immunol 60: 152–158.
7. de Vries N, Tijssen H, van Riel PL, van de Putte LB (2002) Reshaping the shared epitope hypothesis: HLA-associated risk for rheumatoid arthritis is encoded by amino acid substitutions at positions 67–74 of the HLA-DRB1 molecule. Arthritis Rheum 46: 921–928.
8. Mattey DL, Dawes PT, Gonzalez-Gay MA, Garcia-Porrua C, Thomson W, et al. (2001) HLA-DRB1 alleles encoding an aspartic acid at position 70 protect against development of rheumatoid arthritis. J Rheumatol 28: 232–239.
9. Gourraud PA, Dieude P, Boyer JF, Nogueira L, Cambon-Thomsen A, et al. (2007) A new classification of HLA-DRB1 alleles differentiates predisposing and protective alleles for autoantibody production in rheumatoid arthritis. Arthritis Res Ther 9: R27.
10. Mewar D, Marinou I, Coote AL, Moore DJ, Akil M, et al. (2008) Association between radiographic severity of rheumatoid arthritis and shared epitope alleles: differing mechanisms of susceptibility and protection. Ann Rheum Dis 67: 980–983.
11. Lundstrom E, Kallberg H, Smolnikova M, Ding B, Ronnelid J, et al. (2009) Opposing effects of HLA-DRB1*13 alleles on the risk of developing anti-citrullinated protein antibody-positive and anti-citrullinated protein antibody-negative rheumatoid arthritis. Arthritis Rheum 60: 924–930.
12. van der Woude D, Lie BA, Lundstrom E, Balsa A, Feitsma AL, et al. (2010) Protection against anti-citrullinated protein antibody-positive rheumatoid arthritis is predominantly associated with HLA-DRB1*1301: a meta-analysis of HLA-DRB1 associations with anti-citrullinated protein antibody-positive and anti-citrullinated protein antibody-negative rheumatoid arthritis in four European populations. Arthritis Rheum 62: 1236–1245.
13. Wakitani S, Murata N, Toda Y, Ogawa R, Kaneshige T, et al. (1997) The relationship between HLA-DRB1 alleles and disease subsets of rheumatoid arthritis in Japanese. Br J Rheumatol 36: 630–636.
14. Shibue T, Tsuchiya N, Komata T, Matsushita M, Shiota M, et al. (2000) Tumor necrosis factor alpha 5′-flanking region, tumor necrosis factor receptor II, and HLA-DRB1 polymorphisms in Japanese patients with rheumatoid arthritis. Arthritis Rheum 43: 753–757.
15. Liu SC, Chang TY, Lee YJ, Chu CC, Lin M, et al. (2007) Influence of HLA-DRB1 genes and the shared epitope on genetic susceptibility to rheumatoid arthritis in Taiwanese. J Rheumatol 34: 674–680.
16. Mitsunaga S, Suzuki Y, Kuwana M, Sato S, Kaneko Y, et al. (2012) Associations between six classical HLA loci and rheumatoid arthritis: a comprehensive analysis. Tissue Antigens 80: 16–25.
17. Shimane K, Kochi Y, Suzuki A, Okada Y, Ishii T, et al. (2013) An association analysis of HLA-DRB1 with systemic lupus erythematosus and rheumatoid arthritis in a Japanese population: effects of *09:01 allele on disease phenotypes. Rheumatology (Oxford) 52: 1172–1182.
18. Kamatani N, Kawamoto M, Kitamura Y, Harigai M, Okumoto T, et al. (2004) Establishment of B-cell lines derived from 996 Japanese individuals. Tissue Culture Res Commun 23: 71–80.
19. Arnett FC, Edworthy SM, Bloch DA, McShane DJ, Fries JF, et al. (1988) The American Rheumatism Association 1987 revised criteria for the classification of rheumatoid arthritis. Arthritis Rheum 31: 315–324.
20. du Montcel ST, Michou L, Petit-Teixeira E, Osorio J, Lemaire I, et al. (2005) New classification of HLA-DRB1 alleles supports the shared epitope hypothesis of rheumatoid arthritis susceptibility. Arthritis Rheum 52: 1063–1068.
21. Furukawa H, Oka S, Shimada K, Sugii S, Ohashi J, et al. (2012) Association of human leukocyte antigen with interstitial lung disease in rheumatoid arthritis: A protective role for shared epitope. PLoS ONE 7: e33133.
22. Furukawa H, Oka S, Shimada K, Sugii S, Hashimoto A, et al. (2013) Association of increased frequencies of HLA-DPB1*05:01 with the presence of anti-Ro/SS-A and anti-La/SS-B antibodies in Japanese rheumatoid arthritis and systemic lupus erythematosus patients. PLoS ONE 8: e53910.
23. Furukawa H, Oka S, Shimada K, Rheumatoid Arthritis-Interstitial Lung Disease Study Consortium, Tsuchiya N, et al. (2013) HLA-A*31:01 and methotrexate-induced interstitial lung aisease in Japanese rheumatoid arthritis patients: A multi-drug hypersensitivity marker? Ann Rheum Dis 72: 153–155.
24. Rousset F (2008) genepop'007: a complete re-implementation of the genepop software for Windows and Linux. Mol Ecol Resour 8: 103–106.
25. Payami H, Joe S, Farid NR, Stenszky V, Chan SH, et al. (1989) Relative predispositional effects (RPEs) of marker alleles with disease: HLA-DR alleles and Graves disease. Am J Hum Genet 45: 541–546.
26. Steinbrocker O, Traeger CH, Batterman RC (1949) Therapeutic criteria in rheumatoid arthritis. J Am Med Assoc 140: 659–662.
27. Kawashima M, Ohashi J, Nishida N, Tokunaga K (2012) Evolutionary analysis of classical HLA class I and II genes suggests that recent positive selection acted on DPB1*04:01 in Japanese population. PLoS One 7: e46806.
28. Madeleine MM, Johnson LG, Smith AG, Hansen JA, Nisperos BB, et al. (2008) Comprehensive analysis of HLA-A, HLA-B, HLA-C, HLA-DRB1, and HLA-DQB1 loci and squamous cell cervical cancer risk. Cancer Res 68: 3532–3539.
29. Migita K, Arai T, Ishizuka N, Jiuchi Y, Sasaki Y, et al. (2013) Rates of serious intracellular infections in autoimmune disease patients receiving initial glucocorticoid therapy. PLoS One 8: e78699.
30. Kamatani Y, Wattanapokayakit S, Ochi H, Kawaguchi T, Takahashi A, et al. (2009) A genome-wide association study identifies variants in the HLA-DP locus associated with chronic hepatitis B in Asians. Nat Genet 41: 591–595.
31. Terao C, Ohmura K, Ikari K, Kochi Y, Maruya E, et al. (2012) ACPA-negative RA consists of two genetically distinct subsets based on RF positivity in Japanese. PLoS One 7: e40067.
32. Jardetzky TS, Brown JH, Gorga JC, Stern LJ, Urban RG, et al. (1994) Three-dimensional structure of a human class II histocompatibility molecule complexed with superantigen. Nature 368: 711–718.
33. Raychaudhuri S, Sandor C, Stahl EA, Freudenberg J, Lee HS, et al. (2012) Five amino acids in three HLA proteins explain most of the association between MHC and seropositive rheumatoid arthritis. Nat Genet 44: 291–296.

7

Risk of Lymphoma and Solid Cancer among Patients with Rheumatoid Arthritis in a Primary Care Setting

Christen Lykkegaard Andersen[1,2]*, Hanne Lindegaard[3], Hanne Vestergaard[4], Volkert Dirk Siersma[2], Hans Carl Hasselbalch[1], Niels de Fine Olivarius[2], Ole Weis Bjerrum[5], Peter Junker[3]

1 Department of Hematology, Roskilde University Hospital, Roskilde, Denmark, **2** The Research Unit for General Practice and Section of General Practice, Department of Public Health, University of Copenhagen, Copenhagen, Denmark, **3** Department of Rheumatology, Odense University Hospital, Odense, Denmark, **4** Department of Hematology, Odense University Hospital, Odense, Denmark, **5** Department of Hematology, Copenhagen University Hospital, Copenhagen, Denmark

Abstract

Background: Several studies have demonstrated an association between rheumatoid arthritis (RA) and lymphoproliferative malignancies, but pathogenic mechanisms remain unclear. We investigated 1) the risk of lymphoproliferative malignancies and solid tumors in adults with RA identified in primary care and 2) the possible mediating role of blood eosinophilia in the clonal evolution of cancer in these patients.

Methods: From the Copenhagen Primary Care Differential Count (*CopDiff*) Database, we identified 356,196 individuals with at least one differential cell count (DIFF) encompassing the eosinophil count between 2000–2007. From these, one DIFF was randomly chosen (the index DIFF). By linking to the Danish National Patient Register, we categorized the selected individuals according to known longstanding (≥3 years) or recent onset (<3 years) RA prior to the index DIFF. In addition, the cohort was stratified according to management in primary or secondary care. From the Danish Cancer Registry we ascertained malignancies within four years following the index DIFF. Using multivariable logistic regression, odds ratios (OR) were calculated and adjusted for sex, age, year, month, eosinophilia, comorbid conditions and C-reactive protein (CRP).

Results: 921 patients had recent onset RA and 2,578 had longer disease duration. Seventy three percent of RA patients were managed in primary care. After adjustment for sex, age, year, and month, neither recent onset nor long-standing RA was associated with incident lymphoproliferative malignancies or solid cancers. These risk estimates did not change when eosinophilia, CRP, and comorbidities were included in the models.

Conclusions: In this large cohort of patients with RA of short or long duration recruited from a primary care resource, RA was not associated with an increased risk of lymphoproliferative or solid cancers during 4 years of follow-up, when the models were adjusted for confounders. Blood eosinophilia could not be identified as a mediator of cancer development in the present setting.

Editor: Ken Mills, Queen's University Belfast, United Kingdom

Funding: Christen Lykkegaard Andersen wishes to thank The Danish Cancer Society, which has granted a three-year scholarship (2010-2013). The authors would also like to express their gratitude to Eva & Henry Frænkels' memorial foundation and Axel Muusfeldts memorial foundation for financial support. The funders had no role in study design, data collection and analysis, decision to publish, or preparation of the manuscript.

Competing Interests: The authors have declared that no competing interests exist.

* E-mail: christenla@gmail.com

Introduction

The association between rheumatoid arthritis (RA) and cancer has been investigated in several mainly hospital-based studies. These have indicated that the overall cancer occurrence in patients with RA is only marginally higher than in healthy individuals, while elevated risk figures have been reported for several specific cancers including leukemia [1], non-melanoma skin cancers [2], and lung cancer [3,4]. In particular, an excess risk ranging from 50% to 200% of lymphoproliferative malignancies, especially diffuse large B-cell lymphoma, has been consistently reported in previous studies on RA and cancer [5–7]. The relative risks of cancer have been reported to be highest within the first year of follow-up although increased risk figures have been observed after up to 20 years of follow-up [8,9].

Two major pathways have been suggested to account for the association between RA and malignancy: extrinsic pro-oncogenic effects of disease-modifying antirheumatic drugs (DMARDs) [10,11]; and intrinsic pro-oncogenic effects related to disease activity [6–8,12–14]. Recent studies indicate that RA patients with active disease are at increased risk of malignant lymphomas, compared with RA patients with low disease activity or remission [6–8,12–14]. Thus, the pathways by which active RA impose an increased risk of lymphoma are poorly understood. In this context, the eosinophilic granulocyte is a pertinent candidate. Eosinophilia ($\geq 0.5 \times 10^9$ eosinophils/l peripheral blood) may be induced by infections and inflammation, including inflammatory processes accompanying solid and hematological malignancies [15–17]. Activation of eosinophils may lead to organ damage, irrespective of the cause of the eosinophilia [16,18,19]. It has been reported that eosinophilia is a rather common finding among patients in rheumatologic outpatient clinics, with an estimated prevalence of 7.7% [20]. Besides, eosinophilia has been linked to prognosis and severity of extra-articular manifestations in RA [21]. Taken together, these observations support the view that eosinophilia may be associated with cancer risk in RA.

The aim of the present study is twofold: 1) to investigate the risk of lymphoproliferative malignancies and solid tumors in adult RA identified in a primary care setting, and 2) to investigate the possible mediating role of blood eosinophilia in the clonal evolution of cancer in these patients.

Methods

Ethics Statement

The study was approved by The Danish Data Protection Agency (journal no: 2013-54-0507), and did not need approval by an institutional review board or ethical review board according to Danish legislation. Patient information was anonymized and de-identified prior to analysis and no clinical records were used. Patient consent is not mandatory for this type of study in Denmark.

Patients

The Copenhagen General Practitioners' Laboratory (CGPL) (renamed the Elective Laboratory of the Capital Region from 01.01.2013) provides laboratory services to all general practitioners (GPs) in the Copenhagen area, covering approximately 1.2 million inhabitants. CGPL has International Organization for Standardization (ISO) accreditation and has stored all laboratory data since 01.05.2000. The Copenhagen Primary Care Differential Count (*CopDiff*) Database contains results from all differential cell counts (DIFF) requested by GPs in Copenhagen from 01.05.2000 to 25.01.2010. From each of the 359,950 unique, adult individuals (aged 18 to 80 years) with at least one DIFF in the period 01.01.2001 to 31.12.2007, one DIFF (i.e. the index DIFF) encompassing the eosinophil count was chosen by computer-generated random numbers (n = 356,196), see (Figure 1). The selected individuals were categorized according to prevalent blood eosinophilia (Figure 2). Where available, the level of C-reactive-protein (CRP), categorized as "increased" (≥10 mg/L) vs. "normal" (<10 mg/L), was also obtained (n = 229,511). Furthermore, we recorded whether another DIFF had been done within 6 months before the request (n = 32,475) and whether eosinophilia was also present in this DIFF. We found that our strategy of randomly choosing one DIFF per individual to assess incidences of the specified outcomes was feasible for two reasons. First, it meant that we did not to have to control for individuals that entered the cohort multiple times at different points in time. Second, we sought to minimize surveillance bias which seemed more likely to occur if, for example, we had opted for "the first DIFF" or "the DIFF closest to the outcome of interest" [22]. The period we chose for index DIFF selection was from 01.01.2001, rather than from the beginning of the *CopDiff* database (01.05.2000), because we wanted to assess whether a possible eosinophilia was longstanding (within 6 months before the index DIFF). Also, since all individuals were to have a fixed 4-year follow up after the index DIFF, we excluded DIFFs after 31.12.2007 (Figure 2).

In November 2013, the *CopDiff* database was linked to The Danish Cancer Registry (DCR), which contains data on all malignancies in Denmark since 1942 and to which reporting is mandatory [23]; and to The Danish National Patient Register (NPR), which contains information on all contacts with hospitals in Denmark with discharge diagnoses and surgical procedures [24]. The NPR also includes outpatient clinic contacts. To adjust for possible confounding by comorbid conditions, we computed Charlson's Comorbidity Index (CCI) [25] from hospital contacts recorded in the NPR for three years before the index DIFF. Information on occurrence of RA prior to the index DIFF was assessed from hospital contacts in the NPR and based on International Classification of Disease, ICD-8 codes: 712.39 (used from 1977–1993) and ICD-10 codes: M05, M06 (used from 1994-present). RA was categorized as recent (<3 years) or longstanding (≥3 years) according to date of first occurrence (since 1977) prior to the index DIFF. Previously, Pedersen *et al* reported that RA diagnoses in the NPR based on recordings from hospitals can be utilized for epidemiological purposes if inherent data limitations are considered [26]. Patients were defined as having "primary care managed RA" if they had been referred back to primary care at their most recent contact with a rheumatology department prior to the index DIFF.

Outcomes were defined as the incidences of the following diagnoses recorded in DCR over the four-year period following the index DIFF: 1) lymphoproliferative malignancies defined as ICD-10 codes: C81, C82–C85, and C91; and ICD for Oncology (ICD-O) morphological codes within the range: 9590/3/-9729/3/ . Diffuse large B-cell lymphoma defined as ICD-10 code C83.3 and ICD-O morphological codes 96793, 96803, and 96843. Solid cancer defined as: buccal cavity and pharynx (C00-C14; C462), digestive organs (C15–C26), respiratory system including thoracic organs (C30–39; C450), bones, joints and articular cartilage (C40–C41), skin (C43–C44; C460), mesothelium and connective tissue (C451–C459; C461; C463; C467; C468; C469; C47–C49; B210), breast (C50), female genital organs (C51–C58), male genital organs (C60–C63), urinary tract (C64–C68; D090–D091; D301–D309; D411–D419), eye and central nervous system (C69–C72; C751–C753; D32–D33; D352–D354; D42–D43; D443–D445), and endocrine glands (C73–C74; C750; C754–C759).

Statistical analysis

In order to pursue our first aim of investigating the risk of lymphoproliferative malignancies and solid tumors in adults with identified RA, we used multivariable logistic regression to compute odds ratios (ORs) with 95% confidence intervals (CIs) for the four-year incidence of lymphoproliferative malignancies and solid cancers following the index DIFF. The ORs were reported without any adjustment, and again after adjusting for potential confounders (sex, age [quadratic], year, and month of DIFF sampling). Regarding our second aim, to investigate the possible mediating role of blood eosinophilia in the clonal evolution of cancer in RA patients, we used the same model with potential confounders, but adjusted for candidate mediators of disease (eosinophilia, competing comorbid conditions, and inflammation) in a stepwise fashion in order to analyze the impact of the mediators sequentially. An overview of the variables included in the analyses is seen in Figure 3. Individuals who had already been diagnosed with a cancer (recorded in the DCR since 1977) were excluded from risk analyses. To account for multiple statistical testing, P-values less than 0.0033 were regarded as significant, as this controls the false discovery rate at 5% using the Benjamini-Hochberg method [27]. All analyses and calculations were performed with SAS version 9.2 (SAS Institute Inc., Cary, NC, USA).

Results

The mean age (SD) of the entire study population was 48.3 years (16.7) with a female:male ratio of 1.38 (208,691/151,259);

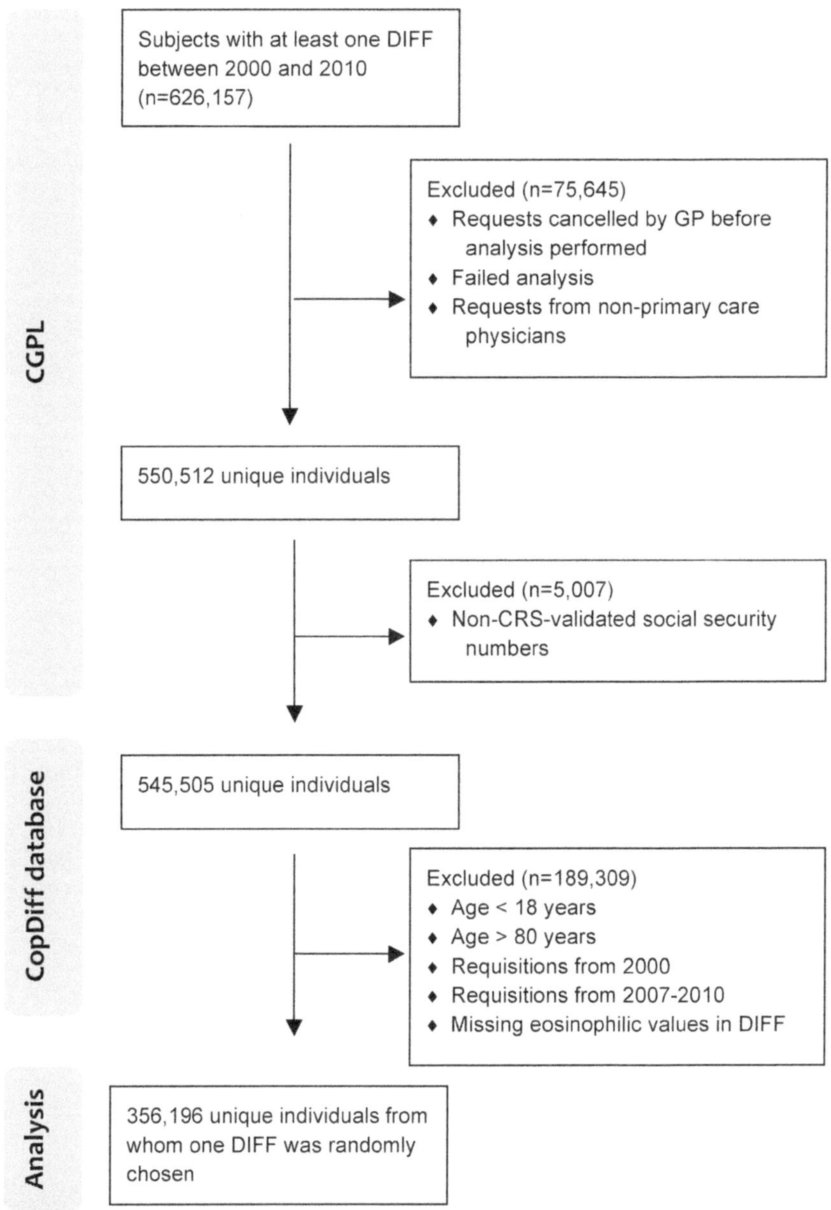

Figure 1. Flowchart for the study population. CGPL, Copenhagen General Practitioners' Laboratory; CopDiff, Copenhagen Primary Care Differential Count Database; CRS, The Danish Civil Registration System; DIFF, differential cell count; GP, general practitioner.

see (Table 1). Since 1977 and before the index DIFF, 1,167 patients (0.3%) had been diagnosed with a lymphoproliferative cancer and 22,541 (6.3%) had experienced a solid cancer. A total of 14.406 patients (4.0%) had eosinophilia.

Of 359,950 individuals, 3,499 (1.0%) had been diagnosed with RA according to the NPR. Of these, 921 were diagnosed during the three years prior to the index DIFF (recent onset), and 2,578 were diagnosed earlier than this (long-standing RA); see (Table 1). The mean age of patients with recent onset and longstanding RA was 56.9 and 60.2 years respectively, with a female:male ratio of 3.15 and 2.95. Seventy-three percent of RA patients were managed in primary care at the time of the index DIFF blood sampling. In the subsequent four-year period, fourteen RA patients developed lymphoproliferative cancer and a solid cancer was diagnosed in 241 RA patients (Table 1). The overall incidences of lymphoproliferative cancer and solid cancers over the four-year period following the index count were 61 and 1,078 per 100,000 person-years, respectively. Additional baseline subject characteristics are presented in Table 1.

In unadjusted analyses, patients with longstanding RA had an increased risk for lymphoproliferative cancer (OR [95% CI] = 1.92 [1.08–3.39]) and solid cancer (1.92 [1.65–2.22]), while the corresponding risk estimates were close to unity among patients with recent onset RA (Table 2). When adjusting for demographic characteristics, neutral ORs for lymphoproliferative or solid cancer were also found for patients with longstanding RA (1.31 [0.74–2.33] and 1.10 [0.94–1.28], respectively). Adjustment for eosinophilia, CRP and comorbidities did not alter any of the risk estimates. When performing subgroup analysis for diffuse large B-cell lymphoma, and including confounders and mediators

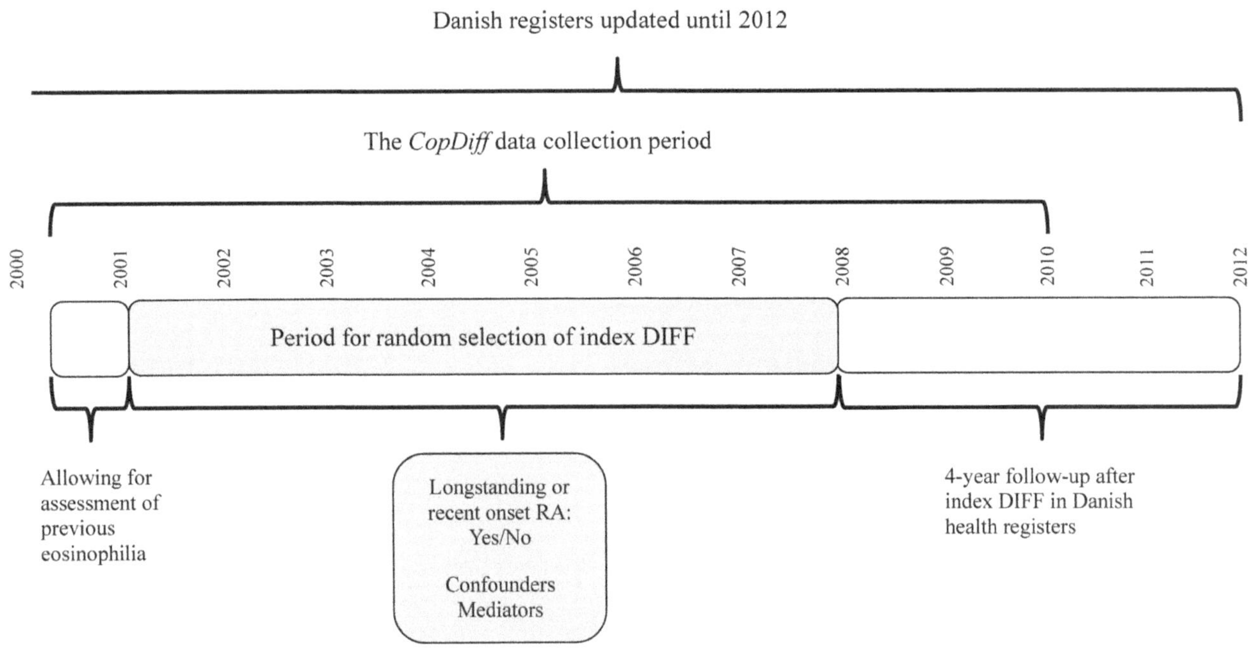

Figure 2. Timeline for index DIFF selection.

in the models, we did not observe any association with RA (ORs of 1.41 [0.44–4.45] and 1.88 [0.25–13.96] for longstanding and recent onset RA, respectively). These estimates did not change when excluding confounders and mediators: ORs were 2.17 (0.69-6.81) and 2.03 (0.28–14.49) for longstanding and recent onset RA, respectively.

Discussion

In this study based on patients in the *CopDiff* database, RA of recent or longstanding duration was not associated with an increased risk of lymphoproliferative malignancies or solid cancer within a 4-year time frame. Adjusting for the anticipated mediators, e.g. eosinophilia, inflammation, and comorbidities yielded similar results. While absence of an association with most solid cancers accords with previous results, the majority of earlier studies reported an excess risk of lymphoproliferative malignancies among RA patients [7–9,12,28–30]. However, the patients included in these studies were recruited on the basis of hospital contacts [4,8,30] or from RA registers [9,12,28,29]. Data from RA registers in particular offer detailed patient data of high quality concerning RA, its course, complications, and comorbidities. Thus, studies based on either of these resources are in danger of reporting associations between RA and malignancies due to further examinations derived from increased awareness of the condition [22]. The *CopDiff* population was sampled continuously without any restrictions as to why the DIFF was requested by the GP which, together with the use of computer-generated random selection of index DIFFs, diminishes surveillance bias. Furthermore, the majority of RA patients in this study were managed in primary care. In Denmark, biological and complex non-biological therapies are offered exclusively in secondary care. Therefore, the majority of patients in the present cohort can be assumed to have mild disease.

The study has limitations. First, the *CopDiff* database is derived from a population which may present with elevated white blood

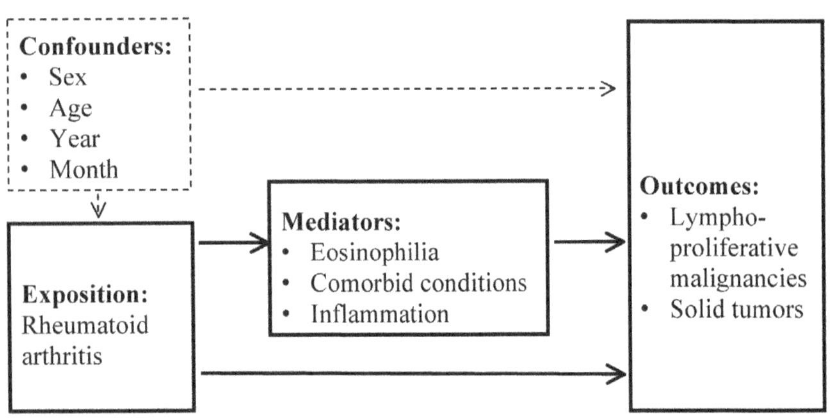

Figure 3. Flowchart illustrating the background for analytical approaches.

Table 1. Baseline subject characteristics.

	Rheumatoid arthritis			
	No, *n = 356,451*	**Longstanding (≥3 years),** *n = 2,578*	**Recent onset (<3 years),** *n = 921*	**Total,** *n = 359,950*
Gender				
Male	150,385 (42,2)	652 (25.3)	222 (24.1)	151,259 (42.0)
Female	206,066 (57.8)	1,926 (74.7)	699 (75.9)	208,691 (58.0)
Age, years	48.2±16.7	60.2±14.0	56.9±14.5	48.3±16.7
Eosinophilia				
No (<0.5•10⁹/L)	338,502 (96.0)	2,414 (94.8)	874 (95.3)	341,790 (96.0)
Yes (≥0.5•10⁹/L)	14,231 (4.0)	132 (5.2)	43 (4.7)	14,406 (4.0)
Previous lymphoproliferative cancer [1]				
No	355,301 (99.7)	2,565 (99.5)	917 (99.6)	358,783 (99.7)
Yes	1,150 (0.3)	13 (0.5)	4 (0.4)	1,167 (0.3)
Previous solid tumor				
No	334,285 (93.8)	2,295 (89.0)	829 (90.0)	337,409 (93.7)
Yes	22,166 (6.2)	283 (10.9)	92 (10.0)	22,541 (6.3)
Charlson's Comorbidity Index [2]	0.21±0.76	0.82±1.22	1.56±1.23	0.22±0.77
C-reactive protein				
No blood test	128,624 (36.2)	836 (32.5)	295 (32.1)	129,755 (36.1)
Normal	179,739 (50.5)	1,019 (39.6)	404 (44.0)	181,162 (50.4)
Increased [3]	47,413 (13.3)	717 (27.8)	219 (23.9)	48,349 (13.5)
Previous eosinophilia (<6 months)				
No blood test	324,665 (91.1)	2,112 (81.8)	698 (75.8)	327,475 (91.0)
Only negative tests	29,465 (8.3)	432 (16.7)	207 (22.5)	30,104 (8.3)
At least one positive test [4]	2,316 (0.6)	39 (1.5)	16 (1.7)	2,371 (0.7)
Incident lymphoproliferative cancer (≤4 years) [1]				
No	354,432 (99.8)	2,553 (99.5)	915 (99.8)	357,900 (99.8)
Yes	869 (0.2)	12 (0.5)	2 (0.2)	883 (0.2)
Incident solid tumor (≤4 years)				
No	319,003 (95.4)	2,102 (91.6)	781 (94.2)	321,886 (95.4)
Yes	15,282 (4.6)	193 (8.4)	48 (5.8)	15,523 (4.6)

Values are number (column-%) or means (SD). [1] Lymphoproliferative cancer defined as Hodgkin's lymphoma, non-Hodgkin lymphoma and chronic lymphocytic leukemia, [2] Calculated on previous hospital contacts (<3 years), [3]>10 mg/L, [4]>0.5·10⁹/L.

cell counts and more background morbidity than the general population. The use of logistic regression analysis on the 4-year incidence, however, ensures that the measures of excess risk (OR) can be interpreted independently of the frequency of the cancers in the study, and the OR can therefore be considered to be a valid estimate of excess risk in the general population as well [31]. Second, the follow-up period of only 4 years was chosen in order to optimize the ability to link RA with incident cancer. Thus, we cannot exclude the view that some RA-related malignancies appeared beyond this time frame due to the latency period for cancer development. Third, information about drug treatment was not available. To our knowledge, only one study has found an association between the use of a specific group of antirheumatic drugs, the TNF-inhibitors, and cancer [10], while all other studies have failed to confirm these results [32,33]. Finally, we did not have access to information on body mass index, smoking, alcohol consumption, exercise patterns, or family history of disease. Smoking is a well-recognized risk factor for the development of RA and lung cancer, and the prevalence of smoking among people with RA is relatively high [3]. However, these risk factors have not been clearly linked to lymphoproliferative malignancies [34,35].

Particular strengths of this study include the fact that all malignant diagnoses were derived from the DCR which was established in 1942 and to which reporting is mandatory. The validity of the DCR is optimized through regular quality control routines applied in daily data production with manual coding and data validation. An incidence of solid cancers of 1.078 per 100.000 person-years also compares with the national incidence of 1.205 per 100.000 person-years [36]. This suggests that the *CopDiff* database participants do not differ significantly from the general population with respect to cancer incidence. In addition, we observed age and gender distributions among RA patients which compare well with figures reported from Nordic countries, thereby adding to the validity of the study [37,38].

In conclusion, based on this large population of individuals identified in a primary care setting, neither early nor longstanding RA was associated with an increased risk of lymphoproliferative or solid cancers within a 4-year time frame. Patients with RA

Table 2. The association between longstanding or recent onset rheumatoid arthritis and 4-year incidence of cancer.

Rheumatoid arthritis	Adjustment	4-year incidence of lymphoproliferative cancer *		4-year incidence of solid cancer	
No	None	1.00	0.13†	1.00	<0.0001†
Longstanding (≥3 years)		1.92 (1.08–3.39)	0.026	1.92 (1.65–2.22)	<0.0001
Recent onset (<3 years)		0.89 (0.22–3.58)	0.87	1.28 (0.96–1.72)	0.094
No	[1]	1.00	0.59†	1.00	0.33†
Longstanding (≥3 years)		1.31 (0.74–2.33)	0.35	1.10 (0.94–1.28)	0.23
Recent onset (<3 years)		0.72 (0.18–2.88)	0.64	0.88 (0.65–1.18)	0.38
No	[1], [2]	1.00	0.64†	1.00	0.26†
Longstanding (≥3 years)		1.29 (0.71–2.34)	0.41	1.10 (0.95–1.28)	0.21
Recent onset (<3 years)		0.72 (0.18–2.88)	0.64	0.86 (0.63–1.15)	0.31
No	[1], [2], [3]	1.00	0.51†	1.00	0.27†
Longstanding (≥3 years)		1.46 (0.80–2.66)	0.22	1.11 (0.96–1.30)	0.17
Recent onset (<3 years)		1.01 (0.25–4.09)	0.99	0.88 (0.65–1.19)	0.40
No	[1], [2], [3], [4]	1.00	0.66†	1.00	0.42†
Longstanding (≥3 years)		1.34 (0.73–2.44)	0.35	1.06 (0.91–1.23)	0.46
Recent onset (<3 years)		0.95 (0.23–3.88)	0.95	0.85 (0.63–1.15)	0.29

Values are odds ratios and *p*-values from multivariable logistic regression analyses for the development of lymphoproliferative cancer and solid tumors for the risk groups: No previous rheumatoid arthritis, Longstanding rheumatoid arthritis, and Recent onset rheumatoid arthritis. Odds ratios are adjusted in a stepwise manner: [1] sex, age (quadratic), year and month; [2] previous and present eosinophilia; [3] Charlson's Comorbidity Index, and [4] C-reactive protein. †*P*-value for the likelihood-ratio test of all categories of eosinophilia simultaneously. * Hodgkin's lymphoma, non-Hodgkin lymphoma and chronic lymphocytic leukemia.

managed in the Danish primary health care system, generally have mild disease which might explain the absence of an association with lymphoproliferative malignancies reported previously among RA patients in secondary care. Blood eosinophilia could not be identified as a mediator of cancer development in the present setting.

Acknowledgments

The authors would also like to express their gratitude to Willy Karlslund, The Research Unit for General Practice in Copenhagen, Denmark for skillful technical assistance.

Author Contributions

Conceived and designed the experiments: CLA NdFO OWB PJ. Performed the experiments: CLA VDS. Analyzed the data: CLA HL HV VDS HCH NdFO OWB PJ. Wrote the paper: CLA HL HV VDS HCH NdFO OWB PJ. Authors who gave final approval of the version to be published: CLA HL HV VDS HCH NdFO OWB PJ.

References

1. Hemminki K, Liu X, Forsti A, Ji J, Sundquist J, et al. (2013) Subsequent leukaemia in autoimmune disease patients. Br J Haematol 161: 677–687.
2. Chakravarty EF, Michaud K, Wolfe F (2005) Skin cancer, rheumatoid arthritis, and tumor necrosis factor inhibitors. J Rheumatol 32: 2130–2135.
3. Khurana R, Wolf R, Berney S, Caldito G, Hayat S, et al. (2008) Risk of development of lung cancer is increased in patients with rheumatoid arthritis: a large case control study in US veterans. J Rheumatol 35: 1704–1708.
4. Mercer LK, Davies R, Galloway JB, Low A, Lunt M, et al. (2013) Risk of cancer in patients receiving non-biologic disease-modifying therapy for rheumatoid arthritis compared with the UK general population. Rheumatology (Oxford) 52: 91–98.
5. Askling J (2007) Malignancy and rheumatoid arthritis. Curr Rheumatol Rep 9: 421–426.
6. Baecklund E, Iliadou A, Askling J, Ekbom A, Backlin C, et al. (2006) Association of chronic inflammation, not its treatment, with increased lymphoma risk in rheumatoid arthritis. Arthritis Rheum 54: 692–701.
7. Baecklund E, Smedby KE, Sutton LA, Askling J, Rosenquist R (2014) Lymphoma development in patients with autoimmune and inflammatory disorders—what are the driving forces? Sem Cancer Biol 24: 61–70.
8. Ekstrom K, Hjalgrim H, Brandt L, Baecklund E, Klareskog L, et al. (2003) Risk of malignant lymphomas in patients with rheumatoid arthritis and in their first-degree relatives. Arthritis Rheum 48: 963–970.
9. Chen YJ, Chang YT, Wang CB, Wu CY (2011) The risk of cancer in patients with rheumatoid arthritis: a nationwide cohort study in Taiwan. Arthritis Rheum 63: 352–358.
10. Bongartz T, Sutton AJ, Sweeting MJ, Buchan I, Matteson EL, et al. (2006) Anti-TNF antibody therapy in rheumatoid arthritis and the risk of serious infections and malignancies: systematic review and meta-analysis of rare harmful effects in randomized controlled trials. JAMA 295: 2275–2285.
11. Cush JJ, Dao KH (2012) Malignancy risks with biologic therapies. Rheum Dis Clin North Am 38: 761–770.
12. Franklin J, Lunt M, Bunn D, Symmons D, Silman A (2006) Incidence of lymphoma in a large primary care derived cohort of cases of inflammatory polyarthritis. Ann Rheum Dis 65: 617–622.
13. Smedby KE, Baecklund E, Askling J (2006) Malignant lymphomas in autoimmunity and inflammation: a review of risks, risk factors, and lymphoma characteristics. Cancer Epidemiol Biomarkers Prevention 15: 2069–2077.
14. Wolfe F, Michaud K (2007) The effect of methotrexate and anti-tumor necrosis factor therapy on the risk of lymphoma in rheumatoid arthritis in 19,562 patients during 89,710 person-years of observation. Arthritis Rheum 56: 1433–1439.
15. Andersen CL, Siersma VD, Hasselbalch HC, Lindegaard H, Vestergaard H, et al. (2013) Eosinophilia in routine blood samples and the subsequent risk of hematological malignancies and death. American journal of hematology 88: 843–847
16. Gotlib J (2014) World Health Organization-defined eosinophilic disorders: 2014 update on diagnosis, risk stratification, and management. Am J Hematol 89: 325–337.
17. Tefferi A, Patnaik MM, Pardanani A (2006) Eosinophilia: secondary, clonal and idiopathic. Br J Haematol 133: 468–492.
18. Cools J (2005) The hypereosinophilic syndrome: idiopathic or not, that is the question. Haematologica 90: 582–584.
19. Jacobsen EA, Helmers RA, Lee JJ, Lee NA (2012) The expanding role(s) of eosinophils in health and disease. Blood 120: 3882–3890.

20. Kargili A, Bavbek N, Kaya A, Kosar A, Karaaslan Y (2004) Eosinophilia in rheumatologic diseases: a prospective study of 1000 cases. Rheumatol Int 24: 321–324.
21. Panush RS, Franco AE, Schur PH (1971) Rheumatoid arthritis associated with eosinophilia. Ann Intern Med 75: 199–205.
22. Haut ER, Pronovost PJ (2011) Surveillance bias in outcomes reporting. JAMA: 305: 2462–2463.
23. Gjerstorff ML (2011) The Danish Cancer Registry. Scand J Public Health 39: 42–45.
24. Lynge E, Sandegaard JL, Rebolj M (2011) The Danish National Patient Register. Scand J Public Health 39: 30–33.
25. Charlson ME, Pompei P, Ales KL, MacKenzie CR (1987) A new method of classifying prognostic comorbidity in longitudinal studies: development and validation. J Chron Dis 40: 373–383.
26. Pedersen M, Klarlund M, Jacobsen S, Svendsen AJ, Frisch M (2004) Validity of rheumatoid arthritis diagnoses in the Danish National Patient Registry. Eur J Epidemiol 19: 1097–1103.
27. Benjamini Y, Hochberg Y (1995) Controlling the False Discovery Rate: a Practical and Powerful Approach to Multiple Testing. J Roy Stat Soc B 57: 289–300.
28. Abasolo L, Judez E, Descalzo MA, Gonzalez-Alvaro I, Jover JA, et al. (2008) Cancer in rheumatoid arthritis: occurrence, mortality, and associated factors in a South European population. Semin Arthritis Rheum 37: 388–397.
29. Geborek P, Bladstrom A, Turesson C, Gulfe A, Petersson IF, et al. (2005) Tumour necrosis factor blockers do not increase overall tumour risk in patients with rheumatoid arthritis, but may be associated with an increased risk of lymphomas. Ann Rheum Dis 64: 699–703.
30. Mellemkjaer L, Linet MS, Gridley G, Frisch M, Moller H, et al. (1996) Rheumatoid arthritis and cancer risk. Eur J Cancer 32A: 1753–1757.
31. Woodward M (2005) Epidemiology: Study Design And Data Analysis. Chapman & Hall/CRC: 278–280.
32. Lopez-Olivo MA, Tayar JH, Martinez-Lopez JA, Pollono EN, Cueto JP, et al. (2012) Risk of malignancies in patients with rheumatoid arthritis treated with biologic therapy: a meta-analysis. JAMA 308: 898–908.
33. Ramiro S, Gaujoux-Viala C, Nam JL, Smolen JS, Buch M, et al. (2014) Safety of synthetic and biological DMARDs: a systematic literature review informing the 2013 update of the EULAR recommendations for management of rheumatoid arthritis. Ann Rheum Dis 73: 529–535.
34. Lichtman MA (2010) Obesity and the risk for a hematological malignancy: leukemia, lymphoma, or myeloma. Oncologist 15: 1083–1101.
35. Morton LM, Hartge P, Holford TR, Holly EA, Chiu BC, et al. (2005) Cigarette smoking and risk of non-Hodgkin lymphoma: a pooled analysis from the International Lymphoma Epidemiology Consortium (interlymph). Cancer Epidemiol Biomarkers Prev 14: 925–933.
36. The Danish Cancer Registry 2010. http://www.sst.dk/publ/Publ2011/DAF/Cancer/Cancerregisteret2010.pdf
37. Simonsson M, Bergman S, Jacobsson LT, Petersson IF, Svensson B (1999) The prevalence of rheumatoid arthritis in Sweden. Scand J Rheumatol 28: 340–343.
38. The nationwide Danish DANBIO registry. https://danbio-online.dk/Danbio-yearly-report-2007-eng.pdf/view

8

Platelet Activation and Anti-Phospholipid Antibodies Collaborate in the Activation of the Complement System on Platelets in Systemic Lupus Erythematosus

Christian Lood[1]*, Helena Tydén[1], Birgitta Gullstrand[2], Gunnar Sturfelt[1], Andreas Jönsen[1], Lennart Truedsson[2], Anders A. Bengtsson[1]

1 Department of Clinical Sciences Lund, Section of Rheumatology, Lund University and Skåne University Hospital, Lund, Sweden, **2** Department of Laboratory Medicine Lund, Section of Microbiology, Immunology and Glycobiology, Lund University, Lund, Sweden

Abstract

Anti-phospholipid (aPL) antibodies are important contributors to development of thrombosis in patients with the autoimmune rheumatic disease systemic lupus erythematosus (SLE). The underlying mechanism of aPL antibody-mediated thrombosis is not fully understood but existing data suggest that platelets and the complement system are key components. Complement activation on platelets is seen in SLE patients, especially in patients with aPL antibodies, and has been related to venous thrombosis and stroke. The aim of this study was to investigate if aPL antibodies could support classical pathway activation on platelets *in vitro* as well as in SLE patients. Furthermore, we investigated if complement deposition on platelets was associated with vascular events, either arterial or venous, when the data had been adjusted for traditional cardiovascular risk factors. Finally, we analyzed if platelet complement deposition, both C1q and C4d, was specific for SLE. We found that aPL antibodies supported C4d deposition on platelets *in vitro* as well as in SLE patients ($p = 0.001$ and $p < 0.05$, respectively). Complement deposition on platelets was increased in SLE patients when compared with healthy individuals ($p < 0.0001$). However, high levels of C4d deposition and a pronounced C1q deposition were also seen in patients with rheumatoid arthritis and systemic sclerosis. In SLE, C4d deposition on platelets was associated with platelet activation, complement consumption, disease activity and venous ($OR = 5.3$, $p = 0.02$), but not arterial, thrombosis, observations which were independent of traditional cardiovascular risk factors. In conclusion, several mechanisms operate in SLE to amplify platelet complement deposition, of which aPL antibodies and platelet activation were identified as important contributors in this investigation. Complement deposition on platelets was identified as a marker of venous, but not arterial thrombosis, in SLE patients independently of traditional risk factors and aPL antibodies. Further studies are needed to elucidate the role of complement deposition on platelets in development of venous thrombosis.

Editor: Gualtiero I. Colombo, Centro Cardiologico Monzino IRCCS, Italy

Funding: This work was supported by grants from the Medical Faculty at Lund University; The Crafoord Foundation; Swedish Combine Projects; Greta and Johan Kock's Foundation; King Gustaf V's 80th Birthday Foundation; Lund University Hospital; the Swedish Rheumatism Association; Swedish Society of Medicine; and the Foundation of the National Board of Health and Welfare and Österlund's Foundation. The funders had no role in study design, data collection and analysis, decision to publish, or preparation of the manuscript.

Competing Interests: The authors have declared that no competing interests exist.

* E-mail: Christian.Lood@med.lu.se

Introduction

Systemic lupus erythematosus (SLE) is an autoimmune rheumatic disease characterized by systemic inflammation affecting several organ systems including joints, kidney, skin and central nervous system [1]. SLE patients have a highly increased cardiovascular morbidity and mortality which can only be partly explained by traditional risk factors [2,3,4,5]. Anti-phospholipid (aPL) antibodies are a group of phospholipid-binding autoantibodies with overlapping, but partly different specificities. There are three main aPL tests used in clinical practice; anti-cardiolipin (aCL) antibodies, anti-beta 2 glycoprotein I (aB2GPI) antibodies and lupus anticoagulans (LA). Positivity in one or more of those assays is associated with development of venous thrombosis and stroke [6,7,8,9]. The underlying mechanism of aPL antibody-mediated thrombosis is not fully understood. It is known that aPL antibodies are able to bind to platelets and amplify platelet activation and aggregation through the p38 MAPK signaling pathway [10,11,12,13,14,15]. Furthermore, investigations in complement deficiency, both in mice and human, suggest that classical pathway activation of the complement system is essential in development of aPL antibody-mediated thrombosis [16,17,18,19,20,21]. Thus, even though the exact underlying mechanism for aPL antibody-mediated development of thrombosis is still not known, existing data suggest that two of the components behind the pro-thrombotic effects are platelets and the complement system.

Data from our group and from others have previously demonstrated that SLE patients have increased complement activation on platelets, especially patients with aPL antibodies [22,23,24]. It is known that some aPL antibodies have complement-fixing activity and allow complement activation through the classical pathway [25]. However, whether aPL antibodies support complement activation specifically on platelets is not known. In addition, complement activation on platelets may be caused by platelet activation and subsequent exposure of C1q binding epitopes on the activated platelet cell surface [23,26]. Currently, it is unclear which of these mechanisms, autoantibody-mediated complement activation or direct binding of C1q due to platelet activation, is operating in SLE to increase platelet complement deposition.

Complement deposition on platelets has been seen in cases of individuals with stroke, but is otherwise thought to be specific for SLE [22,27], although studies have not been extensive in other chronic inflammatory diseases. In SLE, increased C4d deposition on platelets is associated with vascular events [23,24,28]. However, there are discrepancies in the literature as to whether it is venous or arterial vascular events which are associated with complement deposition on platelets. In addition it is also important to note that none of the previous investigations adjusted data for traditional cardiovascular risk factors.

The aim of this study was to investigate if aPL antibodies could support classical pathway activation on platelets *in vitro* as well as in SLE patients. Furthermore, in data which had been adjusted to account for traditional cardiovascular risk factors and aPL antibodies, we investigated with which kind of vascular events, arterial or venous, complement deposition on platelets was associated. Finally, we analyzed if deposition of complement factors C1q and C4d on platelets was specific for SLE or also found in disease controls and healthy individuals. In brief we found that aPL antibodies supported activation of the classical pathway of the complement system on platelets by two separate mechanisms; amplification of platelet activation, and by providing complement-fixing antibodies on the platelet surface. Platelet activation was analyzed by flow cytometry measuring platelet P-selectin and CD69 expression. CD69 is constitutively expressed on platelets, but is increased upon activation and is important for platelet aggregation [29,30]. In SLE patients, deposition on platelets of both complement factor C1q and C4d, was associated with venous, but not arterial, thrombosis when the data was adjusted to account for traditional cardiovascular risk factors and aPL antibodies. These results suggest a possible link between aPL antibodies and development of venous thrombosis through mechanisms involving complement activation on platelets. Finally, complement deposition on platelets was not specific for SLE but high levels of both C1q and C4d on platelets were also found in other disease groups, in particular in patients with rheumatoid arthritis.

Materials and Methods

Patients

Patients with SLE (n = 148), rheumatoid arthritis (n = 20) and systemic sclerosis (n = 20) were recruited to participate in studies related to cardiovascular disease at the Department of Rheumatology, Skåne University Hospital, Lund, Sweden. Healthy volunteers (n = 79) were age- and sex-matched as a group to the SLE patients. Patients who had a recent myocardial infarction (within the previous year) but with no diagnosis of chronic inflammatory diseases (n = 39) were recruited at the Department of Cardiology, Skåne University Hospital, Lund, Sweden. The myocardial infarction patients were treated with Warfarin (n = 3), acetylsalicylic acid (n = 34) and the $P2Y_{12}$ receptor inhibitor Clopidogrel (n = 9). Furthermore, all patients with myocardial infarction used different anti-hypertension treatments, including beta blockers (n = 28). An overview of the clinical characteristics of the patients is presented in Tables 1, 2, and 3. Disease activity was assessed using SLEDAI-2K [31]. All but two individuals fulfilled at least four American College of Rheumatology (ACR) 1982 criteria for SLE [32]. These two patients fulfilled three ACR criteria, had a clinical SLE diagnosis with at least two organ manifestations characteristic of SLE, autoimmune phenomena, and no other diagnosis that could better explain the symptoms. The following treatments were used in the SLE cohort at the time of blood sampling: glucocorticoids (n = 98, median dose = 5 mg, range 1–30 mg), hydroxychloroquine (n = 105), azathioprine (n = 32), mycophenolatmofetil (n = 20), methotrexate (n = 13), intravenous immunoglobulins (n = 2), non-steroidal anti-inflammatory drugs (n = 12), acetylsalicylic acid (n = 44) and Warfarin (n = 23). Previous episodes of myocardial infarction, claudicatio intermittens, cerebrovascular incidents (CVI), angina pectoris, deep venous thrombosis or pulmonary embolisms were defined by the Systemic Lupus International Collaborative Clinics/ACR Damage Index (SLICC/ACR-DI) [33]. Traditional cardiovascular risk factors; age, gender, smoking, diabetes, hypertension (systolic blood pressure equal or higher than 140 at the time of blood sampling or hypertensive treatment due to high blood pressure), body mass index (BMI) and LDL levels, were assessed at the visit to the clinic (Table 3). Complement proteins and autoantibodies were measured by routine standard analyses at the Department of Clinical Immunology and Transfusion Medicine, LabMedicin Skåne, Lund, Sweden.

Ethics statement

The study was approved by the regional ethics board (LU-06014520) and an informed written consent was obtained from all participants.

Complement deposition on platelets in SLE patients

Blood, collected in sodium-citrate tubes (BD Biosciences Pharmingen, Franklin Lakes, NJ, USA), was centrifuged at 280×g for 10 minutes to obtain platelet-rich plasma (PRP). Platelet purity was routinely analyzed by CD42a expression and was found to be more than 98% (mean: 98.8% (range 98.1–99.4%). Ethylenediaminetetraacetic acid (EDTA) was added to PRP to a final concentration of 10 mM to avoid complement activation during the isolation process, and then the platelets were centrifuged at 1125×g for 10 minutes. The platelets were resuspended in 10 mM N-2-hydroxyethylpiperazine-N′-2-ethanesulfonic acid (HEPES) buffer pH 7.4, containing 145 mM NaCl and 5 mM KCl (HEPES buffer) and incubated with fluorescein isocyanate (FITC)-conjugated anti-C1q antibodies (Dako, Glostrup, Denmark) or antibodies against C4d (Quidel, San Diego, CA, USA) for 30 minutes at room temperature. For detection of C4d, the platelets were washed once in HEPES buffer and then incubated with FITC-conjugated rabbit anti-mouse IgG antibodies (Dako) for an additional 30 minutes at 4°C. The platelets were analyzed by flow cytometry on an Accuri C6 (BD).

In vitro complement deposition on activated platelets

PRP, 5 µl, was incubated with 5 µM ADP (Chrono-log, Havertown, PA, USA), for 30 minutes at room temperature in phosphate buffered saline pH 7.4 (PBS). The activation was terminated by incubation with 2% paraformaldehyde for 10 minutes. Activated and fixed platelets were isolated by centrifugation at 1125×g for 10 minutes. Purified platelets were resuspended in veronal buffered saline with 0.15 mM Ca^{2+} and 0.5 mM Mg^{2+} (VBS CaMg) containing 10% normal human serum and human IgG (Immuno AG, Vienna, Austria) or anti-cardiolipin IgG antibodies, at a final concentration of 20 µg/ml, (Antibodies-online.com, Atlanta, GA, USA) and incubated for 60 minutes at 37°C to allow complement activation. The platelets were washed

Table 1. Distribution of American College of Rheumatology (ACR) 1982 classification criteria for the 148 SLE patients.

ACR criteria, median (range)	5 (3–10)
Malar rash %	52
Discoid rash %	20
Photosensitivity %	56
Oral ulcers %	24
Arthritis %	78
Serositis %	39
Renal disease %	33
Neurological disorder %	6
Hematological manifestations %	55
Leukopenia %	37
Lymphopenia %	24
Thrombocytopenia %	14
Immunology %	69
Anti-dsDNA antibodies %	59
ANA %	98

once in PBS and incubated with an anti-C4d antibody (Quidel) for 30 minutes followed by a FITC-conjugated rabbit anti mouse IgG antibody (Dako) for an additional 30 minutes at 4°C. The platelets were analyzed by flow cytometry on an Accuri C6 (BD).

Platelet activation assay

PRP, 5 µl, was incubated with a suboptimal concentration of ADP (0.2 µM, established by titration curve (Figure 1B and Figure S1)), anti-cardiolipin IgG antibodies at a final concentration of 20 µg/ml, human IgG and PE-conjugated antibodies against P-selectin (BD) for 30 minutes at room temperature. The platelets were analyzed by flow cytometry on an Accuri C6 (BD). For detection of CD69, PRP was incubated with monoclonal antibodies against CD69 (Santa Cruz Biotechnology, Santa Cruz, CA, USA), in PBS for 40 min at room temperature. The platelets were washed once in PBS and then incubated with FITC-conjugated rabbit anti-mouse Ig antibodies (Dako) for an additional 30 min at 4°C. The platelets were analyzed by flow cytometry on an Accuri C6 (BD).

Statistics

Spearman's correlation test was used to analyze correlations between C1q and C4d deposition on platelets. For paired analyses, Friedman test was followed by Wilcoxon matched-pairs signed rank test. For group analyses, Kruskal-Wallis test was followed by Mann-Whitney U test. Bonferroni correction was used as a post

Table 2. Clinical characteristics of the SLE patients.

Disease duration, median (range), years	11 (0–46)
SLEDAI score, median (range)	1.5 (0–18)
Serum C3 (g/L), median (range)	1.02 (0.36–2.46)
Serum C4 (g/L), median (range)	0.15 (0.03–0.58)
Serum C1q (%), median (range)	102 (8–200)
Serum C3dg (mg/L), median (range)	0 (0–25.10)
aCL at visit %	5
aCL titer (GPLU/mL)[a], median (range)	60 (42–158)
aCL ever %	28
aB2GP1 at visit %	7
aB2GP1 titer (U/mL)[a], median (range)	28 (16–100)
aB2GP1 ever %	11
Lupus anticoagulans visit %	11
Lupus anticoagulans ever %	11
SLICC/ACR-DI, median (range)	0 (0–8)

[a]Calculation only done for patients with detectable levels of autoantibodies. Abbreviations: SLEDAI; SLE disease activity index, aCL; anti-cardiolipin antibody, aB2GP1; anti-beta 2 glycoprotein 1 antibody.

Table 3. Distribution of traditional cardiovascular risk factors in the different cohorts included in the study.

Patient group	Healthy volunteers	SLE	RA	SSc	MI
Number	79	148	20	20	39
Female %	85	87	75	80	15
Age (median, range)	47 (18–81)	48 (20–82)	56 (28–67)	67 (19–82)	69 (61–77)
LDL concentration (mM), mean and SD	3.16±0.87	3.06±0.95	3.28±0.87	2.91±1.10	2.41±1.08
Smoking %	9	21	30	20	0
Diabetes %	1	3	5	5	15
Hypertension[a] %	18	43	30	35	69
Body mass index	23.5±3.1	25.5±4.9	26.5±4.2	22.5±3.0	25.7±2.9

[a]Hypertension was defined as systolic blood pressure equal or higher than 140 at time point of blood sampling or hypertensive treatment due to high blood pressure.
Abbreviations: LDL; low-density lipoproteins.

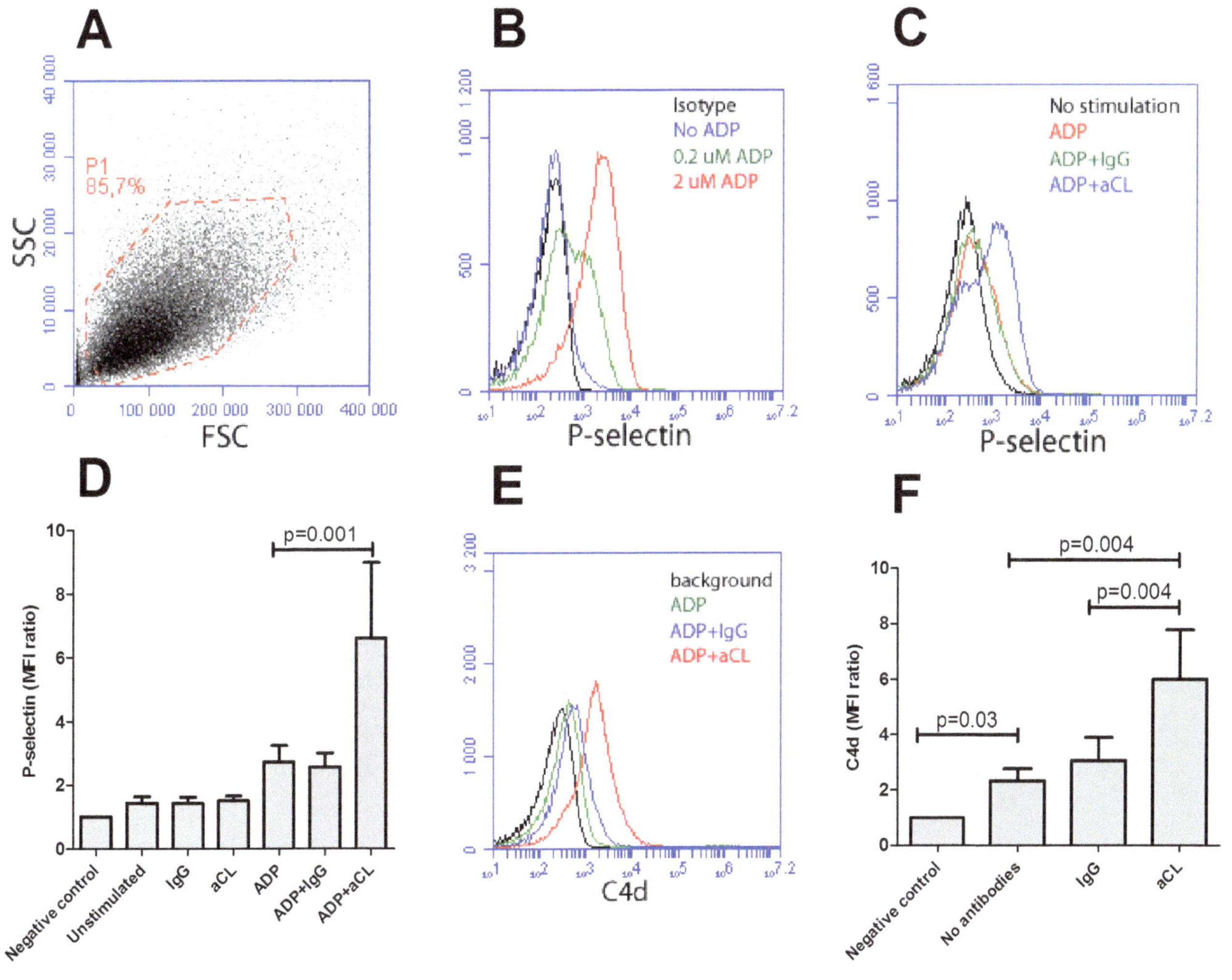

Figure 1. Anti-phospholipid (aPL) antibody-mediated platelet activation and complement deposition. A) Isolated platelets from healthy individuals were gated by flow cytometry (P1) and had consistently purity above 98%. B) Platelet activation after ADP stimulation was detected as P-selectin expression. The lower concentration (0.2 μM) was used for sub-optimal activation. C) Representative figure of P-selectin expression in sub-optimal activated platelets with or without addition of anti-cardiolipin antibodies (aCL). D) A summary of the data presented in Figure 1C. The results are the mean and standard deviation of six or more independent experiments. E–F) Activated and fixed platelets were incubated with or without aCL antibodies in presence of normal human serum. Complement deposition was analyzed with flow cytometry and illustrated as E) a representative histogram and F) a summary of the mean and standard deviation of six or more independent experiments.

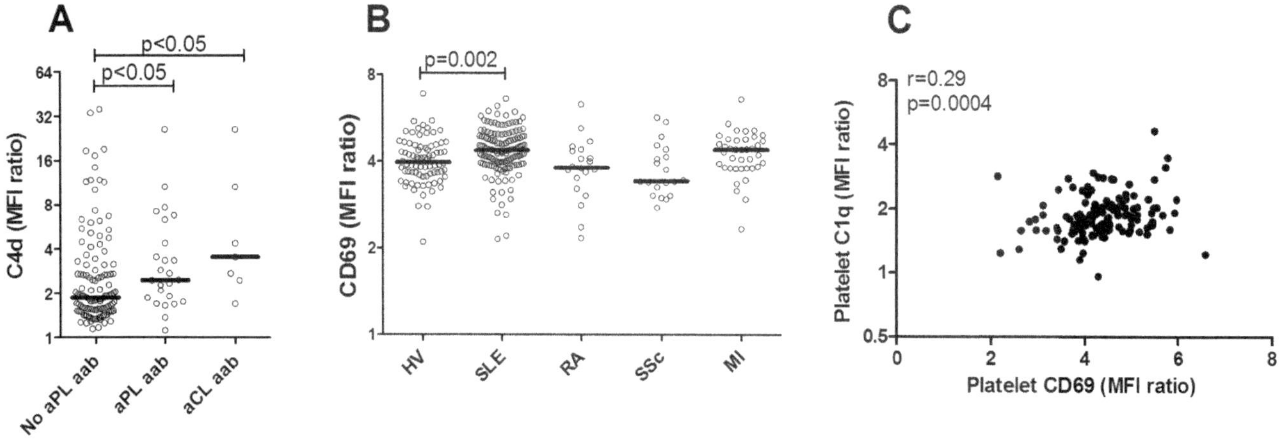

Figure 2. Complement deposition on platelets in SLE patients is associated with aCL antibodies and platelet activation. A) Platelet expression of C4d was analyzed in 148 SLE patients and grouped into patients with or without anti-phospholipid (aPL) or anti-cardiolipin (aCL) antibodies at the time of blood sampling. The line represents the median value in each group. B) Platelet expression of CD69 was measured by flow cytometry in healthy volunteers (HV), patients with systemic lupus erythematosus (SLE), rheumatoid arthritis (RA), systemic sclerosis (SSc) and myocardial infarction (MI). The line represents the median value in each group. C) Correlation analysis between C1q deposition on platelets and platelet activation marker CD69 in the 148 SLE patients.

hoc test for all analyses. Platelet deposition of C1q and C4d did not assume Gaussian distribution why the variables were normalized through logarithms and associations determined by logarithmic regression analysis. The odds ratio (OR) describes the OR for the investigated variable if it increases by one standard deviation. The cut-off for high C1q and C4d deposition on platelets was determined by the 95 percentile of the healthy individuals. A p-value <0.05 was considered statistically significant.

Results

Anti-cardiolipin antibodies mediate platelet activation and complement deposition in vitro

Studies have shown that aPL antibodies can interact with platelets and amplify platelet activation [10,11,12,13,14,15]. However, it is not known whether or not aPL antibodies contribute to complement activation on platelets. In this study, isolated platelets were first incubated with anti-cardiolipin (aCL) antibodies, or human IgG, and P-selectin expression measured by flow cytometry as a marker of platelet activation. Using sub-optimally ADP-activated platelets, this study found that aCL antibodies, but not purified human IgG, were able to amplify platelet activation ($p = 0.001$, Figures 1C and 1D). However, this effect was not seen in non-activated platelets, indicating that low grade platelet activation was necessary to allow aCL antibody interactions with the platelets (Figure 1D). Thus, the data presented herein validated the methodology used and supports the observation that aCL antibodies were able to amplify platelet activation, which is in agreement with previous investigations [10,11,12,13,14,15].

In addition, the ability of aCL antibodies to support complement activation on platelets was tested. Purified platelets were activated with ADP and subsequently fixed with paraformaldehyde to end the activation process. The fixation of the platelets also prevented extensive complement-mediated lysis of the activated platelets during the course of the experiment. Once activated and fixed, serum from a healthy individual supplemented with either human IgG or aCL antibodies was added. Addition of aCL antibodies, but not human IgG, markedly increased the C4d deposition on activated fixed platelets ($p = 0.004$, Figures 1E and 1F). Even in the absence of additional antibodies, using human serum from a healthy individual, the classical pathway of the complement system was activated and C4d was readily measured on the surface of activated platelets ($p = 0.03$, Figure 1F). Thus, in vitro, activated platelets supported classical pathway activation and subsequent deposition of C4d and this process was amplified in the presence of aCL antibodies.

Anti-phospholipid antibody-mediated complement deposition in SLE patients

The presence of aPL antibodies has previously been statistically associated with complement deposition on platelets in SLE patients [22,23,24], but to date it has not been established whether aPL antibodies truly support complement activation on platelets in SLE patients. At the time-point of blood sampling, 25/148 SLE patients (17%) had anti-cardiolipin or anti-B2GP1 antibodies of IgG type, or presence of lupus anticoagulant (LA). Presence of any of these factors was associated with increased C4d deposition on platelets ($p<0.05$, Figure 2A). When analyzed separately, anti-cardiolipin antibodies were associated with increased C4d deposition on platelets ($p<0.05$ Figure 2A). Using a cut-off for high levels of C4d deposition on platelets, presence of anti-cardiolipin antibodies at the time point of blood sampling was highly associated with increased C4d deposition on platelets (OR = 7.1 (1.1–44.3), $p = 0.04$).

However, patients without any detectable levels of aPL antibodies also had high levels of C4d on platelets. Thus, aPL antibodies did not explain all complement deposition on platelets, but clearly other factors also contributed. As described in Figure 1F, as well as previously [23,26], platelet activation, even in the absence of autoantibodies, supported complement activation. SLE patients are known to have increased platelet activation and accordingly, increased platelet expression of CD69 ($p = 0.002$, Figure 2B) was demonstrated in this study, which correlated to complement deposition on platelets ($r = 0.29$, $p = 0.0004$, Figure 2C). Thus, our results suggest that both platelet activation and aPL antibodies can act synergistically to support complement deposition and activation on platelets in SLE patients.

Complement deposition on platelets is associated with venous, but not arterial, thrombosis in SLE patients

In SLE patients, increased C4d deposition on platelets has been suggested to be associated with vascular events [23,24,28]. However, there are discrepancies in these investigations as to which vascular events, venous or arterial, complement deposition on platelets is associated.

In this study we observed no associations between C1q and C4d deposition on platelets and arterial vascular disease including myocardial infarction (OR = 1.2 (0.4–3.9), p = 0.81 and OR = 2.4 (0.7–8.1), p = 0.16, respectively) and cerebrovascular insult (OR = 0.8 (0.4–1.5), p = 0.44 and OR = 0.4 (0.1–1.2), p = 0.09, respectively, Table 4) in SLE patients using a logistic regression model adjusting for traditional cardiovascular risk factors. Not even when combining all arterial vascular diseases (claudicatio intermittens, angina pectoris, myocardial infarction and cerebrovascular insult) could an association with C1q or C4d deposition on platelets be found (OR = 0.8 (0.5–1.4), p = 0.50 and OR = 0.7 (0.4–1.3), p = 0.23, respectively, Table 4). Thus, in this study's SLE cohort, complement deposition on platelets was not associated with arterial vascular events. However, both C1q and C4d deposition on platelets were clearly associated with deep venous thrombosis (OR = 2.3 (1.2–4.2), p = 0.008, and OR = 2.0 (1.2–3.4), p = 0.01, respectively), independent of traditional cardiovascular risk factors: age, gender, smoking, hypertension, hyperglycemia, diabetes and obesity. Combining all venous manifestations the association with C1q and C4d levels on platelets remained statistically significant (p = 0.04 and p = 0.03, respectively, Table 4). For both arterial and venous thrombosis, adjusting for presence of aPL antibodies in the logistic regression model did not affect the results significantly (Table 4).

Whereas our statistical model uses a continuous variable, other investigators have used a cut-off to describe complement deposition on platelets as a dichotomized variable [22,28]. Using the cut-off as described in the material and methods section C4d deposition on platelets still remained highly associated with venous thrombosis (OR = 5.3 (1.3–22.1), p = 0.02) after adjusting for traditional risk factors and aPL antibodies. However, using the same cut-off, C4d deposition on platelets was associated with a decreased frequency of arterial thrombosis (OR = 0.2 (0.1–0.8), p = 0.03) as well as stroke (OR = 0.2 (0.0–1.0), p<0.05), adjusted for traditional cardiovascular risk factors and presence of aPL antibodies. Thus, in SLE patients, increased complement deposition on platelets was clearly associated with venous, and not arterial, thrombosis independently of traditional cardiovascular risk factors and aPL antibodies.

Complement deposition on platelets is not specific for SLE patients

C4d deposition on platelets has been suggested to be highly specific for SLE [22]. However, whether C1q deposition on platelets is specific for SLE had not been investigated previously. Complement deposition of both C1q and C4 on platelets were markedly increased in SLE patients as compared to healthy volunteers (p<0.0001 for both analyses, Figure 3). Patients with rheumatoid arthritis had increased C1q deposition (p = 0.002, Figure 3B) as well as increased C4d deposition (p<0.0001, Figure 3D) whereas patients with systemic sclerosis only were found to have increased C4d deposition (p<0.05, Figure 3D) on platelets as compared to healthy volunteers. Notably, some of the apparently healthy individuals had increased C4d deposition on their platelets. Using the cut-off value for high and low complement deposition on platelets 12% of the SLE patients,

Table 4. Associations between complement deposition on platelets and cardiovascular disease and venous thromboembolism.

Manifestation	N		OR (95% CI)	p-value	OR (95% CI)[a]	p-value[a]	OR (95%CI)[d]	p-value[d]
Arterial[b]	25	C1q	1.0 (0.7–1.5)	0.98	0.8 (0.5–1.4)	0.50	0.8 (0.5–1.4)	0.40
		C4d	0.8 (0.5–1.3)	0.28	0.7 (0.4–1.3)	0.23	0.6 (0.3–1.2)	0.18
CVI	14	C1q	0.9 (0.5–1.6)	0.75	0.8 (0.4–1.5)	0.44	0.7 (0.4–1.3)	0.23
		C4d	0.5 (0.2–1.2)	0.12	0.4 (0.1–1.2)	0.09	0.3 (0.1–1.0)	**<0.05**
MI	8	C1q	1.0 (0.5–2.1)	0.92	1.2 (0.4–3.9)	0.81	2.0 (0.4–11.6)	0.42
		C4d	1.3 (0.7–2.4)	0.44	2.4 (0.7–8.1)	0.16	2.9 (0.8–11.5)	0.12
DVT	12	C1q	2.2 (1.3–3.8)	**0.005**	2.3 (1.2–4.2)	**0.008**	2.2 (1.2–4.2)	**0.01**
		C4d	1.7 (1.0–2.7)	**0.04**	2.0 (1.2–3.4)	**0.01**	2.0 (1.1–3.3)	**0.01**
Venous [c]	17	C1q	1.7 (1.0–2.7)	**0.03**	1.7 (1.0–2.9)	**0.04**	1.7 (1.0–2.9)	**0.04**
		C4d	1.4 (0.9–2.2)	0.11	1.7 (1.1–2.8)	**0.03**	1.7 (1.1–2.8)	**0.03**

[a]Adjusted for traditional risk factors; age, gender, smoking, hypertension, hyperglycemia and diabetes.
[b]Arterial disease includes cerebrovascular insult (CVI), myocardial infarction (MI), angina pectoris and claudicatio intermittens.
[c]Venous thrombosis includes deep venous thrombosis (DVT) and pulmonary embolism.
[d]Further adjusted for presence of aPL antibodies at time-point of blood sampling.

35% of the rheumatoid arthritis patients, 10% of the systemic sclerosis patients, 12% of the myocardial infarction patients and 5% of the healthy individuals were regarded as having high levels of C1q on platelets (Figure 3B). For the C4d deposition on platelets, 35% of the SLE patients, 20% of the rheumatoid arthritis patients, 5% of the systemic sclerosis patients, 8% of the myocardial infarction patients and 4% of the healthy individuals were regarded as having high levels (Figure 3D). There was a correlation between C1q and C4d deposition on platelets ($r = 0.41$, $p<0.0001$, Figure 3E). Only 67% of the SLE patients positive for C1q deposition were also positive for C4d deposition on platelets suggesting that complement activation does not always proceed after C1q binding. Furthermore, of the SLE patients negative for C1q deposition, 31% had increased deposition of C4d on platelets, indicating that small amounts of C1q might be enough to activate C4.

Complement deposition on platelets is associated with disease activity

To investigate the clinical relevance of our findings we first assessed if complement deposition on platelets was associated with disease activity. C4d deposition on platelets, but not C1q deposition, was positively correlated to SLEDAI ($r = 0.27$, $p = 0.001$). Furthermore, patients with active disease (SLEDAI≥ 5) had highly increased C4d deposition on their platelets ($p = 0.008$) compared to SLE patients with no or low disease activity. Patients treated with Prednisone had a higher C4d deposition on platelets ($p = 0.006$), most likely due to increased disease activity seen in this group ($p = 0.01$). None of the other immunosuppressive treatments affected C1q or C4d deposition on platelets in a statistically significant manner. Even though not correlated to disease activity in general, C1q deposition on platelets was increased in SLE patients with ongoing arthritis ($p = 0.01$). For C4d deposition, no associations were found with any specific clinical disease manifestation. Instead C4d deposition correlated with the presence in serum of anti-dsDNA antibodies ($p = 0.03$) and low levels of either C3 or C4 ($p<0.0001$). The deposition of C4d on platelets was inversely correlated with serum levels of both C3 and C4 ($r = -0.38$, $p<0.0001$ for both analyses, Figures 4A and 4B) as well as positively correlated with the complement split product C3dg ($r = 0.44$, $p<0.0001$, Figure 4C). Finally, even when using a modified SLEDAI excluding any score for anti-dsDNA antibodies or low complement levels, C4d deposition on platelets remained statistically significantly correlated to disease activity, even though the association was weak ($r = 0.17$, $p = 0.04$).

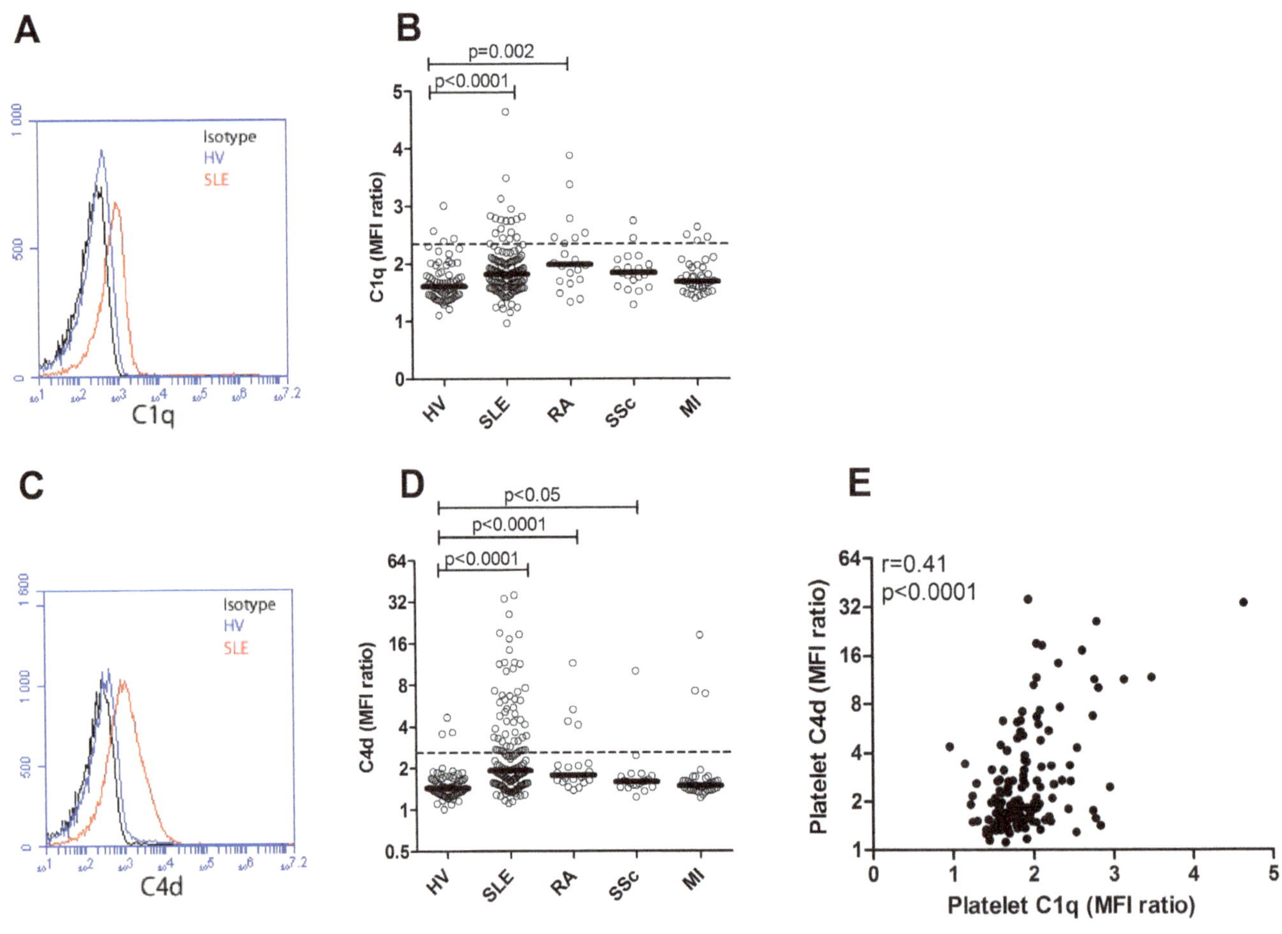

Figure 3. Increased complement deposition on platelets in SLE patients. A) Deposition of C1q and C) C4d was analyzed by flow cytometry and illustrated as representative flow cytometry histograms. Deposition of B) C1q and D) C4d on platelets from healthy volunteers (HV), patients with systemic lupus erythematosus (SLE), rheumatoid arthritis (RA), systemic sclerosis (SSc) and myocardial infarction (MI). The dotted lines represent the 95th percentile of the healthy volunteers and depict the cut-off level for positivity in each analysis. E) Correlation analysis between C1q and C4d deposition on platelets in the SLE patients.

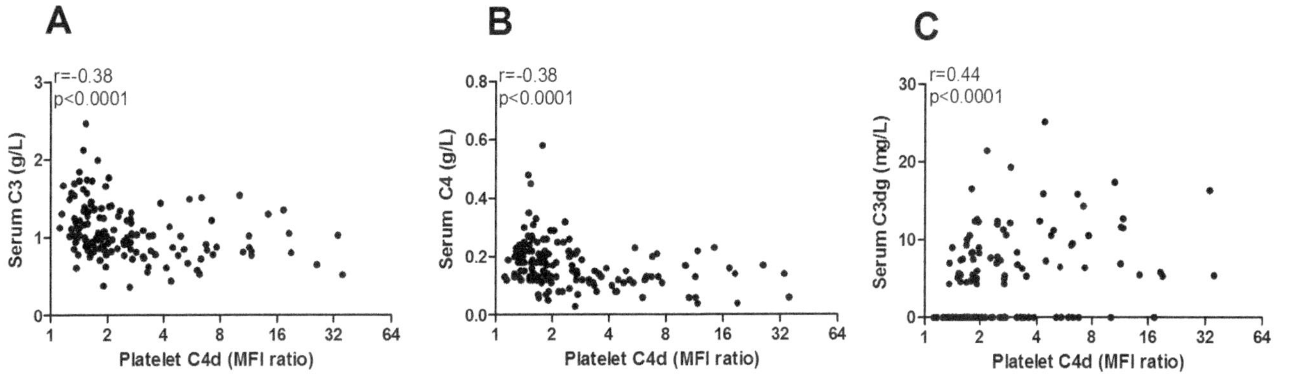

Figure 4. Platelet C4d deposition is associated with complement consumption and activation. C4d deposition on platelets from SLE patients was correlated to A) serum level of C3, B) serum level of C4, and C) the complement activation split fragment C3dg.

Discussion

Anti-phospholipid antibodies are well-known important pro-thrombotic factors contributing to development of venous thrombosis and stroke in SLE patients [9,34,35]. The molecular mechanism of how aPL antibodies mediate development of thrombosis is not fully understood but may involve activation of both platelets and the classical pathway of the complement system [16,17,23]. In human C2 deficiency (C2D), anti-cardiolipin antibodies are frequently seen but virtually never lead to development of venous thrombosis [17]. Furthermore, in mouse, C3, C5a and C6 are all necessary for development of aPL antibody-mediated thrombosis [16,18,19,20,21]. In this investigation we have studied the role of aPL antibodies in mediating complement activation on the surface of platelets and if this could be a possible mechanism linking aPL antibodies, complement activation, platelet activation and vascular events in SLE patients. Furthermore, we present a detailed examination of associations between complement deposition on platelets and other clinical variables.

Increased complement activation has been seen on platelets in SLE patients, especially in patients with aPL antibodies [22,23,24]. However, it was not known if aPL antibodies could support complement activation on platelets. Data presented herein demonstrates that aPL antibodies indeed allow complement activation on platelets by two separate mechanisms, both of which could be operating in SLE patients. Firstly, aPL antibodies contribute to platelet activation-mediated complement deposition. It is well-established that aPL antibodies amplify platelet activation [10,11,12,13,14,15], which was verified in this investigation. Activated platelets expose several molecules including phosphatidylserine and chondroitinsulfate which support binding of C1q and subsequent complement activation [26]. Supporting the hypothesis of platelet activation being sufficient to allow complement activation we observed that sera from healthy individuals supported complement activation on the surface of activated platelets (Figure 1F) also confirming observations in one of our previous studies [23].

Secondly, we hypothesized that the complement-fixing ability of some anti-PL antibodies [25] may allow C1q binding with subsequent activation of the classical pathway on platelets. To test the validity of this model, normal human serum, supplemented with purified aPL antibodies, was added to activated fixed platelets. Using this experimental approach it was found that aPL antibodies also mediated complement activation on platelets independently of their ability to also support platelet activation. Those results are strongly supported by the current as well as previous investigations demonstrating associations between aPL antibodies and complement deposition on platelets [22,23,24]. Thus, we suggest that aPL antibodies, through both platelet activation and binding of complement-fixing antibodies, support complement activation on platelets.

However, aPL antibodies are not indispensable in activating the complement system on platelets, and several mechanisms may operate to mediate complement activation on platelets. This was highlighted by the significant number of SLE patients having no detectable aPL antibodies but still having high levels of both C1q and C4d on platelets. One explanation for this may be presence of other anti-platelet antibodies, including anti-GPIIb/IIIa [36,37,38], but more likely, complement deposition on platelets can be explained by increased platelet activation. In this study we could demonstrate that SLE patients had increased platelet activation and the platelet activation correlated with complement deposition on the platelet surface. The cause for the initial platelet activation in SLE is not known but may include immune complexes, shear stress, type I IFNs or endothelial damage with exposure of extracellular matrix proteins and collagen [39,40,41]. Furthermore, oxidized LDL (oxLDL), which is increased in SLE patients [42], may also participate in the initial platelet activation [43]. Thus, based on our results, we suggest that complement deposition is increased in SLE patients due to ongoing platelet activation and this process, both platelet activation and complement activation on platelets, is amplified in the presence of aPL antibodies.

Earlier studies have established that anti-PL antibodies are associated with development of venous thrombosis and stroke in SLE patients [9], and previous studies have demonstrated an association between increased complement deposition on platelets and vascular events [23,24,28]. However, there are some discrepancies in the literature with regard to which type of vascular event, venous or arterial, complement deposition on platelets is associated with. Furthermore, none of the previous studies have taken into account the role of traditional cardiovascular risk factors in their statistical analyses. In the current investigation we found that complement deposition on platelets was associated with venous, but not arterial, thrombosis, which is in line with our previous study [23]. However, in this study, data demonstrated that the association to venous thrombosis was independent of traditional cardiovascular risk factors and aPL antibodies. Previous studies have suggested that aPL antibodies found in patients with venous thrombosis have increased complement-fixing ability compared to aPL antibodies found in patients with arterial thrombosis [25] and this may be one reason for the increased complement deposition on platelets in patients with aPL antibodies and venous thrombosis.

C4d deposition on platelets has been suggested to be highly specific for SLE [22] but it was not known if C1q deposition on platelets could be seen in inflammatory diseases other than SLE. In contrast to a previous investigation [22] increased C4d and C1q deposition could be readily observed on platelets in patients with rheumatoid arthritis, increased C4d deposition on platelets was found in patients with systemic sclerosis, as well as high levels of complement deposition found on platelets in some apparently healthy individuals. Thus, complement activation on platelets is not specific for SLE but associated with platelet activation in general. However, different patterns of C1q and C4d deposition were found in SLE patients and patients with rheumatoid arthritis. Patients with rheumatoid arthritis had a high frequency of elevated C1q levels on platelets but a relatively low frequency of C4d, whereas SLE patients had the opposite with high frequency of elevated C4d levels compared to a relatively low frequency of C1q. This suggests that different mechanisms of complement activation and regulation might be operating in the two diseases. Interestingly, SLE patients with ongoing arthritis had increased C1q deposition on platelets compared to SLE patients with no arthritis. Even though the pathogenesis of arthritis is different between rheumatoid arthritis and lupus, platelet activation has been demonstrated in the joints of patients with rheumatoid arthritis, but the contribution of complement activation on platelets to this is not known [44]. Further studies are needed to elucidate how complement activation on platelets is regulated in different conditions and contributes to disease manifestations.

In conclusion, we suggest that aPL antibodies are able to amplify C4d deposition on platelets through two separate mechanisms; amplification of platelet activation, and providing complement-fixing antibodies on platelets. Complement deposition on platelets is associated with venous, but not arterial, thrombosis in SLE patients, independent of traditional cardiovascular risk factors and aPL antibodies. Further studies are needed to elucidate the underlying mechanisms linking complement activation on platelets to cardiovascular disease.

Supporting Information

Figure S1 Dose-response curve for ADP. ADP, at different concentrations, was incubated with platelets for 15 minutes at room temperature and platelet activation analyzed by P-selectin expression by flow cytometry. Concentrations ranging between 0.2-0.4 μM ADP were found to induce sub-optimal platelet activation.

Author Contributions

Conceived and designed the experiments: CL HT BG GS AJ LT AAB. Performed the experiments: CL HT BG. Analyzed the data: CL HT BG GS AJ LT AAB. Contributed reagents/materials/analysis tools: HT GS AJ AAB. Wrote the paper: CL AAB. Critically revised the manuscript: HT BG GS AJ LT.

References

1. Crispín JC, Liossis SN, Kis-Toth K, Lieberman LA, Kyttaris VC, et al. (2010) Pathogenesis of human systemic lupus erythematosus: recent advances. Trends Mol Med 16: 47–57.
2. Esdaile JM, Abrahamowicz M, Grodzicky T, Li Y, Panaritis C, et al. (2001) Traditional Framingham risk factors fail to fully account for accelerated atherosclerosis in systemic lupus erythematosus. Arthritis Rheum 44: 2331–2337.
3. Manzi S, Meilahn EN, Rairie JE, Conte CG, Medsger TA Jr, et al. (1997) Age-specific incidence rates of myocardial infarction and angina in women with systemic lupus erythematosus: comparison with the Framingham Study. Am J Epidemiol 145: 408–415.
4. Jonsson H, Nived O, Sturfelt G (1989) Outcome in systemic lupus erythematosus: a prospective study of patients from a defined population. Medicine (Baltimore) 68: 141–150.
5. Rubin LA, Urowitz MB, Gladman DD (1985) Mortality in systemic lupus erythematosus: the bimodal pattern revisited. Q J Med 55: 87–98.
6. Al-Homood IA (2012) Thrombosis in systemic lupus erythematosus: a review article. ISRN Rheumatol 2012: 428269.
7. Koskenmies S, Vaarala O, Widen E, Kere J, Palosuo T, et al. (2004) The association of antibodies to cardiolipin, beta 2-glycoprotein I, prothrombin, and oxidized low-density lipoprotein with thrombosis in 292 patients with familial and sporadic systemic lupus erythematosus. Scand J Rheumatol 33: 246–252.
8. Sallai KK, Nagy E, Bodo I, Mohl A, Gergely P (2007) Thrombosis risk in systemic lupus erythematosus: the role of thrombophilic risk factors. Scand J Rheumatol 36: 198–205.
9. Vikerfors A, Johansson AB, Gustafsson JT, Jonsen A, Leonard D, et al. (2013) Clinical manifestations and anti-phospholipid antibodies in 712 patients with systemic lupus erythematosus: evaluation of two diagnostic assays. Rheumatology (Oxford) 52: 501–509.
10. Betts NA, Ahuja KD, Adams MJ (2013) Anti-beta2GP1 antibodies have variable effects on platelet aggregation. Pathology 45: 155–161.
11. Nojima J, Kuratsune H, Suehisa E, Kitani T, Iwatani Y, et al. (2004) Strong correlation between the prevalence of cerebral infarction and the presence of anti-cardiolipin/beta2-glycoprotein I and anti-phosphatidylserine/prothrombin antibodies—Co-existence of these antibodies enhances ADP-induced platelet activation in vitro. Thromb Haemost 91: 967–976.
12. Wiener HM, Vardinon N, Yust I (1991) Platelet antibody binding and spontaneous aggregation in 21 lupus anticoagulant patients. Vox Sang 61: 111–121.
13. Lin YL, Wang CT (1992) Activation of human platelets by the rabbit anticardiolipin antibodies. Blood 80: 3135–3143.
14. Wang L, Su CY, Chou KY, Wang CT (2002) Enhancement of human platelet activation by the combination of low concentrations of collagen and rabbit anticardiolipin antibodies. Br J Haematol 118: 1152–1162.
15. Vega-Ostertag M, Harris EN, Pierangeli SS (2004) Intracellular events in platelet activation induced by antiphospholipid antibodies in the presence of low doses of thrombin. Arthritis Rheum 50: 2911–2919.
16. Pierangeli SS, Vega-Ostertag M, Liu X, Girardi G (2005) Complement activation: a novel pathogenic mechanism in the antiphospholipid syndrome. Ann N Y Acad Sci 1051: 413–420.
17. Jönsson G, Sjöholm AG, Truedsson L, Bengtsson AA, Braconier JH, et al. (2007) Rheumatological manifestations, organ damage and autoimmunity in hereditary C2 deficiency. Rheumatology (Oxford) 46: 1133–1139.
18. Girardi G, Berman J, Redecha P, Spruce L, Thurman JM, et al. (2003) Complement C5a receptors and neutrophils mediate fetal injury in the antiphospholipid syndrome. J Clin Invest 112: 1644–1654.
19. Salmon JE, de Groot PG (2008) Pathogenic role of antiphospholipid antibodies. Lupus 17: 405–411.
20. Carrera-Marin A, Romay-Penabad Z, Papalardo E, Reyes-Maldonado E, Garcia-Latorre E, et al. (2012) C6 knock-out mice are protected from thrombophilia mediated by antiphospholipid antibodies. Lupus 21: 1497–1505.
21. Holers VM, Girardi G, Mo L, Guthridge JM, Molina H, et al. (2002) Complement C3 activation is required for antiphospholipid antibody-induced fetal loss. J Exp Med 195: 211–220.
22. Navratil JS, Manzi S, Kao AH, Krishnaswami S, Liu CC, et al. (2006) Platelet C4d is highly specific for systemic lupus erythematosus. Arthritis Rheum 54: 670–674.
23. Lood C, Eriksson S, Gullstrand B, Jonsen A, Sturfelt G, et al. (2012) Increased C1q, C4 and C3 deposition on platelets in patients with systemic lupus erythematosus - a possible link to venous thrombosis? Lupus 21: 1423–1432.
24. Peerschke E, Yin W, Alpert D, Roubey R, Salmon J, et al. (2009) Serum complement activation on heterologous platelets is associated with arterial thrombosis in patients with systemic lupus erythematosus and antiphospholipid antibodies. Lupus 18: 530–538.
25. Shinzato MM, Bueno C, Trindade Viana VS, Borba EF, Goncalves CR, et al. (2005) Complement-fixing activity of anticardiolipin antibodies in patients with and without thrombosis. Lupus 14: 953–958.
26. Hamad OA, Ekdahl KN, Nilsson PH, Andersson J, Magotti P, et al. (2008) Complement activation triggered by chondroitin sulfate released by thrombin receptor-activated platelets. J Thromb Haemost 6: 1413–1421.
27. Mehta N, Uchino K, Fakhran S, Sattar MA, Branstetter BFt, et al. (2008) Platelet C4d is associated with acute ischemic stroke and stroke severity. Stroke 39: 3236–3241.

28. Kao AH, McBurney CA, Sattar A, Lertratanakul A, Wilson NL, et al. (2013) Relation of Platelet C4d with All-Cause Mortality and Ischemic Stroke in Patients with Systemic Lupus Erythematosus. Transl Stroke Res.
29. Testi R, Pulcinelli F, Frati L, Gazzaniga PP, Santoni A (1990) CD69 is expressed on platelets and mediates platelet activation and aggregation. J Exp Med 172: 701–707.
30. Testi R, Pulcinelli FM, Cifone MG, Botti D, Del Grosso E, et al. (1992) Preferential involvement of a phospholipase A2-dependent pathway in CD69-mediated platelet activation. J Immunol 148: 2867–2871.
31. Gladman DD, Ibanez D, Urowitz MB (2002) Systemic lupus erythematosus disease activity index 2000. J Rheumatol 29: 288–291.
32. Tan EM, Cohen AS, Fries JF, Masi AT, McShane DJ, et al. (1982) The 1982 revised criteria for the classification of systemic lupus erythematosus. Arthritis Rheum 25: 1271–1277.
33. Gladman D, Ginzler E, Goldsmith C, Fortin P, Liang M, et al. (1996) The development and initial validation of the Systemic Lupus International Collaborating Clinics/American College of Rheumatology damage index for systemic lupus erythematosus. Arthritis Rheum 39: 363–369.
34. Hughes G (2007) Hughes Syndrome: the antiphospholipid syndrome—a clinical overview. Clin Rev Allergy Immunol 32: 3–12.
35. Hughes GR, Khamashta MA (1994) The antiphospholipid syndrome. J R Coll Physicians Lond 28: 301–304.
36. Tsubakio T, Tani P, Curd JG, McMillan R (1986) Complement activation in vitro by antiplatelet antibodies in chronic immune thrombocytopenic purpura. Br J Haematol 63: 293–300.
37. Ziakas PD, Routsias JG, Giannouli S, Tasidou A, Tzioufas AG, et al. (2006) Suspects in the tale of lupus-associated thrombocytopenia. Clin Exp Immunol 145: 71–80.
38. Anderson GP, van de Winkel JG, Anderson CL (1991) Anti-GPIIb/IIIa (CD41) monoclonal antibody-induced platelet activation requires Fc receptor-dependent cell-cell interaction. Br J Haematol 79: 75–83.
39. Lood C, Amisten S, Gullstrand B, Jönsen A, Allhorn M, et al. (2010) Platelet transcriptional profile and protein expression in patients with systemic lupus erythematosus: up-regulation of the type I interferon system is strongly associated with vascular disease. Blood 116: 1951–1957.
40. Larsson A, Egberg N, Lindahl TL (1994) Platelet Activation and Binding of Complement Components to Platelets Induced by Immune-Complexes. Platelets 5: 149–155.
41. Shanmugavelayudam SK, Rubenstein DA, Yin W (2011) Effects of physiologically relevant dynamic shear stress on platelet complement activation. Platelets.
42. Svenungsson E, Jensen-Urstad K, Heimburger M, Silveira A, Hamsten A, et al. (2001) Risk factors for cardiovascular disease in systemic lupus erythematosus. Circulation 104: 1887–1893.
43. Wraith KS, Magwenzi S, Aburima A, Wen Y, Leake D, et al. (2013) Oxidized low-density lipoproteins induce rapid platelet activation and shape change through tyrosine kinase and Rho kinase-signaling pathways. Blood 122: 580–589.
44. Boilard E, Nigrovic PA, Larabee K, Watts GF, Coblyn JS, et al. (2010) Platelets amplify inflammation in arthritis via collagen-dependent microparticle production. Science 327: 580–583.

9

Anti-TNF Treatment Response in Rheumatoid Arthritis Patients Is Associated with Genetic Variation in the NLRP3-Inflammasome

Jacob Sode[1,2,3*], Ulla Vogel[4], Steffen Bank[5,6], Paal Skytt Andersen[7], Marianne Kragh Thomsen[8], Merete Lund Hetland[9,10], Henning Locht[2], Niels H. H. Heegaard[1], Vibeke Andersen[3,5,11,12]

1 Clinical Biochemistry, Immunology & Genetics, Statens Serum Institut, Copenhagen, Denmark, **2** Department of Rheumatology, Frederiksberg Hospital, Frederiksberg, Denmark, **3** Institute of Regional Health Research, University of Southern Denmark, Odense, Denmark, **4** National Research Centre for the Working Environment, Copenhagen, Denmark, **5** Department of Medicine, Viborg Regional Hospital, Viborg, Denmark, **6** Biomedicine, University of Aarhus, Aarhus, Denmark, **7** Department of Microbiology and Infection Control, Statens Serum Institut, Copenhagen, Denmark, **8** Department of Clinical Microbiology, Aarhus University Hospital, Aarhus, Denmark, **9** The DANBIO Registry, Copenhagen Center for Arthritis Research, Center for Rheumatology and Spine Diseases, Glostrup Hospital, Glostrup, Denmark, **10** Department of Clinical Medicine, Faculty of Health and Medical Sciences, University of Copenhagen, Copenhagen, Denmark, **11** Organ Center, Hospital of Southern Jutland, Aabenraa, Denmark, **12** OPEN (Odense Patient data Explorative Network), Odense University Hospital, Odense, Denmark

Abstract

Objective: Many patients with rheumatoid arthritis (RA) benefit from tumor necrosis factor-α blocking treatment (anti-TNF), but about one third do not respond. The objective of this study was to replicate and extend previously found associations between anti-TNF treatment response and genetic variation in the TNF-, NF-κB- and pattern recognition receptor signalling pathways.

Methods: Forty-one single nucleotide polymorphisms (SNPs), including 34 functional, in 28 genes involved in inflammatory pathways were assessed in 538 anti-TNF naive Danish RA patients with clinical data. Multivariable logistic regression analyses were performed to test associations between genotypes and treatment response at 3–6 months using the *European League Against Rheumatism* (EULAR) response criterion. American College of Rheumatology treatment response (ACR50) and relative change in 28-joint disease activity score (relDAS28) were used as secondary outcomes. Subgroup analyses were stratified according to smoking status, type of anti-TNF drug and IgM-Rheumatoid Factor (IgM-RF) status. False discovery rate (FDR) controlling was used to adjust for multiple testing.

Results: Statistically significant associations with EULAR response were found for two SNPs in *NLRP3*(rs4612666) (OR (odds ratio) for good/moderate response = 0.64 (95% confidence interval: 0.44–0.95), p = 0.025, q = 0.95) and *INFG*(rs2430561) (OR = 0.40 (0.21–0.76), p = 0.005, q = 0.18) and among IgM-RF positive patients for *TNFRS1A*(rs4149570) (0.59 (0.36–0.98), p = 0.040, q = 0.76). Current smokers who carried the *NLRP3*(rs4612666) variant allele were less likely to benefit from anti-TNF treatment (OR = 0.24 (0.10–0.56), p = 0.001, q = 0.04).

Conclusions: In a population of Danish RA patients, we confirm the *NLRP3* gene as associated with EULAR anti-TNF response as previously reported. The *NLRP3* variant (T) allele is associated with lower treatment response, in particular among current smokers. Furthermore, we find that a functional polymorphism in the interferon-γ gene is associated with anti-TNF response. All findings should be tested by replication in independent validation cohorts and augmented by assessing cytokine levels and activities of the relevant gene products.

Editor: Amr H. Sawalha, University of Michigan, United States of America

Funding: This study was supported by the Danish Rheumatism Association (www.gigtforeningen.dk), Region of Southern Denmark's PhD Fund (www.regionsyddanmark.dk) and the Department of Rheumatology, Frederiksberg Hospital (www.frederiksberghospital.dk). The funders had no role in study design, data collection and analysis, decision to publish, or preparation of the manuscript.

Competing Interests: The authors have declared that no competing interests exist.

* Email: jaso@ssi.dk

Introduction

Tumour necrosis factor α inhibitors (anti-TNF) have improved the treatment of rheumatoid arthritis (RA); however, the effect varies and approximately one third of patients do not respond [1]. Furthermore, the anti-TNF drugs are expensive and have potentially severe side effects including adverse immunological reactions and increased risk of serious infections [2]. Thus, biomarkers predictive of anti-TNF treatment outcome are likely to improve treatment of patients with RA.

Accordingly, several studies have evaluated biochemical markers, which alone or in combination with clinical parameters are associated with treatment response [3,4]. Until now, a locus in the *PTPRC* gene that was first identified in a genome-wide association study (GWAS) [5,6] is the only confirmed genetic marker that can predict treatment response [7,8]. Recently, polymorphisms in genes encoding the NLRP3-inflammasome (*NLRP3, CARD8*) [9], nuclear factor κ B (NF-κB) and Toll-like receptor (TLR) signalling pathways (*TLR2, TLR4, MyD88, CHUK*) [10] have been associated with *European League Against Rheumatism* (EULAR) response to anti-TNF treatment.

Anti-TNF treatment blocks TNF from binding to TNF receptor 1 (TNFR1), thereby preventing NF-κB signaling. It seems likely that genetic variants in genes encoding proteins in the inflammatory pathways involved in NF-κB activation are involved in the differential response to anti-TNF drugs.

NF-κB is a central regulator of inflammation and regulates the expression of more than 150 genes (http://www.bu.edu/nf-kb/gene-resources/target-genes/) including *TNFA* (TNF-α), *TNFAIP3* (A20), *TLR2, TLR9, CD14, NFKBIA* (IκBα), *NFKB1* (NF-κB1/p50-RelA), *IL1B, IL1RN, IL6, IL10, IL17A* and *IFNG*.

The *NLRP3* gene (cryopyrin/NALP3) encodes one of several proteins forming the NLRP3-inflammasome, an intracellular innate immune sensor that also includes the cysteine protease, caspase-1. Upon inflammasome activation by cellular stress and damage [11], caspase-1 controls activation and cellular release of IL-1β and IL-18, both strong pro-inflammatory cytokines.

NF-κB activation [12] as well as increased TLRs [13] and NLRP3 [14] expression can be detected in synovial tissue from RA patients, but several other molecules activating the pathway (TNF-α, IL-1β) [15] or regulated by the pathway, e.g. IL-17 [15], are central in the pathogenesis of RA.

The objective of this study was to replicate and extend the reported associations between anti-TNF treatment response and genes in the TNF-, NF-κB- and pattern recognition receptor signalling pathways (TLRs and NLRP3). We assessed 41 mainly functional polymorphisms based on available knowledge to allow a biological interpretation of associations with treatment response to anti-TNF, thus potentially adding new knowledge on the underlying causes of treatment success and failure. We used the nationwide Danish database with prospectively collected clinical data of patients with RA (the DANBIO registry).

Methods

Ethics Statement

The study was conducted in accordance with the Declaration of Helsinki and was approved by the Regional Ethics Committee of Central Denmark Region (M-20100153 and S-20120113) and the Danish Data Protection Agency (J. 2010-41-4719). The Regional Ethics Committee of Central Denmark Region gave exemption from informed consent requirements because samples were taken for other reasons and data were not identifiable.

Patients and samples

The DANBIO registry includes data on patients with inflammatory joint diseases, monitored prospectively as part of routine care during treatment with synthetic and biologic disease-modifying anti-rheumatic drugs (DMARDs) [16]. We linked the clinical data from DANBIO with blood samples available from the routine screening for tuberculosis performed prior to treatment with anti-TNF agents.

We included 538 anti-TNF naïve patients with RA in the study. All these patients initiated their first anti-TNF treatment, had clinical variables registered at baseline and follow-up in DANBIO, and had blood samples available.

Biological material (after whole blood analysis for *Mycobacterium tuberculosis* infection) was collected at Statens Serum Institut from September 2009 and at Aarhus University Hospital from January 2011 and until 1st of July 2012.

Candidate gene analyses

We chose to focus on genes involved in the NF-κB, TNF-α and pattern recognition receptor signalling pathways (see full list of polymorphisms in Table S1). Candidate polymorphisms in genes in these pathways were identified by searching for "polymorphism AND Gene name AND (reporter gene OR luciferase OR ELISA OR RT-PCR OR flow cytometry OR EMSA)" in PubMed in August 2011 [17,18]. After an extensive literature search approximately 100 polymorphisms were found and 41 were subsequently chosen primarily based on evidence of biological effect and secondly based on association with autoimmune disease. We screened for linkage disequilibrium (LD) in SNAP, a web-based database based on the International HapMap Project [19]. The selected polymorphisms had expected minor allele frequencies (MAF) ranging from 5% to 48%.

The polymorphisms were genotyped by PCR-based KASP genotyping assay by KBioscience (KBioscience, Hoddesdon, United Kingdom - www.lgcgenomics.com) on extracted DNA (Maxwell 16 LEV Blood DNA Kit, Promega, Madison, Wisconsin, USA) as described by Bank et al. [20]. Genotyping of *TNF* (TNF-α) rs1799724 and rs1800630 failed due to their close proximity to each other, causing bias in genotype failure. All other chosen assays had a call rate exceeding 97%.

Outcome measures, data handling, and statistical methods

Patient data from the DANBIO database included pre-treatment and follow-up data on tender and swollen joint counts (28 joints), C-reactive protein (CRP, mg/l) and patient global score on a 100 mm VAS-scale, which were combined to calculate the disease activity score (DAS28) [21]. Furthermore, data on baseline DMARD treatment (yes/no), type of anti-TNF drug, IgM rheumatoid factor (IgM-RF) status (ICD-10: seropositive RA DM5.9/seronegative RA DM6.0+DM6.9), sex, age, smoking status (never/previous/current) and functional status assessed by the health assessment questionnaire (HAQ, range: 0–3, with 3 being completely disabled), were also drawn from DANBIO. Titers on IgM-RF and anti-citrullinated protein antibodies (ACPA) were not available.

The baseline (pre-treatment) visit was defined as a visit 0–30 days before start of anti-TNF treatment and follow-up as a visit within 60–180 days after treatment onset (at the contact closest to 120 days if more than one visit was registered).

Primary outcome was EULAR response criteria (good, moderate or none) at follow-up [21].

Univariate statistical analysis was used to assess the association between EULAR good/moderate response and genotypes under a dominant model (chi-square tests). Multivariable logistic regression analyses were then performed to investigate association between EULAR good or moderate response and genotype with the variant alleles grouped together (dominant model) and, furthermore, the individual genotypes with the homozygote wildtype as the reference genotype.

The final model included the following baseline covariates: sex, age, HAQ, CRP, baseline DMARD and IgM-RF status. Smoking was not included in the final analyses as data were missing for 15% of patients. However, in patients with available data, we assessed gene-smoking interaction for all polymorphisms by stratifying patients into current-, previous- and never smokers. We also stratified patients into anti-TNF subgroups to check drug specific associations. The remaining variables were also checked for

Table 1. Baseline clinical and demographic characteristics.

	All RA patients	Seropositive RA patients	Seronegative RA patients
No.	538 (–)	407 (75.7%)	131 (24.3%)
Female	407 (75.7%)	303 (74.4%)	105 (80.2%)
Age/years (SD)			
at treatment start	55.0 (13.0)	55.7 (12.8)	53.0 (13.6)
Smoking status			
Current	142 (31.8%)	110 (32.7%)	32 (29.1%)
Previous	151 (33.9%)	120 (35.7%)	31 (28.2%)
Never	153 (34.3%)	106 (31.6%)	47 (42.7%)
Missing data	92 (–)	71 (–)	21 (–)
DMARD	453 (84.2%)	343 (84.3%)	110 (84.0%)
VAS Patient global score (0–100)/Mean (SD)	62.6 (22.6)	60.8 (22.9)	68.5 (20.7)
VAS Physician global score (0–100)/Mean (SD)	38.4 (20.7)	38.0 (20.2)	39.8 (22.3)
VAS pain score (0–100)/Mean (SD)	58.0 (22.8)	55.9 (23.2)	64.4 (20.2)
TJC 0-28/Mean (SD)	9.5 (7.3)	9.0 (7.0)	11.1 (8.1)
SJC 0-28/Mean (SD)	5.4 (4.6)	5.6 (4.5)	4.8 (4.8)
HAQ score/Mean (SD)	1.2 (0.7)	1.2 (0.7)	1.3 (0.7)
CRP/mg/mL (SD)	19.7 (25.5)	20.5 (27.0)	17.2 (20.3)
DAS28/mean (SD)	4.9 (1.2)	4.8 (1.2)	5.0 (1.1)
Anti-TNF drug			
Infliximab (%)	168 (31.2%)	122 (30.0%)	46 (35.1%)
Etanercept (%)	166 (30.8%)	124 (30.5%)	42 (32.1%)
Adalimumab (%)	134 (24.9%)	105 (25.8%)	29 (22.1%)
Golimumab (%)	49 (9.1%)	38 (9.3%)	11 (8.4%)
Certolizumab (%)	21 (3.9%)	18 (4.4%)	3 (2.3%)
EULAR response			
Good (%)	231 (42.9%)	178 (43.7%)	53 (40.5%)
Moderate (%)	148 (27.5%)	108 (26.5%)	40 (30.5%)
None (%)	159 (29.6%)	121 (29.7%)	38 (29.0%)
ACR50 response (%)	170 (31.6%)	131 (32.2%)	39 (29.8%)
RelDAS28 response (SD)	0.28 (0.32)	0.28 (0.34)	0.285 (0.27)

SD: standard deviation, DMARD: disease modifying anti-rheumatic drugs, VAS: visual analogue scale, TJC: tender joint count, SJC: swollen joint count, HAQ: health assessment score, CRP: C-reactive protein, DAS28: disease activity score (28-joints), EULAR: European League Against Rheumatism, ACR50: American College of Rheumatology, 50% improvement, RelDAS28: relative change in DAS28.

interaction with the polymorphisms using Wald's test and likelihood-ratio test.

Secondary outcomes were the relative change in DAS28 (*relDAS28 = (baseline DAS28-follow-upDAS28)/baseline DAS28*) and the American College of Rheumatology outcome measure, ACR50 response. Furthermore, we used ACR70 response in case of statistically significant association for ACR50 response and gene variants. Multivariate linear regression analysis was performed for relDAS28.

All statistical analyses were performed in Stata version 12 (StataCorp, Texas, USA). The Genetic Power Calculator was used for power analysis of discrete traits [22].

At the 5% significance level and MAF of 0.1, 0.25 and 0.4 we had >80% power to detect effect sizes of 1.5, 1.5 and 1.5, respectively, assuming a dominant genetic model. For a recessive model the corresponding effect sizes were 2.9, 1.8 and 1.6, respectively.

We performed correction for multiple testing using False Discovery Rate (FDR) classical one-stage method set at 0.05 (q-value) [23].

Results

Study population

Clinical and demographic baseline characteristics of the 538 patients are presented in Table 1. The patients were treated with the following anti-TNF drugs: infliximab (31.2%), etanercept (30.9%), adalimumab (24.9%), golimumab (9.1%) or certolizumab (3.9%). Overall, EULAR responses (good, moderate, and none) were achieved for 42.9%, 27.5% and 29.6%, respectively.

Primary outcome EULAR response

Statistically significant associations with EULAR response were found for polymorphisms in *NLRP3* (rs4612666), *IFNG* (rs2430561) and *TNFRSF1A* (rs4149570) (Table 2, Table S2).

Table 2. Genotypes of associated polymorphisms and adjusted odds ratios for associations between gene variants and EULAR anti-TNF treatment response.

						EULAR GOOD/MODERATE			EULAR GOOD		
GENE (SNP)	GENOTYPE	FREQ.	NONE	MODERATE	GOOD	ADJ. OR	95% CI	P-VALUE	ADJ. OR	95% CI	P-VALUE
All RA											
IFNG	TT	137	34	37	66	Ref.			Ref.		
rs2430561	TA	263	74	71	118	0.81	(0.50–1.31)	0.395	0.75	(0.45–1.27)	0.285
	AA	114	40	38	36	0.59	(0.34–1.02)	0.059	0.40	(0.21–0.76)	0.005**
	TA or AA	377	114	109	154	0.73	(0.47–1.15)	0.177	0.63	(0.38–1.03)	0.067
NLRP3	CC	275	69	84	122	Ref.			Ref.		
rs4612666	CT	210	73	54	83	0.62	(0.42–0.92)	0.018*	0.62	(0.40–0.97)	0.037*
	TT	31	9	8	14	0.85	(0.37–1.96)	0.707	0.89	(0.36–2.24)	0.808
	CT or TT	241	82	62	97	0.64	0.44–0.95)	0.025*	0.65	(0.43–1.00)	0.050*
Seropositive RA											
IFNG	TT	106	26	30	50	Ref.			Ref.		
rs2430561	TA	205	56	55	94	0.85	(0.49–1.46)	0.547	0.83	(0.43–1.51)	0.544
	AA	78	30	21	27	0.51	(0.26–0.96)	0.038*	0.42	(0.20–0.87)	0.020*
	TA or AA	283	86	76	121	0.73	(0.43–1.22)	0.229	0.69	(0.39–1.21)	0.196
NLRP3	CC	212	51	62	99	Ref.			Ref.		
rs4612666	CT	156	55	39	62	0.58	(0.37–0.92)	0.020*	0.58	(0.35–0.96)	0.035*
	TT	25	9	5	11	0.59	(0.24–1.43)	0.241	0.64	(0.24–1.71)	0.375
	CT or TT	181	64	44	73	0.58	(0.37–0.90)	0.016*	0.59	(0.36–0.96)	0.032*
TNFRSF1A	GG	137	33	40	64	Ref.			Ref.		
rs4149570	GT	196	68	47	81	0.59	(0.36–0.98)	0.040*	0.63	(0.37–1.09)	0.102
	TT	56	15	18	23	0.89	(0.43–1.85)	0.760	0.82	(0.37–1.82)	0.619
	GT or TT	252	83	65	104	0.65	(0.40–1.04)	0.074	0.67	(0.39–1.13)	0.130

Logistic regression, adjusted (Adj.) for sex, age, HAQ, CRP, DMARD at baseline, IgM RF status (seropositive/seronegative). CI: confidence interval, Freq.: Frequency, OR: odds ratio, EULAR: European League Against Rheumatism, P-value: *<0.05, **<0.01.

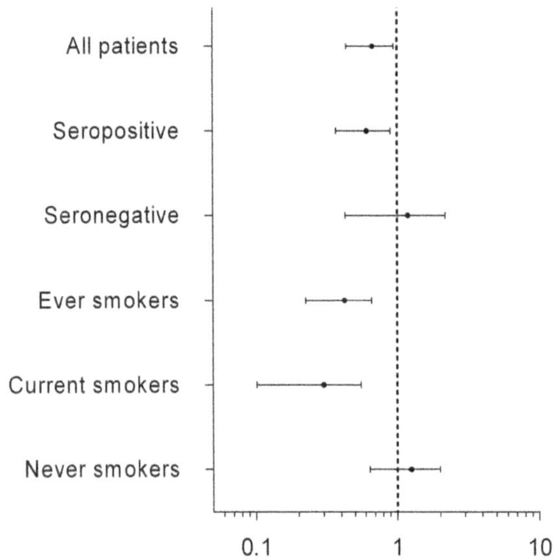

Figure 1. Odds ratio (OR) for association between *NLRP3* (rs4612666) variant allele and EULAR good/moderate response (log scale, 95% confidence interval). Patients stratified on diagnose (seropositive-/seronegative RA) or smoking status. Smoking as independent predictor of EULAR good/moderate response: OR = 1.018, p = 0.941.

NLRP3 rs4612666 variant allele carriers had a significantly lower chance of achieving EULAR good/moderate response (OR = 0.64, p = 0.025, q = 0.95) and EULAR good response (OR = 0.65, p = 0.050, q = 0.97). Stratification according to both smoking status and to IgM RF status revealed even lower OR among seropositive RA patients and current smokers (Table 2, Figure 1).

For *IFNG* rs2430561, the homozygous variant genotype was significantly associated with a lower chance of EULAR good response (OR = 0.40, p = 0.005, q = 0.18), and–among seropositive RA patients–with a lower chance of both EULAR good/moderate response (OR = 0.51, p = 0.038, q = 0.83) and EULAR good response (OR = 0.42, p = 0.020, q = 0.70).

TNFRSF1A rs4149570 was associated with EULAR good/ moderate response (OR = 0.59, p = 0.040, q = 0.760) in the seropositive subgroup analysis, exclusively.

Secondary outcomes relDAS28 and ACR50

Of the three polymorphisms associated with EULAR response, *NLRP3* rs4612666 (seropositive RA: p = 0.024, q = 0.65) and *TNFRSF1A* rs4149570 (seropositive RA: p = 0.034, q = 0.65) were also significantly associated with the relDAS28 (Table 3, Table S3a–b).

Additionally, significant associations with ACR50 outcome (Table 3, Table S3a-c) were found for variant allele carriers of *TLR4* rs5030728 (OR = 1.51, p = 0.033, q = 0.82) and for carriers of the homozygote variant genotype of *IL1B* rs1143623 (OR = 2.14, p = 0.037, q = 0.90) among all RA patients.

Among seropositive RA patients, the variant alleles of *TLR4* rs12377632 (OR = 0.63, p = 0.042, q = 0.61) and *IL17A* rs2275913 (OR = 1.63, p = 0.030, q = 0.61) were significantly associated with ACR50 response.

Statistically significant associations were found between ACR70 response (13.9% of patients) and *IL1B* (rs1143623, rs1143627), and *IL17A* (rs2275913) but not *IL1B* (rs4848306) and *TLR4* (rs12377632, rs1554973, rs5030728) (data not shown).

Smoking and anti-TNF drug stratified analyses

Subgroup analyses stratifying for smoking status and type of anti-TNF drug was performed (Table S4+S5).

Among current smokers, the variant alleles of *NLRP3* rs4612666 (OR = 0.24, p = 0.001, q = 0.04) and *IL4R* rs1805010 (OR = 2.69, p = 0.028, q = 0.56) were significantly associated with EULAR good/moderate response.

In patients treated with infliximab three polymorphisms (*IL1B* (rs4848306) (OR = 2.84, p = 0.004, q = 0.16), *LY96* (rs11465996) (OR = 2.21, p = 0.023, q = 0.45), *NLRP3* (rs4612666) (OR = 0.50, p = 0.041, 0.53)) were associated with EULAR good/moderate response. For etanercept-treated patients, the variant allele of *TNFRSF1A* rs4149570 (OR = 0.40, p = 0.025, q = 0.87) was associated with EULAR good/moderate response. No drug-specific association with any polymorphism was found for adalimumab-treated patients. However, in the seropositive subgroup significant associations with polymorphisms were found for infliximab (*TNF*), etanercept (*LY96, NFKB1, NLRP3, TNFRSF1A*) and adalimumab (*IL23R, CD14, TLR5*) treated patients.

No associations were found for the combined group of anti-TNF drugs based on monoclonal antibodies (all except etanercept).

Summarized effect of polymorphisms

For each seropositive RA patient we counted the alleles (homozygote wildtype or carrier of variant) that were significantly associated with EULAR non-response and calculated a weighted aggregated genetic risk score. The risk of EULAR non response increased *per* associated polymorphism, and patients with five polymorphisms associated had about 15 times higher risk of EULAR non response than did patients with no associated alleles (Figure 2).

Discussion

We assessed the associations between 41 inflammatory pathway-related polymorphisms and the response to treatment with anti-TNF in 538 anti-TNF naive RA patients in a genetically homogeneous and clinically well-characterised and closely monitored cohort of RA patients [7]. The polymorphisms were chosen in genes encoding proteins in the TNF-, NFκB- and pattern recognition receptor signalling pathways (TLRs and NLRP3). Most of the chosen polymorphisms (34/41) were functional, *i.e.,* affecting gene expression or protein function and, thus, allowing biological interpretation of the results.

We analysed treatment response using both EULAR response criteria, relative change in DAS28, and ACR50/ACR70. This enables comparison with other studies.

We were able to confirm the association between the *NLRP3* gene and EULAR anti-TNF response recently reported in a well-powered study on UK RA patients [9]. However, in the UK study the specific *NLRP3* polymorphism (rs4612666) was not reported as associated with EULAR response but three other polymorphisms in *NLRP3* were. Although these three polymorphisms are poor markers for rs4612666 (r^2 for linkage with rs4612666: rs4925659, $r^2 = 0.005$; rs10925026, $r^2 = 0.09$; rs4925648, $r^2 = 0.22$), there is relatively strong linkage disequilibrium between rs4612666 and rs10925026 (D' = 0.81) (Figure S1). Thus, two different polymorphisms in an area of the *NLRP3* gene with low recombination have now been associated EULAR good and moderate response vs no response in two different cohorts treated with anti-TNF. This is a strong indicator of a true association of the gene with treatment response. As indicated, there are contradicting results for rs4612666 between our and the UK study [9]. This may be due

Table 3. Adjusted odds ratio (OR) for associations between gene variants and ACR50 and relDAS28 response to anti-TNF treatment.

			ACR50 response					relDAS28		
***GENE* (SNP)**	**GENOTYPE**	**Freq.**	**No**	**Yes**	**Adj. OR**	**95% CI**	**P-VALUE**	**Adj. Coeff.**	**95% CI**	**P-VALUE**
ALL RA										
IL1B	GG	255	181	74						
rs1143623	GC	223	149	74	1.22	(0.82–1.80)	0.330	0.02	(−0.04–0.08)	0.489
	CC	37	20	17	2.14	(1.05–4.35)	0.037*	0.02	(−0.09–0.13)	0.693
	GC/CC	260	169	91	1.32	(0.91–1.93)	0.145	0.02	(−0.04–0.08)	0.466
TLR4	GG	253	183	70						
rs5030728	GA	215	134	81	1.58	(1.06–2.35)	0.023*	0.01	(−0.05–0.07)	0.786
	AA	46	32	14	1.21	(0.61–2.42)	0.584	0.01	(−0.09–0.11)	0.794
	GA/AA	261	166	95	1.51	(1.03–2.21)	0.033*	0.01	(−0.05–0.06)	0.748
NLRP3	CC	275	183	92						
rs4612666	CT	210	147	63	0.86	(0.58–1.27)	0.434	−0.06	(−0.12–0.00)	0.049*
	TT	31	21	10	0.97	(0.44–2.17)	0.947	−0.04	(−0.16–0.08)	0.524
	CT/TT	241	168	73	0.87	(0.60–1.27)	0.467	−0.06	(−0.11–0.00)	0.050*
SEROPOSITIVE RA										
IL17A	GG	176	127	49						
rs2275913	GA	172	106	66	1.73	(1.09–2.75)	0.021*	0.01	(−0.06–0.08)	0.752
	AA	44	30	14	1.30	(0.63–2.69)	0.471	0.05	(−0.06–0.16)	0.363
	GA/AA	216	136	80	1.63	(1.05–2.54)	0.030*	0.02	(−0.05–0.09)	0.562
NLRP3	CC	212	137	75						
rs4612666	CT	156	109	47	0.80	(0.51–1.25)	0.330	−0.08	(−0.15–0.01)	0.024*
	TT	25	17	8	0.90	(0.37–2.19)	0.813	−0.08	(−0.22–0.06)	0.256
	CT/TT	181	126	55	0.81	(0.53–1.25)	0.345	−0.08	(−0.15–0.01)	0.018*
TLR4	TT	147	90	57						
rs12377632	TC	189	133	56	0.64	(0.40–1.02)	0.061	−0.03	(−0.10–0.04)	0.400
	CC	50	36	14	0.59	(0.29–1.21)	0.152	−0.02	(−0.13–0.09)	0.708
	TC/CC	239	169	70	0.63	(0.41–0.98)	0.042*	−0.03	(−0.10–0.04)	0.412
TNFRSF1A	GG	137	87	50						
rs4149570	GT	196	137	59	0.77	(0.48–1.23)	0.268	−0.08	(−0.15–0.01)	0.034*
	TT	56	38	18	0.81	(0.41–1.60)	0.544	−0.04	(−0.14–0.07)	0.506
	GT/TT	252	175	77	0.78	(0.50–1.21)	0.267	−0.07	(−0.14–0.00)	0.051

Adj. OR: adjusted odds ratio for ACR50 and coefficient (Coeff.) for relative change in DAS28 (relDAS28). Adjusted for gender, age, HAQ-, DMARD at baseline, CRP, IgM RF status (seropositive/seronegative). Freq.: frequency.

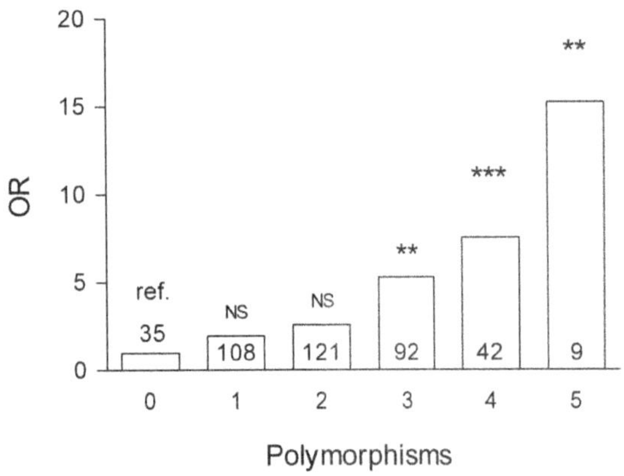

Figure 2. Aggregate genetic risk score. Weighted odds ratio (OR) for seropositive RA patients' risk of EULAR non-response according to the number of associated polymorphisms, relative to patients with zero associated polymorphisms. Number of patients in bars. NS: not significant. P-value: **<0.01, ***<0.001.

to a type 1 error in our study. On the other hand it can also reflect differences in the population of the two cohorts, e.g. the proportion of the specific anti-TNF drugs used for treatment is different in the two studies. Also, geographical/ethnic variation may play a role. Further validation is needed to clear this question.

The data also showed that a polymorphism in *IFNG* and in subgroups, polymorphisms *IL1B, LY96, TLR2* and *TNFRSF1A* were significantly associated with EULAR response to anti-TNF treatment. However, due to the low number of observations in subgroups and the fact that they, to our knowledge, have not earlier been linked to a differentiated anti-TNF response, these results should be considered preliminary.

When analysing the secondary outcome (ACR50), polymorphisms in *IL1B, IL17* and *TLR4* were associated with response to anti-TNF treatment. Another study [10] also found a polymorphism in *TLR4* associated with anti-TNF response, though this study used the EULAR response criterion.

The importance of the NLRP3-inflammasome in RA pathogenesis is illustrated by the findings of increased *NLRP3* mRNA in synovial tissue from RA patients compared to subjects with osteoarthritis [14]. Moreover, another polymorphism in *NLRP3* has been found to be associated with delayed apoptosis of neutrophils suggesting that NLRP3 could influence the resolution of inflammation through a dysregulated innate immune response [24].

Hitomi *et al.* found the rs4612666 variant allele to cause lower mRNA expression by decreasing the transcriptional enhancer activity (in intron 7) of the *NLRP3* gene in a cell expression study [25].

It is premature to give a solid biological interpretation on the association found for *NLRP3* (rs4612666) as the association of this specific polymorphism has not been replicated. However, since the association found in this polymorphism remained statistically significant after correction for multiple testing (among smoking variant allele carriers) it is tempting to hypothesize that this SNP is functionally relevant for the outcome of anti-TNF treatment in RA patients.

Smoking produce exogenous reactive oxygen species (ROS) [26] and ROS has been found to increase expression and activation of the NLRP3-inflammasome [27]. This may explain why the largest ORs were found in the subgroup of current smokers in whom increased activation of a differentially expressed

Table 4. Polymorphisms' effect on anti−/pro-inflammatory signal and chance of good anti-TNF response (EULAR good/moderate or ACR50).

GENE/PROTEIN (SNP)	Protein Inflammatory effect	Variant allele Expected effect on gene expression	Variant allele Association with Anti-TNF response	Subgroup
NLRP3/NLRP3	Pro-	↓ [25]	↓ *	All
rs4612666 C>T				Smokers
				Seropositive
				Infliximab
TNFRS1A/TNFR1	Pro-	↑ [32]	↓ *	Seropositive
rs4149570 G>T				Etanercept
IL17A/IL-17	Pro-	↑ [33]	↑ #	Seropositive
rs2275913 G>A				
TLR4/TLR4	Pro-	Unknown	↑ #	All
rs5030728 G>A				
IL1B/IL-1β	Pro-	↑ [34]	↑ #	All
rs1143623 G>C				Seropositive
IL1B/IL-1β	Pro-	↓ [34]	↑ *	Infliximab
rs4848306				
LY96/MD-2	Pro-	↑ [35]	↑ *	Infliximab
rs11465996 C>G				
INFG/Interferon-γ	Pro−/Anti-	↓ [36]	↓ *	All
rs2430561 T>A				Seropositive

EULAR (*): European League Against Rheumatism ACR50 (#): American College of Rheumatology response criterion (50% improvement).

NLRP3-inflammasome should have the strongest biological effects (carriers of the *NLRP3* variant (T) allele were less likely to benefit from anti-TNF treatment). Taken together, our results indicate a potential impact of smoking on anti-TNF response and suggest that the non-responders may have lower expression of *NLRP3* (Table 4).

This study was not designed to detect effect sizes below 1.5 and had low power to perform subgroup analyses. In the seropositive subgroup there was >80% power to detect effect sizes above 1.7 for polymorphisms with MAFs above 0.25, whereas power in the seronegative subgroup was too low for relevant analyses. Though also limited by low power we found it relevant to analyse associations for individual drugs and monoclonal-based anti-TNFs because of the small differences and similarities which exist between them.

We have chosen to present significant result at the 5% significance level. Though most of these results become insignificant after correction for multiple testing, we also present FDR corrected q-value. We cannot exclude that choosing this level of statistical significance may result in type 1 errors but obviously may too conservative testing result in type 2 errors [28]. Due to the exploratory nature of the study we found it relevant to present even weak genetic associations, which may subsequently be replicated in other studies. Other factors than significance level should be considered when interpreting these results [29]. The prior probability of finding associations in functional polymorphisms is higher since earlier studies have found these to result in an altered expression of their corresponding genes. These genes were chosen based on their expected biological effects in the mechanism of action of the anti-TNF treatment.

Also the presence or absence of systematic bias is important for the risk of type 1 error. In this study, the selection of patients was based on the availability of sufficient clinical data to calculate EULAR responses and this could theoretically create a selection bias. Overall, however, the response rates found in this study are comparable to on the response rates in the complete DANBIO cohort [30] and other comparable studies [10,31]. Genotyping artefacts are theoretically possible and were identified for two polymorphisms but re-genotyping of 94 randomly selected samples in another cohort yielded >99% identical genotypes.

A strength of the study is that the clinical data were collected independently and prospectively as part of routine care.

In conclusion, we confirm the *NLRP3* gene as associated with anti-TNF treatment response based on EULAR criteria in a Danish cohort of RA patients [9]. The *NLRP3* variant (T) allele is associated with a poorer treatment response, in particular among current smokers. Furthermore, we find the homozygous variant genotype of an *IFNG* polymorphism associated with a poorer anti-TNF response.

Results indicating association with other polymorphisms among subgroups in this cohort should be interpreted with care and all findings tested by replication in independent validation cohorts.

Supporting Information

Figure S1 Linkage Disequilibrium Plot for polymorphisms spanning the *NLRP3*-gene. D' values are shown. Darker grey indicates higher r^2.

Table S1 Chosen polymorphisms and corresponding gene. Associated effect of polymorphism.

Table S2 Adjusted odds ratios for associations between gene variants and EULAR anti-TNF treatment response. (a. All RA patients, b. Seropositive RA patients).

Table S3 Adjusted odds ratio (OR)/coefficient for associations between gene variants and ACR50 and relDAS28 response to anti-TNF treatment. (a. All RA patients, b. Seropositive RA patients).

Table S4 Smoking strata: Odds ratio for minor allele carriers achieving EULAR good/moderate response.

Table S5 Anti-tumour necrosis factor (TNF) subgroup odds ratio for EULAR good/moderate response. (a. All RA patients, b. Seropositive RA patients).

Acknowledgments

We thank Hans Jürgen Hoffmann, Department of Respiratory Diseases, Aarhus University Hospital, Aarhus, Denmark; and Vibeke Østergaard Thomsen, International Reference Laboratory of Mycobacteriology, Statens Serum Institut for collecting samples; Andreas Nicolai Andersen, Statens Serum Institut, for statistics support; Elvira Chapka, Statens Serum Institut for laboratory support; and Niels Steen Krogh, Zitelab Aps, Copenhagen, Denmark for database management. We also thank Department of Medicine, Viborg Regional Hospital, Denmark and OPEN (Odense Patient data Explorative Network), Odense University Hospital, Denmark for supporting this work.

Author Contributions

Conceived and designed the experiments: JS UV SB PSA MLH HL NH VA. Performed the experiments: JS SB PSA. Analyzed the data: JS UV NH VA. Contributed reagents/materials/analysis tools: JS UV SB PSA MKT MLH HL NH VA. Wrote the paper: JS UV SB PSA MKT MLH HL NH VA.

References

1. Hetland ML, Christensen IJ, Tarp U, Dreyer L, Hansen A, et al. (2010) Direct comparison of treatment responses, remission rates, and drug adherence in patients with rheumatoid arthritis treated with adalimumab, etanercept, or infliximab: results from eight years of surveillance of clinical practice in the nationwide Danish DANBIO registry. Arthritis Rheum 62: 22–32. 10.1002/art.27227 [doi].
2. Rosenblum H, Amital H (2011) Anti-TNF therapy: safety aspects of taking the risk. Autoimmun Rev 10: 563–568. 10.1016/j.autrev.2011.04.010 [doi].
3. Emery P, Dorner T (2011) Optimising treatment in rheumatoid arthritis: a review of potential biological markers of response. Ann Rheum Dis 70: 2063–2070. 10.1136/ard.2010.148015 [doi].
4. Toonen EJ, Gilissen C, Franke B, Kievit W, Eijsbouts AM, et al. (2012) Validation study of existing gene expression signatures for anti-TNF treatment in patients with rheumatoid arthritis. PLoS One 7: e33199. 10.1371/journal.-pone.0033199 [doi];PONE-D-11-21951 [pii].
5. Cui J, Saevarsdottir S, Thomson B, Padyukov L, van der Helm-van Mil AH, et al. (2010) Rheumatoid arthritis risk allele PTPRC is also associated with response to anti-tumor necrosis factor alpha therapy. Arthritis Rheum 62: 1849–1861. 10.1002/art.27457 [doi].
6. Plant D, Prajapati R, Hyrich KL, Morgan AW, Wilson AG, et al. (2012) Replication of association of the PTPRC gene with response to anti-tumor necrosis factor therapy in a large UK cohort. Arthritis Rheum 64: 665–670. 10.1002/art.33381 [doi].
7. Krintel SB, Palermo G, Johansen JS, Germer S, Essioux L, et al. (2012) Investigation of single nucleotide polymorphisms and biological pathways associated with response to TNFalpha inhibitors in patients with rheumatoid arthritis. Pharmacogenet Genomics 22: 577–589. 10.1097/FPC.0b013e3283544043 [doi].
8. Umicevic MM, Cui J, Vermeulen SH, Stahl EA, Toonen EJ, et al. (2012) Genome-wide association analysis of anti-TNF drug response in patients with

rheumatoid arthritis. Ann Rheum Dis 0: 1–7. annrheumdis-2012-202405 [pii];10.1136/annrheumdis-2012-202405 [doi].
9. Mathews RJ, Robinson JI, Battellino M, Wong C, Taylor JC, et al. (2013) Evidence of NLRP3-inflammasome activation in rheumatoid arthritis (RA); genetic variants within the NLRP3-inflammasome complex in relation to susceptibility to RA and response to anti-TNF treatment. Ann Rheum Dis 0: 1–9. annrheumdis-2013-203276 [pii];10.1136/annrheumdis-2013-203276 [doi].
10. Potter C, Cordell HJ, Barton A, Daly AK, Hyrich KL, et al. (2010) Association between anti-tumour necrosis factor treatment response and genetic variants within the TLR and NF{kappa}B signalling pathways. Ann Rheum Dis 69: 1315–1320. ard.2009.117309 [pii];10.1136/ard.2009.117309 [doi].
11. Strowig T, Henao-Mejia J, Elinav E, Flavell R (2012) Inflammasomes in health and disease. Nature 481: 278–286. 10.1038/nature10759 [doi].
12. van LG, Beyaert R (2011) Negative regulation of NF-kappaB and its involvement in rheumatoid arthritis. Arthritis Res Ther 13: 221. ar3324 [pii];10.1186/ar3324 [doi].
13. Goh FG, Midwood KS (2012) Intrinsic danger: activation of Toll-like receptors in rheumatoid arthritis. Rheumatology (Oxford) 51: 7–23. ker257 [pii];10.1093/rheumatology/ker257 [doi].
14. Rosengren S, Hoffman HM, Bugbee W, Boyle DL (2005) Expression and regulation of cryopyrin and related proteins in rheumatoid arthritis synovium. Ann Rheum Dis 64: 708–714. ard.2004.025577 [pii];10.1136/ard.2004.025577 [doi].
15. Klareskog L, Catrina AI, Paget S (2009) Rheumatoid arthritis. Lancet 373: 659–672. S0140-6736(09)60008-8 [pii];10.1016/S0140-6736(09)60008-8 [doi].
16. Hetland ML (2011) DANBIO–powerful research database and electronic patient record. Rheumatology (Oxford) 50: 69–77. keq309 [pii];10.1093/rheumatology/keq309 [doi].
17. Bank S, Andersen PS, Burisch J, Pedersen N, Roug S, et al. (2014) Associations between functional polymorphisms in the NFkappaB signaling pathway and response to anti-TNF treatment in Danish patients with inflammatory bowel disease. Pharmacogenomics J. tpj201419 [pii];10.1038/tpj.2014.19 [doi].
18. Bank S, Andersen PS, Nexo BA, Sode J, Vogel U, et al. (2014) Polymorphisms in the inflammatory pathway genes TLR2, TLR4, TLR9, LY96, NFKBIA, NFKB1, TNFA, TNFRSF1A, IL6R, IL10, IL23R, PTPN22, and PPARG are associated with susceptibility of inflammatory bowel disease in a Danish cohort. PLoS ONE (Accepted for publication).
19. Johnson AD, Handsaker RE, Pulit SL, Nizzari MM, O'Donnell CJ, et al. (2008) SNAP: a web-based tool for identification and annotation of proxy SNPs using HapMap. Bioinformatics 24: 2938–2939. btn564 [pii];10.1093/bioinformatics/btn564 [doi].
20. Bank S, Nexo BA, Andersen V, Vogel U, Andersen PS (2013) High-Quality and -Quantity DNA Extraction from Frozen Archival Blood Clots for Genotyping of Single-Nucleotide Polymorphisms. Genet Test Mol Biomarkers 17: 501–503. 10.1089/gtmb.2012.0429 [doi].
21. Fransen J, van Riel PL (2005) The Disease Activity Score and the EULAR response criteria. Clin Exp Rheumatol 23: S93–S99.
22. Purcell S, Cherny SS, Sham PC (2003) Genetic Power Calculator: design of linkage and association genetic mapping studies of complex traits. Bioinformatics 19: 149–150.
23. Benjamini Y, Hochberg Y (1995) Controlling the false discovery rate: a practical and powerful approach to multiple testing. J R Stat Soc Series B 57: 289–300.
24. Blomgran R, Patcha BV, Verma D, Bergstrom I, Soderkvist P, et al. (2012) Common genetic variations in the NALP3 inflammasome are associated with delayed apoptosis of human neutrophils. PLoS One 7: e31326. 10.1371/journal.pone.0031326 [doi];PONE-D-10-02541 [pii].
25. Hitomi Y, Ebisawa M, Tomikawa M, Imai T, Komata T, et al. (2009) Associations of functional NLRP3 polymorphisms with susceptibility to food-induced anaphylaxis and aspirin-induced asthma. J Allergy Clin Immunol 124: 779–785.
26. Valavanidis A, Vlachogianni T, Fiotakis K (2009) Tobacco smoke: involvement of reactive oxygen species and stable free radicals in mechanisms of oxidative damage, carcinogenesis and synergistic effects with other respirable particles. Int J Environ Res Public Health 6: 445–462. 10.3390/ijerph6020445 [doi].
27. Simard JC, Cesaro A, Chapeton-Montes J, Tardif M, Antoine F, et al. (2013) S100A8 and S100A9 Induce Cytokine Expression and Regulate the NLRP3 Inflammasome via ROS-Dependent Activation of NF-κB. PLoS ONE 8: e72138. doi:10.1371/journal.pone.0072138.
28. Perneger TV (1998) What's wrong with Bonferroni adjustments. BMJ 316: 1236–1238.
29. Plenge RM, Bridges SL, Huizinga TWJ, Criswell LA, Gregersen PK (2011) Recommendations for publication of genetic association studies in Arthritis & Rheumatism. Arthritis & Rheumatism 63: 2839–2847.
30. Hetland ML, Lindegaard HM, Hansen A, Podenphant J, Unkerskov J, et al. (2008) Do changes in prescription practice in patients with rheumatoid arthritis treated with biological agents affect treatment response and adherence to therapy? Results from the nationwide Danish DANBIO Registry. Ann Rheum Dis 67: 1023–1026. ard.2007.087262 [pii];10.1136/ard.2007.087262 [doi].
31. Coenen MJ, Enevold C, Barrera P, Schijvenaars MM, Toonen EJ, et al. (2010) Genetic variants in toll-like receptors are not associated with rheumatoid arthritis susceptibility or anti-tumour necrosis factor treatment outcome. PLoS One 5: e14326. 10.1371/journal.pone.0014326 [doi].
32. Wang GB, Li CR, Yang J, Wen PQ, Jia SL (2011) A regulatory polymorphism in promoter region of TNFR1 gene is associated with Kawasaki disease in Chinese individuals. Hum Immunol 72: 451–457. S0198-8859(11)00032-2 [pii];10.1016/j.humimm.2011.02.004 [doi].
33. Espinoza JL, Takami A, Nakata K, Onizuka M, Kawase T, et al. (2011) A genetic variant in the IL-17 promoter is functionally associated with acute graft-versus-host disease after unrelated bone marrow transplantation. PLoS One 6: e26229. 10.1371/journal.pone.0026229 [doi];PONE-D-11-15752 [pii].
34. Chen H, Wilkins LM, Aziz N, Cannings C, Wyllie DH, et al. (2006) Single nucleotide polymorphisms in the human interleukin-1B gene affect transcription according to haplotype context. Hum Mol Genet 15: 519–529. ddi469 [pii];10.1093/hmg/ddi469 [doi].
35. Gu W, Shan YA, Zhou J, Jiang DP, Zhang L, et al. (2007) Functional significance of gene polymorphisms in the promoter of myeloid differentiation-2. Ann Surg 246: 151–158. 10.1097/01.sla.0000262788.67171.3f [doi];00000658-200707000-00023 [pii].
36. Pravica V, Perrey C, Stevens A, Lee JH, Hutchinson IV (2000) A single nucleotide polymorphism in the first intron of the human IFN-gamma gene: Absolute correlation with a polymorphic CA microsatellite marker of high IFN-gamma production. Human Immunology 61: 863–866. 10.1016/S0198-8859(00)00167-1 [doi].

Clinicopathological Correlations of Podoplanin (gp38) Expression in Rheumatoid Synovium and Its Potential Contribution to Fibroblast Platelet Crosstalk

Manuel J. Del Rey[1]‡, Regina Faré[1]‡, Elena Izquierdo[2], Alicia Usategui[1], José L. Rodríguez-Fernández[2], Abel Suárez-Fueyo[1], Juan D. Cañete[3], José L. Pablos[1]*

1 Servicio de Reumatología, Instituto de Investigación Hospital 12 de Octubre (i+12), Madrid, Spain, 2 Centro de Investigaciones Biológicas, Consejo Superior de Investigaciones Científicas, Madrid, Spain, 3 Unitat d'Artritis, Servei de Reumatologia, Hospital Clínic de Barcelona and Institut d'Investigacions Biomèdiques August Pí i Sunyer, Barcelona, Spain

Abstract

Introduction: Synovial fibroblasts (SF) undergo phenotypic changes in rheumatoid arthritis (RA) that contribute to inflammatory joint destruction. This study was undertaken to evaluate the clinical and functional significance of ectopic podoplanin (gp38) expression by RA SF.

Methods: Expression of gp38 and its CLEC2 receptor was analyzed by immunohistochemistry in synovial arthroscopic biopsies from RA patients and normal and osteoarthritic controls. Correlation between gp38 expression and RA clinicopathological variables was analyzed. In patients rebiopsied after anti-TNF-α therapy, changes in gp38 expression were determined. Platelet-SF coculture and gp38 silencing in SF were used to analyze the functional contribution of gp38 to SF migratory and invasive properties, and to SF platelet crosstalk.

Results: gp38 was abundantly but variably expressed in RA, and it was undetectable in normal synovial tissues. Among clinicopathologigal RA variables, significantly increased gp38 expression was only found in patients with lymphoid neogenesis (LN), and RF or ACPA autoantibodies. Cultured synovial but not dermal fibroblasts showed strong constitutive gp38 expression that was further induced by TNF-α. In RA patients, anti-TNF-α therapy significantly reduced synovial gp38 expression. In RA synovium, CLEC2 receptor expression was only observed in platelets. gp38 silencing in cultured SF did not modify their migratory and invasive properties but reduced the expression of IL-6 and IL-8 genes induced by SF-platelet interaction.

Conclusions: In RA, synovial expression of gp38 is strongly associated to LN and it is reduced after anti-TNF-α therapy. Interaction between gp38 and CLEC2 platelet receptor is feasible in RA synovium *in vivo* and can specifically contribute to gene expression by SF.

Editor: Kathleen Freson, University of Leuven, Belgium

Funding: This study was supported by Instituto de Salud Carlos III (FIS 12/439, RETICS RD12/0009 RIER, and Río Hortega program to R. F.), and Comunidad de Madrid (S2010/BMD2350, RAPHYME). The funders had no role in study design, data collection and analysis, decision to publish, or preparation of the manuscript.

Competing Interests: The authors have declared that no competing interests exist.

* E-mail: jlpablos@h12o.es

‡ These authors contributed equally to this work.

Introduction

Synovial fibroblasts (SF) are a heterogeneous cell population that represents the main resident cell component of synovial tissue. In rheumatoid arthritis (RA), SF expand and undergo phenotypic changes that contribute to the pathogenesis of chronic arthritis [1–3]. SF can respond to cytokines and, they maintain prolonged changes on the expression of genes involved in persistent inflammation and joint destruction in RA [4–6]. Crosstalk between SF and myeloid and lymphoid cell seems critical for persistent recruitment, survival and activation in chronic inflammation. These functions are associated to specific SF properties that resemble those of stromal cells in lymphoid tissues [7–10]. Lymphoid stromal cells play critical roles for the physiological trafficking and anatomico-functional compartmentalization of immune cells that supports normal immune responses [11,12].

Among the shared lymphoid and RA stromal features, the expression of the surface glycoprotein podoplanin or gp38 has been reported [12–14]. gp38 expression is normally restricted to lymphatic endothelium and in lymphoid organs, to stromal cells of the T-cell zone. Aberrant expression of gp38 in fibroblasts has also been observed in other pathological tissues where fibroblasts play diverse roles in cancer progression or fibrosis [12,15,16]. gp38(+) fibroblasts might emerge in inflammatory tissues due to either specific cell proliferation of local gp38(+) progenitors or to induced expression in gp38(−) fibroblasts by inflammatory cytokines [14,16,17]. In a murine model of experimental autoimmune encephalomyelitis, a gp38 antagonist reduced inflammation-associated lymphoid neogenesis (LN) pointing to additional functions for gp38 in inflammation, although the precise mechanism remains unknown [18].

In cancer epithelial cells undergoing epithelial-mesenchymal transformation, gp38 expression confers enhanced cell migration and tumour invasiveness, consistently with the observation of gp38 up-regulation on the invasive front of tumors [19,20]. In cultured lymphatic endothelium gp38 knockdown has also shown to reduce cell migration by regulating the activities of RhoA and Cdc42 GTPases [21]. This effect has been studied *ex vivo* and it seems mediated by indirect mechanisms of intracellular interaction between gp38 intracellular domains and ERM proteins ezrin and moesin that result in modification of small GTPase activities involved in cancer cell motility. Whether gp38 can modify cell motility in stromal cells of lymphoid organs or in inflammatory fibroblasts is not known.

The physiological and developmental functions of gp38 have been dissected in knockout mice. gp38 lacks intracellular signalling domains and its function seems to depend on its monogamous signalling receptor CLEC2. gp38 and CLEC2 knockout mice display an identical phenotype characterized by an embryonary defect in blood-lymphatic vascular separation [22–24]. In mice, CLEC2 is only expressed by platelets and some myeloid cell types, notably dendritic cells (DC) [25]. gp38 triggering of CLEC2 receptor induces platelet activation through Syk and SLP-76 signaling and this pathway seems critical for blood-lymphatic vessels partitioning during development [26,27]. Crosstalk between lymphoid endothelial cells and platelets involves CLEC2 receptor triggering by gp38 and the release of specific platelet mediators that induce paracrine effects on endothelial cells [27].

To analyze the significance of increased gp38 expression in RA, we analyzed its correlation with clinical and pathological variables of the disease in a series of RA synovial tissues, including serial samples obtained before and after anti-TNF-α therapy. We also investigated the function of gp38 in SF by mean of RNA interference in different models of cell migration and platelet interaction relevant to RA pathogenesis.

Material and Methods

Patients and synovial biopsies

Synovial tissues were obtained from arthroscopic biopsies from the knee of patients who fulfilled the American Rheumatism Association revised criteria for RA (n = 38) [28]. All patients had active disease characterized by inflammation of at least one knee joint. Patients characteristics at biopsy were recorded and are shown in Table 1.

Osteoarthritis (OA) synovial tissues were obtained by synovectomy at prostetic join replacement surgery (n = 15, age: 68±21, 60% female) and histologically normal synovial tissues were obtained from healthy individuals without joint disease at elective arthroscopy for minor traumatic lesions (n = 6, age 59±19, 60% female). In a subgroup of patients (n = 16), a second biopsy was obtained after at least 6 months of anti-TNF-α therapy. The study was approved by ethics committees of Hospital Clinic, Barcelona, and Hospital 12 de Octubre, Madrid, and a written informed consent was obtained from all patients.

Immunolabeling of cells and synovial tissues

Immunohistochemical (IHC) staining was performed using a standard indirect avidin-biotin peroxidase method (ABC standard; Vector Laboratories, Burlingame, CA, USA) and developed by diaminobenzidine chromogen. The following antibodies and matched isotype controls were used: anti-gp38 mAb (D2/40 IgG1 clone, Dako, Glostrup, Denmark) [29], anti-CD61 mAb (SZ21 IgG1clone, Immunotech, Marseille, France), and anti-CLEC2 polyclonal goat Ab (R&D Systems, Minneapolis, MN, USA). Pretreatments included 10 μg/ml proteinase K (Sigma-Aldrich Quimica SA, Madrid, Spain) for CD61 detection, and microwave heating in 1 mM EDTA pH 8 for gp38 and CLEC2 detection. Double CLEC2 and CD61 immunofluorescent labeling was performed using sequential incubation with anti-goat IgG Alexa-Fluor 488 (green) and anti-mouse IgG_1 Alexa-Fluor 594 (red) secondary antibodies (Invitrogen Molecular Probes, Eugene, OR, USA).

Synovial tissue sections were photographed and digitalized using a Spot RT CCD camera and Spot 4.0.4 software (Diagnostic Instruments, Sterling Heights, Michigan) on a Zeiss Axioplan-2 fluorescence microscope (Zeiss, Jena, Germany). gp38 immunoperoxidase stainned fractional area was quantified using ImageJ software (http://rsb.info.nih.gov/ij). IHC analysis and quantification of CD3, CD20 CD68, hsp47, CD31 in RA synovial biopsies as well as characterization of lymphoid neogenesis was performed as previously described [30,31].

Fibroblasts grown on glass coverslips were immunolabeled with anti-gp38 mAb (D2/40 clone, Dako). Detection was performed with goat anti-mouse IgG_1 Alexa-Fluor 594 labeled antibody and DAPI counterstaining. Photographs were obtained on a Zeiss LSM 510 META confocal microscopy (Zeiss).

Flow cytometric analysis of gp38 expression in cultured fibroblasts was performed with anti-gp38 mAb (clone 18H5, Santa Cruz Biotechnology Inc, Santa Cruz, CA, USA) [32] and goat anti-mouse IgG Alexa-Fluor 647 (Invitrogen Molecular Probes). Cells were analyzed on a BD FACSCalibur instrument (Becton Dickinson, San José, CA, USA).

SF cultures and lentiviral siRNA transduction of fibroblasts

SF and normal dermal fibroblast (DF) cultures were established by explant growth of small biopsy fragments in Dulbecco's modified Eagle's medium (DMEM) supplemented with 10% heat inactivated fetal bovine serum (FBS) (Lonza, Verviers, Belgium) and used after 3rd passage.

A small-interfering RNA (siRNA) targeting human gp38 and a scrambled non-silencing construction in pGIPz vector lentiviral were purchased from Open Biosystems (Thermo Fisher Scientific, Waltham, MA, USA). Lentiviral particles were obtained by co-transfection of 293T cells with pGIPz transfer vector, pPAX2 packaging vector, and pMD2-VSVg envelope vector as previously described [33]. Supernatants were harvested 48 hours after transfection, filtrated through a 0.45 μm filter and diluted 1/2 in DMEM medium for fibroblast transduction. Silencing efficiency was monitored by analyzing gp38 mRNA and protein expression by qRT-PCR and flow cytometry.

SF migration and invasiveness studies

SF migration was analyzed in wound-healing assays. Cells were grown to confluence on culture chambered coverglasses (Lab-Tek II 4, NUNC, Rochester, NY, USA) and a wound was made by a single scrape using a sterile pipette tip. The wound area was sequentially photographed at 0, 18 and 24 h. The area covered by

Table 1. Clinicopathological data of RA patients at biopsy.*

RA characteristics	
Age, years	60.6±12.5 [40–89]
Female	61.8%
RA duration, months	103.2±111.4 [4–441]
CD3+T cells/mm2	736±557 [9–2374] 2374 range]
CD20+B cells/mm	282±265 [2–1040]
CD68+cells/mm2	2267±1416 [45–1016]
DAS28	5.2±1.5 [2.34–8.35]
Lymphoid neogenesis positive (%)	63.9%
CRP (mg/dl)	3.5±2.8 [0.1–10.1]
Erosive disease	79.4%
RF positive†	61.2%
ACPA positive†	80.6%
Previous DMARD	100%
Previous anti-TNF-α	48.6%

*Quantitative data are expressed as mean±SD and [range]. CRP, C-reactive protein; DAS28, 28-joint Disease Activity Score; DMARD, disease-modifying antirheumatic drug; †RF>30 IU/ml; anti-citrullinated protein antibodies ACPA>50 IU/ml.

cells migrating into the wound area was determined using ImageJ software as the average closed area of the wound at 18 and 24 h after scraping.

The invasive capability of RA SF was analyzed using a matrigel coated transwell system (BioCoat Growth Factor Reduced Matrigel Invasion Chamber, Becton Dickinson). SF were resuspended in DMEM 0.1% BSA, plated on the upper chamber of the transwell insert (8 μm pores) and allowed to migrate through the matrigel matrix membrane for 4 days. DMEM with 10% FBS and 10% human serum was added to the bottom well and used as chemoattractant. The membrane was fixed with 4% paraformaldehyde and stained with DAPI for direct fluorescent microscopy. Ten random fields per membrane were photographed and digitalized and the number of cells per area was counted using ImageJ software.

The capacity of SF to invade cartilage was indirectly determined as the release of glycosaminoglycan (GAG) degradation products from cartilage SF cocultures. Fresh frozen human cartilage slices of fixed diameter and height (6×2 mm) were collected from cartilage obtained during joint replacement surgery for hip fracture and attached to 24-well plates. SF were dropwise added on top of the slices. After incubation for 3 h at 37°C and 5% CO_2, wells were filled with 1 ml DMEM 10% FBS. Supernatants were removed after 4 and 7 days of culture and GAG determined using Blyscan assay (Biocolor Ltd, Belfast, N. Ireland) according to the manufacturer's protocols.

SF platelet co-cultures

Platelets were isolated from peripheral whole blood in EDTA from healthy donors. Platelet-rich plasma (PRP) was obtained by centrifugation at 150 g at room temperature for 10 minutes. Platelets were pelleted, resuspended on DMEM and added to SF cultures at 1:1000 ratio (SF:Platelets). SF were seeded into 6-well plates in 1% FBS DMEM one day before platelet co-culture. Co-cultures were maintained at 37°C for 5 h. Cells and supernatants were collected for RNA and protein quantification. Parallel SF cultures without platelets were established and used as controls.

Quantitative Real Time-PCR (qRT-PCR) of RNA extracts from SF was carried out on Applied Biosystems 7500 Fast Real-Time PCR System using either Power Sybr Green PCR Master Mix or TaqMan Gene Expression assays (Applied Biosystems). The sequences of PCR primers used are listed in Table S1. For relative quantification, we calculated the amount of target gene normalized to the endogenous reference gene (β-actin) using $2^{-\Delta\Delta Ct}$ formula, where Ct is the mean of threshold cycle at which the amplification of the PCR product is first detected. We performed a previous validation experiment comparing the standard curve of the reference and the target to demonstrate that the primers efficiencies were approximately equal.

IL-6 concentration in supernatants from SF platelets co-cultures was determined by ELISA (Biolegend Inc, San Diego, CA, USA).

Statistical Analysis

Data were analyzed using Prism software v5.0 (GraphPad Software, San Diego, CA, USA). Results are expressed as mean±SD and means were compared by Student's *t*-test, Mann-Whitney U-test, and Wilcoxon tests as appropriate. Correlation between different numerical variables was analyzed by Spearman's or Pearson's tests as appropriate. Categorical variables were analyzed by Chi-square test. In all experiments, p value <0.05 was considered statistically significant.

Results

Clinicopathological correlates of gp38 expression in RA synovial tissues

To extend previous observations by Ekwall *et al* in advanced RA disease undergoing joint replacement [14], to RA patients biopsied at earlier stages, we performed quantitative IHC analyses in arthroscopic biopsies from a series of RA patients with active arthritis of the knee, heterogeneous regarding other characteristics of the disease (Table 1). Abundant gp38 expression was observed in synovial lining and sublining fibroblasts in RA biopsies (n = 38), whereas minimal expression was observed in OA (n = 15), and it was undetectable in normal synovial tissues (n = 6). In all RA

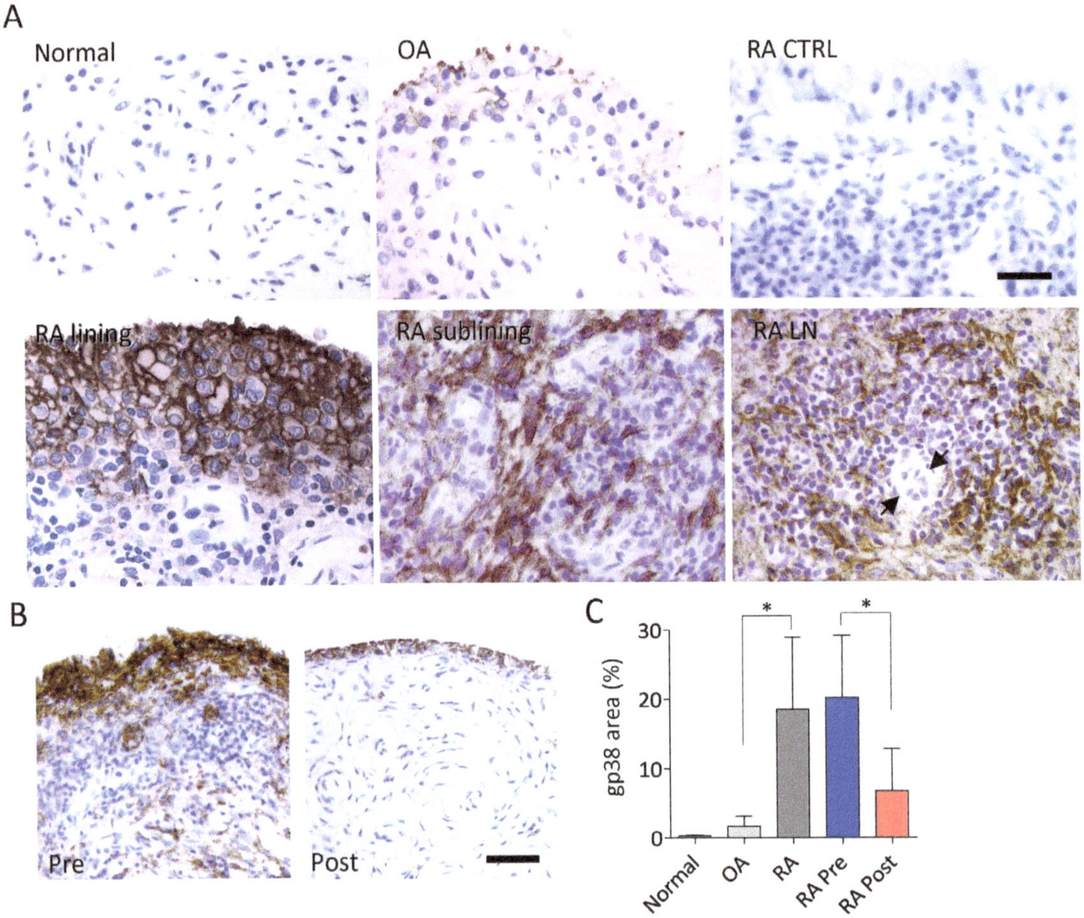

Figure 1. Expression of gp38 in synovial tissues. (A) IHC immunoperoxidase labelling of gp38 expression in normal, OA and RA tissues. RA CTRL: IgG1 isotype control. Lining and sublining areas, and a large lymphoid aggregate centered by a HEV (arrows) are shown. Bar: 50 μm. Original magnification 400x **(B)** Changes in gp38 expression after anti-TNF therapy. Representative imunoperoxidase labeling of gp38 of a single patient pre- and post-treatment. Bar: 100 μm. Original magnification 200x **(C)** Mean±SD gp38 immunostained fractional area in the different groups (OA vs RA Mann Whitney test *$p<0.0001$), and in basal (Pre) and post-anti-TNF-α therapy (Post) in 16 patients (RA Pre vs RA Post Wilcoxon matched-pairs signed rank test *$p<0.0001$).

tissues, gp38 was observed in lining cells, whereas in 54% of the cases it extended to sublining fibroblasts, and stromal cells within LN structures (Figure 1A). Lymphatic gp38(+) vessels were extremely rare in the superficial lining and sublining areas used for quantitative evaluation, but were readily observed in deeper tissues.

The level of gp38 expression in RA, expressed as the fractional labeled area, did not correlate with age, disease duration, activity evaluated as DAS28, C-reactive protein, macrophagic, T-cell or B-cell infiltration, and fibroblast or vascular density (data not shown). gp38 expression was found significantly increased in the group of patients (64%) with ectopic LN (Table 2). We also found significantly increased gp38 expression in the groups of patients with rheumatoid factor or anti-citrullinated protein (ACPA) autoantibodies compared to seronegative patients (Table 2). No correlation between LN and the presence of autoantibodies was found.

In a subgroup of 16 patients that initiated therapy with a TNF-α antagonist after biopsy, we analyzed the changes in gp38 expression after therapy. In synovial tissues obtained after 12.3±14.1 months of anti-TNF-α therapy, a significant reduction in gp38 expression compared to pretreatment tissues was observed (20.2±9.0% to 6.9±6.0%, $p=0.0001$) (Figure 1B). EULAR good or moderate responses [34] had been achieved in 12 of 16 patients at second biopsy. A lower decrease on gp38 expression in the second biopsy was observed in non-responders but the difference was not statistically significant.

gp38 expression and function in cultured fibroblasts

Cultured SF displayed abundant gp38 expression irrespective of their source (RA, OA or healthy synovium) but this was not a general feature of cultured human fibroblasts since DF did not show gp38 expression (Figure 2). Membrane expression of gp38 was also confirmed by labeling of unpermeabilized SF by flow cytometry and confocal microscopy (Figure 2). Treatment of cultured SF with TNF-α induced a significant up-regulation of gp38 mRNA and protein expression, as determined by qRT-PCR (data not shown) and flow cytometry (Figure 2). In cultured DF, TNF-α also induced gp38 mRNA and protein expression but to a lower extent compared to SF.

To analyze the potential role of gp38 on the cell behaviour of SF, we performed RNA interference experiments in cultured RA fibroblasts. In SF transduced with a lentiviral gp38-specific siRNA construct, a profound downregulation of gp38 mRNA and

Table 2. Clinicopathological correlations of gp38 expression* in RA synovial tissue.

RA variables	gp38 expression*	p value
RF(+/−)	20.1±10.6/13.0±7.9	0.0078
ACPA(+/−)	20.4±10.2/12.3±7.9	0.0450
LN(+/−)	21.9±10.4/10.6±5.6	0.0004
Erosive disease(+/−)	18.9±10.6/15.0±8.0	0.22
Earlier disease¶(+/−)	19.5±7.4/18.2±10.8	0.55

*Fractional immunolabeled gp38 area (%, mean±SD). RF, rheumatoid factor; ACPA; Anti-citrullinated protein antibodies; LN, lymphoid neogenesis. ¶Patients with RA duration less than 1 year. Mean±SD.

membrane protein was observed compared to control siRNA transduced SF (Figure S1A). Cell viability was similar in gp38 (82.51±15.29%) and control (84.09±11.88%) transduced cells.

Since the best described function of gp38 is a gain of function in cell migratory and invasive properties of epithelial cancer cells [19,20], we compared cell migration and invasive capacities of SF transduced with gp38 or control siRNA lentivirus. Cell migration through matrigel coated transwells was similar in gp38 silenced and control SF (Figure S1B). Invasion of wound area on plastic monolayer was also similar in gp38 silenced or control SF (Figure S1C), therefore excluding a relevant function for gp38 in cell adhesion and motility on matrigel or plastic surfaces in SF.

Previous studies have shown that RA SF attach and invade the cartilage causing degradation of the extracellular matrix. Therefore, to analyze the invasive capacity of SF in a model relevant to RA, SF were seed onto human cartilage slices [35,36]. Transduced RA SF expressing GFP and siRNA efficiently attached and invaded cartilage *ex vivo*, as observed by direct fluorescent microscopy, and induced an increase on GAG release to the media. GAG release at 4 and 7 days after SF seeding was similar in gp38 silenced compared to control RA SF, excluding an important role for gp38 membrane expression in this process (Figure S1D).

CLEC2 expression in RA synovial tissues

To identify expression of CLEC2 receptor in cells potentially interacting with gp38(+)SF, we performed IHC studies in RA synovial tissues. CLEC2 expression was only detected in small particles or aggregates lacking nuclei located in intra- and perivascular areas of the sublining area. In some cases, CLEC2 positive aggregates were associated to amorphous fibrin deposits attached to the lining surface. In these locations we demonstrated the presence of platelets by specific CD61 IHC (Figure 3). Double immunofluorescent labeling confirmed colocalization of CLEC2 and CD61(+) platelets (Figure S2).

Although IHC observations did not support CLEC2 expression by myeloid cells, to exclude lower levels of gp38 signalling receptor CLEC2 expression in human myeloid DC as recently described in murine DC [21], we performed western blot analysis of platelet and human DC under different maturation and activation status. Our data confirmed CLEC2 expression in platelet extracts but failed to detect CLEC2 in human DC (Figure S3). By flow

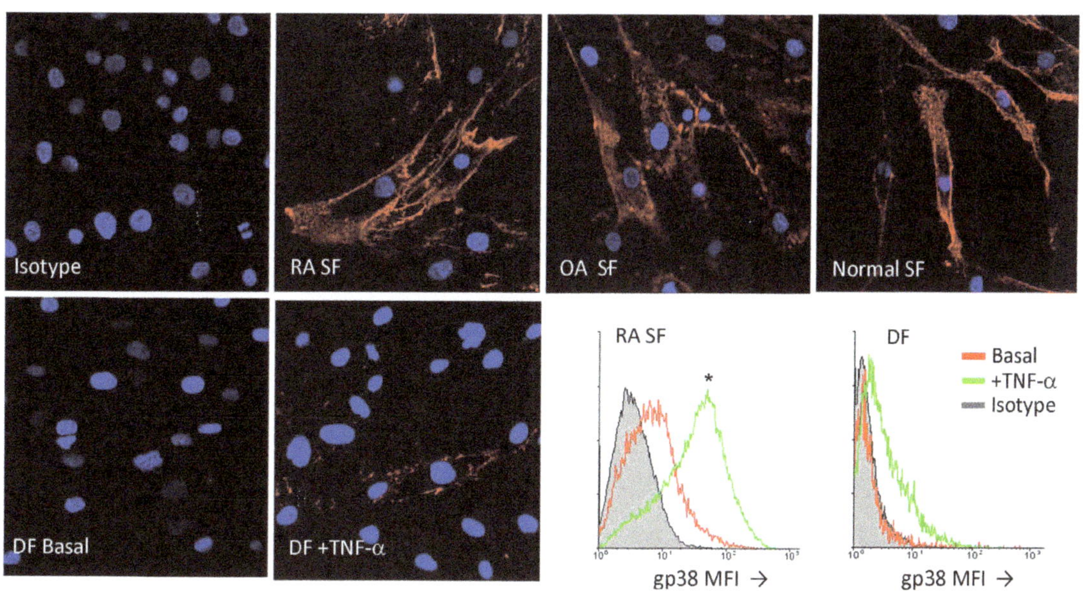

Figure 2. gp38 expression of cultured synovial fibroblasts. SF from RA, OA and normal synovial tissues, and normal skin dermal fibroblasts (DF) were cultured on glass coverslips and immunolabeled (red) for gp38 expression. TNF-α treated DF cultures are also shown (DAPI nuclear counterstaining). Flow cytometric detection of surface gp38 by in RA SF and DF untreated (basal) or treated with TNF-α for 24h. Data are representative of 6 SF and 3 DF lines (*p = 0.03 basal vs TNF-α treated). MFI: Mean fluorescence intensity.

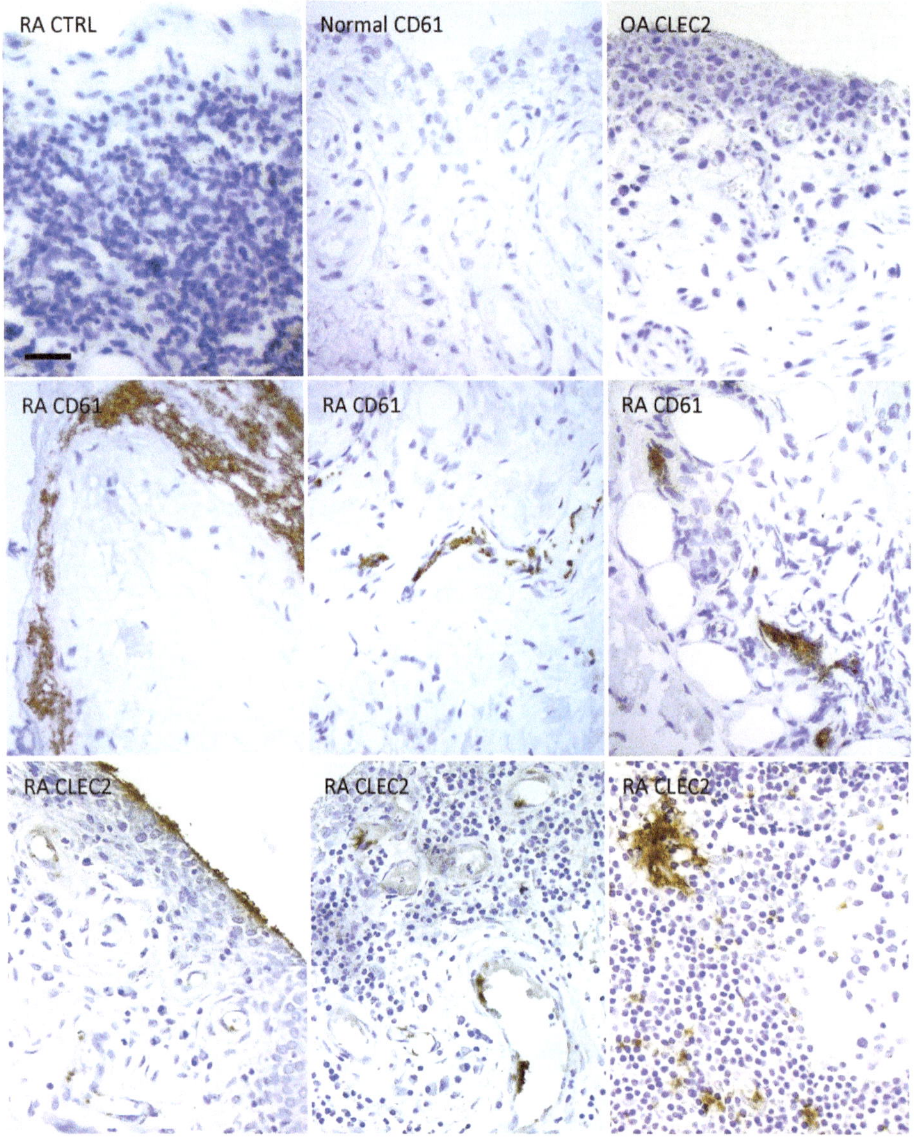

Figure 3. Detection of CLEC2 expression in synovial tissues. IHC immunoperoxidase labelling of CLEC2 receptor and CD61 (platelets) in OA, RA and normal synovial tissues as indicated. Non immune serum control for anti-CLEC2 IHC is also shown (RA CTRL). Bar: 50 μm. Original magnification 400x.

cytometry, we also failed to detect binding of gp38-Fc protein to mature or immature DC (data not shown).

gp38 function in fibroblast CLEC2 platelet interaction

Since CLEC2 was not detected in any other cellular element of RA synovium, we focused on platelet SF functional interactions to analyze the potential function of gp38 in this system. Gene expression of cytokines, chemokines and metalloproteinases factors previously associated to proinflammatory or tissue destructive functions of RA SF was analyzed in SF platelet co-cultures compared to parallel SF cultures in the absence of platelets. Platelet co-culture induced a strong increase in the expression of IL-6 and the chemokines IL-8, CXCL2 and CXCL3 mRNA (Figure 4A), whereas MMP (MMP-1, MMP-3 and MMP-9 mRNA) and LN stroma related factors were non-significantly increased (IL-7, CXCL13 mRNA) or decreased (CCL21 mRNA) (data not shown).

In platelet cocultured SF, gp38 silencing significantly reduced IL-6 and IL-8 mRNA expression, whereas CXCL2 and CXCL3 mRNA expression was not significantly modified (Figure 4A). Protein levels of IL-6 in the supernatant of SF platelet co-cultures were also significantly reduced in gp38 silenced SF compared to non-silenced controls (Figure 4B).

Discussion

Our data confirm that fibroblast gp38 expression is characteristic of RA inflammatory tissue, in contrast to normal synovial tissue, where it is undetectable. Interestingly, regardless *in vivo* expression, both normal and arthritic SF acquire similar membrane gp38 expression in culture. Therefore, exposure to growth factors and tissue culture conditions seem to induce gp38 in normal SF that do not express the protein *in vivo* but not in normal DF pointing to different tissue-specific fibroblast pheno-

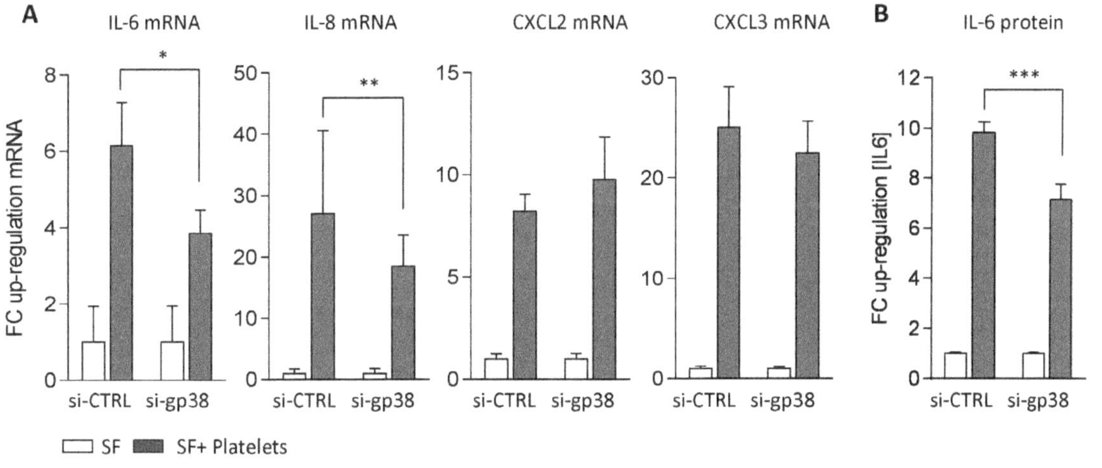

Figure 4. Expression of cytokines and chemokines in gp38 silenced RA SF platelet co-cultures. (A) Magnitude of the up-regulation on IL-6, IL-8, CXCL2 and CXCL3 mRNA expression induced by platelets and expressed as the ratio (FC) between SF and platelet co-cultures compared to parallel SF only cultures in gp38 siRNA silenced SF and non-silenced controls (si-CTRL) as measured by qRT-PCR. **(B)** IL-6 protein levels in supernatants of platelet cocultured gp38 siRNA silenced SF compared to non-silenced controls as measured by ELISA. Mean±SD data are representative of 3 independent experiments (*p = 0.0002, **p = 0.01, ***p<0.0001).

types. TNF-α and inflammatory cytokines may also induce gp38 expression in SF as previously reported [14] but again at much higher levels in SF compared to DF. Therefore, the higher capacity of SF to express gp38 represents a tissue specific property potentially relevant to their participation in joint specific inflammatory diseases. Recent studies have identified the proliferation of specific perivascular stromal precursors characterized by constitutive expression of gp38 and ADAM12 as the source of gp38 fibroblasts in different inflammatory mouse models [16,17]. We failed to detect perivascular gp38(+) cells in human healthy skin (data not shown) and normal synovium. This observation, together with the uniform acquisition of gp38 expression by cultured SF and its induction by TNF-α, suggest that growth factor or cytokine induced expression may underlie the observed gp38 stromal expansion in RA synovium. In addition, gp38 was significantly downregulated in patients treated with TNF-α antagonists further supporting this mechanism.

The expression of gp38 in RA tissues from patients with advanced destructive disease had suggested its potential role in structural damage [14]. We have also identified high gp38 expression in patients at earlier phases of the disease, excluding a correlation between disease progression and the level of gp38 expression and indicating that gp38 expression may be an early feature in RA. No significant correlations between the level of gp38 expression and most clinical or pathological RA features were found, with the striking exceptions of LN and RA autoantibodies positive groups. The finding of increased gp38 expression in patients with synovial LN, together with the previous observation of defective lymphoid development in gp38 deficient mice, point to a mechanistic link between both processes [18]. In several mouse models of inflammation also characterized by LN, the expansion of gp38(+) fibroblasts has been demonstrated [17]. The dependence of inflammatory LN on gp38 has been demonstrated in the mouse model of autoimmune encephalomyelitis, where anti-gp38 antibodies abrogated LN development [18]. However, the role of gp38(+)stromal cells is uncertain in that study, since gp38 expression and function was attributed to Th17 cells.

Whether ontogenic or pathological LN is dependent on functional gp38/CLEC2 receptor interaction is unknown. Such interaction is feasible in RA, where we observed both gp38(+) SF and CLEC2(+) platelets in the synovial tissue. Previous studies had also demonstrated the presence of abundant platelet microparticles in the synovial fluid of patients with RA ant their capacity to induce potent paracrine proinflammatory effects on SF [37,38]. Platelets respond to CLEC2 triggering by phosphorylating its cytoplasmic immunoreceptor tyrosine-based activation motifs (ITAM) which, in turn, recruits and activates tyrosin kinases Syk/Btk resulting in platelet activation. This process leads to the generation of platelet microparticles and the release of mediators stored in platelet granules such as IL-1 with potent paracrine effects on SF [27,38]. ITAM-dependent platelet activation may also be induced by GPVI receptor and therefore, both pathways might participate in platelet-stromal inflammatory crosstalk. CLEC2 specific effects, not triggered by GPVI receptor activation, have been proposed using CLEC2 deficient platelets but are difficult to dissect out in inflammatory models where platelet activation is required to maintain vascular integrity [27,39].

Our data confirm that platelet-SF co-culture induces strong changes in the expression of multiple genes by SF, similar to those induced by platelet microparticles [37,38]. Among these genes, IL-6 and IL-8 were specifically reduced by gp38 silencing in SF in contrast with other platelet-induced genes, providing evidence of a contribution of CLEC2 to proinflammatory platelet-SF crosstalk. IL-6 plays a pivotal role in RA pathogenesis and its therapeutic targeting is highly effective in modifying the course of the disease [40]. Although macrophagic cytokines IL-1β and TNF-α are also potent stimuli for IL-6 expression in RA SF, our and previous data suggest that platelets may also play an important role [37]. However, the link between this observation and the potential role of gp38 expression in rheumatoid LN is unclear. IL-6 has pleiotropic functions on lymphoid cells including the development of Th17 cells as well as T follicular helper and B cells involved in the development of orthotopic germinal centres in autoimmune arthritis but its influence on ectopic LN development is unknown [41-43]. We did not detect gp38 dependent changes on the expression of stromal factors associated to ontogenic or inflammatory LN such as IL-7 or lymphoid homing chemokines CXCL13 or CCL21 [10,44].

We failed to confirm an intrinsic role for gp38 in an *ex vivo* model of SF invasion and cartilage degradation, in contrast to that observed in cancer cells [19,20]. In cancer epithelial cells, gp38 is associated to EMT, a process that provides mesenchymal cell migratory properties to epithelial cells otherwise lacking motile or invasive capacity. It is therefore possible that gp38 does not provide these functionalities to fibroblasts which are highly mobile cells. An alternative explanation is that siRNA silencing of gp38 expression is not complete and remaining gp38 expression might be sufficient to maintain its function.

In conclusion, our study shows a new mechanism involved in platelet-SF proinflammatory interactions in RA synovium, supporting an important role for the acquisition of gp38 expression in SF. We also identify a strong association between gp38 expression and synovial LN, consistent with its reported role in developmental and experimental LN, but the mechanistic basis of this association requires further studies.

Supporting Information

Figure S1 Migratory and invasive capabilities of gp38 silenced RA SF. (A) Silencing efficiency of siRNA lentiviral transduction of RA SF as analyzed by qRT-PCR (si-CTRL mRNA gp38/β-actin ratio set to 100%) and flow cytometry (percentage of gp38(+) RA SF is indicated, *p = 0.03). MFI: Mean fluorescence intensity. **(B)** Invasive capability of RA SF on matrigel coated transwells expressed as the number of cells per field that migrated through the matrigel at 4 days. **(C)** SF migration in wound assays expressed as the percentual closure of the wound area 18 h and 24 h after scraping. A representative image is shown (100x). **(D)** GAG release into the supernatant at 4 and 7 days of RA SF cartilage co-culture. Basal: GAG release by cartilage in the absence of SF. A representative image of siRNA GFP transduced SF attached to cartilage is shown (200x). Results are representative of three independent experiments (NS: not significant).

Figure S2 Double CLEC2 and CD61 platelet labeling in RA synovial tissues. Double green (CLEC2) red (CD61) labeling with DAPI counterstaining is shown is shown in upper row as indicated. Controls (CTRL) including only anti-CLEC or only CD61 primary antibody and both secondary antibodies are shown in lower rows as indicated. Bar 20 μm.

Figure S3 Western blot analysis of CLEC2 expression. Platelets were obtained from healthy donors peripheral blood. Immature DC (imDC) were derived from buffy coat monocytes cultured for 7 days in complete RPMI medium containing GM-CSF (1000 U/ml) and IL-4 (1000 U/ml). For maduration, imDC were treated with LPS (1 μg/ml) or TNF-α (50 ng/ml) for 24 or 72 h respectively. Protein extracts (30 μg) are analyzed by western blotting with anti-CLEC2 polyclonal antibody (R&D Systems) or anti-β-actin mAb (Sigma), developed by peroxidase-conjugated secondary antibodies and ECL system.

Table S1 Primer sequences used for quantitative real-time PCR analysis.

Acknowledgments

We are grateful to the Servicio de Traumatología y Cirugía Ortopédica (Hospital 12 de Octubre) for providing normal and osteoarthritic synovial tissues. We also acknowledge Jordi Monfort (IMIM, Barcelona) for providing human healthy cartilage slices, and Vanesa Miranda and Juan Carlos Armas (Hospital 12 de Octubre) for excellent technical assistance.

Author Contributions

Conceived and designed the experiments: MJD RF JLP. Performed the experiments: MJD RF EI AU JLR ASF. Analyzed the data: MJD RF JDC JLP. Wrote the paper: MJD RF JLP.

References

1. Bartok B, Firestein GS (2010) Fibroblast-like synoviocytes: key effector cells in rheumatoid arthritis. Immunol Rev 233: 233–255.
2. Naylor AJ, Filer A, Buckley CD (2013) The role of stromal cells in the persistence of chronic inflammation. Clin Exp Immunol 171: 30–35.
3. Neumann E, Lefèvre S, Zimmermann B, Gay S, Müller-Ladner U (2010) Rheumatoid arthritis progression mediated by activated synovial fibroblasts. Trends Mol Med 16: 458–468.
4. Lee A, Qiao Y, Grigoriev G, Chen J, Park-Min KH, et al. (2013) Tumor necrosis factor α induces sustained signaling and a prolonged and unremitting inflammatory response in rheumatoid arthritis synovial fibroblasts. Arthritis Rheum 65: 928–938.
5. Müller-Ladner U, Kriegsmann J, Franklin BN, Matsumoto S, Geiler T, et al. (1996) Synovial fibroblasts of patients with rheumatoid arthritis attach to and invade normal human cartilage when engrafted into SCID mice. Am J Pathol 149: 1607–1615.
6. del Rey MJ, Izquierdo E, Caja S, Usategui A, Santiago B, et al. (2009) Human inflammatory synovial fibroblasts induce enhanced myeloid cell recruitment and angiogenesis through a hypoxia-inducible transcription factor 1alpha/vascular endothelial growth factor-mediated pathway in immunodeficient mice. Arthritis Rheum 60: 2926–2934.
7. Bradfield PF, Amft N, Vernon-Wilson E, Exley AE, Parsonage G, et al. (2003) Rheumatoid fibroblast-like synoviocytes overexpress the chemokine stromal cell-derived factor 1 (CXCL12), which supports distinct patterns and rates of CD4+ and CD8+ T cell migration within synovial tissue. Arthritis Rheum 48: 2472–2482.
8. Benito-Miguel M, García-Carmona Y, Balsa A, Bautista-Caro MB, Arroyo-Villa I, et al. (2012) IL-15 expression on RA synovial fibroblasts promotes B cell survival. PLoS One 2012, 7: e40620.
9. Lindhout E, van Eijk M, van Pel M, Lindeman J, Dinant HJ, et al. (1999) Fibroblast-like synoviocytes from rheumatoid arthritis patients have intrinsic properties of follicular dendritic cells. J Immunol 162: 5949–5956.
10. Manzo A, Paoletti S, Carulli M, Blades MC, Barone F, et al. (2005) Systematic microanatomical analysis of CXCL13 and CCL21 in situ production and progressive lymphoid organization in rheumatoid synovitis. Eur J Immunol 35: 1347–1359.
11. Bajénoff M, Egen JG, Koo LY, Laugier JP, Brau F, et al. (2006) Stromal cell networks regulate lymphocyte entry, migration, and territoriality in lymph nodes. Immunity 25: 989–1001.
12. Link A, Hardie DL, Favre S, Britschgi MR, Adams DH, et al. (2011) Association of T-zone reticular networks and conduits with ectopic lymphoid tissues in mice and humans. Am J Pathol 178: 1662–1675.
13. Farr AG, Berry ML, Kim A, Nelson AJ, Welch MP, et al. (1992) Characterization and cloning of a novel glycoprotein expressed by stromal cells in T-dependent areas of peripheral lymphoid tissues. J Exp Med 176: 1477–1482.
14. Ekwall AK, Eisler T, Anderberg C, Jin C, Karlsson N, et al. (2011) The tumour-associated glycoprotein podoplanin is expressed in fibroblast-like synoviocytes of the hyperplastic synovial lining layer in rheumatoid arthritis. Arthritis Res Ther 13: R40
15. Kawase A, Ishii G, Nagai K, Ito T, Nagano T, et al. (2008) Podoplanin expression by cancer associated fibroblasts predicts poor prognosis of lung adenocarcinoma. Int J Cancer 123: 1053–1059.
16. Dulauroy S, Di Carlo SE, Langa F, Eberl G, Peduto L (2012) Lineage tracing and genetic ablation of ADAM12(+) perivascular cells identify a major source of profibrotic cells during acute tissue injury. Nat Med 18: 1262–1270.
17. Peduto L, Dulauroy S, Lochner M, Späth GF, Morales MA, et al. (2009) Inflammation recapitulates the ontogeny of lymphoid stromal cells. J Immunol 182: 5789–5799.
18. Peters A, Pitcher LA, Sullivan JM, Mitsdoerffer M, Acton SE, et al. (2011) Th17 cells induce ectopic lymphoid follicles in central nervous system tissue inflammation. Immunity 35: 986–996.
19. Wicki A, Lehembre F, Wick N, Hantusch B, Kerjaschki D, et al. (2006) Tumor invasion in the absence of epithelial-mesenchymal transition: podoplanin-mediated remodeling of the actin cytoskeleton. Cancer Cell 9: 261–272.
20. Martín-Villar E, Megías D, Castel S, Yurrita MM, Vilaró S, et al. (2006) Podoplanin binds ERM proteins to activate RhoA and promote epithelial-mesenchymal transition. J Cell Sci 119: 4541–4553.

21. Navarro A, Perez RE, Rezaiekhaligh MH, Mabry SM, Ekekezie II (2011) Polarized migration of lymphatic endothelial cells is critically dependent on podoplanin regulation of Cdc42. Am J Physiol Lung Cell Mol Physiol 300: L32–42.
22. Schacht V, Ramirez MI, Hong YK, Hirakawa S, Feng D, et al. (2003) T1alpha/podoplanin deficiency disrupts normal lymphatic vasculature formation and causes lymphedema. EMBO J 22: 3546–3556.
23. Uhrin P, Zaujec J, Breuss JM, Olcaydu D, Chrenek P, et al. (2010) Novel function for blood platelets and podoplanin in developmental separation of blood and lymphatic circulation. Blood 115: 3997–4005.
24. Suzuki-Inoue K, Inoue O, Ding G, Nishimura S, Hokamura K, et al. (2010) Essential in vivo roles of the C-type lectin receptor CLEC-2: embryonic/neonatal lethality of CLEC-2-deficient mice by blood/lymphatic misconnections and impaired thrombus formation of CLEC-2-deficient platelets. J Biol Chem 285: 24494–24507.
25. Acton SE, Astarita JL, Malhotra D, Lukacs-Kornek V, Franz B, et al. (2012) Podoplanin-rich stromal networks induce dendritic cell motility via activation of the C-type lectin receptor CLEC-2. Immunity 37: 276–289.
26. Bertozzi CC, Schmaier AA, Mericko P, Hess PR, Zou Z, et al. (2010) Platelets regulate lymphatic vascular development through CLEC-2-SLP-76 signaling. Blood 116: 661-670.
27. Osada M, Inoue O, Ding G, Shirai T, Ichise H, et al. (2012) Platelet activation receptor CLEC-2 regulates blood/lymphatic vessel separation by inhibiting proliferation, migration, and tube formation of lymphatic endothelial cells. J Biol Chem 287: 22241–22252.
28. Arnett FC, Edworthy SM, Bloch DA, McShane DJ, Fries JF, et al. (1988) The American Rheumatism Association 1987 revised criteria for the classification of rheumatoid arthritis. Arthritis Rheum 31: 315–324.
29. Zimmer G, Oeffner F, Von Messling V, Tschernig T, Gröness HJ, et al. (1999) Cloning and characterization of gp36, a human mucin-type glycoprotein preferentially expressed in vascular endothelium. Biochem J 341 (Pt 2): 277–284.
30. Cañete JD, Celis R, Moll C, Izquierdo E, Marsal S, et al. (2009) Clinical significance of synovial lymphoid neogenesis and its reversal after anti-tumour necrosis factor alpha therapy in rheumatoid arthritis. Ann Rheum Dis 68: 751–756.
31. Izquierdo E, Cañete JD, Celis R, Del Rey MJ, Usategui A, et al. (2011) Synovial fibroblast hyperplasia in rheumatoid arthritis: clinicopathologic correlations and partial reversal by anti-tumor necrosis factor therapy. Arthritis Rheum 63: 2575–2583.
32. Schacht V, Dadras SS, Johnson LA, Jackson DG, Hong YK, et al. (2005) Up-regulation of the lymphatic marker podoplanin, a mucin-type transmembrane glycoprotein, in human squamous cell carcinomas and germ cell tumors. Am J Pathol 166: 913–921.
33. Zufferey R, Dull T, Mandel RJ, Bukovsky A, Quiroz D, et al. (1998) Self-inactivating lentivirus vector for safe and efficient in vivo gene delivery. J Virol 72: 9873–9880.
34. Van Gestel AM, Prevoo ML, van't Hof MA, van Rijswijk MH, van de Putte LB, et al. (1996) Development and validation of the European League Against Rheumatism response criteria for rheumatoid arthritis: comparison with the preliminary American College of Rheumatology and the World Health Organization/International League Against Rheumatism criteria. Arthritis Rheum 39: 34–40.
35. Neidhart M, Seemayer CA, Hummel KM, Michel BA, Gay RE, et al. (2003) Functional characterization of adherent synovial fluid cells in rheumatoid arthritis: destructive potential in vitro and in vivo. Arthritis Rheum 48: 1873–1880.
36. Pretzel D, Pohlers D, Weinert S, Kinne RW (2009) In vitro model for the analysis of synovial fibroblast-mediated degradation of intact cartilage. Arthritis Res Ther 11: R25.
37. Boilard E, Nigrovic PA, Larabee K, Watts GF, Coblyn JS (2010) Platelets amplify inflammation in arthritis via collagen-dependent microparticle production. Science 327: 580–583.
38. Hsu J, Gu Y, Tan SL, Narula S, DeMartino JA, et al. (2013) Bruton's Tyrosine Kinase mediates platelet receptor-induced generation of microparticles: a potential mechanism for amplification of inflammatory responses in rheumatoid arthritis synovial joints. Immunol Lett 150: 97-104.
39. Boulaftali Y, Hess PR, Getz TM, Cholka A, Stolla M, et al. (2013) Platelet ITAM signaling is critical for vascular integrity in inflammation. J Clin Invest 123: 908–916.
40. Genovese MC, Rubbert-Roth A, Smolen JS, Kremer J, Khraishi M, et al. (2013) Longterm Safety and Efficacy of Tocilizumab in Patients with Rheumatoid Arthritis: A Cumulative Analysis of Up to 4.6 Years of Exposure. J Rheumatol 40: 768–780.
41. Kopf M, Herren S, Wiles MV, Pepys MB, Kosco-Vilbois MH (1998) Interleukin 6 influences germinal center development and antibody production via a contribution of C3 complement component. J Exp Med 188: 1895–1906.
42. Choi YS, Eto D, Yang JA, Lao C, Crotty S (2013) Cutting edge: STAT1 is required for IL-6-mediated Bcl6 induction for early follicular helper cell differentiation. J Immunol 190: 3049–3053.
43. Victoratos P, Kollias G (2009) Induction of autoantibody-mediated spontaneous arthritis critically depends on follicular dendritic cells. Immunity 30: 130–142.
44. Timmer TC, Baltus B, Vondenhoff M, Huizinga TW, Tak PP, et al. (2007) Inflammation and ectopic lymphoid structures in rheumatoid arthritis synovial tissues dissected by genomics technology: identification of the interleukin-7 signaling pathway in tissues with lymphoid neogenesis. Arthritis Rheum 56: 2492–2502.

Bacteria in the Adventitia of Cardiovascular Disease Patients with and without Rheumatoid Arthritis

Samuel A. Curran[1], Ivana Hollan[2], Clett Erridge[3], David F. Lappin[1], Colin A. Murray[1], Gunnar Sturfelt[4], Knut Mikkelsen[5], Oystein T. Førre[6], Sven M. Almdahl[7], Magne K. Fagerhol[8], Carl S. Goodyear[9]*, Marcello P. Riggio[1]*

1 Dental School, University of Glasgow, Glasgow, United Kingdom, **2** Hospital for Rheumatic Diseases, Lillehammer, Norway, and Feiring Heart Clinic, Feiring, Norway, **3** Department of Cardiovascular Sciences, University of Leicester, Glenfield General Hospital, Leicester, United Kingdom, **4** Department of Rheumatology, Lund University Hospital, Lund, Sweden, **5** Hospital for Rheumatic Diseases, Lillehammer, Norway, **6** Department of Rheumatology, Oslo University Hospital, Rikshospitalet, Oslo, Norway, **7** Department of Surgery, University Hospital of North Norway, Tromsø, Norway, **8** Department of Immunology and Transfusion Medicine, Ullevaal University Hospital, Oslo, Norway, **9** Institute of Infection Immunity and Inflammation, University of Glasgow, Glasgow, United Kingdom

Abstract

The incidence of atherosclerosis is significantly increased in rheumatoid arthritis (RA). Infection is one factor that may be involved in the pathogenesis of both diseases. The cause of RA and atherosclerosis is unknown, and infection is one of the factors that may be involved in the pathogenesis of both diseases. The aims of this study were to identify bacteria in the aortic adventitia of patients with cardiovascular disease (CVD) in the presence and absence of RA, and to determine the effect of identified candidate pathogens on Toll-like receptor (TLR)-dependent signalling and the proinflammatory response. The aortic adventitia of 11 CVD patients with RA (RA+CVD) and 11 CVD patients without RA (CVD) were collected during coronary artery bypass graft surgery. Bacteria were detected in four samples from CVD patients and three samples from RA+CVD patients and identified by 16S rRNA gene sequencing. *Methylobacterium oryzae* was identified in all three RA+CVD samples, representing 44.1% of the bacterial flora. The effect of *M. oryzae* on TLR-dependent signalling was determined by transfection of HEK-293 cells. Although mild TLR2 signalling was observed, TLR4 was insensitive to *M. oryzae*. Human primary macrophages were infected with *M. oryzae*, and a TLDA qPCR array targeting 90 genes involved in inflammation and immune regulation was used to profile the transcriptional response. A significant proinflammatory response was observed, with many of the up-regulated genes encoding proinflammatory cytokines (IL-1α, IL-1β, IL-6, TNF-α) and chemokines (CCR7, IL-8). The aortic adventitia of CVD patients contains a wide range of bacterial species, and the bacterial flora is significantly less diverse in RA+CVD than CVD patients. *M. oryzae* may stimulate an proinflammatory response that may aggravate and perpetuate the pathological processes underlying atherosclerosis in RA patients.

Editor: Peter Szodoray, Institute of Immunology, Rikshospitalet, Norway

Funding: This study was funded a PhD scholarship from Medical Research Council (United Kingdom) and administered through the University of Glasgow. The funders had no role in study design, data collection and analysis, decision to publish, or preparation of the manuscript.

Competing Interests: The authors have declared that no competing interests exist.

* E-mail: Marcello.Riggio@glasgow.ac.uk (MPR); Carl.Goodyear@glasgow.ac.uk (CSG)

These authors contributed equally to this work.

Introduction

Premature cardiovascular disease (CVD), as a result of atherosclerosis, is the leading cause of mortality among rheumatoid arthritis (RA) patients [1]. The incidence of CVD is reported to be up to four-fold greater in RA patients, compared to age- and sex-matched controls [1–2]. Several traditional risk factors are common to both CVD and RA e.g. obesity, smoking, dyslipidaemia [3], however these cannot fully account for the increased CVD burden observed in RA [2], suggesting that alternative mechanisms are at least partly responsible.

Atherosclerosis and RA are both complex conditions with a strikingly similar autoimmune and inflammatory pathophysiology [4]. Elevated levels of activated T cells and B cells have been observed in both the RA synovium and the atherosclerotic lesion. The persistent 'high-grade' systemic inflammation manifest in RA has been suggested to contribute to the elevated atherosclerotic burden [3,5]. In RA, inflammatory markers are principally expressed in the synovial tissue. Consequently, a variety of over-expressed cytokines such as tumour necrosis factor-α (TNF-α), interleukin-6 (IL-6) and IL-1β, may enter the systemic circulation and alter numerous pathways that potentiate the onset of atherosclerosis [6].

Infection as a contributing factor to both atherosclerosis and RA has received much attention. To date, most studies have concentrated on *Chlamydia pneumoniae* as a possible aetiological agent in atherosclerosis [7]. However, several periodontal bacteria (*Porphyromonas gingivalis*, *Treponema denticola*, *Prevotella intermedia* and *Tannerella forsythia*) have also been isolated from atherosclerotic plaques [8,9]. Nevertheless, the potential aetiological roles of such bacteria are unknown. Furthermore, data from longitudinal cohort studies have demonstrated that patients with RA are at increased risk of developing infections compared to non-RA subjects [10], and that higher disease activity is associated with a higher probability of developing infections [11]. Moreover, elevated levels of calprotectin (a peptide with antimicrobial and pro-apoptotic effects that is predominantly produced by neutrophils) has been observed in RA serum [12] and atherosclerotic lesions [13]. Additionally, plasma levels of calprotectin in RA have been demonstrated to positively correlate with erythrocyte sedimentation rate, C-reactive protein (CRP) and IgM rheumatoid factor [14].

Accumulating evidence suggests that alterations to the host microbiome precedes RA and may play a key role in pathogenesis [15], however it is equally plausible that alteration to the microbiome follows RA and may lead to vascular co-morbidity. Intriguingly, RA patients exhibit elevated levels of T_H17 cells (and their signature cytokine, IL-17) in the serum and although normal levels of circulating regulatory T-cells are expressed, they exhibit decreased functionality *ex vivo* [16]. Conceivably, altered T cell functionality in parallel with the elevation of systemic pro-inflammatory mediators characteristic to RA supports a hypothesis of RA-driven dysbiosis and vulnerability to infection by a few select organisms.

A growing body of research supports a novel 'outside-in' hypothesis in which vascular inflammation is initiated in the aortic adventitia and progresses inwards to the luminal surface [17]. Furthermore, the aortic adventitia is an area of considerable immunological interest, exhibiting large areas of diffuse inflammatory infiltrate [18]. However, studies carried out to date have not identified potential immunological triggers. In the current study, we explore the hypothesis that the aortic adventitia contains potentially pro-atherosclerotic bacteria and that the microbiome is altered in patients with RA.

Materials and Methods

Subjects

The study was undertaken with prior approval of the Regional Ethics Committee for Medical Research (Feiring, Norway), and all patients gave written informed consent before participating. None of the patients were on antibiotic therapy prior to recruitment to the study, but were administered 2 g cefalotin intravenously 15 minutes before surgery.

Aortic samples were collected during coronary artery bypass graft (CABG) surgery of patients with RA (RA+CVD) and without RA (CVD). Study cohorts were enrolled at Feiring Heart Clinic, Feiring, Norway and were age- and gender-matched. All patients were screened for the presence of RA and were evaluated pre-operatively by a single rheumatologist to verify the rheumatologic diagnosis and to assess disease severity and activity. Inclusion criteria for the RA+CVD group were age older than 18 years, a confirmed diagnosis of RA according to accepted criteria [19] and absence of clinically significant malignancy and infection. Inclusion criteria for the CVD group were age older than 18 years and absence of inflammatory rheumatic disease, psoriasis and clinically significant malignancy and infection [18].

Collection of aortic biopsies

Part of the adventitia covered by the epicardium, from the ventral part of the ascending aorta in connection with the establishment of the proximal aortocoronary anastomoses, was collected as described previously [18]. To avoid thromboembolic complications, the anastomoses were established in areas with less pronounced gross signs of atherosclerosis. Biopsies were snap frozen at time of surgery and stored at −80°C prior to analysis.

DNA extraction from tissue samples

At all stages strict aseptic techniques were used. Tissue samples were homogenised on dry ice in 1 mL TRIzol (Invitrogen, Paisley, United Kingdom) using a TissueRuptor kit and sterile probe (Qiagen, Crawley, United Kingdom). 200 μL of chloroform was added, followed by incubation at room temperature for 15 minutes then centrifugation at 12x*g* for 15 minutes at 4°C. The aqueous phase was removed and the remaining interphase and organic phases were suspended in 300 μL of 100% ethanol and the sample centrifuged at 12x*g* for 5 minutes to pellet the DNA. The pellet was washed twice in 1 mL 100 mM sodium citrate before re-suspension in 1 mL 75% ethanol. This was then centrifuged at 12x*g* for 5 minutes at room temperature and the supernatant removed. The remaining pellet was dissolved in 100 μL of sterile water, and the DNA containing supernatant removed and stored at −20°C. Control samples containing sterile water instead of tissue were run in parallel to monitor for sterility of reagents and apparatus.

PCR amplification

PCR amplification of the 16S rRNA gene was performed using the universal primer pair 5′-CAGGCCTAACACATGCAAGTC-3′ (63f) and 5′-GGGCGGWGTGTACAAGGC-3′ (1387r), which amplified a 1325 bp segment of the 16S rRNA gene. PCR reactions were performed in a total volume of 50 μL containing 5 μL of the extracted DNA and 45 μL of reaction mixture comprising 1x GoTaq PCR buffer (Promega, Southampton, United Kingdom) 1.25 units GoTaq polymerase (Promega, Southampton, United Kingdom), 1.5 mM $MgCl_2$, 0.2 mM dNTPs (New England Biolabs, Hitchin, United Kingdom), and each primer at a concentration of 0.2 μM. Thermal cycling comprised one cycle of 95°C for 2 minutes, followed by 35 cycles of 95°C for 1 minutes, 60°C for 1 minutes and 72°C for 1.5 minutes, followed by a final extension cycle at 72°C for 10 minutes.

PCR quality control

When performing PCR, stringent procedures were employed to prevent contamination. Negative and positive controls were included with each batch of samples being analysed. The positive control comprised a standard PCR reaction mixture containing 10 ng of *Escherichia coli* genomic DNA instead of sample, whereas the negative control contained sterile water instead of sample. Each PCR product (10 μL) was subjected to electrophoresis on a 2% agarose gel, and amplified DNA was detected by staining with ethidium bromide (0.5 μg/mL) and examination under ultraviolet illumination.

Cloning of PCR products

PCR products were cloned into the StrataClone PCR cloning vector pSC-A-amp/kan (Agilent Technologies, Wokingham, United Kingdom) in accordance with the manufacturer's instructions.

PCR amplification of 16S rRNA gene inserts

Following cloning of the 16S rRNA gene products amplified by PCR for each sample, approximately 50 clones from each generated library were randomly selected. The 16S rRNA gene insert from each clone was amplified by PCR with the primer pair 5′-TGTAAAACGACGGCCAGT-3′ (M13 forward) and 5′-GAGCGGATAACAATTTCACACAGG - 3′ (M13 reverse).

Restriction enzyme analysis

Each re-amplified 16S rRNA gene insert was subjected to restriction enzyme analysis. 0.5 μg of each PCR product was digested in a total volume of 20 μL with 2.0 units of each of the restriction enzymes *Rsa*I and *Mnl*I (Fermentas Life Sciences, York, United Kingdom) at 37°C for 2 hours. Restriction fragments were visualised by agarose gel electrophoresis. For each library, clones were initially segregated into groups based upon their *Rsa*I restriction digestion profiles. Further discrimination was achieved by digestion of clones with *Mnl*I, and clones with identical restriction profiles for both enzymes were finally grouped together in distinct restriction fragment length polymorphism (RFLP) groups.

DNA sequencing

16S rRNA gene PCR products insert of a single representative clone from each RFLP group were sequenced. Sequencing was performed using the SequiTherm EXCEL II DNA Sequencing Kit (Cambio, Cambridge, United Kingdom) and IRD800-labelled 357f sequencing primer (5′-CTCCTACGGGAGGCAGCAG-3′). The following cycling parameters were used: (i) initial denaturation at 95°C for 30 seconds; (ii) 10 seconds at 95°C and 30 seconds at 70°C for 15 cycles. Formamide loading dye (6 μL) was added to each reaction mixture after thermal cycling and 1.5 μL of each reaction mixture was run on a LI-COR Gene ReadIR 4200S automated DNA sequencing system.

DNA sequence analysis

Sequencing data were converted to FASTA format and compared with bacterial 16S rRNA gene sequences from the EMBL and GenBank sequence databases using the BLAST program [20]. The program was run through the National Centre for Biotechnology Information website (http://www.ncbi.nlm.nih.gov/BLAST). Clone sequences that demonstrated at least 98% identity with a known sequence from the database were considered to be the same species as the matching sequence with the highest score. Clone sequences possessing less than 98% identity were classified as potentially novel phylotypes.

16S rRNA clone sequences have been deposited in GenBank with the following accession numbers:

BankIt1722590 SEQ1 KJ767741
BankIt1722590 SEQ2 KJ767742
BankIt1722590 SEQ3 KJ767743
BankIt1722590 SEQ4 KJ767744
BankIt1722590 SEQ5 KJ767745
BankIt1722590 SEQ6 KJ767746
BankIt1722590 SEQ7 KJ767747
BankIt1722590 SEQ8 KJ767748
BankIt1722590 SEQ9 KJ767749
BankIt1722591 SEQ1 KJ767750
BankIt1722591 SEQ2 KJ767751
BankIt1722591 SEQ3 KJ767752
BankIt1722591 SEQ4 KJ767753
BankIt1722591 SEQ5 KJ767754
BankIt1722591 SEQ6 KJ767755
BankIt1722591 SEQ7 KJ767756
BankIt1722591 SEQ8 KJ767757
BankIt1722591 SEQ9 KJ767758
BankIt1722591 SEQ10 KJ767759
BankIt1722591 SEQ11 KJ767760
BankIt1722591 SEQ12 KJ767761
BankIt1722591 SEQ13 KJ767762
BankIt1722591 SEQ14 KJ767763
BankIt1722591 SEQ15 KJ767764
BankIt1722591 SEQ16 KJ767765
BankIt1722591 SEQ17 KJ767766
BankIt1722591 SEQ18 KJ767767
BankIt1722591 SEQ19 KJ767768
BankIt1722591 SEQ20 KJ767769
BankIt1722591 SEQ21 KJ767770
BankIt1722591 SEQ22 KJ767771
BankIt1722591 SEQ23 KJ767772
BankIt1722591 SEQ24 KJ767773
BankIt1722591 SEQ25 KJ767774
BankIt1722591 SEQ26 KJ767775
BankIt1722591 SEQ27 KJ767776
BankIt1722591 SEQ28 KJ767777

Calprotectin immunohistochemistry.

Slides were prepared as previously described [18]. Briefly, citrate heat antigen retrieval was performed followed by blocking with 2.5% normal horse serum. Tissue sections were then incubated with monoclonal rabbit anti-human calprotectin primary antibody, or an isotype control, overnight at 4°C, followed by incubation with 0.5% hydrogen peroxide. Secondary HRP-conjugate secondary antibodies were incubated for 1 hour. Binding was visualised with ImmPACT DAB peroxidase substrate (Vector Labs, Peterborough, United Kingdom). Slides were counterstained with hematoxylin. The main negative control used was an isotype control antibody plus the secondary antibody.

Culture of Methylobacterium oryzae

Methylobacterium oryzae 18207^{T} was obtained from the DSMZ culture collection (DSMZ, Braunschweig, Germany) and cultured at 30°C in nutrient agar (0.5% peptone, 0.3% meat extract, 1.5% agar, pH 7.0).

Isolation and culture of CD14+ monocytes

CD14+ monocytes were isolated from human buffy coats using the EasySep positive selection kit (StemCell Technologies, Grenoble, France) in accordance with the manufacturer's instructions. Isolated cells were tested for purity by FACS analysis. CD14+ monocytes were then cultured for seven days at 37°C in 5% CO2 in RPMI-1640 medium (Sigma-Aldrich, Poole, United Kingdom) supplemented with 200 mM L-glutamine (Life Technologies, Paisley, United Kingdom), 10000 units Pen-strep (Life Technologies, Paisley, United Kingdom) and 10% foetal calf serum (Sigma-Aldrich, Poole, United Kingdom). CD14+ monocytes were differentiated into macrophages in the presence of 15 ng/mL human M-CSF (Peprotech, London, United Kingdom).

Primary macrophage challenge with *M. oryzae*, RNA isolation and cDNA synthesis

Macrophages were cultured until 70% confluence was achieved and then challenged with exponentially growing *M. oryzae* (multiplicity of infection 200) or vehicle control. Cells were harvested at four and eight hours post-infection and total cellular RNA purified using the RNeasy Kit (Qiagen, Crawley, United Kingdom). cDNA was prepared by reverse transcription of RNA (500 ng) using a High Capacity RNA-to-cDNA Kit (Life Technologies, Paisley, United Kingdom).

TaqMan mRNA analysis

Transcriptional activity of primary human macrophages following infection with *M. oryzae* was determined using Human Immune TaqMan Low Density Arrays (Life Technologies, Paisley, United Kingdom) in accordance with the manufacturer's instructions. 400 ng of DNase-treated cDNA was used in each sample. Gene expression was quantified using the comparative threshold (C_T) method with GAPDH as the endogenous control.

TLR transfection assay

HEK-293 cells were plated in 96-well plates at 8×10^3 cells per well and transfected after 24 hours using GeneJuice (Novagen, Watford, United Kingdom) with 30 ng of human TLR2, TLR4 (co-expressing MD-2), 30 ng pCD14, 20 ng renilla luciferase-reporter construct (pRL-TK) and 10 ng firefly luciferase-reporter construct driven by the NF*k*B dependent E-selectin promoter (pELAM) cloned into pGL3 (Promega, Southampton, United Kingdom). Cells were grown for two to three days post-transfection prior to 18-hour challenge. Reporter levels were normalised to co-transfected renilla luciferase and represented as fold induction relative to cells cultured in medium alone.

Results

Patient characteristics

The characteristics of each study population are shown in **Table 1**. The RA+CVD group had increased levels of inflammatory biomarkers i.e., CRP, history of myocardial infarction and use of oral steroids, Cox2 inhibitors and disease-modifying anti-rheumatic drugs. However, use of other medication was similar between the groups. Conversely, patients without RA (CVD group) had an increased familial history of CVD.

Evaluation of calprotectin in the aortic adventitia

Detection of calprotectin was conducted on 19 RA+CVD samples and 20 CVD samples. Immunohistochemical staining demonstrated that calprotectin was expressed in areas of mononuclear cell infiltration and was detectable in 8 of the 19 RA+CVD patients (42.1%) and 9 of the 20 CVD patients (45%) (**Figure 1**). There was no significant difference in either the number of patients expressing calprotectin or the intensity of calprotectin expressed across the two cohorts.

Molecular detection of bacteria in the aortic adventitia

16S PCR confirmed that 4 of 11 CVD and 3 of 11 RA+CVD patients had detectable levels of bacteria present in the aortic adventitia. A total of 273 clones from the seven 16S rRNA PCR-positive samples were subjected to RFLP analysis and a single representative clone from each RFLP group was sequenced. Subsequent NCBI BLAST gene alignments revealed a broad range of bacterial species. The bacteria identified in each of the 3 RA+CVD and 4 CVD 16S rRNA PCR-positive samples and their relative prevalence in each sample is shown in **Figure 2**.

The four samples from CVD patients contained 31 different bacterial phylotypes and the three positive samples from RA+CVD patients contained nine different bacterial phylotypes. This difference in the heterogeneity of bacteria between RA+CVD and CVD patients was statistically significant ($p<0.00001$).

In the CVD group the predominant species were uncultured *Stenotrophomonas* sp. (14.6% of clones analysed), uncultured eubacterium clone (12.9%) and *Haemophilus* sp. oral clone (12.9%). In the RA+CVD group the predominant species were *Methylobacterium oryzae* (44.1%), which was present in all three 16S rRNA PCR-positive RA+CVD samples, and uncultured *Stenotrophomonas* sp. (32.4%).

Effect of *M. oryzae* on TLR-dependent signaling

While whole *E. coli* and purified lipopolysaccharide (LPS) were able to stimulate nuclear factor kappa B (NFκB) signalling via TLR4 in transfected HEK-293 cells, whole *M. oryzae* failed to do so (**Figure 3**). However, *M. oryzae* was able to stimulate TLR2-mediated NFκB signalling albeit at a lower level than Pam3SK4 or whole *E. coli*. Subsequent hot phenol extraction followed by sodium dodecyl sulphate polyacrylamide gel electrophoresis confirmed the absence of the TLR4 ligands LPS and lipopolyo-ligosaccharide (LOS) in *M. oryzae* (data not shown).

Proinflammatory responses to *M. oryzae* infection in human primary macrophages

We have evidence that the human aortic adventitia possesses significant numbers of CD68$^+$ macrophages (Carl Goodyear, unpublished data). Although, macrophages express both TLR2 and TLR4 on their cell surface, a range of other non-opsonic pattern recognition receptors also support their recognition of pathogens. To further characterise the potential atherogenic role of *M. oryzae* we infected human primary macrophages and determined the relative expression of 90 genes involved in inflammation and immune regulation. Following four and eight hours of infection with *M. oryzae*, macrophages displayed an excessive pro-inflammatory response. After both 4 and 8 hours of infection, many of the up-regulated genes were those that encode pro-inflammatory cytokines (IL-1α, IL-1β, IL-6 and TNF-α) and chemokines (CCR7 and IL-8) (**Figure 4**), all of which have been

Table 1. Patient characteristics.

Characteristics	16S rRNA gene sequencing		Histology	
	CVD (n = 11)	RA+CVD (n = 11)	CVD (n = 20)	RA+CVD (n = 19)
Age, years	68±8	66±9	68±9	69±9
Males (%)	4 (36)	4 (36)	14 (70)	12 (63)
Current smokers (previous smokers)	0 (6)	2 (5)	1 (12)	2 (11)
CRP, mg/L	3.3±2	10±9	3±3	23±40
Duration of coronary artery disease, years	5.1±4	2.6±4	7.2±6.6	6.3±8.7
Time from angiography to CABG, days	6.7±8	9.7±8	31±60	17±30
Acute coronary syndrome (%)	1 (9)	4 (36)	4 (20)	9 (47)
Hypertension (%)	8 (72)	4 (36)	9 (45)	13 (68)

Demographic and clinical characteristics of patient from whom samples were analysed by histology and 16S rRNA gene sequencing. Where applicable, values represent mean ± SD.

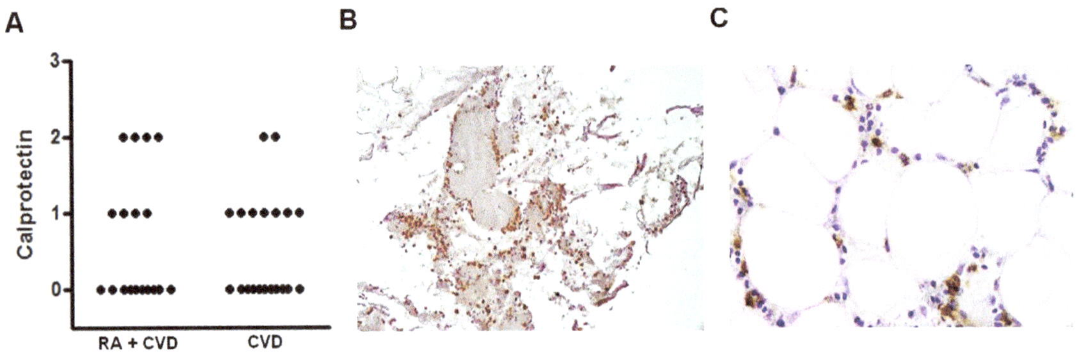

Figure 1. Calprotectin presence in the inflammatory infiltrate of the aortic adventitia of late stage CVD patients. (A) Immunohistological quantification of calprotectin in the aortic adventitia of RA+CVD (n = 19) or CVD (n = 20) patients. The number of inflammatory cells was counted and each section was scored according to the percentage of cells expressing calprotectin. 0, negative; 1, >0%<10%; 2, 10–25%; 3, >25%. Representative images show calprotectin staining within the inflammatory infiltrate at (B) 10x and (C) 40x magnifications.

implicated in RA and CVD pathogenesis. This inflammatory milieu may aggravate and perpetuate the pathological processes underlying atherosclerosis in RA patients.

Discussion

This novel study demonstrated the presence of bacterial DNA in aortic adventitia of patients with CVD. A mixed bacterial population was detected in the aortic adventitia in both RA+CVD and CVD patients, but it was less heterogeneous in the RA+CVD group. In RA+CVD, *M. oryzae* appeared in all samples positive for bacterial DNA presence. Further investigation confirmed that this bacterial species triggers a robust pro-inflammatory response by macrophages following infection. Taken together, these data suggest that the aortic adventitia environment is susceptible to microbial colonisation and that RA pathophysiology selects for specific bacterial species, or *vice versa.*

Atherosclerosis pathogenesis has been independently suggested to originate from both the intima and the adventitia, but is now recognised as a disease of the entire vessel [17]. However, an understanding of how the adventitial microenvironment functions

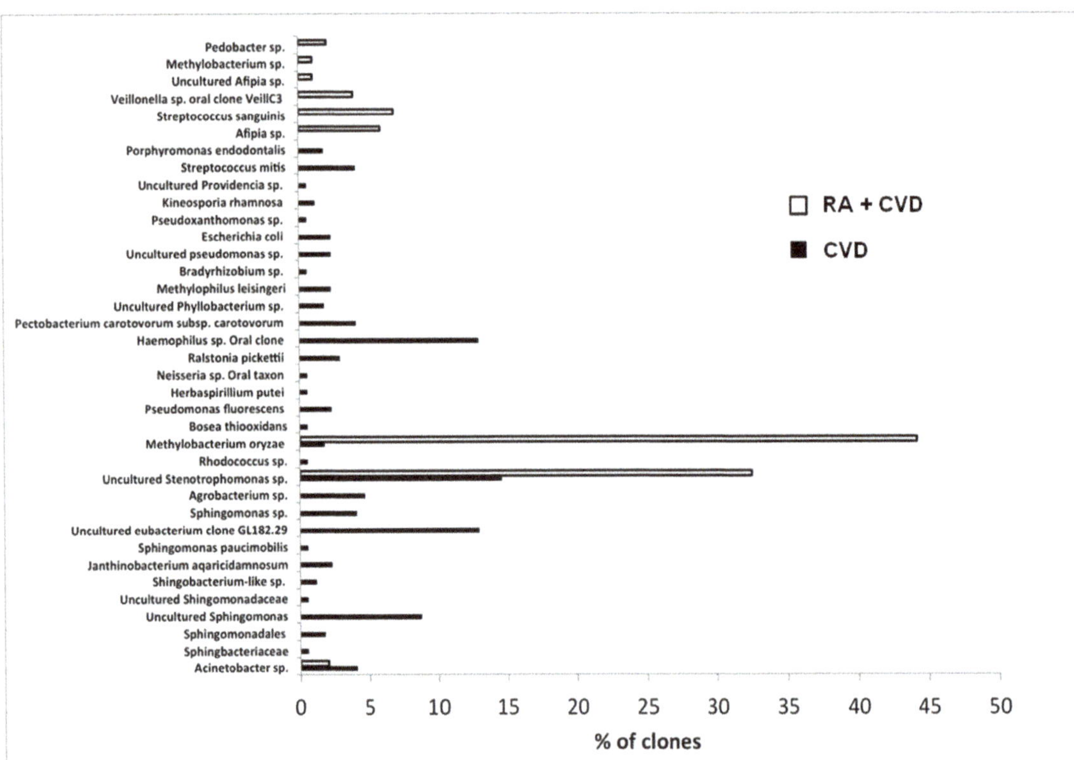

Figure 2. Bacterial species identified by 16S rRNA gene sequencing. Overall prevalence of bacterial species identified in all samples from the RA+CVD and CVD cohorts is shown. Bars depict the overall % of clones representing each bacterial species from the aortic adventitia of three RA+CVD patients (white bars) and four CVD patients (black bars).

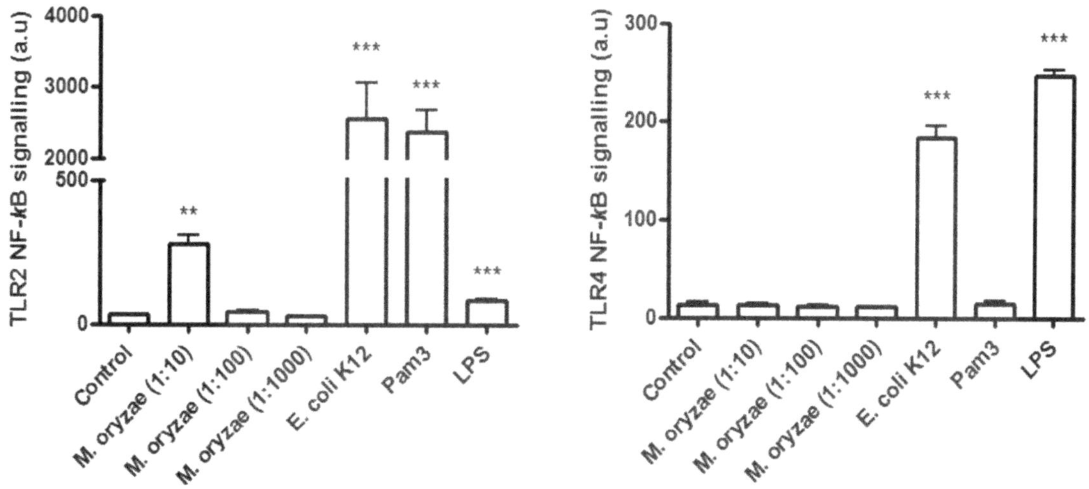

Figure 3. Effect of *M. oryzae* on TLR-dependent signaling. HEK-293 cells co-transfected with NFkB sensitive reporter (pELAM) and TLR2 and TLR4 were challenged for 18 hours with *M. oryzae* (1:10 dilution equivalent to 1×10^7 cells/mL), *E. coli* K12 (1×10^7 cells/mL), pam3CSK4 (10 ng/mL) and LPS (10 ng/mL). The vehicle control was treated with medium only. Arbitrary units (a.u.) represents mean fluorescent intensity of the reporter construct normalised to co-transfected renilla. Data are representative of three experiments ± S.D. $^{**}p<0.01$ vs. control; $^{***}p<0.001$ vs. control.

in atherosclerosis pathology and how co-morbidities such as RA influence this site has received little attention.

In the current study we demonstrate for the first time that the anti-microbial peptide calprotectin, an inflammatory biomarker released from neutrophils, is expressed within the human aortic adventitia of CVD patients with and without RA. Calprotectin is involved in inflammation and in the response to infection. Calprotectin-expressing monocytes identified in the ascending aorta of $ApoE^{-/-}$ mice have been suggested to regulate monocyte transmigration and endothelial activation [21]. Importantly, calprotectin expression resided in areas of diffuse inflammation within the adventitia. A number of potential triggers, including hypertension, lipoproteins, smoking and oxidative stress, are capable of inducing a vascular pro-inflammatory response, However, an interesting hypothesis is that infectious agents may play a role in atherosclerosis, either through a direct pro-inflammatory role on the vessel wall or through a less specific, systemic pro-inflammatory effect [22]. In theory, calprotectin may play a role in antimicrobial defence in the vessel wall.

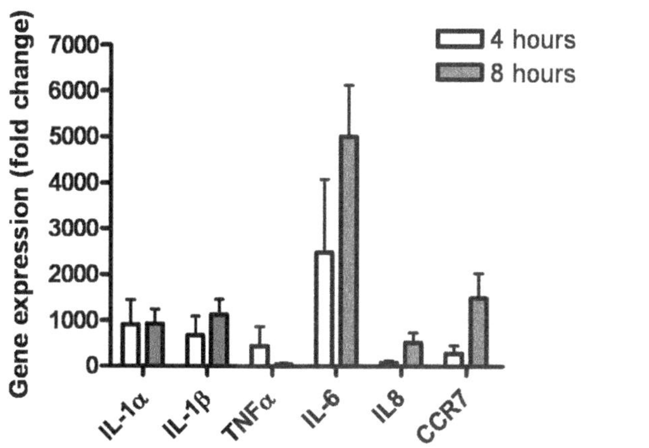

Figure 4. Response of human primary macrophages following *M. oryzae* infection. Primary macrophages were infected with exponentially growing *M. oryzae* (MOI 200) for four and eight hours. Each column represents the mean ± standard error of three experiments.

The ability of a diverse range of bacterial species to infect atherosclerotic tissue has been well documented [8,23,24]. However, it has been proposed that atherosclerotic tissue may act as a 'mechanical sieve' trapping bacteria present in blood circulation and that detected bacteria, although present, may have no pathological significance [24]. In contrast, our study was confined to the adventitia and was from areas of minimal macroscopic signs of atherosclerosis.

The current study supports the hypothesis that bacterial infection may contribute to the pathophysiology of atherosclerosis. The bacteria identified included an array of environmental and oral species. Most of these species have previously been reported as opportunistic or nosocomial pathogens. For example, members of the *Stenotrophomonas* genus, which were detected in both RA+CVD and CVD patients, have recently emerged as important opportunistic pathogens in debilitated individuals [25], and have been reported to infect immunocompromised individuals with increasing frequency [26]. *Stenotrophomonas maltophilia* has been demonstrated to cause blood-stream infections [27]. Furthermore, several species of *Stenotrophomonas* including *S. maltophilia*, express a protease (*StmPr1*) capable of breaking down fibrinogen, fibronectin and collagen [28], which could cause local tissue damage and as such may be a potential atherogenic trigger.

M. oryzae was detected in the adventitia of all three 16S rRNA gene-positive RA+CVD patients, and may act as a primary pathogen. However, eight samples did not appear to harbour bacterial DNA (as evidenced by a negative 16S rRNA PCR result). This could be due to bacteria being present at a level below that detectable by the standard PCR detection method used. It could be also be possible that bacteria contributed to disease pathology at a time prior to sampling. The occurrence of *M. oryzae* in vessels may occur in a patchy pattern and differs in segments of the vascular tree, thus it is possible that we did not detect all cases with *M. oryzae* in the aorta since we examined only a small aortic specimen and not the whole aorta. Alternatively, the pathology in these eight non-infected samples could be driven by other unknown mechanisms. Interestingly, *Methylobacterium* sp. has previously been identified in human aortic aneurysm samples

[29]. Although knowledge of *M. oryzae* is lacking, insight may be gained from considering its closest known relative, *M. mesophilicum* [30]. Interestingly, *M. mesophilicum* has been reported as a cause of opportunistic infections in immunocompromised hosts [31] and has been isolated from several clinical sites, including blood, synovial, and cerebral spinal fluid [32–34]. Although the source of infection remains unclear, infection has been associated with environmental exposure. In particular, *M. mesophilicum* contamination of hospital tap water has been implicated as the source of an isolated nosocomial outbreak [35].

Previous studies have demonstrated that TLR2 and TLR4 are the most abundant TLRs in human atherosclerotic lesions [36]. TLR2 mediates host responses to bacteria principally by recognition of the lipopeptides (e.g. PAM3), and TLR4 mediates host responses to bacteria by recognition of LPS. In the current study we demonstrated that although *M. oryzae* does not activate TLR4 signalling (due to non-detectable levels of LPS) and stimulates only mild TLR2 signalling, this bacterium can trigger an aggressive macrophage-mediated pro-inflammatory response that may potentiate atherosclerosis.

It has been suggested that RA patients exhibit a distinctive oral enterotype, characterised by the overabundance of a single and virulent *Porphyromonas* species [37]. It can be speculated that a reduction in oral bacterial heterogeneity may reduce the diversity of microbes entering the bloodstream. Furthermore, RA is characterised by a chronic systemic T-cell response [38–39] and increased expression of pro-inflammatory mediators and cytokines such as TNF-α, IL-17 and IL-1. This may explain the reduction in bacterial heterogeneity in the adventitia of RA+CVD patients observed in the present study. Conceivably, the increased systemic inflammatory state associated with RA may reduce the ability of certain bacteria to invade the body and enter systemic circulation, although this remains to be established. Also, anti-rheumatic treatment may contribute to an imbalance in the immune system, resulting in the different bacterial populations observed between RA+CVD and CVD patients.

Complement C2-deficient individuals have a high frequency of severe infections and systemic lupus erythematosus-like disorders [40]. Interestingly they also have a very high frequency of CVD, as has been shown for RA patients in our current study.

Although our current study is relatively small, it is still important as no similar studies have been performed earlier and, due to feasibility, studies on surgical vascular specimens in RA are often lacking or small [41].

In conclusion, our study suggests that bacterial colonisation of the aortic adventitia might contribute to the development of atherosclerotic disease. Furthermore, the immunological and pathological alterations that accompany RA may coincide with a reduced bacterial heterogeneity, allowing only a few select organisms to successfully colonise. One such organism may be *M. oryzae*. However, further studies are required to investigate a potential role for this microorganism in atherosclerotic pathology.

Author Contributions

Conceived and designed the experiments: MPR CSG CE SAC DFL CAM. Performed the experiments: SAC CE. Analyzed the data: SAC MPR CSG CE DFL. Contributed reagents/materials/analysis tools: CSG DFL MKF. Wrote the paper: SAC MPR CSG IH. Contributed clinical material: IH GS KM OTF SMA. Recruited patients: IH GS KM OTF SMA.

References

1. Solomon DH, Karlson EW, Rimm EB, Cannuscio CC, Mandl LA, et al. (2003) Cardiovascular morbidity and mortality in women diagnosed with rheumatoid arthritis. Circ 107: 1303–1307.
2. del Rincón I, Williams K, Stern MP, Freeman GL, Escalante A (2001) High incidence of cardiovascular events in a rheumatoid arthritis cohort not explained by traditional cardiac risk factors. Arthritis Rheum 44: 2737–2745.
3. Sattar N, McCarey DW, Capell H, McInnes IB (2003) Explaining how "high-grade" systemic inflammation accelerates vascular risk in rheumatoid arthritis. Circ 108: 2957–2963.
4. Snow MH, Mikuls TR (2005) Rheumatoid arthritis and cardiovascular disease: the role of systemic inflammation and evolving strategies of prevention. Curr Opin Rheumatol 17: 234–241.
5. Pearson TA, Mensah GA, Alexander RW, Anderson JL, Cannon RO, et al. (2003) Markers of inflammation and cardiovascular disease application to clinical and public health practice - A statement for healthcare professionals from the Centers for Disease Control and Prevention and the American Heart Association. Circ 107: 499–511.
6. Young JL, Libby P, Schönbeck U (2002) Cytokines in the pathogenesis of atherosclerosis. Thromb Haemost 88: 554–567.
7. Deniset JF, Cheung PKM, Dibrov E, Lee K, Steigerwald S, et al. (2010) *Chlamydophila pneumoniae* infection leads to smooth muscle cell proliferation and thickening in the coronary artery without contributions from a host immune response. Am J Pathol 176: 1028–1037.
8. Haraszthy VI, Zambon JJ, Trevisan M, Zeid M, Genco RJ (2000) Identification of periodontal pathogens in atheromatous plaques. J Periodontol 71: 1554–1560.
9. Toyofuku T, Inoue Y, Kurihara N, Kudo T, Jibiki M, et al. (2011) Differential detection rate of periodontopathic bacteria in atherosclerosis. Surg Today 41: 1395–1400.
10. Doran MF, Crowson CS, Pond GR, O'Fallon WM, Gabriel SE (2002) Frequency of infection in patients with rheumatoid arthritis compared with controls. A population-based study. Arthritis Rheum 46: 2287–2293.
11. Au K, Reed G, Curtis JR, Kremer JM, Greenberg JD, et al. (2011) High risk disease activity is associated with an increased risk of infection in patients with rheumatoid arthritis. Ann Rheum Dis 70: 785–791.
12. Hammer HB, Ødegård S, Fagerhol MK, Landewé R, van der Heijde D, et al. (2007) Calprotectin (a major leucocyte protein) is strongly and independently correlated with joint inflammation and damage in rheumatoid arthritis. Ann Rheum Dis 66: 1093–1097.
13. McCormick MM, Rahimi F, Bobryshev YV, Gaus K, Zreiqat H, et al. (2005) S100A8 and S100A9 in human arterial wall. Implications for atherogenesis. J Biol Chem 280: 41521–41529.
14. Brun JG, Haga HJ, Bøe E, Kallay I, Lekven C, et al. (1992) Calprotectin in patients with rheumatoid arthritis: relation to clinical and laboratory variables of disease activity. J Rheumatol 19: 859–862.
15. Wu H-J, Ivanov II, Darce J, Hattori K, Shima T, et al. (2010) Gut-residing segmented filamentous bacteria drive autoimmune arthritis via T helper 17 cells. Immunity 32: 815–827.
16. Valencia X, Stephens G, Goldbach-Mansky R, Wilson M, Shevach EM, et al. (2006) TNF downmodulates the function of human $CD4^{+}CD25^{hi}$ T-regulatory cells. Blood 108: 253–261.
17. Maiellaro K, Taylor WR (2007) The role of the adventitia in vascular inflammation. Cardiovasc Res 75: 640–648.
18. Hollan I, Scott H, Saatvedt K, Prayson R, Mikkelsen K, et al. (2007) Inflammatory rheumatic disease and smoking are predictors of aortic inflammation. A controlled study of biopsy specimens obtained at coronary artery surgery. Arthritis Rheum 56: 2072–2079.
19. Arnett FC, Edworthy SM, Bloch DA, McShane DJ, Fries JF, et al. (1988) The American Rheumatism Association 1987 revised criteria for the classification of rheumatoid arthritis. Arthritis Rheum 31: 315–324.
20. Altschul SF, Madden TL, Schäffer AA, Zhang J, Zhang Z, et al. (1997) Gapped BLAST and PSI-BLAST: a new generation of protein database search programs. Nucleic Acids Res 25: 3389–3402.
21. Eue I, Langer C, Eckardstein A, Sorg C (2000) Myeloid related protein (MRP) 14 expressing monocytes infiltrate atherosclerotic lesions of ApoE null mice. Atherosclerosis 151: 593–597.
22. Shah PK (2001) Link between infection and atherosclerosis. Who are the culprits: viruses, bacteria, both, or neither? Circ 103: 5–6.
23. Chiu B, Viira E, Tucker W, Fong IW (1997) *Chlamydia pneumonia*, cytomegalovirus, and herpes simplex virus in atherosclerosis of the carotid artery. Circ 96: 2144–2148.
24. Lehtiniemi J, Karhunen PJ, Goebeler S, Nikkari S, Nikkari ST (2005) Identification of different bacterial DNAs in human coronary arteries. Eur J Clin Invest 35: 13–16.
25. Looney WJ, Narita M, Mühlemann K (2009) *Stenotrophomonas maltophilia*: an emerging opportunist human pathogen. Lancet Infect Dis 9: 312–323.
26. Rolston KVI, Kontoyiannis DP, Yadegarynia D, Raad II (2005) Nonfermentative gram-negative bacilli in cancer patients: increasing frequency of infection and antimicrobial susceptibility of clinical isolates to fluoroquinolones. Diagn Microbiol Infect Dis 51: 215–218.
27. Park YS, Kim S-Y, Park SY, Kang J-H, Lee HS, et al. (2008) Pseudooutbreak of *Stenotrophomonas maltophilia* bacteremia in a general ward. Am J Infect Control 36: 29–32.

28. Windhorst S, Frank E, Georgieva DN, Genov N, Buck F, et al. (2002) The major extracellular protease of the nosocomial pathogen *Stenotrophomonas maltophilia*. J Biol Chem 277: 11042–11049.
29. Marques da Silva R, Caugant DA, Eribe ERK, Aas JA, Lingaas PS, et al. (2006) Bacterial diversity in aortic aneurysms determined by 16S ribosomal RNA gene analysis. J Vasc Surg 44: 1055–1060.
30. Madhaiyan M, Kim B-Y, Poonguzhali S, Kwon S-W, Song M-H, et al. (2007) *Methylobacterium oryzae* sp. nov., an aerobic, pink-pigmented, facultatively methylotrophic, 1-aminocyclopropane-1-carboxylate deaminase-producing bacterium isolated from rice. Int J Syst Evol Microbiol 57: 326–331.
31. Sanders JW, Martin JW, Hooke M, Hooke J (2000) *Methylobacterium mesophilicum* infection: case report and literature review of an unusual opportunistic pathogen. Clin Infect Dis 30: 936–938.
32. Gilardi GL, Faur YC (1984) *Pseudomonas mesophilica* and an unnamed taxon, clinical isolates of pink-pigmented oxidative bacteria. J Clin Microbiol 20: 626–629.
33. Kaye KM, Macone A, Kazanjian PH (1992) Catheter infection caused by *Methylobacterium* in immunocompromised hosts: report of three cases and review of the literature. Clin Infect Dis 14: 1010–1014.
34. Liu J-W, Wu J-J, Chen H-M, Huang A-H, Ko W-C, et al. (1997) *Methylobacterium mesophilicum* synovitis in an alcoholic. Clin Infect Dis 24: 1008–1009.
35. Gilchrist MJR, Kraft JA, Hammond JG, Connelly BL, Myers MG (1986) Detection of *Pseudomonas mesophilica* as a source of nosocomial infections in a bone marrow transplant unit. J Clin Microbiol 23: 1052–1055.
36. Edfeldt K, Swedenborg J, Hansson GK, Yan ZQ (2002) Expression of toll-like receptors in human atherosclerotic lesions: a possible pathway for plaque activation. Circ 105: 1158–1161.
37. Scher JU, Ubeda C, Bretz W, Pillinger MH, Buischi Y, et al. (2011) A distinctive oral microbiome characterizes periodontitis in patients with early rheumatoid arthritis. Arthritis Rheum 63 Suppl 10: S985–S986.
38. Weyand CM, Gorozny JJ (1999) T-cell responses in rheumatoid arthritis: systemic abnormalities-local disease. Curr Opin Rheumatol 11: 210–217.
39. Ma J, Zhu C, Ma B, Tian J, Baidoo SE, et al. (2012) Increased frequency of circulating follicular helper T cells in patients with rheumatoid arthritis. Clin Dev Immunol doi:10.1155/2012/827480.
40. Jönsson G, Sjöholm AG, Truedsson L, Bengtsson AA, Braconier JH, et al. (2007) Rheumatological manifestations, organ damage and autoimmunity in hereditary C2 deficiency. Rheumatol 46: 1133–1139.
41. Aubry MC, Riehle DL, Edwards WD, Maradit-Kremers H, Roger VL, et al. (2004) B-Lymphocytes in plaque and adventitia of coronary arteries in two patients with rheumatoid arthritis and coronary atherosclerosis: preliminary observations. Cardiovasc Pathol 13: 233–236.

12

Circadian Timekeeping Is Disturbed in Rheumatoid Arthritis at Molecular Level

Vesa-Petteri Kouri[1,2], Juri Olkkonen[1], Emilia Kaivosoja[1], Mari Ainola[1,3], Juuso Juhila[4], Iiris Hovatta[4,5], Yrjö T. Konttinen[1,3,6,7], Jami Mandelin[1,3,6]*

1 Department of Medicine, Institute of Clinical Medicine, University of Helsinki, Helsinki, Finland, **2** Department of Anatomy, Institute of Biomedicine, University of Helsinki, Helsinki, Finland, **3** Department of Medicine/invärtes medicin, Helsinki University Central Hospital, Helsinki, Finland, **4** Research Program of Molecular Neurology and Department of Medical Genetics, Haartman Institute, University of Helsinki, Helsinki, Finland, **5** Department of Mental Health and Substance Abuse Services, National Institute for Health and Welfare, Helsinki, Finland, **6** ORTON Orthopedic Hospital of the ORTON Foundation, Helsinki, Finland, **7** COXA Hospital for Joint Replacement, Tampere, Finland

Abstract

Introduction: Patients with rheumatoid arthritis (RA) have disturbances in the hypothalamic-pituitary-adrenal (HPA) axis. These are reflected in altered circadian rhythm of circulating serum cortisol, melatonin and IL-6 levels and in chronic fatigue. We hypothesized that the molecular machinery responsible for the circadian timekeeping is perturbed in RA. The aim of this study was to investigate the expression of circadian clock in RA.

Methods: Gene expression of thirteen clock genes was analyzed in the synovial membrane of RA and control osteoarthritis (OA) patients. BMAL1 protein was detected using immunohistochemistry. Cell autonomous clock oscillation was started in RA and OA synovial fibroblasts using serum shock. The effect of pro-inflammatory stimulus on clock gene expression in synovial fibroblasts was studied using IL-6 and TNF-α.

Results: Gene expression analysis disclosed disconcerted circadian timekeeping and immunohistochemistry revealed strong cytoplasmic localization of BMAL1 in RA patients. Perturbed circadian timekeeping is at least in part inflammation independent and cell autonomous, because RA synovial fibroblasts display altered circadian expression of several clock components, and perturbed circadian production of IL-6 and IL-1β after clock resetting. However, inflammatory stimulus disturbs the rhythm in cultured fibroblasts. Throughout the experiments *ARNTL2* and *NPAS2* appeared to be the most affected clock genes in human immune-inflammatory conditions.

Conclusion: We conclude that the molecular machinery controlling the circadian rhythm is disturbed in RA patients.

Editor: Oliver Frey, University Hospital Jena, Germany

Funding: This work was supported by the Academy of Finland, Finnish Society for Rheumatology, Finska Läkaresällskapet, ORTON Orthopaedic Hospital of the ORTON Foundation, Danish Council for Strategic Research, Scandinavian Rheumatology Research Foundation, Paulo Foundation, University of Helsinki, National Graduate School of Musculoskeletal Disorders and Biomaterials and Orion-Farmos Research Fund. The funders had no role in study design, data collection and analysis, decision to publish, or preparation of the manuscript.

Competing Interests: The authors have declared that no competing interests exist.

* E-mail: jami.mandelin@helsinki.fi

These authors contributed equally to this work.

Introduction

Endogenous circadian rhythm is maintained by the central circadian timekeeper, the suprachiasmatic nuclei of the hypothalamus. The clock machinery is composed of heterodimeric transcription factors and transcription regulatory proteins. The expression of these factors oscillates rhythmically over 24-hour cycles [1–3]. The rhythm of the central master clock is transferred to cells in the peripheral organs through hormonal and neuronal connections [2,4]. The de-synchronization of endogenous and geophysical time leads to fatigue as in jet lag. Altered circadian rhythm can cause e.g., cancer and obesity [5,6].

The molecular core of the circadian machinery is composed of transcription factors Aryl hydrocarbon Receptor Nuclear Translocator-Like (*ARNTL/BMAL1*) and Circadian Locomotor Output Cycles Kaput (*CLOCK*), which heterodimerize and activate transcription from E-box elements located in the promoters of clock controlled genes. Their paralogs *ARNTL2* (*BMAL2*) and Neuronal PAS domain-containing protein 2 (*NPAS2*), respectively, may functionally replace them. These transcription factors drive the expression of clock output genes, for example albumin D-box binding protein (*DBP*) but also their own repressors cryptochrome (*CRY1*, *CRY2*) and period (*PER1*, *PER2* and *PER3*) proteins. CRY and PER proteins form heterodimers and translocate to nucleus, in which they inhibit the function of DNA bound BMAL1:CLOCK heterodimer. Thus, CRY and PER proteins inhibit their own expression but also the expression of other clock controlled genes composing a negative regulatory limb of the circadian clock. RAR-related Orphan Receptor proteins RORs and REV-ERBs effect on the positive limb of circadian machinery. RORs bind into the promoter region and drive the expression of *BMAL1*. By competing of this binding site REV-ERBs inhibit ROR activity. This network of feedback loops affecting on the positive and negative sites around the core drives the usually extremely accurate self-sustained rhythmic expression of the circadian clock genes. Basic helix–loop–helix (bHLH) transcription factors *BHLHE40* (*DEC1*) and *BHLHE41* (*DEC2*) directly inhibit BMAL1:CLOCK by competing in binding of E-box elements in DNA. Thus, they form still another layer of the control mechanisms. This complex system of transcriptional regulation forms the molecular clockwork of the circadian timekeeper and creates the rhythmic expression of its output genes [1,2,4].

Rheumatoid arthritis (RA; MIM 180300) is a chronic inflammatory joint disease, a progressive destructive and debilitating arthritis caused by an invasive infiltrate composed of inflammatory cells and synoviocytes. Patients suffering from RA as well as other autoimmune diseases display blunted hypothalamic-pituitary-adrenal (HPA) axis reactions to inflammation [7], altered rhythm of circulating cortisol, melatonin and IL-6 levels [8,9]. Remarkably, up to 80% of patients experience chronic fatigue [10,11].

The function of T- and B-cells is perturbed in RA. This is seen e.g., in autoantibody production and in the fact that therapeutic targeting of either T- or B-cells is an effective treatment for RA. Interestingly, the same molecules that function in the intact clock controlling circadian rhythm e.g., rhythmic cortisol production [12] also control the development and function of immune cells. For example, *Dec1* deficient animals develop systemic autoimmunity [13], *Dec2* affects the development of Th2 cells [14], *Rorc* the development of Th17 cells [15] and *Rora* is a negative regulator of NF-κB signaling pathway [16].

It also appears that there are bidirectional links between the circadian time keeping and TNF-α production. For example, *Cry1/Cry2* deficiency in mice affects TNF-α production and exacerbates arthritis [17]. Conversely, TNF-α can alter the expression of clock genes and inflammation modifies the endogenous rhythm [18,19].

Because RA patients suffer from chronic fatigue, have immune cell dysfunction, and pathogenic production of TNF-α, all of which are affected by the molecular clock, we hypothesized that the circadian timekeeping is perturbed in RA. Thus, we analyzed the function of the circadian clock in RA patients and compared that to the function of clock in osteoarthritis (OA) patients, who have cartilage deterioration without autoimmunity and chronic fatigue. By doing so, we revealed clearly abnormal molecular clockwork in the synovial membrane tissue of the patients as well as in the cells derived from the synovial membrane.

Methods

Subjects

The research plan was approved by the ethical committee of the Helsinki University Central Hospital. Guidelines of the Declaration of Helsinki were followed. RA patients fulfilled the 1987 revised criteria of the American College of Rheumatology. Tissue samples (n = 10 for both RA and OA patients) were taken at 10 a.m. ±2 h during synovectomy or operation for total joint replacement. Samples were divided so that one half was formalin fixed and embedded in paraffin and the other half was immediately snap-frozen in isopentane precooled by dry ice and stored at −70°C.

Immunohistochemistry

Serial 3 μm thick paraffin tissue sections from the formalin fixed synovial membrane samples were stained using Bond MaX fully automated IHC and ISH Staining System (Leica Microsystems) using programs and Bond reagents for Dewax solution for deparaffinization, Epitope Retrieval solution 1 for antigen retrieval and Bond Polymer Refine kit for antigen detection. Briefly, slides were deparaffinised followed by one wash in absolute ethanol. Antigens were retrieved following endogenous peroxidase quenching. Sections were incubated in 1 μg/ml rabbit anti-MOP3 (anti-Bmal1; AB4140, Chemicon). Rabbit IgG at the same concentration was used for negative staining control. After secondary antibody containing the HRP polymer, color was developed using H_2O_2 and DAB. Between each step slides were washed at least three times. Finally, slides were dehydrated, cleared and coverslips were mounted using Mountex (Histolab).

RNA Isolation, cDNA Synthesis and Quantitative Real-time PCR

RNA was isolated using RNeasy Mini Kit according to the manufacturer's instructions. RNA concentrations were measured using NanoDrop ND-1000 instrument (Thermo Fisher Scientific). The cDNA synthesis was performed using 500 ng of total RNA and iScript™cDNA Synthesis Kit (Bio-Rad) in a 20 μl reaction volume. Quantitative real-time PCR was performed from 1:5 diluted cDNA in iQ™ SYBR® Green Supermix (Bio-Rad) using gene specific primers (Table 1) in 20 μl reaction volume. The PCR was performed in iQ5 real-time PCR detection system (Bio-Rad).

Cell Culture

Synovial fibroblasts from RA (n = 3) and OA (n = 3) patients were established using explant culture method. Tissue samples were cut into pieces with a sterile scalpel in a laminar flow hood. The explants were left overnight in RPMI-1640 medium (Lonza) containing 10% fetal bovine serum (Lonza) with 1000 U/ml penicillin and 0.1 mg/ml streptomycin (10×) solution. The next day, the media were changed to basal RPMI with 10% FBS media and 100 U penicillin and 0.1 mg streptomycin (1× solution). The medium was changed twice a week for 3 weeks. After roughly 80% monolayer confluence was reached, the explants were removed, and the cells were subcultured 1:3 until confluent. Passages 2–4 were used for subsequent experiments.

Clock Resetting with Serum Shock

The clock resetting in RA and OA fibroblasts was performed as reported earlier [20]. Briefly, cells were cultured in RPMI including supplements until ready for the serum shock. For the serum shock 150 000 cells were plated on 6-well plates. The cells were grown to confluence. At TIME = -2, the medium was replaced to RPMI containing penicillin/streptomycin and 50% horse serum (GIBCO). Samples to determine baseline were also collected at this point. After 2 hours, the medium was replaced with serum-free RPMI containing the antibiotics (TIME = 0). Exactly at the indicated times, the wells were washed with PBS and lyzed with 350 μl RLT lysis buffer (Qiagen). The lysates were stored at −70°C until RNA isolation was performed.

TNF-α and IL-6 Stimulation

OA fibroblasts were cultured in RPMI including supplements until ready for the stimulations. For the stimulations 80 000 cells were plated on 12-well plates. The cells were grown to confluence. Before stimulations the cells were synchronized with

Table 1. Primers.

Gene	GeneBank Accession	5′ Primer	3′ Primer	Length
BMAL1	NM_001178	CTGGAGAAGGTGGCCCAAAGAG	CCACTGGAAGGAATGTCTGGAGTC	250
ARNTL2	NM_020183	GCTAGAGGCTACCAGGCAAAACC	GGTCCACTGGATGTCACTGAAGTC	193
CLOCK	NM_004898	TTCTGCCTCTTCTCGGAGTTCAAG	CCTGGGTGGAGTGCTCGTATC	103
NPAS2	NM_002518	CTTCCCTGCCTCCCAACCATC	GGTCCCTGGCTGTTGTGAGTAG	151
BHLHE40	NM_003670	TCAGCAGCAGCAGAAAATCATTGC	GTGGGTGACAAGCTGCGAAGAC	187
BHLHE41	NM_030762	TGCTTTACAGAATGGGGAGCGATC	CCCTGGGTGTCCAGCTCTCAAAC	134
PER1	NM_002616	CTCCAATCAGGACGCACTTTC	GCTGCCAAAGTATTTGCTTGTG	211
PER2	NM_022817	TGTAGGGGCGGACTGCAAAC	TGCTGGTATGACTTGTGTCACTAC	251
PER3	NM_016831	TGAAGAATCCATCCCATCCTACTG	TATACTGCTGTCGCTGCTTCC	218
CRY1	NM_004075	TCTGGCATCAGTACCTTCTAATCC	CTGTGTGTCCTCTTCCTGACTAG	226
CRY2	NM_021117	GGTGAAGAACTCAGCAAACGG	ACACACATGCTCGCTCTATCTC	189
RORA	NM_134262.2	CCAGCCCCGACGTCTTCAAAT	GCCATGAGCGATCTGCTGACA	150
RORB	NM_006914.3	ACCGTTGCCAACACTGCCGA	GCTGGTGCTTCTGCACCTCA	126
RORC	NM_001001523.1	GGGCTGCAGCGAGCTCATCA	TCTCTTGGAGCCCTGGCCGA	134
NR1D1	NM_021724	CTTGGCTGCCCAGCGTCATAAC	CCAGATCTCCTGCACCGTTCG	274
DBP	NM_001352	CTTAAGCCCCAGCCAATCATGAAG	CCGCCCGCACCGATATCTG	160
IL-1β	NM_000576	TGGCAATGAGGATGACTTGT	GGAAAGAAGGTGCTCAGGTC	237
IL-6	NM_000600.3	AGGAGACTTGCCTGGTGAAA	GAGGTGCCCATGCTACATTT	329
β-act	NM_001101.3	TCACCCACACTGTGCCCATCTACGA	CAGCGGAACCGCTCATTGCCAATGG	295
PBGD	NM_000190.3	ACATGCCCTGGAGAAGAATG	AGATGCGGGAACTTTCTCTG	237
RPLPO	NM_001002	GGCGACCTGGAAGTCCAACT	CCATCAGCACCACAGCCTTC	149

18 hours serum starvation using RPMI containing penicillin/streptomycin and 1% fetal bovine serum. At TIME = 0, the media were replaced with RPMI media containing penicillin/streptomycin, 1% fetal bovine serum and TNF-α (10 ng/ml; R&D Systems), IL-6 (10 ng/ml; R&D Systems) or no cytokines (negative control). At the indicated times, the wells were washed with PBS and lyzed with 350 μl RLT lysis buffer (Qiagen). The lysates were stored at −70°C until RNA isolation was performed.

Statistical Analysis

The data from tissues were analyzed using Student's t-test and Pearson correlation test with SPSS 15.0 for Windows. The data from clock reset experiment were fitted to a sine wave equation, y(x) = BaseLine+Amplitude sin (frequency x+PhaseShift) in Matlab (The MathWorks Inc., Natick, MA, USA). The frequency was fixed to 24 hours. From IL-1β, IL-6 and Per1, the first time point (TIME = 0) was excluded from the fit, to avoid errors generated by the initial high expression peak caused by the stimulus. A Student's t-test was applied to determine, whether or not the phase, baseline (general expression level) or amplitude (peak expression) was shifted between RA and OA samples.

Results

Clock Gene Expression is Disturbed in RA Synovium

Driven by our hypothesis that the circadian timekeeping is perturbed in RA, we analyzed expression levels of clock genes in the synovial membrane of RA patients in comparison to OA patients. The expression levels of *BHLHE40* and *NR1D1* (*REV-ERBα*) were significantly increased in RA synovium compared to OA synovium (Figure 1a).

To overcome the variation of sampling time between individuals we reasoned that the best indication of the subjective (endogenous) time would be the correlation of the expression of *BMAL1* and *PER1*, which are normally in antiphase against each other. Due to the negative feedback loop, the peak expression of *BMAL1* and *PER1* should definitely not occur at the same time. Indeed, this was true in the control synovial membranes obtained from OA patients: high *BMAL1* expression coexisted with low *PER1* expression and *vice versa* (Figure 1). RA patients, in contrast, did not have this kind of anti-phase *BMAL1* and *PER1* expression (Figure 1). Similarly, high *ARNTL2* and *NPAS2* expression occurred simultaneously with the inhibitory clock components only in RA. Most striking was the significant positive correlation of *NPAS2* and *PER1* expression in RA (Figure 1), while it as expected was significantly negative in OA (Figure 1). Further, *ARNTL2* expression correlated positively with the expression of *CRY1* (.715; $p<0.05$), *CRY2* (.951; $p<0.001$), *PER2* (.862; $p<0.01$), *BHLHE40* (.936; $p<0.001$) and *BHLHE41* (.785; $p<0.01$) only in RA.

Ectopic Sub-cellular BMAL1 Protein Localization in RA Synovium

After revealing that the expression of clock genes is disturbed in the RA patients, we sought for confirmation to this observation on the protein level. We used immunohistochemistry to localize the limiting core clock component BMAL1 in the synovial tissues of RA and OA patients. The intense cytoplasmic BMAL1 protein staining in RA tissues draws attention to another major aberration. Not only are the phases of *ARNTLs* and *NPAS2* relative to *CRYs*

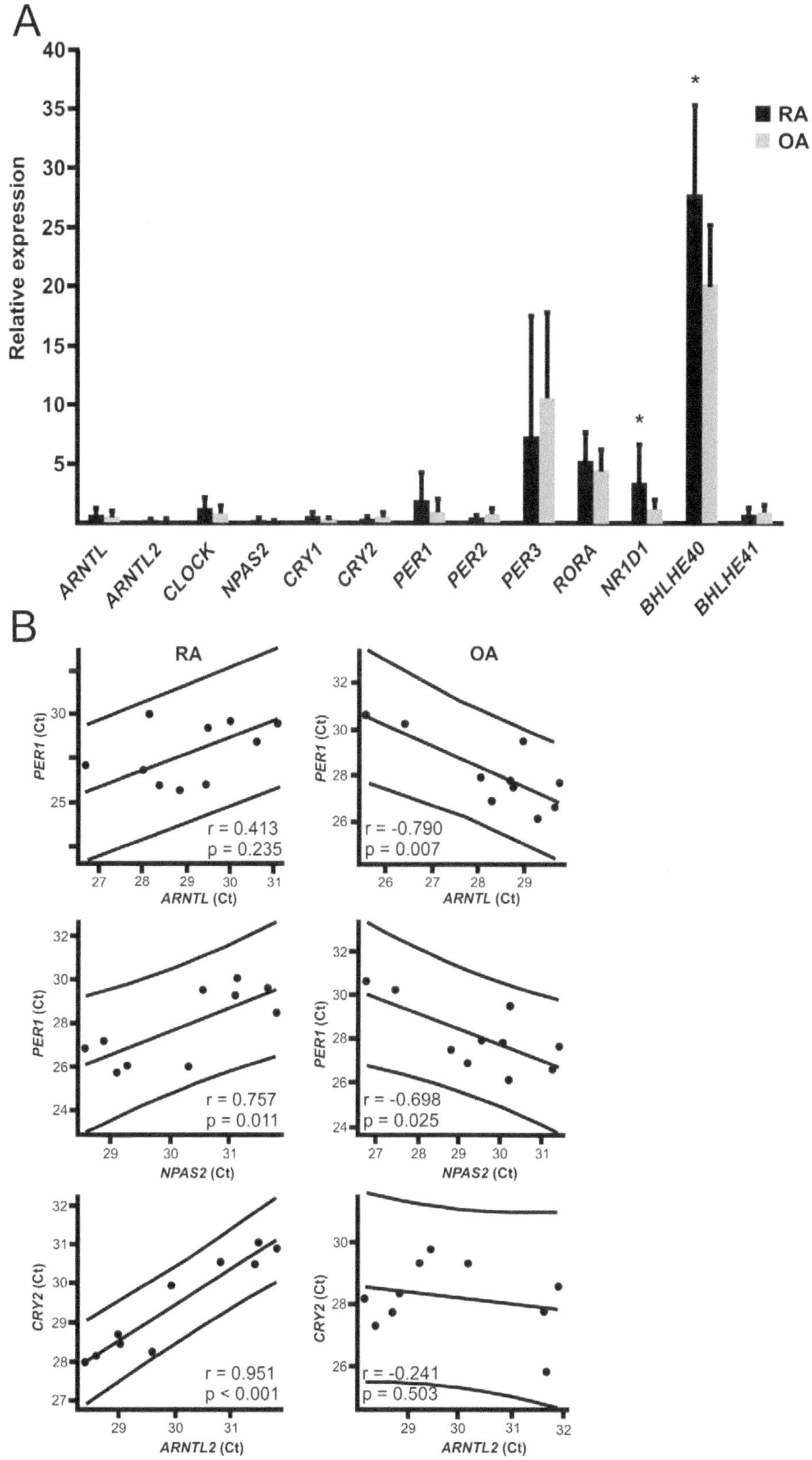

Figure 1. The expression of circadian genes in RA and OA patients. A. Synovial membrane samples were collected from RA and OA patients (n = 10 for each) and analyzed for circadian gene expression. The relative expression of each gene is expressed as mean ± SD. B. The expression of *BMAL1* and *PER1* should be in anti-phase. Pearson correlation and the linear fit for the expression of *BMAL1* and *PER1* in the synovial membrane of RA patients reveals that high expression of *BMAL1* correlates with high *PER1* expression and *vice versa*, low *BMAL1* expression correlates with low *PER1* expression. In contrast to synovium of RA patients, the high expression of *BMAL1* was associated with low *PER1* expression and conversely, low *BMAL1*

expression was coupled with high *PER1* expression in the synovial membrane of OA patients. Similar findings were observed with *NPAS2* and *PER1* as well as with *ARNTL2* and *CRY2*. Each dot indicates the Ct value of *BMAL1*, *NPAS2* or *ARNTL2* in the x-axis and *PER1* or *CRY2* in the y-axis in the synovial membrane sample of an individual patient. *p<0.05.

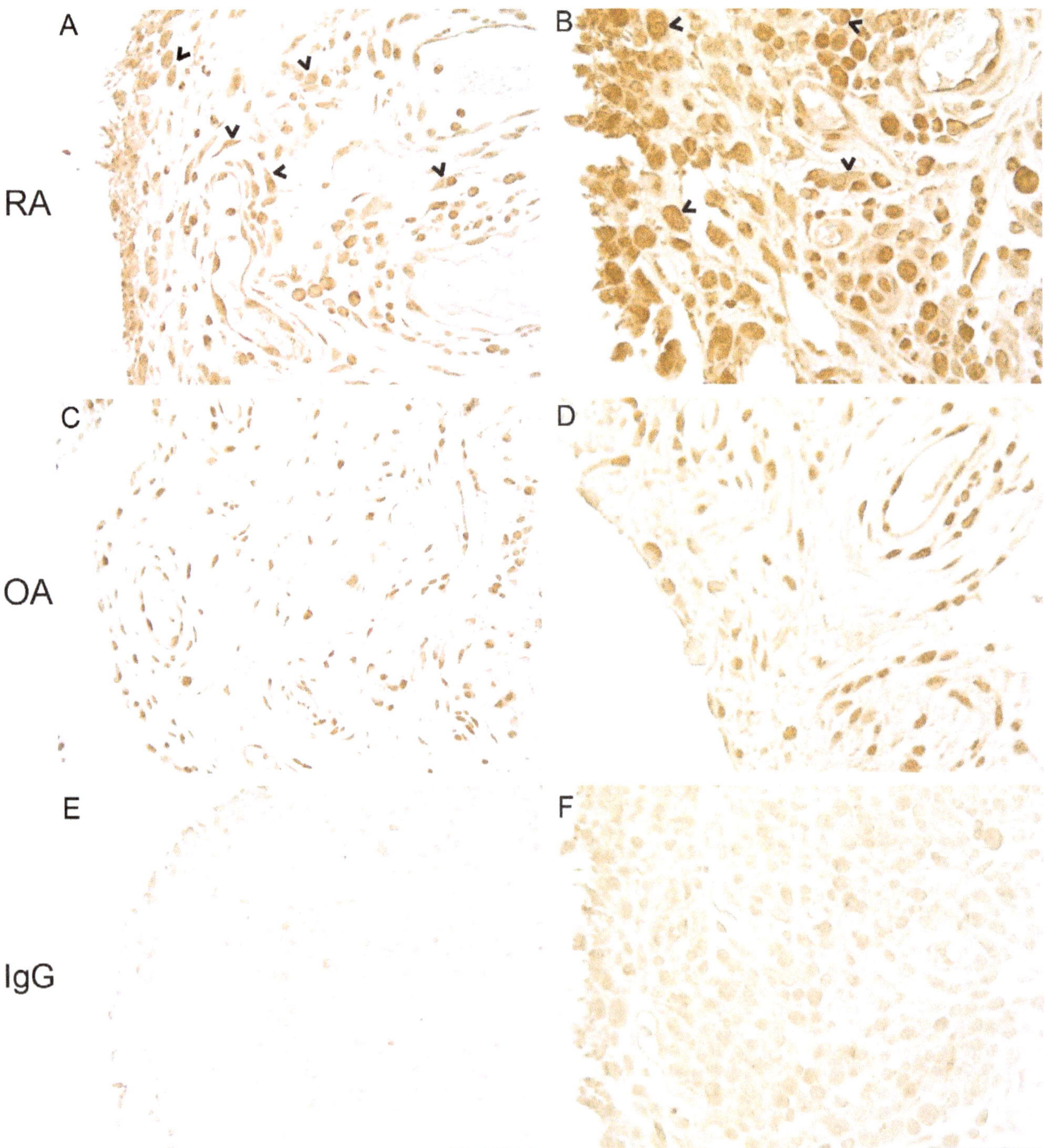

Figure 2. Localization of BMAL1 protein in RA and OA synovium. Tissue sections were incubated in rabbit anti-BMAL1 (anti-MOP3). In RA (A and B), relatively strong immunoreactivity was detected in the nuclei (arrows) of the immune cells and fibroblasts, but even stronger immunoreactivity was observed in the cytoplasm of the cells (arrowheads). In contrast to RA, BMAL1 protein was localized only in the nuclei (arrows) of OA synovium (C and D). Irrelevant rabbit IgG was used to confirm the specificity of the BMAL1 antibody (E and F). Scale bar 100 μm.

and *PER*s disturbed in RA, but this is also accompanied by ectopic localization of a core clock component (Figure 2).

Cell Autonomous Defect of Clock Function in RA

To rule out the possibility that inflammation, medication or some endocrine factors in the patients is the reason for the perturbed expression of circadian genes in RA synovium, we induced clock resetting with serum [20] in synovial fibroblasts isolated from RA and OA tissue samples. Immediately after resetting the expression pattern of *BMAL1* was delayed 0.5 hours ($p = 0.05$) in RA fibroblasts compared to OA fibroblasts, i.e. the expression of *BMAL1* in RA cells peaked 30 minutes later that OA cells. In addition to this, the expression level of *BMAL1* in RA cells never reached the level of OA ($p = 0.05$). The expression peak of *ARNTL2* was delayed 1.1 hours ($p<0.05$) and the level was throughout the experiment significantly lower ($p<0.05$) in RA cells compared to OA cells. Similarly, *CLOCK* expression was delayed 1.4 hours ($p<0.05$) in RA fibroblasts and the relative expression was constantly lower ($p<0.05$) in RA cells and *NPAS2* expression was delayed 1.9 hours ($p = 0.05$) but was constantly higher in RA fibroblast ($p = 0.01$) than in OA fibroblasts. Based on the delayed expression of the core clock, one would expect that the expression of clock driven circadian genes would lag in RA cells compared to OA cells. In contrast, the expression of *PER1* increased 0.5 hours earlier ($p = 0.05$), and the expression of *CRY2* was constantly higher in RA than OA cells after serum shock. Also *CRY1* expression increased earlier in RA cells than in OA cells, indicating that expression of the negative feedback loop is activated faster in RA than in OA. On the positive limb of the circadian machinery, *RORA* expression was 1.2 hours ($p<0.05$) ahead and constantly higher ($p = 0.01$) in RA cells than in OA cells, and *NR1D1* expression was exactly the same in both cell types (Figure 3). *RORB* and *RORC* were not expressed.

Altered Circadian IL-1β and IL-6 Expression in RA Fibroblasts

RA patients display altered circadian hormonal and cytokine profiles. For example, the circulating concentration of IL-6 in RA patients differs from that of healthy individuals [8]. We tested the possibility that the perturbed clock function is also reflected in disturbed *IL-6* expression after clock resetting. Fibroblasts derived from RA displayed significantly weaker rhythmic expression of *IL-6* after clock resetting than cells from OA synovium (Figure 4). Both the general expression as well as the peak expression was higher in OA cells ($p<0.05$ for both). Because of this observation, we analyzed if this is the case also for *IL-1β* or *TNF-α* expression, which are also rhythmically produced pro-inflammatory cytokines [21,22]. Similar to *IL-6* expression, RA fibroblasts displayed significantly weaker rhythmic expression of *IL-1β* than OA fibroblasts ($p<0.05$) Also *TNF-α* expression was rhythmic over time. In contrast to the expression of *IL-1β* and *IL-6*, the general expression level of *TNF-α* was higher ($p = 0.05$) in RA cells than in OA cells. Like in the expression of *IL-1β*, both the phase ($p<0.05$) and the amplitude ($p<0.05$) in *TNF-α* expression were different between the cells derived from RA and OA synovium (Figure 4) confirming the near absent and misaligned self-sustained rhythmic expression of pro-inflammatory cytokines in RA cells.

Inflammation Changes the Expression of Clock Genes In Vitro

Due to the bidirectionally maintained control of clock and inflammation, we investigated the effect TNF-α on human fibroblasts. A strong response in the expression of *IL-1β* (Figure 5) was evident confirming the effect of TNF-α on the cells. The most significantly affected clock genes after stimulation with TNF-α were *ARNTL2* and *NPAS2*. Unlike earlier observations in mouse cells [18], TNF-α did not affect the expression of *PER1*. However, the inhibitory (anti-phase) effect of TNF-α on the expression of clock controlled genes *DBP* and *PER3* was clear (Figure 5). IL-6 did not markedly alter the expression of clock genes.

Discussion

Abnormal fatigue, morning stiffness and altered circadian hormone and cytokine production suggest that the internal neuroimmunoendocrine milieu and the activity of daily living may be desynchronized in RA patients [7,8,10] i.e., the body is adjusted for activity (subjective day) during sleep (geophysical night), but meets the challenges of the day when geared for sleep and rest. Central molecular clock in the hypothalamus normally synchronizes body functions and entrains the circadian clocks in all cells of the peripheral tissues [2,4]. According to our findings the clock is dysfunctional in the joints of RA patients. Our results suggest that inflammation may initially disturb circadian timekeeping and that a cell autonomous defect prevents accurate clock function in the synovial fibroblasts of RA patients.

The variation in the expression of circadian genes at a defined and very narrow time point used for sample collection was evident between different individuals. Due to the characteristic oscillation of the expression of clock genes [1–3] leading to individual sleeping habits of each subject this was expected. To overcome the problem, we utilized the characteristic property of the clock and analyzed the endogenous (subjective) time using the expected anti-phase expression of inhibitory circadian genes in RA synovium and in OA synovium, i.e. checked the circadian time. This anti-phase expression of inhibitory circadian components, which forms the very basis for the circadian timekeeping, was totally lost in RA synovium i.e., the endogenous circadian time is clearly perturbed in the synovial membrane tissue of RA patients.

The perturbed expression of the machinery is also reflected in the amount and sub-cellular localization of BMAL1 protein. Apparently, there is much higher levels of BMAL1 protein in RA than OA while at RNA levels the difference is not significant. Of the core clock genes the expression of *BMAL1* varies the most during the day. Due to this oscillation of the expression, however, we may have not detected the highest differences in the gene expression. The most dramatic differences in the gene expression may well be seen at different time points whereas the amount of protein in the tissue may reflect the differences in the expression or different kinetics in the posttranslational mechanisms that regulate the degradation of the core clock proteins [23,24]. This may well explain why the gene expression and protein amounts do not correlate. However, the result reinforces the finding of a disturbed clock in RA tissue.

RA patients suffer from chronic inflammation and altered glucocorticoid signaling, both of which affect the circadian timekeeping effectively [18,25]. Thus, these factors or medication might explain altered clock gene expression in the synovium of RA patients. This possibility was excluded using cultured synovial fibroblast derived from RA and OA patients. Clock gene oscillation in fibroblasts can be started with serum, which activates several intracellular pathways. Due to the intrinsic character of the clock the cells maintain the rhythm several days without any external time cues and further activation of the signaling pathways [20]. This phenomenon thus reflects the normal function of the endogenous timekeeping molecular machinery. Using this system

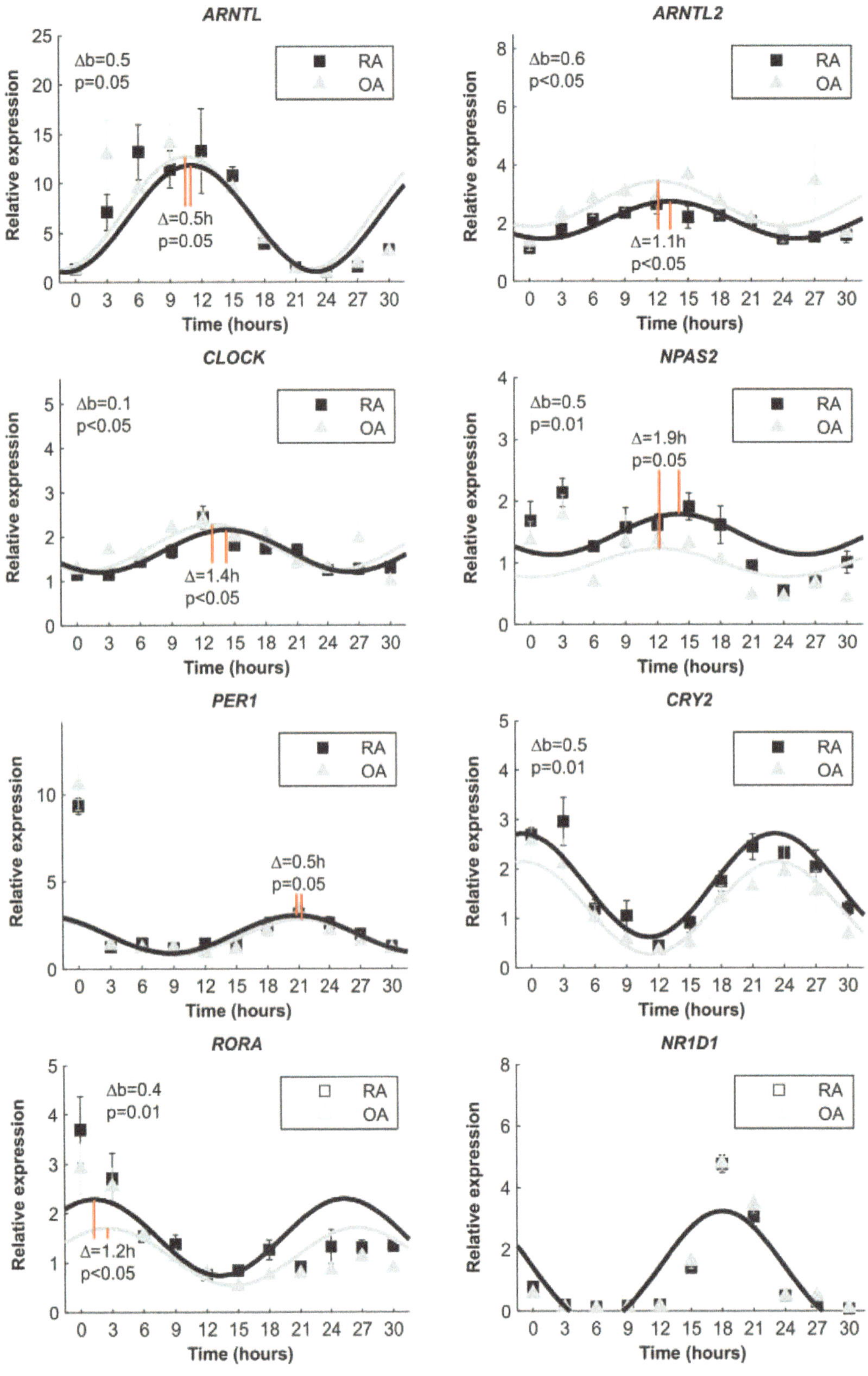

Figure 3. Relative clock gene expression over time after serum shocked primary fibroblasts. Fitted sin graphs of the expression and mean ± SD of the mean from three individual patients per group are shown. The time of serum removal is 0 in the graphs and the relative expression is normalized to the expression before serum (at time = −2). Δb indicates the general difference in the expression i.e., the baseline of the expression. Phase differences are marked as red solid lines and the difference is indicated in hours.

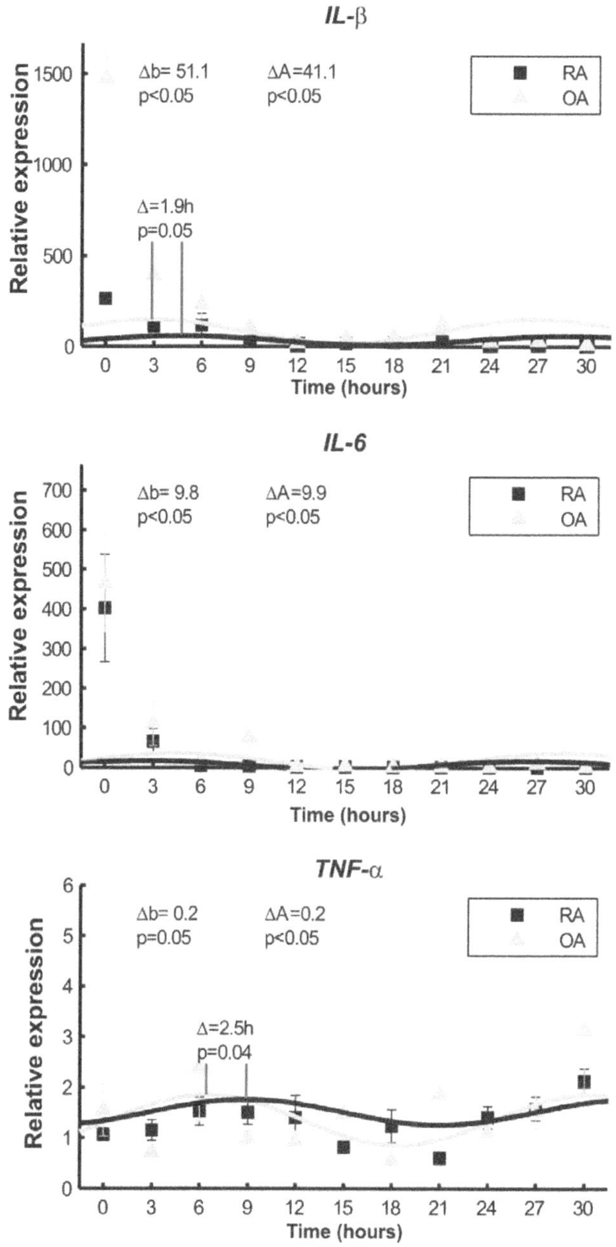

Figure 4. The oscillation of *IL-1β*, *IL-6* and *TNF-α* in RA and OA cells after serum shock. Relative gene expression over time is displayed. Fibroblasts derived from RA synovium display weaker rhythmic expression of *IL-1β*, *IL-6* and *TNF-α* after clock resetting than cells from OA synovium. Fitted sin graphs of the expression and mean ± SD of the mean from three individual patients per group is shown. The time of serum removal is 0 in the graphs and the relative expression is normalized to the expression before serum (at time = −2). Δb indicates the general difference in the expression i.e., the baseline of the expression. ΔA indicates the differences in the peak amplitude. Phase differences are marked as red solid lines and the difference is indicated in hours.

we observed near two-hour phase differences between RA and OA in the circadian gene expression already short after clock resetting. This is remarkable, because normally the self-sustained rhythm varies only 0.32 hours per day [26] and patients from whom these fibroblasts were isolated were randomly selected i.e., they were not selected by chronotype or any other factor that may impact the results. Thus, our results most likely reflect true differences between RA and OA patients. Importantly, the expression of *PER1*, for example, increased equally in RA and OA cells immediately after clock resetting, but the self-sustained rhythm was divergent. This excludes the effect of the initial serum shock, inflammation or other endocrine factors as the sole reasons for the disturbed clock gene expression in RA synovium and underlines a primary, cell autonomous defect in the control of the biorhythm in RA, i.e. a defect in the circadian clockwork itself.

Because RORs drive the expression of *BMAL1* [27,28], lag of *BMAL1* expression suggests delayed or diminished expression of *ROR* genes or a low ratio between the expression of *ROR* genes and their competitor *REV-ERBα* in RA cells. However, early and increased *RORA* expression in RA cells and equal *REV-ERBα* expression in RA and OA cells exclude this possibility. The expression of *ARNTL2* and *NPAS2* were also different in RA and OA. This is particularly important based on the fact that *ARNTL2* and *NPAS2*, not *PER1*, react to inflammation in human fibroblasts and some mouse tissues (data not shown).

RA patients have HPA-axis dysfunction in response to inflammation [7,8]. Due to the bidirectional links between inflammation and clock, we wanted to investigate the effect of inflammation on clock gene expression. IL-6 did not affect significantly the expression of clock genes. Thus, the purpose of robust oscillation of IL-6 levels in the blood most likely is not to synchronize peripheral clocks. However, TNF-α affected clock gene expression in the cultured synovial fibroblasts, indicating that inflammation can disturb normal circadian rhythm rapidly in the peripheral tissues.

Accurate circadian clock allows orchestrated proactive rather than reactive bodily functions. The data presented here clearly show that RA patients have a deficiency in the function of the clock. It must be emphasized that it is not the synovium or synovial fibroblasts that may cause these disturbances. Rather this cell autonomous phenomenon reflects the behavior of all molecular clocks in the body including the central clock, because circadian clock has virtually the same molecular makeup in the central timekeeper and different peripheral cells [29]. Based on this, our *in vitro* results suggest that RA patients, despite obtaining resetting stimuli every day, tend to lose the rhythm relatively fast due to a cell autonomous defect in their circadian clock. This may explain why the patients experience the fatigue as if they would be in a constant jet lag. The clock not only controls the circadian rhythm but also affects the development and function of immune cells. Thus, the immunological, neuronal and endocrine problems observed in the RA patients may be caused by cell autonomous dysfunction of the clock. This is further reinforced by the fact that novel biotherapies (anti-TNF, anti-B cell, anti T-cell, or anti-IL-6) have only limited impact on chronic fatigue in RA [30] at least partly excluding the possibility that inflammatory factors directly cause this severe problem in RA. Notably, *ARNTL2* and *NPAS2* are the clock genes that throughout different experiments were the most disturbed.

Conclusion

Herein, we show that RA patients display cell autonomous disconcerted circadian timekeeping. Throughout the analysis *ARNTL2* and *NPAS2* were the genes revealed to be most associated with human inflammatory conditions. Strikingly, *PER1* did not react to inflammatory stimulation in human fibroblasts. It appears that RA patients may experience the fatigue as if they would be in constant jet lag. Thus, chronotherapy that takes this altered

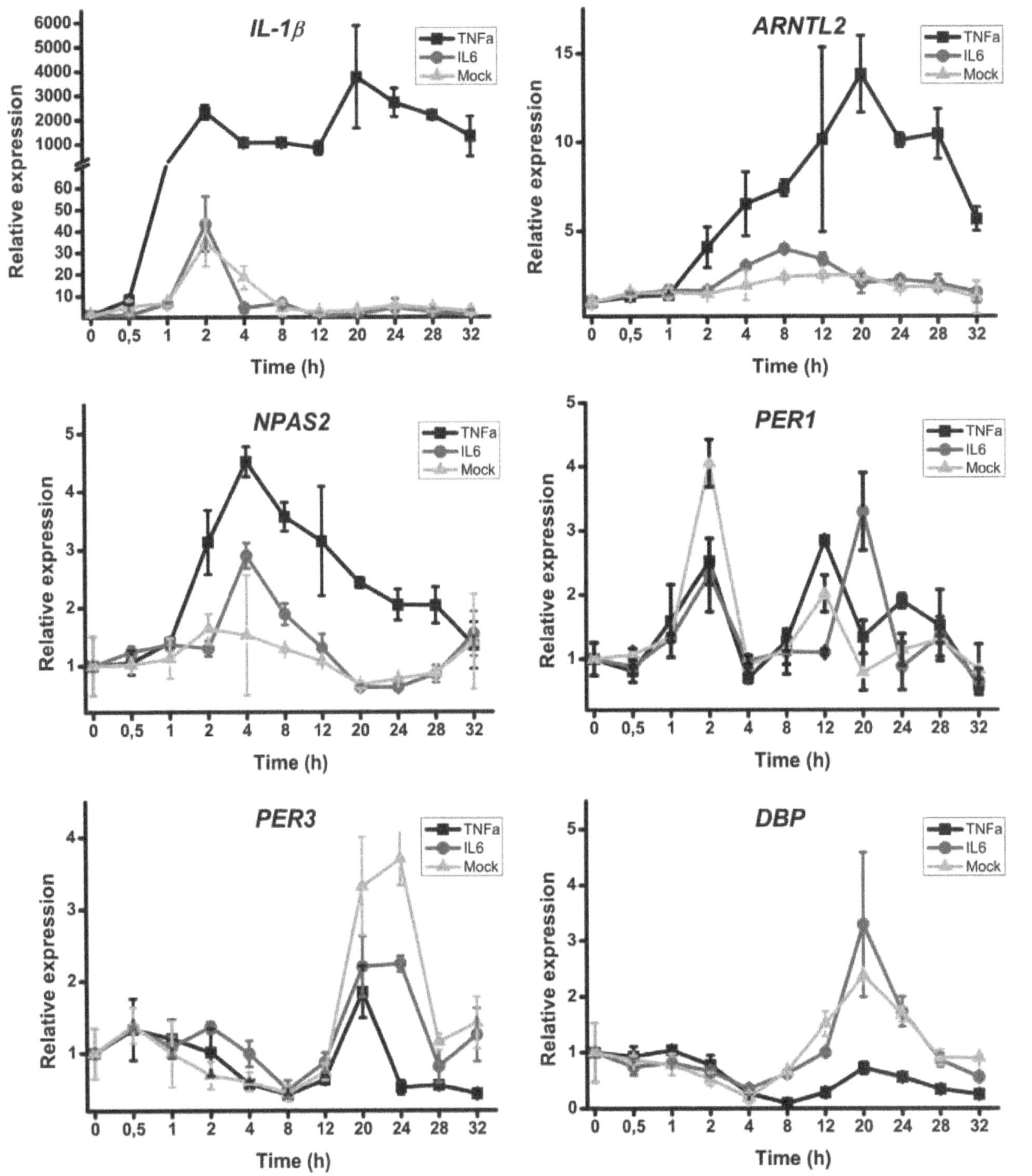

Figure 5. TNF-α increased *ARNTL2* and *NPAS2*, and suppresses *PER3* and *DBP* expression but IL-6 did not. Relative gene expression over time is displayed. Representative data from one experiment is shown. The experiment was repeated five times using fibroblasts from different OA patients. The time of TNF-α or IL-6 addition is 0 in the graphs.

rhythm into account and/or tries to correct it could be beneficial for the patients.

Acknowledgments

We thank Mr. Erkki Hänninen for expert technical help.

Author Contributions

Conceived and designed the experiments: VPK JO JJ IH JM. Performed the experiments: VPK JO JJ JM. Analyzed the data: VPK JO MA EK YTK JM. Contributed reagents/materials/analysis tools: EK MA YTK JM. Wrote the paper: IH YTK JM.

References

1. Welsh DK, Takahashi JS, Kay SA (2010) Suprachiasmatic nucleus: Cell autonomy and network properties. Annu Rev Physiol 72: 551–577.
2. Takahashi JS, Hong HK, Ko CH, McDearmon EL (2008) The genetics of mammalian circadian order and disorder: Implications for physiology and disease. Nat Rev Genet 9: 764–775.
3. Stetson MH, Watson-Whitmyre M (1976) Nucleus suprachiasmaticus: The biological clock in the hamster? Science 191: 197–199.
4. Dibner C, Schibler U, Albrecht U (2010) The mammalian circadian timing system: Organization and coordination of central and peripheral clocks. Annu Rev Physiol 72: 517–549.
5. Turek FW, Joshu C, Kohsaka A, Lin E, Ivanova G, et al. (2005) Obesity and metabolic syndrome in circadian clock mutant mice. Science 308: 1043–1045.
6. Fu L, Pelicano H, Liu J, Huang P, Lee C (2002) The circadian gene Period2 plays an important role in tumor suppression and DNA damage response in vivo. Cell 111: 41–50.
7. Chikanza IC, Petrou P, Kingsley G, Chrousos G, Panayi GS (1992) Defective hypothalamic response to immune and inflammatory stimuli in patients with rheumatoid arthritis. Arthritis Rheum 35: 1281–1288.
8. Cutolo M, Villaggio B, Otsa K, Aakre O, Sulli A, et al. (2005) Altered circadian rhythms in rheumatoid arthritis patients play a role in the disease's symptoms. 4: 497–502.
9. Kowanko IC, Pownall R, Knapp MS, Swannell AJ, Mahoney PG (1981) Circadian variations in the signs and symptoms of rheumatoid arthritis and in the therapeutic effectiveness of flurbiprofen at different times of day. Br J Clin Pharmacol 11: 477–484.
10. Hewlett S, Cockshott Z, Byron M, Kitchen K, Tipler S, et al. (2005) Patients' perceptions of fatigue in rheumatoid arthritis: Overwhelming, uncontrollable, ignored. 53: 697–702.
11. Repping-Wuts H, van Riel P, van Achterberg T (2009) Fatigue in patients with rheumatoid arthritis: What is known and what is needed. Rheumatology (Oxford) 48: 207–209.
12. Ishida A, Mutoh T, Ueyama T, Bando H, Masubuchi S, et al. (2005) Light activates the adrenal gland: Timing of gene expression and glucocorticoid release. Cell Metab 2: 297–307.
13. Sun H, Lu B, Li RQ, Flavell RA, Taneja R (2001) Defective T cell activation and autoimmune disorder in Stra13-deficient mice. Nat Immunol 2: 1040–1047.
14. Yang XO, Angkasekwinai P, Zhu J, Peng J, Liu Z, et al. (2009) Requirement for the basic helix-loop-helix transcription factor Dec2 in initial TH2 lineage commitment. Nat Immunol 10: 1260–1266.
15. Ivanov II, McKenzie BS, Zhou L, Tadokoro CE, Lepelley A, et al. (2006) The orphan nuclear receptor RORgammat directs the differentiation program of proinflammatory IL-17+ T helper cells. Cell 126: 1121–1133.
16. Delerive P, Monte D, Dubois G, Trottein F, Fruchart-Najib J, et al. (2001) The orphan nuclear receptor ROR alpha is a negative regulator of the inflammatory response. EMBO Rep 2: 42–48.
17. Hashiramoto A, Yamane T, Tsumiyama K, Yoshida K, Komai K, et al. (2010) Mammalian clock gene cryptochrome regulates arthritis via proinflammatory cytokine TNF-alpha. J Immunol 184: 1560–1565.
18. Cavadini G, Petrzilka S, Kohler P, Jud C, Tobler I, et al. (2007) TNF-alpha suppresses the expression of clock genes by interfering with E-box-mediated transcription. Proc Natl Acad Sci U S A 104: 12843–12848.
19. Durum SK, Schmidt JA, Oppenheim JJ (1985) Interleukin 1: An immunological perspective. Annu Rev Immunol 3: 263–287.
20. Balsalobre A, Damiola F, Schibler U (1998) A serum shock induces circadian gene expression in mammalian tissue culture cells. Cell 93: 929–937.
21. Gudewill S, Pollmacher T, Vedder H, Schreiber W, Fassbender K, et al. (1992) Nocturnal plasma levels of cytokines in healthy men. Eur Arch Psychiatry Clin Neurosci 242: 53–56.
22. Lange T, Dimitrov S, Born J (2010) Effects of sleep and circadian rhythm on the human immune system. Ann N Y Acad Sci 1193: 48–59.
23. Lee C, Etchegaray JP, Cagampang FR, Loudon AS, Reppert SM (2001) Posttranslational mechanisms regulate the mammalian circadian clock. Cell 107: 855–867.
24. Kwon I, Lee J, Chang SH, Jung NC, Lee BJ, et al. (2006) BMAL1 shuttling controls transactivation and degradation of the CLOCK/BMAL1 heterodimer. Mol Cell Biol 26: 7318–7330.
25. Balsalobre A, Brown SA, Marcacci L, Tronche F, Kellendonk C, et al. (2000) Resetting of circadian time in peripheral tissues by glucocorticoid signaling. Science 289: 2344–2347.
26. Herzog ED, Aton SJ, Numano R, Sakaki Y, Tei H (2004) Temporal precision in the mammalian circadian system: A reliable clock from less reliable neurons. J Biol Rhythms 19: 35–46.
27. Preitner N, Damiola F, Lopez-Molina L, Zakany J, Duboule D, et al. (2002) The orphan nuclear receptor REV-ERBalpha controls circadian transcription within the positive limb of the mammalian circadian oscillator. Cell 110: 251–260.
28. Sato TK, Panda S, Miraglia LJ, Reyes TM, Rudic RD, et al. (2004) A functional genomics strategy reveals rora as a component of the mammalian circadian clock. Neuron 43: 527–537.
29. Asher G, Schibler U (2011) Crosstalk between components of circadian and metabolic cycles in mammals. Cell Metab 13: 125–137.
30. Tak PP, Kalden JR (2011) Advances in rheumatology: New targeted therapeutics. Arthritis Res Ther 13 Suppl 1: S5.

13

Novel Insights into the Regulatory Architecture of CD4+ T Cells in Rheumatoid Arthritis

Adrià Aterido[1], Carlos Palacio[2], Sara Marsal[1]*, Gabriela Ávila[1], Antonio Julià[1]*

1 Rheumatology Research Group, Vall d'Hebron Hospital Research Institute, Barcelona, Spain, **2** Department of Hematology, Hospital Universitari Vall d'Hebron, Barcelona, Spain

Abstract

Rheumatoid arthritis (RA) is the most frequent autoimmune chronic inflammatory disease of the joints and it is characterized by the inflammation of the synovial membrane and the subsequent destruction of the joints. In RA, CD4+ T cells are the main drivers of disease initiation and the perpetuation of the damaging inflammatory process. To date, however, the genetic regulatory mechanisms of CD4+ T cells associated with RA etiology are poorly understood. The genome-wide analysis of expression quantitative trait loci (eQTL) in disease-relevant cell types is a recent genomic integration approach that is providing significant insights into the genetic regulatory mechanisms of many human pathologies. The objective of the present study was to analyze, for the first time, the genome-wide genetic regulatory mechanisms associated with the gene expression of CD4+ T cells in RA. Whole genome gene expression profiling of CD4+ T cells and the genome-wide genotyping (598,258 SNPs) of 29 RA patients with an active disease were performed. In order to avoid the excessive burden of multiple testing associated with genome-wide *trans*-eQTL analysis, we developed and implemented a novel systems genetics approach. Finally, we compared the genomic regulation pattern of CD4+ T cells in RA with the genomic regulation observed in reference lymphoblastoid cell lines (LCLs). We identified a genome-wide significant *cis*-eQTL associated with the expression of *FAM66C* gene ($P = 6.51e-9$). Using our new systems genetics approach we identified six statistically significant *trans*-eQTLs associated with the expression of *KIAA0101* ($P < 7.4e-8$) and *BIRC5* ($P = 5.35e-8$) genes. Finally, comparing the genomic regulation profiles between RA CD4+ T cells and control LCLs we found 20 genes showing differential regulatory patterns between both cell types. The present genome-wide eQTL analysis has identified new genetic regulatory elements that are key to the activity of CD4+ T cells in RA.

Editor: Kottarappat N. Dileepan, University of Kansas Medical Center, United States of America

Funding: This work was supported by the Spanish Ministry of Economy and Competitiveness grants [PSE-010000-2006-6 and IPT-010000-2010-36] and the Fondo de Investigación Sanitaria grant [PI040720]. The funders had no role in study design, data collection and analysis, decision to publish, or preparation of the manuscript.

Competing Interests: The authors have declared that no competing interests exist.

* Email: toni.julia@vhir.org (AJ); sara.marsal@vhir.org (SM)

Introduction

Rheumatoid arthritis (RA) is the most frequent autoimmune chronic inflammatory disease of the joints and affects up to 1% of the World population. RA is characterized by synovial membrane hyperplasia, increased vascularity and chronic immune cell infiltration that lead to joint destruction and pain [1]. The predominant immune cell type that infiltrates RA synovial joints is the CD4+ T lymphocyte and, for many years, it has been considered a T-cell driven disease [2]. Consequently, treatments targeting the activation of CD4+ T cells have proven successful in the control of disease activity in RA [3,4]. This evidence, together with the strong genetic association of the molecules that mediate antigen presentation to CD4+ T cells in RA, clearly indicate that the characterization of the regulatory elements of this cell type will be key to completely understand the disease pathogenesis [5]. To date, however, a global analysis of the regulatory mechanisms of CD4+ T cells in RA has not been performed.

Genome-wide association studies (GWAS), in which common genetic variants are tested for association with complex traits, have revolutionized the identification of genetic risk factors for many common diseases [6]. More recently, the integration of GWAS with gene expression data to identify quantitative trait loci (eQTLs) is starting to provide significant insights into the genetic architecture of human diseases [7]. The number of transcripts expressed by a gene is modified by the variation in genetic regulatory elements. RNA levels can therefore be considered as a quantitative trait and used to map these crucial regulatory elements in the genome [8]. Gene expression microarrays and more recently ultra-high throughput RNA sequencing systems coupled with genome-wide genotyping assays are allowing to scan the whole genome variation to identify trait-specific eQTLs [9]. eQTL studies are leading to the characterization of functional sequence variation as well as the understanding of basic genetic regulatory mechanisms [10]. So far, one of the most important discoveries of genome-wide eQTL mapping has been the finding that a substantial fraction of the gene expression regulation is cell type-specific [11]. Consequently, the understanding of the genomic regulatory basis that underlies a complex disease like RA will only be possible if it is performed at the cell type level, in particular analyzing those cell types that play a crucial role in the disease onset and progression [12,13].

Recently, studies have been reported that characterize regulatory variants that operate in a cell type-specific manner [11,14,15]. However, most of these studies focused only on *cis*-acting elements rather than identifying *trans*-acting elements. While *cis*-eQTLs are likely to influence molecular mechanisms involved in transcription, splicing or mRNA decay [16], *trans*-eQTLs are more likely to perturb entire pathways and mediate complex epistatic and gene-environment interactions and, therefore, are of particular interest in the study of prevalent diseases with a complex genetic basis like RA [17,18]. Importantly, while *cis*-eQTLs are often conserved among different cell types, *trans*-eQTLs tend to be cell type-specific [19]. The genome-wide analysis of *trans*-eQTLs, however, requires the analysis of an exponential number of transcript-SNP pairs, resulting in a prohibitive multiple testing problem. As a consequence, very few studies have explored the presence of *trans*-eQTLs in human traits [20], and new strategies to reduce the burden of multiple testing in these studies must be devised.

In this study, we have analyzed, for the first time, the regulatory variation associated with the gene expression of CD4+ T cells in RA. To do so, we have performed a genome-wide *cis*-eQTL analysis and we have implemented a robust systems genetic approach to perform the *trans*-eQTL analysis. In this approach we exploit the presence of cell-specific gene expression networks, together with the power of biological knowledge and the statistical analysis of networks, to efficiently reduce the high dimensionality associated with the global analysis of *trans*-eQTLs. Finally, in order to identify additional specific gene expression regulation, we have compared the regulatory patterns observed in CD4+ T cells to those of lymphoblastoid cell lines (LCLs), a well-characterized reference cell type. Taken together, the results of this study provide new insights into the key regulatory elements of CD4+ T cells in RA.

Materials and Methods

Patients and samples

A total of 29 patients with rheumatoid arthritis from the Rheumatology Unit of the Vall d'Hebron University Hospital (Barcelona, Spain) were recruited. All patients had been diagnosed as RA following the 1987 *American College Rheumatology* criteria [21]. In order to obtain a gene expression profile more representative of the disease, all patients had to have a high disease activity at the moment of sample collection. In this study, high disease activity was defined as an European League against Rheumatoid Arthritis (EULAR) Disease Activity Score (DAS28) [22] higher than 3.2. The DAS28 score efficiently reflects the disease activity of the RA patient by combining the evidence of tenderness and swelling in 28 joints together with the patient's global assessment and a systemic marker of inflammation (erythrocyte sedimentation rate or C-reactive protein levels). In order to avoid the influence of treatment over the gene expression patterns in RA, all patients were receiving the same treatment (≤20 mg/wk metothrexate) and were all naïve to biological immunomodulating agents like anti-TNF agents. Patients suspected to have a concomitant infection or were positive for hepatitis B or C viruses (active or inactive) were also not included in this study. The main features of the RA patient cohort used in this study are shown in Table S1. From each patient, 30 mL of venous blood was obtained, from which 5 mL were used for genomic DNA isolation and 25 mL for CD4+ T cell RNA isolation. Genomic DNA was isolated using the Chemagic Magnetic Separation Module I (PerkinElmer, USA). In order to obtain the total RNA from CD4+ T cells, we first isolated the CD4+ lymphocytes from whole blood using the *RossetteSep* negative selection kit (Stem Cell Technologies, Canada). Isolated cells were immediately preserved in RNA stabilization reagent RNAlater (Qiagen, Hilden, Germany) and frozen at −80°C. In order to determine the level of cell purity, FACS flow cytometry analysis was performed on CD4+ T cells. The CD45+, CD4+, CD3+ and CD8+ T cells were stained by direct immune fluorescence using monoclonal antibodies conjugated with fluorochromes fluorescein isothiocyanate, phycoerythrin, pycoerythrin-cyanin-5 and Phycoerythrin-Texas (all antibodies from Beckman Coulter, FL, USA), respectively. Isotype-matched immunoglobulins with no reactivity against surface markers and the fluorochrome combination were used as negative controls to determine fluorescence background. Acquisition of flow data was performed using an EPICS-XL˙MCL cytometer and Expo32 software (Beckman-Coulter, FL, USA) after antibody incubation followed by erythrocyte lysis. This analysis was carried out on the same day of blood extraction in all RA patients and >95% CD4+ T cell purity from all samples was confirmed. RNA extraction from the isolated CD4+ T cells was performed with the *RNeasy* extraction kit (Qiagen, Hilden, Germany) and its quality determined using the *2100 BioAnalyzer* system (Agilent technologies, Waldbronn, Germany).

All the procedures followed were in compliance with the principles of the Declaration of Helsinki. All patients provided written informed consent. The study and the consent procedure were approved by the Institut de Recerca Hospital Universitari Vall d'Hebron ethics committee.

Gene expression profiling

Whole genome transcript abundance from the CD4+ T cells of patients with RA was performed using the Illumina Human-6 v1 Beadchip array system (Illumina, San Diego, CA, USA). This microarray platform measures the gene expression levels of more than 47,000 different transcripts. In order to update the probe annotation for this microarray, we used the NCBI RefSeq database [23]. Matching the microarray probe sequence to the latest RefSeq database version (2nd May 2013) we found that 13,555 probes perfectly mapped to unique transcripts, 26,729 probes that did not map any transcript and 8,013 probes that mapped more than one transcript from which 7,565 mapped to the same gene. Consequently, the updated microarray probe annotation was composed by 21,120 probes matching to known transcripts. Data preprocessing was conducted using the R statistical software [24]. The raw expression intensities of the 29 microarrays were processed using background adjustment. One sample showed intensity dependent biases and it was finally removed. The gene expression intensities were normalized on the log2-scale using the quantile normalization method [25]. In order to remove the potential variability introduced by the presence of different microarray processing batches, we used the ComBat empirical Bayes method [26]. The data discussed in this publication have been deposited in NCBI's Gene Expression Omnibus [27] and are accessible through GEO Series accession number GSE55468.

Whole genome genotyping

The genome-wide genotyping of the 29 RA patients was performed using the Illumina Quad610 Beadchips (Illumina, San Diego, California, USA). The Quad610 genotyping arrays scan 618,150 polymorphisms (598,258 SNPs and 19,892 CNV probes). Genotype calling was performed using the GenomeStudio data analysis software (v2011.1, Illumina, San Diego, California, USA). The quality control evaluation was performed using PLINK software [28]. All the autosomal SNPs were initially selected (n = 582,539). A total of 7,886 markers showing >10% missing data were excluded, as well as 1,724 SNPs with P<1e-5 for test of deviance from Hardy-Weinberg equilibrium. After all quality control steps, a final number of 572,980 SNPs were used for the eQTL analysis in CD4+ T cells. In order to compare the exact same polymorphisms in the CD4+ T cell and LCL eQTL analyses, 6,962 SNPs had to be excluded from the initial dataset. In this case, a final number of 566,018 SNPs were used for the comparative eQTL analysis between both cell types. The presence of population stratification in the study samples was estimated using principal component analysis (PCA) implemented in EIGENSOFT (v4.2) software [29]. Using the top ten principal components over ten iterations and using a threshold of six standard deviations, we excluded two samples showing an outlier genetic background.

Statistical association analysis

Cis- and *trans*-eQTL analyses were performed using Matrix eQTL software [30]. Matrix eQTL efficiently performs large numbers of eQTL analyses by the use of large matrix multiplications. Most gene regulatory elements that act in *cis* have been previously reported to be located in close proximity to the gene [31]. However, there is clear evidence that *cis* regulatory elements like enhancers can be located as far as 1 Mb from the gene they regulate [32]. Consequently, we used 1 Mb as the maximal distance at which *cis* regulation can occur. This distance is in accordance to most recent studies on genome-wide eQTLs [10]. For each transcript-SNP pair, we fitted the following linear model assuming additive effect of genotype on gene expression:

$$Y_i = \gamma + \beta \cdot X_i + \varepsilon_i$$

The genotype X_i of individual i at given SNP is encoded by 0, 1 and 2 according to the number of minor alleles present in the genotype of the individual. The gene expression Y_i is the normalized log-expression level of the probe for individual i. The ε_i captures all other factors which influence the gene expression. The null hypothesis of the statistical test was that there is no association between the genotype and the gene expression ($\beta = 0$). In the present study, we included gender as a covariate. In order to avoid false positives due to low allele frequency, we filtered those SNPs with a minor allele frequency < 10%. Multiple testing correction was performed using the False Discovery Rate (FDR) method [33]. A total of 21,120 transcripts and 572,980 SNPs measured in 26 individuals were finally used for the *cis*-eQTL analysis in CD4+ T cells.

Novel systems genetics approach for *trans*-eQTL identification

We present a novel systems genetics approach to address the dimensionality problem present in *trans*-eQTL analyses. The pipeline of this approach is composed by five consecutive steps (Figure 1).

In the first step, the gene expression modules that characterize the cell type of interest are identified using the genome-wide expression data. There are several methods that can be used for this objective. In our study, we used the weighted correlation network analysis implemented in the WGCNA R software package [34]. In this method, the correlation between genes is used to compute a network adjacency matrix, which fully determines the gene co-expression networks. From this network adjacency matrix, WGCNA then uses an unsupervised clustering approach to identify the gene expression modules that best characterize the gene expression of the cell or tissue of interest.

In the second step, the gene expression modules that characterize the cell type of interest are analyzed for enrichment of a specific biological process that is related to the disease or trait of interest (i.e. cell cycle in cancer studies). For this objective, a biological annotation database like the gene ontology (GO) database [35] is used. The enrichment can then be quantitatively measured using well-known statistical methods. In our study, we assessed the statistical significance of the GO functional enrichment using the Fisher's exact test as described previously [36]. Only those gene expression modules that are significantly enriched by the biological process of interest are selected for the next step.

In the third step, the biological knowledge is used to build functional-based networks from the gene expression modules of interest. In these functional-based networks, the nodes are the genes from the selected gene expression modules. Then, according to the presence or absence of biological evidence between each gene pair, the edges of the network are established. For this objective, a complete and updated database of functional associations is required. In our study, we used STRING (v9.1, 2013) software tool [37]. STRING is a powerful bioinformatics database that integrates five different sources of functional associations between genes in more than 1,100 organisms. These sources are i) physical interactions, ii) curated biological pathway knowledge, iii) computational predictions, iv) text-mining and v) association transfer between organisms. The association transfer between organisms is based on the principle of interaction conservation, which means that a pair of proteins binding in one organism is expected to be binding in another organism if both genes are present in both genomes. Therefore, the functional associations in one organism can be transferred to another organism using comparative genomics.

In the fourth step of this approach, network analysis methods are used to identify those genes that are likely to play a central role in the previously identified functional-based networks. In network analysis, the most influential genes are those that show either many connections to other genes and/or that exert an essential connection between gene (node) subnetworks. These two features are commonly known as degree centrality (DC) and betweenness centrality (BC), respectively. Genes with high DC are defined as hubs and may also be more evolutionary conserved than non-hubs [38]. Bottlenecks, that is genes with high BC, are more likely to be essential than proteins with low BC [39,40]. In our study, the network analysis was performed using the Cytoscape v3.0.1 software [41].

In the last step of this systems genetics method, only those genes that are more likely to play a central role in the cell-specific network are selected and analyzed for the *trans*-eQTL analysis. These genes are selected according to their DC and BC values obtained in the previous step and, therefore, will have a higher probability to be associated to an influential genetic variation in the cell type of interest.

With this systems genetics approach, biological and network information is efficiently used to objectively reduce the number of genes included in the *trans*-eQTL analysis to those with highest influence on the cell type of interest and, therefore, increase the likelihood of identifying relevant *trans*-eQTL associations.

Analysis of differential genomic regulation profiles

In order to compare the genomic regulation profiles of CD4+ T cells and LCL cells, we focused on the study of *cis*- and *trans*-eQTL associations of two different groups of genes. In the first group, we

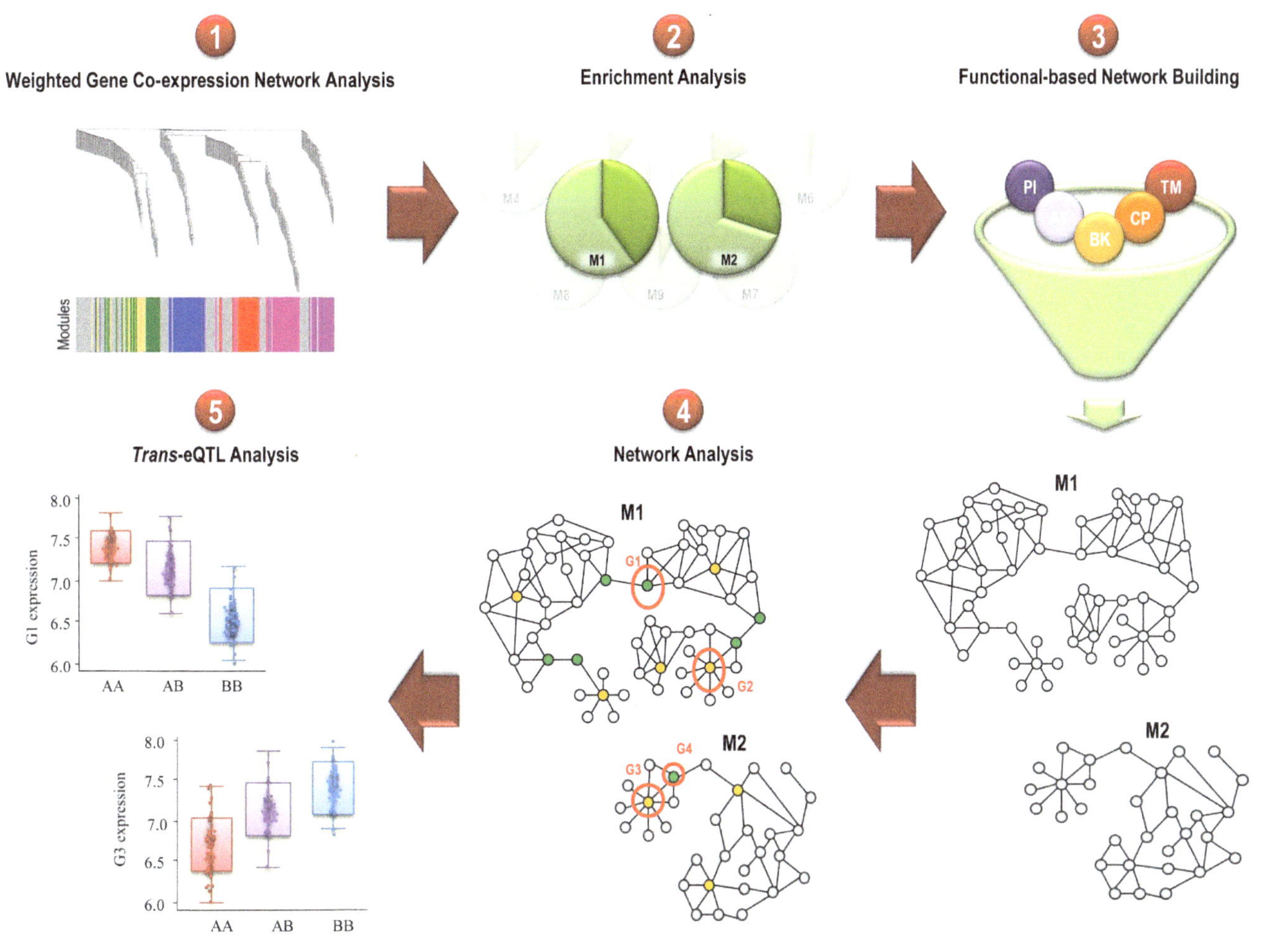

Figure 1. Workflow of the systems genetics approach for *trans*-eQTL identification. The new systems genetics approach is based on four steps that are performed before the *trans*-eQTL analysis in order to efficiently reduce the number of analyzed genes: 1) Identification of the gene expression modules (M) that characterize CD4+ T cell gene expression 2) Enrichment analysis of a specific biological process that is related to the trait of interest 3) Construction of the functional-based networks using biological knowledge within the significantly enriched modules 4) Network analysis to identify those genes that are likely to play a central role in the functional-based networks 5) *Trans*-eQTL analysis using the subset of genes that show the highest centrality in each module. Abbreviations: AT, association transfer between organisms; BK, curated biological pathway knowledge; CP, computational predictions; G, gene; M, module; PI, physical interactions; TM, text-mining.

analyzed those genes previously associated with RA risk and belonging to known biological pathways [42]. In the second group, we analyzed those genes associated with the T cell differentiation into different CD4+ T cell subtypes, including T helper 1 (Th1), T helper 2 (Th2), T helper 17 (Th17) and T regulatory (Treg) subtypes. This last set of genes was extracted from the Kyoto Encyclopedia of Genes and Genomes (KEGG) database [43]. In total, the comparative eQTL analysis between CD4+ T cells and LCL cells was performed using 145 transcripts, corresponding to 113 different genes (Table S2). The LCL gene expression profiles and the corresponding whole genome genotype data were obtained from 26 unrelated Caucasian European (CEU) individuals from the HapMap reference project [44].

In order to avoid the study of redundant eQTLs (i.e. neighboring SNPs in high linkage disequilibrium associated to one single transcript), we divided the autosomal chromosomes into 32,962 independent loci according to the localization of high recombination sites (i.e. *hotspots*) [45]. The whole set of SNPs were mapped to these independent loci in order to be able to determine the Transcript Complexity Value (TCV). The TCV represents the number of independent loci that are associated to the expression of one particular gene. Using the *cis*- ($P<0.05$) and *trans*-eQTLs ($P<1e-5$) identified in the CD4+ T cells and LCLs analyses, we computed the TCV for each of the 113 selected genes. The statistical significance of the differences in TCVs between both cell types was assessed using the Fisher's exact test.

Results

Genome-wide *cis*-eQTL analysis in RA CD4+ T cells

After performing the *cis*-eQTL analysis of the gene expression of CD4+ T cell from RA patients having an active disease ($n = 8{,}747{,}394$ tests), we detected two genome-wide significant associations with *FAM66C* gene: SNP rs7976243 (chromosome 12p13.3, $P_{FDR} = 2.85e-2$) and SNP rs2244822 (chromosome 12p13.3, $P_{FDR} = 2.85e-2$). Both genome-wide significant *cis*-eQTLs are only 2.14 Kb apart and, as expected, they are in high linkage disequilibrium ($r^2 = 0.95$, HapMap Caucasian European samples) and consequently, they represent the same association signal. A complete list of *cis*-eQTLs from RA CD4+ T cells having a $P_{FDR}<0.5$ is shown in Table S3.

Trans-eQTL analysis in RA CD4+ T cells using the novel systems genetics approach

A total of 16 gene expression modules were found to characterize the CD4+ T cell gene expression of RA patients with active disease (Table 1). Given that RA is an autoimmune disease characterized by the chronic activity of inflammatory cells, we performed the functional enrichment analysis of the CD4+ T cell modules over GO terms related to the immune system. From the 16 gene expression modules identified in RA CD4+ T cells, we found two modules to be highly significantly enriched in genes related to the immune system ($P=9.23e-21$ and $P=9.14e-5$ for modules 9 and 12, respectively). Using these two immune-related gene expression modules, we built their corresponding functional-based networks. The M9 CD4+ T cell module functional analysis revealed a network of 15 interconnected genes (Figure 2 A). The analysis of the M12 gene-expression module showed larger and more complex network involving 247 genes. The topological structure of the M12 functional network (Figure 2 B) suggests the existence of different subnetworks that are connected by a few genes (i.e. genes showing high BC).

After computing the network properties of each gene in the identified M9 and M12 functional networks (Table 2), we selected those genes showing the highest centrality measures. A total of 13 genes showing either high connectivity with other genes ($DC_{M9}\geq 5$, $DC_{M12}\geq 51$) or high connectivity between node subnetworks ($BC_{M9}\geq 0.26$, $BC_{M12}\geq 0.05$) were selected. These selected genes were *IL4, MS4A2, CCR3, IL8* and *FCER1A* genes from M9 module and *TSPO, CDK1, RPS3, TYROBP, CD4, BIRC5, CDC45 and KIAA0101* genes from M12 module (Figure 3). Using this set of genes that have a very high probability of being relevant in the CD4+ T cell pathophysiology in RA, we finally performed the *trans*-eQTL analysis ($N_{M9}=3{,}435{,}556$ tests, $N_{M12}=5{,}725{,}245$ tests). After multiple test correction, we identified six statistically significant *trans*-eQTLs (Table 3). A complete list of the *trans*-eQTLs having a nominal P-value<1e-5 in modules M9 and M12 is shown in Tables S4 and S5, respectively.

The statistically significant *trans*-eQTLs identified with our novel systems genetics approach were associated to the expression of *KIAA0101* and *BIRC5* genes, both central genes of the M12 CD4+ T cell network. Five of the significant *trans*-eQTLs were associated to the expression of *KIAA0101* and are located in different chromosomic regions: SNP rs3862556 (intergenic variant, chromosome 10q22.2, $P_{FDR}=4.6e-2$), SNPS rs711114 (intergenic variant, chromosome 12q21.1, $P_{FDR}=4.8e-2$), SNP rs9561023 (*GPC5* locus, chromosome 13q31.3, $P_{FDR}=4.8e-2$), SNP rs2513046 (*AHNAK* locus, chromosome 11q12.1, $P_{FDR}=4.8e-2$) and SNP rs17009383 (*ZNF385D* locus, chromosome 3p24.3, $P_{FDR}=4.8e-2$). The remaining *trans*-eQTL was established between the genetic variation at SNP rs10283761 (intergenic variant, chromosome 9p21.2, $P_{FDR}=4.8e\text{-}2$) and the expression levels of the *BIRC5* gene.

Analysis of differential genomic regulation profiles

The comparison of the genomic regulation profiles of CD4+ T cells and LCL cells revealed several genes showing significantly different genetic regulatory mechanisms between both cell types.

In the RA risk gene group, three genes showing a highly differential genomic regulation between CD4+ T cells and LCLs were identified (Figure 4). In the T cell receptor signaling pathway, *PRKCQ* gene had similar TCVs in LCLs *cis*- and *trans*-eQTLs while CD4+ T cells had a high *cis*-TCV and a practically absent *trans*-TCV ($P=4.1e-3$). In this same pathway, *RASGRP1* gene showed an opposite regulatory pattern in both cell types, with a predominant *trans*-TCV in CD4+ T cells and a predominant *cis*-TCV in LCLs ($P=7.3e-3$). Finally, *PRDM1* gene, belonging to the B cell development pathway, was found to be mainly *cis*-

Table 1. Gene expression modules identified in RA CD4+ T cells.

Module	Number of Transcripts	Immune System Process	P-value
M1	288	NS	3.69e-01
M2	2326	Underrepresented	5.00e-03*
M3	1682	Underrepresented	3.41e-06*
M4	83	Underrepresented	1.26e-02*
M5	755	NS	2.64e-01
M6	155	NS	3.69e-01
M7	10003	NS	7.71e-01
M8	199	NS	4.94e-01
M9	75	Overrepresented	9.23e-21*
M10	253	NS	1.36e-01
M11	157	NS	7.50e-01
M12	402	Overrepresented	9.14e-05*
M13	124	Underrepresented	5.34e-23*
M14	136	Underrepresented	2.82e-06*
M15	2904	NS	7.90e-02
M16	1578	Underrepresented	3.50e-05*

Applying the new systems genetics approach for *trans*-eQTL identification in RA CD4+ T cells and using WGCNA, 16 genes expression modules (M) that characterize the CD4+ T cells were identified. For each gene expression module, the number of gene transcripts representing each module is shown, as well as the results of the immunological enrichment analysis.
Abbreviations: NS, No Significant.
* Significant (P<0.05).

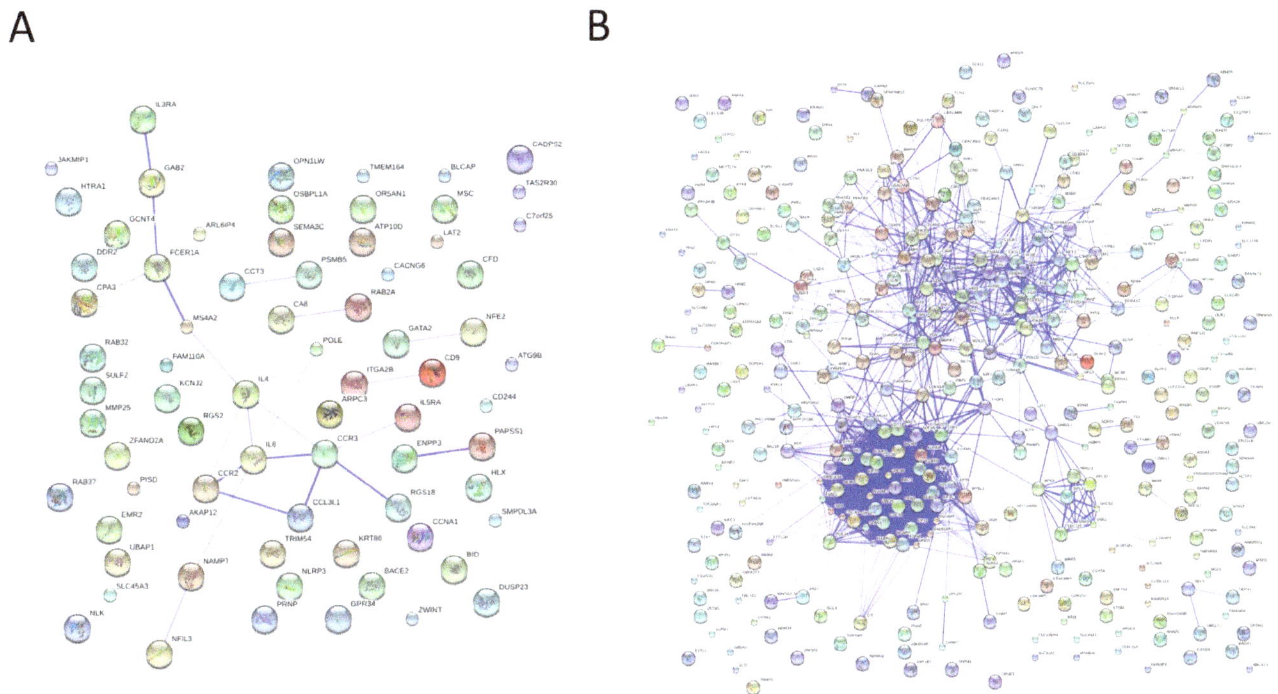

Figure 2. Building of functional-based networks for M9 and M12 CD4+ gene expression modules using biological knowledge. A: Functional-based network obtained from the immunologically enriched M9 gene expression module where 15 genes display a connected network. **B**: Functional-based network obtained from the immunologically enriched M12 gene expression module, which shows a complex network structure with different subnetworks involving 247 interconnected genes.

regulated in CD4+ T cells and *trans*-regulated in LCLs (P = 4.9e−3).

Among those genes involved in T cell differentiation pathways, we found a total of 17 genes showing a differential regulatory profile between both cell types. Taking into account that CD4+ T cell differentiation pathways can share several genes, we found a differential regulation in 13, 5, 3 and 1 genes from the Th1, Th2, Th17 and Treg differentiation pathways, respectively (Figure 5).

NFKB (P = 8.0e−3), *ICAM1* (P = 1.9e−2), *UBE2D* (P = 3.5e−2) and *TGFB2* (P = 4.6e−2) genes showed opposite regulatory

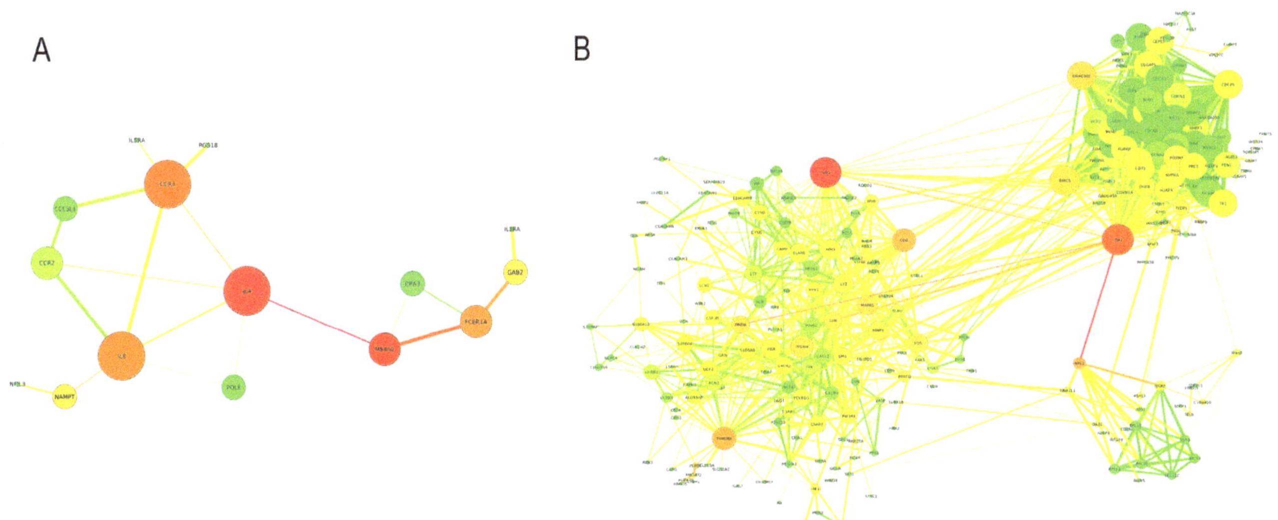

Figure 3. Functional-based networks analyzed in each enriched CD4+ T cell gene expression module. A: Functional-based network obtained from the immunologically enriched M9 gene expression module. **B**: Functional-based network obtained from the immunologically enriched M12 gene expression module. The dimensions of each node (i.e. gene) are proportional to its DC value and its color is based on its BC value, ranging from green (lowest BC values) to red (highest BC values). The edge width is proportional to the strength of the functional association evidences between two genes. The edge betweenness determines the edge color, ranging from green (edges connecting nodes with the lowest BC values) to red (edges connecting nodes with the highest BC values).

Table 2. Network statistics of M9 and M12 RA CD4+ gene expression modules.

Module	Gene Symbol	BC	DC	Module	Gene Symbol	DC	BC
M9	*IL4*	0.5329	5	M9	*IL4*	5	0.5329
M9	*MS4A2*	0.4395	3	M9	*CCR3*	5	0.3297
M9	*CCR3*	0.3297	5	M9	*IL8*	5	0.3021
M9	*IL8*	0.3021	5	M9	*MS4A2*	3	0.4395
M9	*FCER1A*	0.2637	3	M9	*FCER1A*	3	0.2637
M9	*NAMPT*	0.1429	2	M9	*CCR2*	3	0.0549
M9	*GAB2*	0.1429	2	M9	*NAMPT*	2	0.1429
M9	*CCR2*	0.0549	3	M9	*GAB2*	2	0.1429
M9	*CCL3L1*	0.0110	2	M9	*CCL3L1*	2	0.0110
M9	*RGS18*	0.0000	1	M9	*POLE*	2	0.0000
M12	*TSPO*	0.2436	55	M12	*CDK1*	57	0.1717
M12	*CDK1*	0.1717	57	M12	*TSPO*	55	0.2436
M12	*RPS3*	0.0905	11	M12	*BIRC5*	53	0.0432
M12	*TYROBP*	0.0836	35	M12	*CDC45*	51	0.0138
M12	*CD4*	0.0738	36	M12	*KIAA0101*	50	0.0515
M12	*KIAA0101*	0.0515	50	M12	*TOP2A*	50	0.0156
M12	*MNDA*	0.0472	20	M12	*CCNA2*	50	0.0036
M12	*MAPK1*	0.0455	25	M12	*TK1*	49	0.0246
M12	*BIRC5*	0.0432	53	M12	*CDT1*	49	0.0156
M12	*ITGAM*	0.0425	34	M12	*DLGAP5*	49	0.0103

Applying the new systems genetics approach for *trans*-eQTL identification in RA CD4+ T cells, the BC and DC values were computed for each particular gene of M9 and M12 immunity-enriched modules. On the left side of the table, the top 10 genes showing the highest BC values in each module are sorted by BC in decreasing order. On the right side of the table, the top 10 genes showing the highest DC values in each module are sorted by DC in decreasing order.

Abbreviations: BC, Betweenness centrality; DC, Degree centrality.

Table 3. *Trans*-eQTL associations revealed by the application of the systems genetics approach.

Module	SNP	Gene	SNP Coordinates (bp)	Gene Coordinates (bp)	β	P-value	P_{FDR}
M9	rs9293162	*FCER1A*	chr5:25065470	chr1:159253678–159278014	1,851	1.1927e-07	0.077
M9	rs978897	*FCER1A*	chr7:15598156	chr1:159253678–159278014	1,670	3.2865e-07	0.094
M12	rs3862556	*KIAA0101*	chr10:76540987	chr15:64657210–64673702	−0,924	2.4332e-08	0.046*
M12	rs711114	*KIAA0101*	chr12:78003541	chr15:64657210–64673702	−0,848	5.0807e-08	0.048*
M12	rs10283761	*BIRC5*	chr9:26755930	chr17:76210276–76221716	−0,345	5.3493e-08	0.048*
M12	rs9561023	*KIAA0101*	chr13:93022401	chr15:64657210–64673702	−0,999	6.0208e-08	0.048*
M12	rs2513046	*KIAA0101*	chr11:62236094	chr15:64657210–64673702	−0,999	6.0208e-08	0.048*
M12	rs17009383	*KIAA0101*	chr3:21771769	chr15:64657210–64673702	−0,573	7.3813e-08	0.048*
M12	rs4806933	*KIAA0101*	chr19:3414020	chr15:64657210–64673702	−0,727	1.6853e-07	0.079
M12	rs4745758	*KIAA0101*	chr10:76568257	chr15:64657210–64673702	−0,814	4.7989e-07	0.095
M12	rs11001178	*KIAA0101*	chr10:76601805	chr15:64657210–64673702	−0,814	4.7989e-07	0.095
M12	rs10824245	*KIAA0101*	chr10:76666799	chr15:64657210–64673702	−0,814	4.7989e-07	0.095
M12	rs736086	*KIAA0101*	chr10:76683785	chr15:64657210–64673702	−0,814	4.7989e-07	0.095
M12	rs4746248	*KIAA0101*	chr10:76705881	chr15:64657210–64673702	−0,814	4.7989e-07	0.095
M12	rs7046685	*KIAA0101*	chr9:28659143	chr15:64657210–64673702	−0,873	5.0499e-07	0.095
M12	rs12341535	*KIAA0101*	chr9:28663042	chr15:64657210–64673702	−0,873	5.0499e-07	0.095
M12	rs17101861	*KIAA0101*	chr14:34232772	chr15:64657210–64673702	−0,873	5.0499e-07	0.095
M12	rs6756606	*CDK1*	chr2:178700057	chr10:62538211–62554610	−0,688	5.2009e-07	0.095
M12	rs10497482	*CDK1*	chr2:178805428	chr10:62538211–62554610	−0,688	5.2009e-07	0.095
M12	rs6756606	*KIAA0101*	chr2:178700057	chr15:64657210–64673702	−0,955	5.5269e-07	0.095
M12	rs10497482	*KIAA0101*	chr2:178805428	chr15:64657210–64673702	−0,955	5.5269e-07	0.095
M12	rs2714384	*BIRC5*	chr18:25302948	chr17:76210276–76221716	−0,348	6.4318e-07	0.098
M12	rs2617950	*BIRC5*	chr18:25309414	chr17:76210276–76221716	−0,348	6.4318e-07	0.098
M12	rs2851757	*BIRC5*	chr18:25313101	chr17:76210276–76221716	−0,348	6.4318e-07	0.098

Applying the new systems genetics approach for *trans*-eQTL identification in RA CD4+ T cells, the associations obtained after performing the *trans*-eQTL analysis are displayed for each immunity-enriched module ($P_{FDR}<0.01$).
Abbreviations: Bp, Base pair; β, Slope coefficient; P_{FDR}, P-value False Discovery Rate.
* Significant ($P_{FDR}<0.05$).

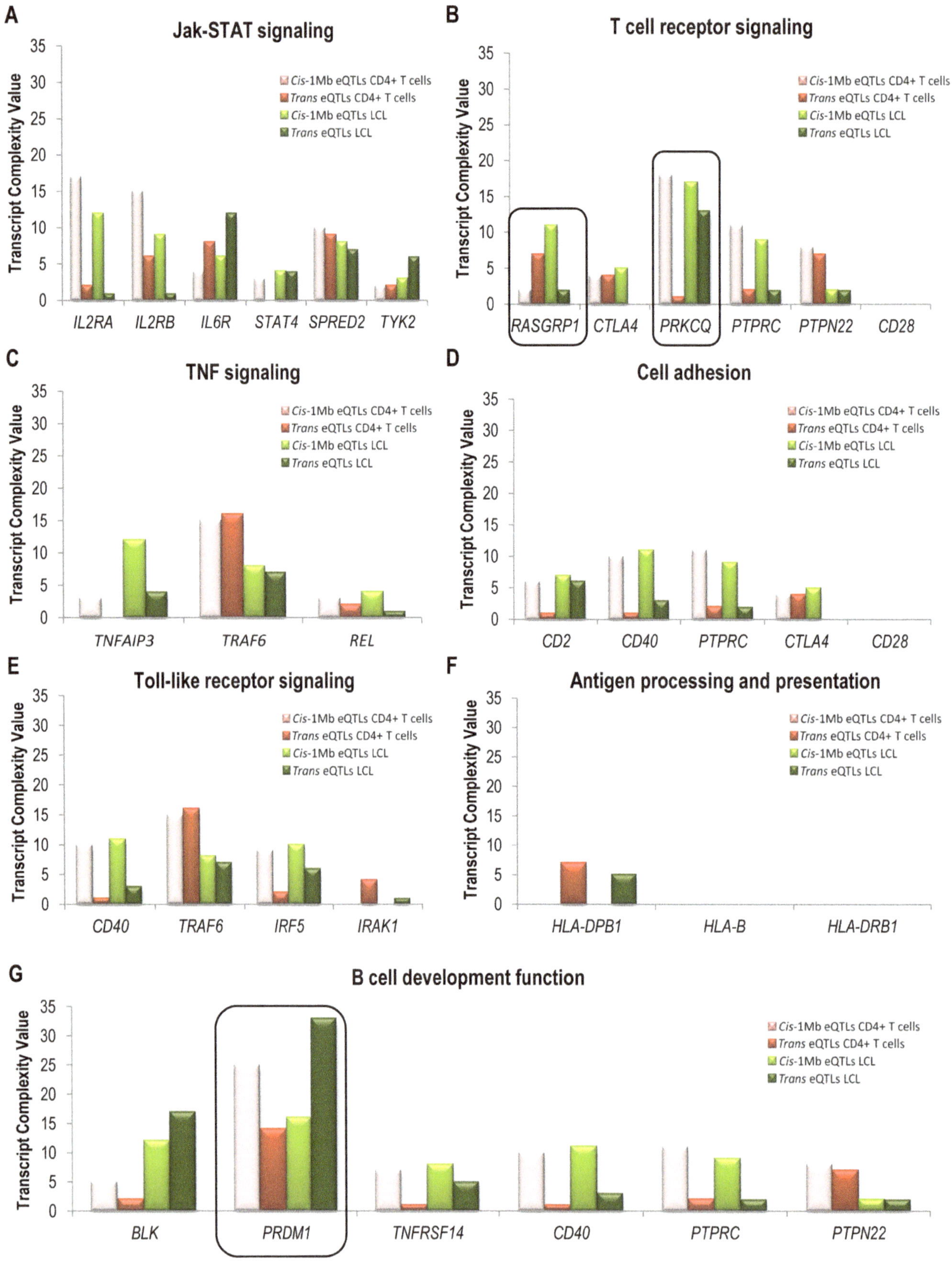
A
Jak-STAT signaling
Transcript Complexity Value
Cis-1Mb eQTLs CD4+ T cells
Trans eQTLs CD4+ T cells
Cis-1Mb eQTLs LCL
Trans eQTLs LCL
IL2RA IL2RB IL6R STAT4 SPRED2 TYK2
B
T cell receptor signaling
RASGRP1 CTLA4 PRKCQ PTPRC PTPN22 CD28
C
TNF signaling
TNFAIP3 TRAF6 REL
D
Cell adhesion
CD2 CD40 PTPRC CTLA4 CD28
E
Toll-like receptor signaling
CD40 TRAF6 IRF5 IRAK1
F
Antigen processing and presentation
HLA-DPB1 HLA-B HLA-DRB1
G
B cell development function
BLK PRDM1 TNFRSF14 CD40 PTPRC PTPN22

Figure 4. Transcript Complexity Value analysis of RA risk genes. TCV from the RA CD4+ T cell and control LCLs analyzed in RA risk genes. **A**: JAK-STAT signaling pathway. **B**: T cell receptor signaling pathway. **C**: TNF signaling pathway. **D**: Cell adhesion pathway. **E**: Toll-like receptor signaling pathway. **F**: Antigen processing and presentation pathway. **G**: B cell development function pathway. The genes that are framed represent those genes showing significant genomic regulation profiles between RA CD4+ T cells and LCLs (P<0.05).

profiles between both cell types, with a higher contribution of *trans* regulation in CD4+ T cells and a higher contribution of *cis* regulation in LCLs. Conversely, we found that the expression of *IRF9* (P = 7.9e−6), *IL12RB2* (P = 4.9e−3), *SHC4* (P = 5.6e−3), *IL12B* (P = 9.5e−3), *IL13* (P = 1.3e−2), *ITPR2* (P = 1.4e−2), *PTPN11* (P = 1.7e−2), *STAT5* (P = 2.3e−2) and *IL4* (P = 3.7e−2) genes were predominantly regulated by *cis*-acting elements in CD4+ T cells from RA patients.

The *IRF1* gene expression, whose *cis*- and *trans*- regulation was clearly found to be similar in RA CD4+ T cells, showed a markedly higher *trans*-eQTL regulation and almost absent *cis*-eQTL evidence of regulation in LCLs (P = 4.4e−2). *PLCG2* gene expression regulation was also similar in CD4+ T cells, but had a markedly high *cis* regulation and almost absent *trans* regulation in LCLs (P = 6.2e−3). Finally, the regulatory profile of *CEBPB* gene expression was characterized by the absence of a *trans* regulation in RA CD4+ T cells and the clear effect of *trans*-acting regulatory elements in LCLs (P = 3.3e−4).

The complete list of *cis*- and *trans*-eQTLs in CD4+ T cells and LCLs that were used to characterize these regulatory profiles are shown in Table S6, Table S7, Table S8 and Table S9.

Discussion

In the present study we have performed a genome-wide analysis of eQTLs in CD4+ T cells and we have identified new genetic regulatory variants associated with the gene expression of this key cell type in RA. Analyzing the transcriptome of CD4+ T cells from RA patients with active disease we found a genome-wide significant *cis*-eQTL regulating the expression of *FAM66C* gene. In order to detect significant *trans*-eQTLs, we developed a novel systems genetics approach that integrates gene expression and network biology information to reduce the multiple test burden associated with this type of analysis. Using this new approach, we found statistically significant *trans*-eQTLs regulating the expression of *BIRC5* and *KIAA0101* genes in CD4+ T cells in RA. Finally, comparing the genetic regulatory patterns of RA CD4+ T cells with control LCLs, we found several differential regulatory patterns. This study represents the first global analysis of the CD4+ T cell regulatory architecture associated with RA.

FAM66C is a long non-coding RNA (lncRNA) gene, whose biological functionality is still unknown. LncRNAs genes are transcribed into non-protein coding transcripts that are longer than 200 nucleotides and have been shown to act as modulators of the gene expression through epigenetic changes, transcriptional regulation and post-transcriptional regulation [46]. To our knowledge, the *FAM66C* lncRNA gene has not been previously associated with the pathophysiology of RA or any other complex disease. Recently, lncRNAs have emerged as possible contributors to the basis of human diseases by regulating the expression of neighbouring protein-coding genes [46,47]. Interestingly, *FAM66C* lncRNA gene maps near *C3AR1* gene (<115 Kb), which encodes a complement receptor that has been shown to be crucial in the modulation of the function of CD4+ T cell subtypes [48]. *C3AR1* expression promotes the proinflammatory activity of CD4+ T cells by enhancing the survival and function of Th1 and Th17 cells, while its inhibition leads to the induction of Treg CD4+ cells [49]. Additional studies will need to be carried out to determine if this or other biological mechanisms are responsible for the observed *FAM66C* association in the RA CD4+ T cell transcriptome.

Genes that encode proteins with high DC and BC values are likely to have a high impact in the network functionality. Consequently, the characterization of such central genes in the functional networks of specific cell types can be a powerful strategy to identify regulatory variants that contribute to disease [50,51]. Based on this assumption we developed a new dimensionality reduction approach that allowed us to determine the most influential genes in the CD4+ T cell specific networks and identify significant *trans*-eQTL associations with two of these genes, *BIRC5* and *KIAA0101*. These cell type-specific regulatory mechanisms are

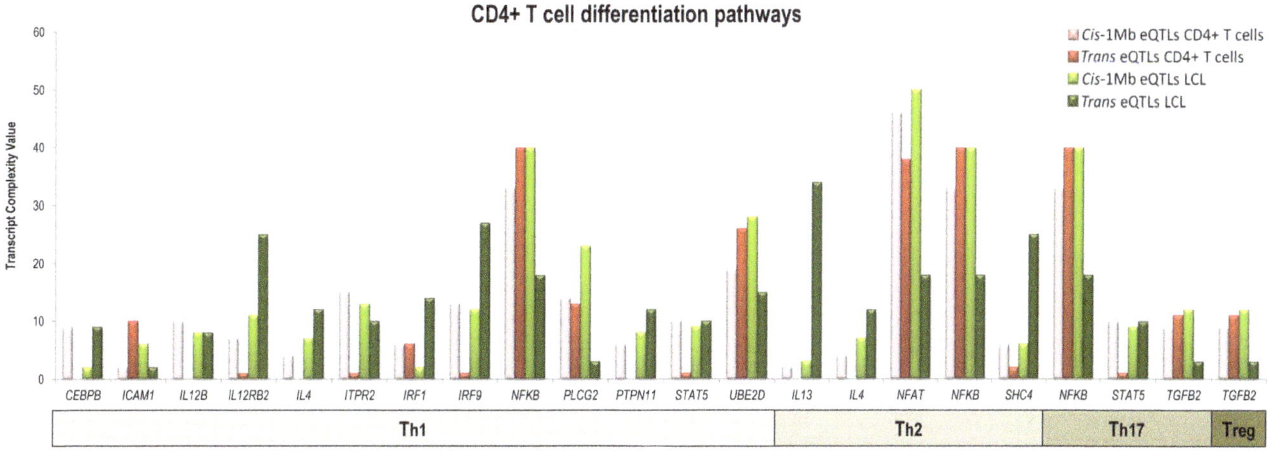

Figure 5. Transcript Complexity Value analysis of T cell differentiation genes. The type and quantity of significant eQTLs in RA CD4+ T cells and LCL cells are compared in the genes from the Th1, Th2, Th17 and Treg differentiation pathways. Only those genes showing a significantly different genomic regulation profile (P<0.05) are shown.

therefore likely to be of high importance in the activity of CD4+ T cells associated with RA pathology.

BIRC5 gene encodes survivin, an antiapoptotic protein that has been strongly associated to RA pathogenesis [52,53,54]. Survivin mRNA levels in peripherial blood mononuclear cells have been significantly associated with disease activity and the extent of joint damage in RA [55]. Importantly, survivin expression has been shown to be a key promoter of T cell proliferation after antigen presentation as well as a powerful antagonizer of apoptosis in activated T cells [56,57]. Increased proliferation and reduced cell death are two of the main characteristics of the CD4+ T cell population infiltrating the synovial membrane in RA [58,59]. Survivin-mediated cell survival could therefore have a major role in maintaining this pathogenic CD4+ T cell features. Additionally, there is recent evidence demonstrating that survivin expression in CD4+ T cells is activated by TNF-α cytokine which is the key regulator of the inflammatory and tissue-destructive pathways in RA [56].

KIAA0101 gene encodes for the Proliferating Cell Nuclear Antigen (PCNA) associated factor that acts as a regulator of DNA repair during DNA replication [60]. Importantly, PCNA-associated factor interacts with PCNA which increases the DNA polymerase's processivity during elongation of the leading strand and, therefore, accelerates the cell cycle progression [61]. In RA, an increased rate of cell proliferation has been shown to be associated with high levels of PCNA in synovial fibroblasts [62]. Accordingly, we suggest that the increased proliferation and reduced apoptosis of CD4+ T cells in the synovial membrane in RA is also regulated by the expression of *KIAA0101* gene.

The main goal of the new systems genetics approach described in this study is to objectively reduce the multiple test problem associated with the genome-wide analysis of *trans*-eQTLs. An exhaustive *trans*-eQTL analysis at a genome-wide scale would have required to perform approximately 12,000e6 association tests. This extremely high number of tests would have lead to an excessive penalization for multiple testing and, consequently, the inability to detect true associations. Using the new systems genetics approach we reduced this number of tests to 3.4e6 and 5.7e6 trans-eQTL analyses for M9 and M12 functional networks, respectively. Clearly, our study demonstrates that this methodological approach can be useful to identify significant *trans*-eQTLs without the need to explore all the combinatorial space. Importantly, the proposed systems genetics workflow includes several steps that can be easily customized to incorporate new or alternative bioinformatics methodologies. For example, in the functional enrichment analysis we used the gene ontology database but other functional annotation databases like the KEGG database can be used instead. The flexibility of this systems genetics approach workflow also makes this method a powerful strategy to uncover the relevant *trans*-eQTLs associated with human traits or diseases, including the upcoming studies based on RNA-seq technologies.

Trans-eQTL associations present in CD4+ T cells and absent in LCLs could be indicative of cell-specific regulatory processes that are specifically activated in RA. In the group of genes associated with RA risk, we found *RASGRP1* and *PRDM1* genes to have a differential regulation between both cell types. *RASGRP1* has been shown to be a critical regulator of the ERK/MAP signaling pathway which is crucial for T cell development, homeostasis and differentiation. T cells from patients with RA have been shown to have hyperresponsive ERK activity upon TCR stimulation [63]. Consequently, *RASGRP1* expression could be a specific modulator of the CD4+ T cell hyperresponsiveness to autoantigens associated with RA. *PRDM1* gene, instead, has been shown to drive the maturation of B-lymphocytes into immunoglobulin-secreting cells [64]. Consistently, we found a predominant *trans* regulation of *PRDM1* gene expression in LCLs, which are cell lines originally generated from B cells.

Among those genes involved in the CD4+ T cell differentiation pathways, we found a markedly differential regulatory profile of *Nuclear Factor Kappa B* (*NFKB*) and *Transforming Growth Factor Beta 2* (*TGFB2*) genes. NKFB is a well known transcription factor that has been associated with the T cell differentiation into Th1, Th2 and Th17 subtypes [65] and is a pivotal regulator of the inflammatory process present in rheumatoid arthritis [66,67,68]. The identification of the genetic variants that control *NFKB* gene expression in CD4+ T cells could lead to a better understanding of the biological mechanisms that are more relevant in the regulation of this cell type in RA.

TGFB2 is a Transforming Growth Factor family cytokine that has been associated with immunological tolerance and Treg and Th17 pathways [69]. Previous studies have shown that normal Treg/Th17 cell balance is not maintained in RA, with an increase in the differentiation of CD4+ T cells into the proinflammatory CD4+ Th17 phenotype and a decrease in the production of anti-inflammatory CD4+ Tregs [70,71,72]. Therefore, the increased *trans*-eQTLs associated with CD4+ T cells compared to LCLs, could indicate a specific regulatory mechanism associated with the increase of T cell autoreactivity observed in RA pathophysiology.

The different methodologies used in this study for the characterization of the CD4+ T cell-specific genetic regulation in RA have nonetheless some limitations. The CD4+ T cell population is highly heterogeneous with different subtypes exerting sometimes opposing regulatory activities in inflammation. Therefore, a more comprehensive analysis would have required the isolation and separate analysis of each CD4+ subpopulation. However, by using a homogeneous cohort of RA patients with a high level of disease activity, we favored the collection of a highly similar gene expression profile representative of the pathogenic regulation of CD4+ T cells in RA. Also, the comparison of the CD4+ regulatory pattern against LCLs of control individuals could have limited the identification of additional relevant regulatory mechanisms. As more eQTL data on different cell subtypes becomes available, more cell-to-cell comparisons can be performed in order to completely characterize the specific regulatory mechanisms of CD4+ T cells in RA.

In the analysis of differential genomic regulation profiles we focused on genes associated with the susceptibility to develop RA as well as genes associated with T cell differentiation. Another potential limitation of this approach is that other genes that encode proteins associated with RA pathophysiology are not included. From these, the pro-inflammatory cytokines TNF-α [73], IL-1β [74] and IFN-γ [75] and the anti-inflammatory cytokine IL-10 [76] have shown to be key in the development and chronification of RA. However, analyzing the regulatory profiles for these genes only a significant differential regulation for IL-1β is observed (data not shown). This association is due to a predominant *cis*-regulation in CD4+ T cells compared to an increased *trans*-regulation in LCLs. This result is consistent with the high level of expression of this cytokine observed in different immune and non-immune cell types like monocytes, tissue macrophages or synovial fibroblasts [77,78]. Together, the results of our study support the use of this methodology to characterize the functionality of disease risk genes as well as genes annotated to the cell type of interest.

One of the most important challenges ahead in human genetics is to identify the regulatory elements that control the gene expression and how they contribute to disease. This study is the first approach to the characterization of the CD4+ T cell regulatory profile associated with RA. In this comprehensive genetic study we report genetic regulatory variants that are significantly associated with the expression of *FAM66C* lncRNA, *BIRC5* and *KIAA0101* genes in RA CD4+ T cells. These results highlight the importance of the cell cycle processes in the pathological activity of RA CD4+ T cells infiltrating the synovial membrane, as well as the potential implication of lncRNA in the genetic regulatory basis of RA. This study represents a significant progress in the characterization of the genetic regulation of the main immune cell type involved in the pathogenesis of RA.

Supporting Information

Table S1 Main epidemiological and clinical features of the RA patients included in this study. Abbreviations: DAS28, Disease Activity Score.

Table S2 Total genes used in the comparative eQTL analysis between RA CD4+ T cells and LCLs.

Table S3 *Cis*-1Mb associations obtained in the genome-wide *cis*-eQTL analysis in RA CD4+ T cells (P_{FDR}<0.5). Abbreviations: Gene chr, Chromosomal location of the expressed gene; Gene coord, Coordinates of the expressed gene; Bp, Base pair; SNP chr, Chromosomal location of the SNP; SNP coord, Coordinates of the SNP; FDR, P-value False Discovery Rate.

Table S4 *Trans* associations in CD4+ T cells for M9 module genes (P<1e-5). Abbreviations: Gene chr, Chromosomal location of the expressed gene; Gene coord, Coordinates of the expressed gene; Bp, Base pair; SNP chr, Chromosomal location of the SNP; SNP coord, Coordinates of the SNP; Beta, Slope coefficient; FDR, P-value False Discovery Rate.

Table S5 *Trans* associations in CD4+ T cells for M12 module genes (P<1e-5). Abbreviations: Gene chr, Chromosomal location of the expressed gene; Gene coord, Coordinates of the expressed gene; Bp, Base pair; SNP chr, Chromosomal location of the SNP; SNP coord, Coordinates of the SNP; Beta, Slope coefficient; FDR, P-value False Discovery Rate.

Table S6 *Cis*-1Mb associations in CD4+ T cells (P<5e-2) that were used to characterize the gene regulatory profiles. Abbreviations: Gene chr, Chromosomal location of the expressed gene; Gene coord, Coordinates of the expressed gene; Bp, Base pair; SNP chr, Chromosomal location of the SNP; SNP coord, Coordinates of the SNP; Beta, Slope coefficient; FDR, P-value False Discovery Rate.

Table S7 *Trans* associations in CD4+ T cells (P<1e-5) that were used to characterize the gene regulatory profiles. Abbreviations: Gene chr, Chromosomal location of the expressed gene; Gene coord, Coordinates of the expressed gene; Bp, Base pair; SNP chr, Chromosomal location of the SNP; SNP coord, Coordinates of the SNP; Beta, Slope coefficient; FDR, P-value False Discovery Rate.

Table S8 *Cis*-1Mb associations in LCLs (P<5e-2) that were used to characterize the gene regulatory profiles. Abbreviations: Gene chr, Chromosomal location of the expressed gene; Gene coord, Coordinates of the expressed gene; Bp, Base pair; SNP chr, Chromosomal location of the SNP; SNP coord, Coordinates of the SNP; Beta, Slope coefficient; FDR, P-value False Discovery Rate.

Table S9 *Trans* associations in LCLs (P<1e-5) that were used to characterize the gene regulatory profiles. Abbreviations: Gene chr, Chromosomal location of the expressed gene; Gene coord, Coordinates of the expressed gene; Bp, Base pair; SNP chr, Chromosomal location of the SNP; SNP coord, Coordinates of the SNP; Beta, Slope coefficient; FDR, P-value False Discovery Rate.

Acknowledgments

We thank Joachim L. Schultze and Svenja Debey-Pascher from the LIMES Institute (Bönn, Germany) for technical support in microarray analysis.

We thank Devin Absher from the HudsonAlpha Institute for Biotechnology (Alabama, United States) for technical support in GWAS genotyping.

Author Contributions

Conceived and designed the experiments: AA SM AJ. Performed the experiments: AA AJ CP. Analyzed the data: AA AJ. Contributed reagents/materials/analysis tools: CP GÁ AJ AA. Contributed to the writing of the manuscript: AA SM AJ.

References

1. Choy EH, Panayi GS (2001) Cytokine pathways and joint inflammation in rheumatoid arthritis. N Engl J Med 344: 907–916.
2. Firestein GS (2003) Evolving concepts of rheumatoid arthritis. Nature 423: 356–361.
3. Maxwell L, Singh JA (2009) Abatacept for rheumatoid arthritis. Cochrane Database Syst Rev: CD007277. doi: 007210.001002/14651858.CD14007277. pub14651852.
4. Pieper J, Herrath J, Raghavan S, Muhammad K, Vollenhoven R, et al. (2013) CTLA4-Ig (abatacept) therapy modulates T cell effector functions in autoantibody-positive rheumatoid arthritis patients. BMC Immunol 14:34: 10.1186/1471-2172-1114-1134.
5. Skapenko A, Leipe J, Lipsky PE, Schulze-Koops H (2005) The role of the T cell in autoimmune inflammation. Arthritis Res Ther 7: S4–14. Epub 2005 Mar 2016.
6. Manolio TA (2010) Genomewide association studies and assessment of the risk of disease. N Engl J Med 363: 166–176. doi: 110.1056/NEJMra0905980.
7. Montgomery SB, Dermitzakis ET (2011) From expression QTLs to personalized transcriptomics. Nat Rev Genet 12: 277–282. doi: 210.1038/nrg2969. Epub 2011 Mar 1039.
8. Cookson W, Liang L, Abecasis G, Moffatt M, Lathrop M (2009) Mapping complex disease traits with global gene expression. Nat Rev Genet 10: 184–194. doi: 110.1038/nrg2537.
9. Majewski J, Pastinen T (2011) The study of eQTL variations by RNA-seq: from SNPs to phenotypes. Trends Genet 27: 72–79. doi: 10.1016/j.tig.2010.1010.1006. Epub 2010 Nov 1029.
10. Nica AC, Dermitzakis ET (2013) Expression quantitative trait loci: present and future. Philos Trans R Soc Lond B Biol Sci 368: 20120362. doi: 20120310.20121098/rstb.20122012.20120362. Print 20122013.
11. Dimas AS, Deutsch S, Stranger BE, Montgomery SB, Borel C, et al. (2009) Common regulatory variation impacts gene expression in a cell type-dependent manner. Science 325: 1246–1250. doi: 1210.1126/science.1174148. Epub 1172009 Jul 1174130.
12. Heintzman ND, Hon GC, Hawkins RD, Kheradpour P, Stark A, et al. (2009) Histone modifications at human enhancers reflect global cell-type-specific gene expression. Nature 459: 108–112. doi: 110.1038/nature07829. Epub 02009 Mar 07818.
13. Ackermann M, Sikora-Wohlfeld W, Beyer A (2013) Impact of natural genetic variation on gene expression dynamics. PLoS Genet 9: e1003514. doi: 1003510.1001371/journal.pgen.1003514. Epub 1002013 Jun 1003516.

14. Heinzen EL, Ge D, Cronin KD, Maia JM, Shianna KV, et al. (2008) Tissue-specific genetic control of splicing: implications for the study of complex traits. PLoS Biol 6: e1. doi: 10.1371/journal.pbio.1000001.
15. Grundberg E, Kwan T, Ge B, Lam KC, Koka V, et al. (2009) Population genomics in a disease targeted primary cell model. Genome Res 19: 1942–1952. doi: 1910.1101/gr.095224.095109. Epub 092009 Aug 095224.
16. Doss S, Schadt EE, Drake TA, Lusis AJ (2005) Cis-acting expression quantitative trait loci in mice. Genome Res 15: 681–691. Epub 2005 Apr 2018.
17. van Nas A, Ingram-Drake L, Sinsheimer JS, Wang SS, Schadt EE, et al. (2010) Expression quantitative trait loci: replication, tissue- and sex-specificity in mice. Genetics 185: 1059–1068. doi: 1010.1534/genetics.1110.116087. Epub 112010 May 116083.
18. Fehrmann RS, Jansen RC, Veldink JH, Westra HJ, Arends D, et al. (2011) Trans-eQTLs reveal that independent genetic variants associated with a complex phenotype converge on intermediate genes, with a major role for the HLA. PLoS Genet 7: e1002197. doi: 1002110.1001371/journal.pgen.1002197. Epub 1002011 Aug 1002194.
19. Civelek M, Lusis AJ (2013) Systems genetics approaches to understand complex traits. Nat Rev Genet 3.
20. Small KS, Hedman AK, Grundberg E, Nica AC, Thorleifsson G, et al. (2011) Identification of an imprinted master trans regulator at the KLF14 locus related to multiple metabolic phenotypes. Nat Genet 43: 561–564. doi: 510.1038/ng.1833. Epub 2011 May 1015.
21. Arnett FC, Edworthy SM, Bloch DA, McShane DJ, Fries JF, et al. (1988) The American Rheumatism Association 1987 revised criteria for the classification of rheumatoid arthritis. Arthritis Rheum 31: 315–324.
22. Prevoo ML, van 't Hof MA, Kuper HH, van Leeuwen MA, van de Putte LB, et al. (1995) Modified disease activity scores that include twenty-eight-joint counts. Development and validation in a prospective longitudinal study of patients with rheumatoid arthritis. Arthritis Rheum 38: 44–48.
23. Pruitt KD, Tatusova T, Brown GR, Maglott DR (2012) NCBI Reference Sequences (RefSeq): current status, new features and genome annotation policy. Nucleic Acids Res 40: D130–135. doi: 110.1093/nar/gkr1079. Epub 2011 Nov 1024.
24. Ihaka R, Gentleman RC (1996) R: A language for data analysis and graphics. Journal of Computational and Graphical Statistics 5: 299–314.
25. Bolstad BM, Irizarry RA, Astrand M, Speed TP (2003) A comparison of normalization methods for high density oligonucleotide array data based on variance and bias. Bioinformatics 19: 185–193.
26. Johnson WE, Li C, Rabinovic A (2007) Adjusting batch effects in microarray expression data using empirical Bayes methods. Biostatistics 8: 118–127. Epub 2006 Apr 2021.
27. Edgar R, Domrachev M, Lash AE (2002) Gene Expression Omnibus: NCBI gene expression and hybridization array data repository. Nucleic Acids Res 30: 207–210.
28. Purcell S, Neale B, Todd-Brown K, Thomas L, Ferreira MA, et al. (2007) PLINK: a tool set for whole-genome association and population-based linkage analyses. Am J Hum Genet 81: 559–575. Epub 2007 Jul 2025.
29. Price AL, Patterson NJ, Plenge RM, Weinblatt ME, Shadick NA, et al. (2006) Principal components analysis corrects for stratification in genome-wide association studies. Nat Genet 38: 904–909. Epub 2006 Jul 2023.
30. Shabalin AA (2012) Matrix eQTL: ultra fast eQTL analysis via large matrix operations. Bioinformatics 28: 1353-1358. doi: 1310.1093/bioinformatics/bts1163. Epub 2012 Apr 1356.
31. Stranger BE, Forrest MS, Clark AG, Minichiello MJ, Deutsch S, et al. (2005) Genome-wide associations of gene expression variation in humans. PLoS Genet 1: e78. Epub 2005 Dec 2016.
32. Lettice LA, Heaney SJ, Purdie LA, Li L, de Beer P, et al. (2003) A long-range Shh enhancer regulates expression in the developing limb and fin and is associated with preaxial polydactyly. Hum Mol Genet 12: 1725–1735.
33. Storey JD, Tibshirani R (2003) Statistical significance for genomewide studies. Proc Natl Acad Sci U S A 100: 9440–9445. Epub 2003 Jul 9425.
34. Langfelder P, Horvath S (2008) WGCNA: an R package for weighted correlation network analysis. BMC Bioinformatics 9:559: 10.1186/1471-2105-1189-1559.
35. Ashburner M, Ball CA, Blake JA, Botstein D, Butler H, et al. (2000) Gene ontology: tool for the unification of biology. The Gene Ontology Consortium. Nat Genet 25: 25–29.
36. Huang da W, Sherman BT, Lempicki RA (2009) Systematic and integrative analysis of large gene lists using DAVID bioinformatics resources. Nat Protoc 4: 44–57. doi: 10.1038/nprot.2008.1211.
37. Franceschini A, Szklarczyk D, Frankild S, Kuhn M, Simonovic M, et al. (2013) STRING v9.1: protein-protein interaction networks, with increased coverage and integration. Nucleic Acids Res 41: D808–815. doi: 810.1093/nar/gks1094. Epub 2012 Nov 1029.
38. Vallabhajosyula RR, Chakravarti D, Lutfeali S, Ray A, Raval A (2009) Identifying hubs in protein interaction networks. PLoS One 4: e5344.
39. Hahn MW, Kern AD (2005) Comparative genomics of centrality and essentiality in three eukaryotic protein-interaction networks. Mol Biol Evol 22: 803–806. Epub 2004 Dec 2022.
40. Joy MP, Brock A, Ingber DE, Huang S (2005) High-betweenness proteins in the yeast protein interaction network. J Biomed Biotechnol 2005: 96–103.
41. Shannon P, Markiel A, Ozier O, Baliga NS, Wang JT, et al. (2003) Cytoscape: a software environment for integrated models of biomolecular interaction networks. Genome Res 13: 2498–2504.
42. Julia A, Marsal S (2013) The genetic architecture of rheumatoid arthritis: from susceptibility to clinical subphenotype associations. Curr Top Med Chem 13: 720–731.
43. Ogata H, Goto S, Sato K, Fujibuchi W, Bono H, et al. (1999) KEGG: Kyoto Encyclopedia of Genes and Genomes. Nucleic Acids Res 27: 29–34.
44. (2003) The International HapMap Project. Nature 426: 789–796.
45. Myers S, Bottolo L, Freeman C, McVean G, Donnelly P (2005) A fine-scale map of recombination rates and hotspots across the human genome. Science 310: 321–324.
46. Mercer TR, Dinger ME, Mattick JS (2009) Long non-coding RNAs: insights into functions. Nat Rev Genet 10: 155–159. doi: 110.1038/nrg2521.
47. Esteller M (2011) Non-coding RNAs in human disease. Nat Rev Genet 12: 861–874. doi: 810.1038/nrg3074.
48. Kolev M, Le Friec G, Kemper C (2013) The role of complement in CD4(+) T cell homeostasis and effector functions. Semin Immunol 25: 12–19. doi: 10.1016/j.smim.2013.1004.1012. Epub 2013 May 1029.
49. Strainic MG, Shevach EM, An F, Lin F, Medof ME (2013) Absence of signaling into CD4(+) cells via C3aR and C5aR enables autoinductive TGF-beta1 signaling and induction of Foxp3(+) regulatory T cells. Nat Immunol 14: 162–171. doi: 110.1038/ni.2499. Epub 2012 Dec 1023.
50. Han JD, Bertin N, Hao T, Goldberg DS, Berriz GF, et al. (2004) Evidence for dynamically organized modularity in the yeast protein-protein interaction network. Nature 430: 88–93. Epub 2004 Jun 2009.
51. Zhu M, Gao L, Li X, Liu Z, Xu C, et al. (2009) The analysis of the drug-targets based on the topological properties in the human protein-protein interaction network. J Drug Target 17: 524–532. doi: 510.1080/10611860903046610.
52. Svensson B, Hafstrom I, Forslind K, Albertsson K, Tarkowski A, et al. (2010) Increased expression of proto-oncogene survivin predicts Joint destruction and persistent disease activity in early rheumatoid arthritis. Ann Med 42: 45–54. doi: 10.3109/07853890903376280.
53. Andersson SE, Svensson MN, Erlandsson MC, Dehlin M, Andersson KM, et al. (2012) Activation of Fms-like tyrosine kinase 3 signaling enhances survivin expression in a mouse model of rheumatoid arthritis. PLoS One 7: e47668. doi: 47610.41371/journal.pone.0047668. Epub 0042012 Oct 0047617.
54. Bokarewa M, Brink M, Erlandsson M, Rantapaa Dahlqvist S (2014) Survivin but not Fms-like tyrosine kinase 3 ligand is up-regulated before the onset of rheumatoid arthritis: a pilot study. Arthritis Res Ther 16: R45.
55. Ahn JK, Oh JM, Lee J, Bae EK, Ahn KS, et al. (2010) Increased extracellular survivin in the synovial fluid of rheumatoid arthritis patients: fibroblast-like synoviocytes as a potential source of extracellular survivin. Inflammation 33: 381–388. doi: 310.1007/s10753-10010-19196-10751.
56. Song J, So T, Cheng M, Tang X, Croft M (2005) Sustained survivin expression from OX40 costimulatory signals drives T cell clonal expansion. Immunity 22: 621–631.
57. Song J, Salek-Ardakani S, So T, Croft M (2007) The kinases aurora B and mTOR regulate the G1-S cell cycle progression of T lymphocytes. Nat Immunol 8: 64–73. Epub 2006 Nov 2026.
58. Salmon M, Scheel-Toellner D, Huissoon AP, Pilling D, Shamsadeen N, et al. (1997) Inhibition of T cell apoptosis in the rheumatoid synovium. J Clin Invest 99: 439–446.
59. Liu H, Pope RM (2003) The role of apoptosis in rheumatoid arthritis. Curr Opin Pharmacol 3: 317–322.
60. Kais Z, Barsky SH, Mathsyaraja H, Zha A, Ransburgh DJ, et al. (2011) KIAA0101 interacts with BRCA1 and regulates centrosome number. Mol Cancer Res 9: 1091–1099. doi: 1010.1158/1541-7786.MCR-1010-0503. Epub 2011 Jun 1014.
61. Burkovics P, Hajdu I, Szukacsov V, Unk I, Haracska L (2009) Role of PCNA-dependent stimulation of 3′-phosphodiesterase and 3′-5′ exonuclease activities of human Ape2 in repair of oxidative DNA damage. Nucleic Acids Res 37: 4247–4255. doi: 4210.1093/nar/gkp4357. Epub 2009 May 4213.
62. Karouzakis E, Gay RE, Michel BA, Gay S, Neidhart M (2009) DNA hypomethylation in rheumatoid arthritis synovial fibroblasts. Arthritis Rheum 60: 3613–3622. doi: 3610.1002/art.25018.
63. Deshpande P, Cavanagh MM, Le Saux S, Singh K, Weyand CM, et al. (2013) IL-7- and IL-15-mediated TCR sensitization enables T cell responses to self-antigens. J Immunol 190: 1416–1423. doi: 1410.4049/jimmunol.1201620. Epub 1202013 Jan 1201616.
64. Shapiro-Shelef M, Lin KI, McHeyzer-Williams LJ, Liao J, McHeyzer-Williams MG, et al. (2003) Blimp-1 is required for the formation of immunoglobulin secreting plasma cells and pre-plasma memory B cells. Immunity 19: 607–620.
65. Oh H, Ghosh S (2013) NF-kappaB: roles and regulation in different CD4(+) T-cell subsets. Immunol Rev 252: 41–51. doi: 10.1111/imr.12033.
66. Makarov SS (2001) NF-kappa B in rheumatoid arthritis: a pivotal regulator of inflammation, hyperplasia, and tissue destruction. Arthritis Res 3: 200–206. Epub 2001 Mar 2026.
67. Feldmann M, Andreakos E, Smith C, Bondeson J, Yoshimura S, et al. (2002) Is NF-kappaB a useful therapeutic target in rheumatoid arthritis? Ann Rheum Dis 61: ii13-18.
68. Simmonds RE, Foxwell BM (2008) Signalling, inflammation and arthritis: NF-kappaB and its relevance to arthritis and inflammation. Rheumatology (Oxford) 47: 584–590. doi: 510.1093/rheumatology/kem1298. Epub 2008 Jan 1029.

69. Li MO, Sanjabi S, Flavell RA (2006) Transforming growth factor-beta controls development, homeostasis, and tolerance of T cells by regulatory T cell-dependent and -independent mechanisms. Immunity 25: 455–471.
70. Eisenstein EM, Williams CB (2009) The T(reg)/Th17 cell balance: a new paradigm for autoimmunity. Pediatr Res 65: 26R–31R. doi: 10.1203/PDR.1200b1013e31819e31876c31817.
71. Noack M, Miossec P (2014) Th17 and regulatory T cell balance in autoimmune and inflammatory diseases. Autoimmun Rev 11: 00008-00001.
72. Wang W, Shao S, Jiao Z, Guo M, Xu H, et al. (2012) The Th17/Treg imbalance and cytokine environment in peripheral blood of patients with rheumatoid arthritis. Rheumatol Int 32: 887–893. doi: 810.1007/s00296-00010-01710-00290. Epub 02011 Jan 00211.
73. Vasanthi P, Nalini G, Rajasekhar G Role of tumor necrosis factor-alpha in rheumatoid arthritis: a review.
74. Contassot E, Beer HD, French LE (2012) Interleukin-1, inflammasomes, autoinflammation and the skin. Swiss Med Wkly 142:w13590: 10.4414/smw.2012.13590.
75. Page CE, Smale S, Carty SM, Amos N, Lauder SN, et al. (2010) Interferon-gamma inhibits interleukin-1beta-induced matrix metalloproteinase production by synovial fibroblasts and protects articular cartilage in early arthritis. Arthritis Res Ther 12: R49. doi: 10.1186/ar2960. Epub 2010 Mar 1122.
76. Fu LH, Ma CL, Cong B, Li SJ, Chen HY, et al. (2011) Hypomethylation of proximal CpG motif of interleukin-10 promoter regulates its expression in human rheumatoid arthritis. Acta Pharmacol Sin 32: 1373–1380. doi: 1310.1038/aps.2011.1398. Epub 2011 Oct 1310.
77. Smolen JS, Aletaha D, Redlich K (2012) The pathogenesis of rheumatoid arthritis: new insights from old clinical data? Nat Rev Rheumatol 8: 235–243. doi: 210.1038/nrrheum.2012.1023.
78. Pope RM, Shahrara S (2013) Possible roles of IL-12-family cytokines in rheumatoid arthritis. Nat Rev Rheumatol 9: 252–256. doi: 210.1038/nrrheum.2012.1170. Epub 2012 Oct 1023.

14

Further Optimization of the Reliability of the 28-Joint Disease Activity Score in Patients with Early Rheumatoid Arthritis

Liseth Siemons[1]*, Peter M. ten Klooster[1], Harald E. Vonkeman[1,2], Mart A. F. J. van de Laar[1,2], Cees A. W. Glas[3]

1 Arthritis Center Twente, Department of Psychology, Health & Technology, University of Twente, Enschede, the Netherlands, **2** Arthritis Center Twente, Department of Rheumatology, Medisch Spectrum Twente, Enschede, the Netherlands, **3** Department of Research Methodology, Measurement and Data Analysis, University of Twente, Enschede, the Netherlands

Abstract

Background: The 28-joint Disease Activity Score (DAS28) combines scores on a 28-tender and swollen joint count (TJC28 and SJC28), a patient-reported measure for general health (GH), and an inflammatory marker (either the erythrocyte sedimentation rate [ESR] or the C-reactive protein [CRP]) into a composite measure of disease activity in rheumatoid arthritis (RA). This study examined the reliability of the DAS28 in patients with early RA using principles from generalizability theory and evaluated whether it could be increased by adjusting individual DAS28 component weights.

Methods: Patients were drawn from the DREAM registry and classified into a "fast response" group (N = 466) and "slow response" group (N = 80), depending on their pace of reaching remission. Composite reliabilities of the DAS28-ESR and DAS28-CRP were determined with the individual components' reliability, weights, variances, error variances, correlations and covariances. Weight optimization was performed by minimizing the error variance of the index.

Results: Composite reliabilities of 0.85 and 0.86 were found for the DAS28-ESR and DAS28-CRP, respectively, and were approximately equal across patients groups. Component reliabilities, however, varied widely both within and between sub-groups, ranging from 0.614 for GH ("slow response" group) to 0.912 for ESR ("fast response" group). Weight optimization increased composite reliability even further. In the total and "fast response" groups, this was achieved mostly by decreasing the weight of the TJC28 and GH. In the "slow response" group, though, the weights of the TJC28 and SJC28 were increased, while those of the inflammatory markers and GH were substantially decreased.

Conclusions: The DAS28-ESR and the DAS28-CRP are reliable instruments for assessing disease activity in early RA and reliability can be increased even further by adjusting component weights. Given the low reliability and weightings of the general health component across subgroups it is recommended to explore alternative patient-reported outcome measures for inclusion in the DAS28.

Editor: Chi Zhang, University of Texas Southwestern Medical Center, United States of America

Funding: There was no involvement of study sponsors, so there were no funders with a role in study design, data collection and analysis, decision to publish, or preparation of the manuscript.

Competing Interests: The authors have declared that no competing interests exist.

* Email: L.siemons@utwente.nl

Introduction

If a concept or condition is too complex to measure with a single instrument, multiple measurements are often combined into a linear composite score (i.e. an index measure). For rheumatoid arthritis (RA) the 28-joint Disease Activity Score (DAS28) is such an index measure, widely used for determining a patient's degree of disease activity [1]. It consists of 4 different individual components: a 28-tender joint count, a 28-swollen joint count, a patient-reported rating of general health, and a non-specific acute phase reactant of systemic inflammation which can be either the erythrocyte sedimentation rate (ESR) or the C-reactive protein (CRP). Each component has its own specific weight in the composite score, based on canonical discriminant functions for classifying high and low disease activity.

The DAS28 has received much attention over the years and has been shown to be a valid measure [1,2]. However, since reliability is a prerequisite for validity [3], the index should be reliable as well. While several studies have already determined the reliability of the DAS28 using Cronbach's Alpha [2,4,5], it is not appropriate to use this internal consistency measure with an index measure, as opposed to scales. Where a scale consists of correlated items which all measure the same construct, an index consists of items which are not necessarily highly correlated but which are considered indicators because they themselves define the construct [6]. As a result, the components might measure completely different aspects of disease activity, which is also the case with the DAS28. This poses significant methodological challenges for reliability testing. To overcome these challenges, generalizability theory [7,8] can be used to estimate the reliability of an index score by disentangling different sources of error.

As such, the first aim of this study was to determine the reliability of the DAS28 using generalizability theory. Since reliability is a concept defined relative to a specific population of patients [9], the second aim of this study was to examine whether the reliability of the index is acceptably high in relevant subpopulations and whether this reliability can be increased by adjusting the weightings of the individual component scores within the DAS28, which was shown to be the case.

Methods

Ethics Statement

As evaluated by the ethics committees of the participating hospitals, and in accordance with Dutch law, no ethical approval was required because data collection took place in daily clinical practice. Nevertheless, informed consent was obtained from each patient.

Patients

Patients were drawn from the remission induction cohort of the Dutch Rheumatoid Arthritis Monitoring (DREAM) registry [10]. This observational multicenter cohort started in 2006 and, although patient recruitment for this cohort has stopped in 2012, data collection of included patients is still ongoing. For this study, all data available at 0, 3, 6, 9, and 12 months were accessible for analyses. To be eligible for inclusion in the cohort, patients were DMARD and prednisolone naïve, they were allowed to have a maximum symptom duration of 1 year, and they needed to be 18 years or older. Additionally, they were not in remission, as measured with the DAS28. Early RA classification was based on a clinical diagnosis by the rheumatologist. For the present study, patients were classified into 2 groups as identified in the study by Siemons et al. [11]: a "fast response" group of patients quickly reaching remission and a "slow response" group of patients reaching remission at a slower pace. Because reliability calculations are sample dependent slight differences can be expected between the two response groups.

Measures

The primary measures of interest were the 28-tender joint count (TJC28), the 28-swollen joint count (SJC28), a 100 millimeter visual analogue scale on general health (GH: where 0 = very good and 100 = very bad), the erythrocyte sedimentation rate (ESR), and the C-reactive protein (CRP). Using these variables, the DAS28-ESR and DAS28-CRP were calculated as follows [12]:

$$DAS28-ESR=0.56*\sqrt{TJC28}+0.28*\sqrt{SJC28}+0.70*Ln(ESR)+0.014*GH \quad (1)$$

$$DAS28-CRP=0.56*\sqrt{TJC28}+0.28*\sqrt{SJC28}+0.36*Ln(CRP+1)+0.014*GH+0.96 \quad (2)$$

Patients additionally completed the Health Assessment Questionnaire (HAQ) which measures physical functioning [13] and the 36-item Short Form Health Survey (SF-36) which assesses physical and mental health status [14].

Statistical analyses

Baseline between-group comparisons were made using independent t-tests for normally distributed continuous variables, Kruskal Wallis tests for variables with skewed distributions, and Chi-Square tests for dichotomous variables.

Although a DAS28 score is assumed to represent a patient's disease activity, in reality this score consists of two parts: 1) the actual (true) score of that patient's disease activity, and 2) random measurement errors [3]. Errors give rise to an under- or overestimation of the true score. This might be due to, among others, certain distractions during test administration, the patient's mood while filling out the test, or a misreading of the items. Reliability is a representation of measurement consistency; it is the ratio between true score variance and observed total score variance, where the latter consists of a true score part and an error part [3]. Higher error variance leads to lower reliability. However, although these basic principles do apply to the individual components of the DAS28, the composite reliability of an index also depends on the interrelationships of its components. Composite reliability is a function of the reliability of the individual components, the weights that are assigned to the components as reflected in the DAS28 formulas, the variances and error variances of the component scores, and the correlations and covariances between the different components. All this can be combined into the following formula [8,15]:

$$r=1-\frac{\sum_{i=1}^{n}(w_i^2\sigma_{e,Xi}^2)}{\sum_{i=1}^{n}(w_i^2\sigma_{Xi}^2)+\sum_{i=1}^{n}\sum_{j(\neq i)=1}^{n}(w_iw_j\sigma_{Xi,Xj})} \quad (3)$$

Where:

I. w_i is the weight of component i, as defined in the DAS28 formulas 1 and 2 described above;
II. σ_{Xi}^2 is the observed variance of component i;
III. $\sigma_{e,Xi}^2$ is the error variance of component i, which is a function of the component reliability and the observed variance: $\sigma_{e,Xi}^2$ = (1 - reliability of component i) * σ_{Xi}^2;
IV. $\sigma_{Xi,Xj}$ is the covariance between the two components, which can be rewritten as: *Correlation* $_{Xi,Xj}$* *Standard deviation* $_{Xi}$* *Standard deviation* $_{Xj}$.

Note that the nominator of the ratio in formula 3 is the error variance of the index, while the denominator is the total variance.

In this study, the error variances of joint count components were calculated from their observed variance and reliability levels, whereas the error variances of GH and both inflammatory measures were obtained from univariate linear regression analyses. However, two significant problems arose during component reliability computations.

First, it was not appropriate to calculate the reliabilities of the joint count components with Cronbach's Alpha, since Cronbach's Alpha assumes the total score to be a linear combination of all items (i.e. each item is regarded as a parallel test of the other component items) whereas the joint count components are square root transformed in the DAS28. Consequently, split-half reliabilities were determined instead. As demonstrated by Siemons et al. [16], RA is characterized by a definite left-right symmetry of joint involvement. Consequently, the square root sum scores of the left and right joints were considered to represent two parallel tests and their correlation was used as an estimate of reliability.

Second, given the structure of the cohort, with time frames of several weeks or even months between consecutive measurements, it was not possible to perform proper test-retest reliabilities for the single-item components (i.e. ESR, CRP, and GH). Therefore, a generalizability theory principle was used to determine reliability. After running a univariate general linear model analysis on a longitudinal dataset (including all available data at 0, 3, 6, 9, and 12 months) the person variance could be separated from the time variance and reliability could be calculated as the ratio between person variance and total variance.

All computations of reliabilities were performed on the total patient group as well as on the two identified subgroups using SPSS version 21.0.

After calculating the composite reliabilities, it was investigated whether the reliability in both the total as well as the specific patient groups could be optimized by adjusting the component's weights. Optimal weights were computed by minimizing the error variance of the index, that is, the nominator of the ratio in formula 3, subject to the constraint that the total variance of the index does not change. The resulting quadratic optimization problem under quadratic constraints was solved using a procedure developed by Albers, Critchley, and Gower [17]. For more applications, refer to Albers, Critchley, and Gower [18].

Results

Patients

A total of 565 patients were included for analysis; 466 from the "fast response" group and 80 from the "slow response" group. Overall, they had a mean age of approximately 58 years, the majority were women (63%) and rheumatoid factor positive (54%), and their baseline disease was characterized by several tender and swollen joints as well as by a diminished physical health status (Table 1).

No significant differences were found in age, mental health, or rheumatoid factor positivity between the fast and slow response group, but the slow response group did contain significantly more women. Additionally, the slow response group had a significantly worse disease condition, characterized by higher DAS28 scores, a poorer state of general and physical health, higher levels of inflammatory markers, and a higher number of tender and swollen joints, as compared to the fast response group.

Reliability calculations

Tables 2–4 show the variances, error variances and reliabilities of the individual components together with their correlations and covariances. All correlations were small to moderate, as is not unusual in index measures. Component reliabilities varied widely both within and between sub-groups, ranging from 0.614 for GH in the "slow response" group to 0.912 for ESR in the "fast response" group. Furthermore, ESR component reliabilities were highest and the TJC28 outperformed the SJC28 across all groups.

Using formula 3 resulted in overall reliabilities of 0.85 and 0.86 for the DAS28-ESR and DAS28-CRP composites, respectively. Sub-analyses showed DAS28-ESR reliabilities of 0.85 and 0.82 and DAS28-CRP reliabilities of 0.85 and 0.84 for the "fast response" and "slow response" group, respectively. These results demonstrate that both DAS28 scores are approximately equally reliable across patient groups, that is, the differences were only small and all reliability levels were high (>0.80).

Optimizing reliability

The results of the optimization of composite reliability by adjusting the weights are shown in Table 5. The original weights are given in the third column. The next three columns give the estimated optimal weights in the total group and in the "fast response" and "slow response" groups, respectively. Further, in

Table 1. Patient characteristics and group comparisons at inclusion.

Variable	Mean (SD) or Median (range)* Total group	Mean (SD) or Median (range)* "Fast response" group	Mean (SD) or Median (range)* "Slow response" group	Significance (p) group comparisons
Gender (female)	342/546 (62.6%)	283/466 (60.7%)	59/80 (73.8%)	0.026~
Age (years)	57.96 (14.31)	57.85 (14.62)	58.59 (12.41)	0.672¶
DAS28-ESR	4.28 (1.45)	4.11 (1.42)	5.22 (1.29)	<0.001¶
DAS28-CRP	4.02 (1.31)	3.88 (1.28)	4.79 (1.24)	<0.001¶
28-Tender joint count	3 (0–28)	3 (0–28)	6 (0–28)	<0.001#
28-Swollen joint count	5 (0–24)	4 (0–24)	6.50 (0–24)	0.001#
GH	44.32 (26.11)	42.52 (25.76)	54.82 (25.83)	<0.001¶
ESR (mm/hour)	21.50 (1–120)	20 (1–111)	30 (7–120)	<0.001#
CRP (mg/l)	9.00 (1–158)	6 (1–158)	11 (1–115)	0.004#
Rheumatoid factor +	274/506 (54.2%)	233/431 (54.1%)	41/75 (54.7%)	0.923~
SF36 – physical health	37.17 (9.09)	37.93 (9.09)	32.91 (7.88)	0.001¶
SF36 – mental health	48.16 (11.67)	48.55 (11.37)	45.99 (13.07)	0.094¶
HAQ	1.00 (0.72)	0.92 (0.70)	1.41 (0.66)	0.001¶

*The values for gender and rheumatoid factor positivity are the number of patients/number of patients assessed (%).
#Group comparisons performed with Kruskall Wallis tests.
~Group comparisons performed with Chi-Square tests.
¶Group comparisons performed with independent t-tests.
DAS28 = disease activity score for 28 joints, GH = general health, ESR = erythrocyte sedimentation rate, CRP = C-Reactive Protein, SF36 = Short Form Health Survey with 36 items, HAQ = Health Assessment Questionnaire.

Table 2. Variances, error variances and reliabilities of the DAS-28 components.

	Total patient group (N=546)			"Fast response" group (N=466)			"Slow response" group (N=80)		
Component	Variance	Error variance	Component Reliability	Variance	Error variance	Component Reliability	Variance	Error variance	Component Reliability
$\sqrt{TJC28}$	1.756	0.400	0.772	1.580	0.409	0.741	2.085	0.325	0.844
$\sqrt{SJC28}$	1.521	0.420	0.724	1.522	0.425	0.721	1.342	0.394	0.706
GH	681.624	269.687	0.783	663.439	247.769	0.766	666.917	359.309	0.614
LN(ESR)	0.779	0.193	0.913	0.807	0.191	0.912	0.477	0.191	0.878
LN(CRP)	0.909	0.246	0.805	0.920	0.231	0.806	0.771	0.335	0.773

TJC28 = 28-tender joint count, SJC28 = 28-swollen joint count, GH = general health, ESR = erythrocyte sedimentation rate, CRP = C-Reactive Protein.

Table 3. Pearson's correlations and covariances of DAS-28 components in total patient sample.

	Covariance	$\sqrt{TJC28}$	$\sqrt{SJC28}$	GH	LN(ESR)	LN(CRP)
Pearson's Correlation						
$\sqrt{TJC28}$		----	0.909	14.818	0.152	0.207
$\sqrt{SJC28}$		0.555**	----	8.467	0.337	0.402
GH		0.427**	0.262**	----	4.129	5.181
LN(ESR)		0.131**	0.309**	0.179**	----	0.488
LN(CRP)		0.164**	0.343**	0.207**	0.581**	----

**$p<0.01$, TJC28 = 28-tender joint count, SJC28 = 28-swollen joint count, GH = general health, ESR = erythrocyte sedimentation rate, CRP = C-Reactive Protein.

the rows labeled "Reliability", the reliabilities using the original weights and the optimal weights are given.

In all groups, reliabilities increased after weight optimization. The largest gains were obtained in the total and "fast response" groups by decreasing the weight of the TJC and GH. In the smaller slow response group, on the other hand, the weights of the TJC28 and SJC28 were increased, while the weights of the inflammatory markers and GH were substantially decreased.

Discussion

Overall, composite reliability levels of 0.85 and 0.86 were found for the DAS28-ESR and DAS28-CRP, respectively. This is sufficiently high for group use and around common thresholds considered sufficient for individual use [19,20], justifying the use of the DAS28 in both clinical research and clinical practice. Moreover, reliability could be increased even further by optimizing the component weights.

Table 4. Pearson's correlations of the DAS-28 components in the "fast response" group and "slow response" group.

	Pearson's correlation group 2 (N=80)	$\sqrt{TJC28}$	$\sqrt{SJC28}$	GH	LN(ESR)	LN(CRP)
Pearson's correlation group 1 (N=466)						
$\sqrt{TJC28}$		1	0.547**	0.313**	−0.09	−0.032
$\sqrt{SJC28}$		0.545**	1	0.288*	0.143	0.263*
GH		0.423**	0.239**	1	0.067	0.104
LN(ESR)		0.125**	0.312**	0.166**	1	0.578**
LN(CRP)		0.171**	0.342**	0.205**	0.574**	1

**$p<0.01$, TJC28 = 28-tender joint count, SJC28 = 28-swollen joint count, GH = general health, ESR = erythrocyte sedimentation rate, CRP = C-Reactive Protein.

Table 5. Reliabilities of the index measures and optimal weights in subpopulations.

Index measure	Component *	Original Weight	Total patient group (N = 546)	"Fast response" group (N = 466)	"Slow response" group (N = 80)
DAS28-ESR	$\sqrt{TJC28}$	0.560 (0.742)	0.226 (0.299)	0.156 (0.196)	0.739 (1.067)
	$\sqrt{SJC28}$	0.280 (0.345)	0.271 (0.334)	0.226 (0.279)	0.355 (0.411)
	GH	0.014 (0.366)	0.004 (0.104)	0.004 (0.103)	0.004 (0.103)
	LN(ESR)	0.700 (0.618)	0.663 (0.585)	0.650 (0.584)	0.052 (0.036)
Reliability	**Original Weights**		0.854	0.848	0.821
	Optimal Weights		0.933	0.942	0.859
DAS28-CRP	$\sqrt{TJC28}$	0.560 (0.742)	0.374 (0.496)	0.247 (0.310)	0.720 (1.040)
	$\sqrt{SJC28}$	0.280 (0.345)	0.378 (0.466)	0.298 (0.368)	0.356 (0.412)
	GH	0.014 (0.366)	0.006 (0.157)	0.005 (0.129)	0.004 (0.103)
	LN(CRP)	0.360 (0.343)	0.522 (0.498)	0.571 (0.548)	0.028 (0.025)
Reliability	**Original Weights**		0.858	0.852	0.845
	Optimal Weights		0.888	0.911	0.858

The weights between brackets are the standardized values by fixing the component variances at 1.
*TJC28 = 28-tender joint count, SJC28 = 28-swollen joint count, GH = general health, ESR = erythrocyte sedimentation rate, CRP = C-Reactive Protein.

Several findings are worth mentioning when comparing the individual component reliabilities or when optimizing the component weights. At first, it can be observed that ESR had the highest reliability of all DAS28 components. The finding that this measure of inflammation was also more reliable than the CRP measure might be explained by their different responsiveness to changes in inflammatory stimuli. While the ESR is a relatively stable measure over time, which responds slowly to changes and reflects the disease activity of the past few weeks, the CRP fluctuates more heavily due to a more rapid response to short-term changes in the inflammatory stimuli [12,21,22]. The ESR is also given a higher weighting than the CRP in the DAS28 formulas and that remained to be the case after weight optimization.

When looking at the joint count reliabilities, the swollen joint count had a lower reliability than the tender joint count, consistent with findings from previous studies [9,23,24]. Joint counts are sometimes referred to as a semi-objective clinical measures [1] and, as discussed by Pincus [25], they have been shown to be poorly reproducible. Large intra- and interobserver variability is commonly found especially in the swollen joint count [24]. This might be explained by a higher dependency of the swollen joint assessment on factors like the assessors' levels of training and experience, a lack of standardization in examination methods, unclear definitions of swelling, or the degree of joint deformity [24,25,26]. After weight optimization, however, the weight of the tender joint count was substantially lowered, even below the weight of the swollen joint count. This corresponds with the common clinical perspective of disease activity in RA. Joint swelling is usually considered to be a more representative measure of inflammation than joint tenderness [27] and has been shown to play a major role in the physician's assessment of disease activity [28].

Finally, it can be observed that the patient reported degree of GH in the "slow response" group had the lowest reliability of all components, even below the recommended reliability threshold for group use (r>0.70). Its weight was also substantially decreased after weight optimization. This could be a confirmation of the weakness of this component, as the inclusion of GH in the DAS28 has been often criticized. For instance, previous studies have shown elevated GH scores while none of the other DAS28 components showed any sign of an active disease, possibly due to effects beyond the clinical inflammatory processes of RA [29]. Also, GH ratings have been shown to be different across patients with similar DAS28 scores, dependent on the moment of administration, possibly caused by a response shift [30]. The GH component is also the most subjective component of the DAS28 and, therefore, more susceptible to measurement error. Although it could be argued to solely include the more objective clinical measures, the inclusion of a patient-driven component is desirable given the increased awareness of the importance of the patient perspective in assessing disease activity since the 1980s [31] as reflected by their inclusion in the provisional ACR/EULAR definition of remission in RA [32] as well as in the preliminary core set of disease activity measures [33]. Disease activity in RA is a multifactorial concept and appears to be best measured by both objective clinical measures and patient-reported outcomes as they each address a different aspect of disease activity [27]. Therefore, it would be interesting to explore other, more reliable, patient-reported outcome measures for inclusion in the DAS28. What measure would be best warrants further research. Measures of pain or fatigue appear to be promising alternatives, given the recognition of pain as one of the most important determinants of a patient's global assessment of disease activity [34,35,36] and the recommendation to measure fatigue in addition to the other core set measures of RA [37]. But, of course, other patient-reported measures can also be explored.

A possible limitation of the current study is the difference in sample size between the fast response and slow response group. Though this might cause the results of the "fast response" group to be more robust than the results of the "slow response" group, the importance of the tender joint count in the slow response group is consistent with the general belief that approximately 10-20% of patients with RA have secondary fibromyalgia (FM) [38,39]. FM patients tend to have a lower pain threshold [38,39] which might explain the higher relevance of the TJC28 rating in this patient group, increasing our confidence in the robustness of the results.

Conclusions

The DAS28-ESR and the DAS28-CRP are both reliable instruments for assessing disease activity in early RA although reliability can be increased even further by adjusting the individual component weights. Overall, the findings suggest that the largest gains in reliability can be achieved by substantially lowering the weights of the tender joint count and patient-reported general health. Future studies should explore the possibilities of including a better indicator of the patient perspective in the disease activity score.

Author Contributions

Conceived and designed the experiments: LS PTK HV MVDL CG. Performed the experiments: LS CG. Analyzed the data: LS CG. Contributed reagents/materials/analysis tools: LS PTK HV MVDL CG. Wrote the paper: LS PTK HV MVDL CG.

References

1. Prevoo ML, van 't Hof MA, Kuper HH, van Leeuwen MA, van de Putte LB, et al. (1995) Modified disease activity scores that include twenty-eight-joint counts: development and validation in a prospective longitudinal study of patients with rheumatoid arthritis. Arthritis Rheum 38: 44–48.
2. Salaffi F, Cimmino MA, Leardini G, Gasparini S, Grassi W (2009) Disease activity assessment of rheumatoid arthritis in daily practice: validity, internal consistency, reliability and congruency of the Disease Activity Score including 28 joints (DAS28) compared with the Clinical Disease Activity Index (CDAI). Clin Exp Rheumatol 27: 552–559.
3. Lord FM, Novick MR (1968) Statistical theories of mental test scores. Reading, MA: Addison-Welsley Publishing Company.
4. Leeb BF, Andel I, Sautner J, Bogdan M, Maktari A, et al. (2005) Disease activity measurement of rheumatoid arthritis: Comparison of the simplified disease activity index (SDAI) and the disease activity score including 28 joints (DAS28) in daily routine. Arthritis Rheum 53: 56–60.
5. Leeb BF, Sautner J, Mai HT, Haindl PM, Deutsch C, et al. (2009) A comparison of patient questionnaires and composite indexes in routine care of rheumatoid arthritis patients. Joint Bone Spine 76: 658–664.
6. Crosby RA, DiClemente RJ, Salazar LF (2006) Research methods in health promotion. San Francisco, CA: Jossey-Bass.
7. Brennan RL (1992) Generalizability theory. Instructional Topics in Educational Measurement 11: 225–232.
8. He Q (2009) Estimating the reliability of composite scores. Coventry: Ofqual.
9. Lassere MN, van der Heijde D, Johnson KR, Boers M, Edmonds J (2001) Reliability of measures of disease activity and disease damage in rheumatoid arthritis: implications for smallest detectable difference, minimal clinically important difference, and analysis of treatment effects in randomized controlled trials. J Rheumatol 28: 892–903.
10. Vermeer M, Kuper HH, Hoekstra M, Haagsma CJ, Posthumus MD, et al. (2011) Implementation of a treat-to-target strategy in very early rheumatoid arthritis: results of the Dutch Rheumatoid Arthritis Monitoring remission induction cohort study. Arthritis Rheum 63: 2865–2872.
11. Siemons L, ten Klooster PM, Vonkeman HE, Glas CAW, van de Laar MAFJ (In press) Distinct trajectories of disease activity over the first year in early rheumatoid arthritis patients following a treat-to-target strategy. Arthritis Care Res.
12. Van Riel PL, Fransen J, Scott DL (2004) EULAR handbook of clinical assessments in rheumatoid arthritis. Alphen aan den Rijn: van Zuiden Communications.
13. Fries JF, Spitz P, Kraines RG, Holman HR (1980) Measurement of patient outcome in arthritis. Arthritis Rheum 23: 137–145.
14. Ware JE, Kosinski M, Dewey JE (2000) How to Score Version Two of the SF-36 Health Survey. Lincoln, RI: QualityMetric, Incorporated.
15. Mosier CI (1943) On the reliability of a weighted composite. Psychometrika 8: 161–168.
16. Siemons L, ten Klooster PM, Taal E, Kuper IH, van Riel PLCM, et al. (2011) Validating the 28-tender joint count using item response theory. J Rheumatol 38: 2557–2564.
17. Albers CJ, Critchley F, Gower JC (2011) Quadratic minimisation problems in statistics. Journal of Multivariate Analysis 102: 698–713.
18. Albers CJ, Critchley F, Gower JC (2011) Applications of quadratic minimisation problems in statistics. Journal of Multivariate Analysis 102.
19. Tennant A, Conaghan PG (2007) The rasch measurement model in rheumatology: What is it and why use it? When should it be applied, and what should one look for in a rasch paper? Arthritis Rheum 57: 1358–1362.
20. Terwee CB, Bot SD, de Boer MR, van der Windt DA, Knol DL, et al. (2007) Quality criteria were proposed for measurement properties of health status questionnaires. J Clin Epidemiol 60: 34–42.
21. Firestein GS, Budd RC, Harris Jr ED, McInnes IB, Ruddy S, et al. (2009) Kelly's textbook of rheumatology. Philadelphia: Saunders Elsevier.
22. Kushner I (1991) C-reactive protein in rheumatology. Arthritis Rheum 34: 1065–1068.
23. Siemons L, Ten Klooster PM, Taal E, Kuper IH, van Riel PLCM, et al. (2013) Contribution of assessing forefoot joints in early rheumatoid arthritis patients: insights from item response theory. Arthritis Care Res 65: 212–219.
24. Cheung PP, Gossec L, Mak A, March L (In press) Reliability of joint count assessment in rheumatoid arthritis: A systematic literature review. Semin Arthritis Rheum.
25. Pincus T (2008) Limitations of a quantitative swollen and tender joint count to assess and monitor patients with rheumatoid arthritis. Bull NYU Hosp Jt Dis 66: 216–223.
26. Marhadour T, Jousse-Joulin S, Chalès G, Grange L, Hacquard C, et al. (2010) Reproducibility of joint swelling assessments in long-lasting rheumatoid arthritis: influence on Disease Activity Score-28 values (SEA-Repro study part I). J Rheumatol 37: 932–937.
27. Wolfe F (1997) The prognosis of rheumatoid arthritis: Assessment of disease activity and disease severity in the clinic. Am J Med 103: 12S–18S.
28. Soubrier M, Zerkak D, Gossec L, Ayral X, Roux C, et al. (2006) Which variables best predict change in rheumatoid arthritis therapy in daily clinical practice? J Rheumatol 33: 1243–1246.
29. Vermeer M, Kuper HH, van der Bijl AE, Baan H, Posthumus MD, et al. (2012) The provisional ACR/EULAR definition of remission in RA: a comment on the patient global assessment criterion. Rheumatology (Oxford) 51: 1076–1080.
30. Kievit W, Welsing PMJ, Adang EMM, Eijsbouts AM, Krabbe PFM, et al. (2006) Comment on the use of self-reporting instruments to assess patients with rheumatoid arthritis: the longitudinal association between the DAS28 and the VAS general health. Arthritis Rheum 55: 745–750.
31. Fries JF, Bruce B, Cella D (2005) The promise of PROMIS: Using item response theory to improve assessment of patient-reported outcomes. Clin Exp Rheumatol 23: S53–S57.
32. Felson DT, Smolen JS, Wells G, Zhang B, van Tuyl LHD, et al. (2011) American College of Rheumatology/European League Against Rheumatism provisional definition of remission in rheumatoid arthritis for clinical trials. Arthritis Rheum 63: 573–586.
33. Felson DT, Anderson JJ, Boers M, Bombardier C, Chernoff M, et al. (1993) The American College of Rheumatology preliminary core set of disease activity measures for rheumatoid arthritis clinical trials. The Committee on Outcome Measures in Rheumatoid Arthritis Clinical Trials. Arthritis Rheum 36: 729–740.
34. Studenic P, Radner H, Smolen JS, Aletaha D (2012) Discrepancies between patients and physicians in their perceptions of rheumatoid arthritis disease activity. Arthritis Rheum 64: 2814–2823.
35. Khan NA, Spencer HJ, Abda E, Aggarwal A, Alten R, et al. (2012) Determinants of discordance in patients' and physicians' rating of rheumatoid arthritis disease activity. Arthritis Care Res 64: 206–214.
36. Markenson JA, Koenig AS, Feng JY, Chaudhari S, Zack DJ, et al. (2013) Comparison of physician and patient global assessments over time in patients with rheumatoid arthritis: a retrospective analysis from the RADIUS cohort. J Clin Rheumatol 19: 317–323.
37. Kirwan JR, Minnock P, Adebajo A, Bresnihan B, Choy E, et al. (2007) Patient perspective: fatigue as a recommended patient centered outcome measure in rheumatoid arthritis. J Rheumatol 34: 1174–1177.
38. Coury F, Rossat A, Tebib A, Letroublon MC, Gagnard A, et al. (2009) Rheumatoid arthritis and fibromyalgia: a frequent unrelated association complicating disease management. J Rheumatol 36: 58–62.
39. Leeb BF, Andel I, Sautner J, Nothnagl T, Rintelen B (2004) The DAS28 in rheumatoid arthritis and fibromyalgia patients. Rheumatology 43: 1504–1507.

15

Porphyromonas gingivalis Peptidylarginine Deiminase, a Key Contributor in the Pathogenesis of Experimental Periodontal Disease and Experimental Arthritis

Neville Gully[1], Richard Bright[1], Victor Marino[1], Ceilidh Marchant[1], Melissa Cantley[2], David Haynes[2], Catherine Butler[3], Stuart Dashper[3], Eric Reynolds[3], Mark Bartold[1]*

1 Colgate Australian Clinical Dental Research, School of Dentistry, University of Adelaide, Adelaide, South Australia, Australia, **2** Discipline of Anatomy and Pathology, School of Medical Sciences, University of Adelaide, Adelaide, South Australia, Australia, **3** Oral Health Collaborative Research Centre, Melbourne Dental School, The University of Melbourne, Melbourne, Victoria, Australia

Abstract

Objectives: To investigate the suggested role of *Porphyromonas gingivalis* peptidylarginine deiminase (PAD) in the relationship between the aetiology of periodontal disease and experimentally induced arthritis and the possible association between these two conditions.

Methods: A genetically modified PAD-deficient strain of *P. gingivalis* W50 was produced. The effect of this strain, compared to the wild type, in an established murine model for experimental periodontitis and experimental arthritis was assessed. Experimental periodontitis was induced following oral inoculation with the PAD-deficient and wild type strains of *P. gingivalis*. Experimental arthritis was induced via the collagen antibody induction process and was monitored by assessment of paw swelling and micro-CT analysis of the radio-carpal joints. Experimental periodontitis was monitored by micro CT scans of the mandible and histological assessment of the periodontal tissues around the mandibular molars. Serum levels of anti-citrullinated protein antibodies (ACPA) and *P. gingivalis* were assessed by ELISA.

Results: The development of experimental periodontitis was significantly reduced in the presence of the PAD-deficient *P. gingivalis* strain. When experimental arthritis was induced in the presence of the PAD-deficient strain there was less paw swelling, less erosive bone damage to the joints and reduced serum ACPA levels when compared to the wild type *P. gingivalis* inoculated group.

Conclusion: This study has demonstrated that a PAD-deficient strain of *P. gingivalis* was associated with significantly reduced periodontal inflammation. In addition the extent of experimental arthritis was significantly reduced in animals exposed to prior induction of periodontal disease through oral inoculation of the PAD-deficient strain versus the wild type. This adds further evidence to the potential role for *P. gingivalis* and its PAD in the pathogenesis of periodontitis and exacerbation of arthritis. Further studies are now needed to elucidate the mechanisms which drive these processes.

Editor: Özlem Yilmaz, University of Florida, United States of America

Funding: This study was supported in part by research grants from the Australian Dental Research Fund (ADRF 56/2010) and the National Health & Medical Council of Australia (NHMRC 1023747). The funders had no role in study design, data collection and analysis, decision to publish, or preparation of the manuscript.

Competing Interests: The authors have declared that no competing interests exist.

* Email: mark.bartold@adelaide.edu.au

Introduction

The endogenous microbes inhabiting humans often interact in complex ways with their hosts. Changes in the local environment can lead to qualitative and/or quantitative changes in commensal microbial communities that, if left unchecked, can result in disease. Chronic periodontitis is a common inflammatory condition affecting the tissues surrounding teeth. A prolonged, uncontrolled inflammatory response to the sub-gingival microbial load may lead to loss of periodontal ligament attachment and the adjacent alveolar bone [1]. In recent years periodontitis has been linked to the development of other disorders, such as coronary heart disease, diabetes mellitus and low birth weight [2]. While these associations are largely based on epidemiological evidence and for most there is currently no apparent common underlying cause, dysregulation of the inflammatory response seems to be a common underlying feature [3]. Two of the most prevalent chronic inflammatory conditions affecting humans that share many common features, including destruction of both fibrous connective tissue and bone, osteoclast activation and many common risk factors, are periodontitis and rheumatoid arthritis (RA) [4,5].

While elevated microbial load is an important factor in the initiation of periodontitis, it is the increase in proportion of specific microbial pathogens that is likely to be the crucial factor in the subsequent progression of this condition [6]. Periodontitis, particularly in its more severe form, has been linked to a biofilm that contains a consortium of oral pathogens that includes the Gram negative anaerobe *Porphyromonas gingivalis*. [7,8]. *P. gingivalis* expresses a peptidylarginine deiminase (PAD) known as PPAD, an enzyme that modifies peptidylarginine residues to citrulline and is unique in this regard amongst prokaryotes [9]. PPAD is not evolutionarily related to the mammalian PADs that catalyse the same reaction, which is the modification of the guanidino group of arginine residues to produce peptidyl-citrulline and ammonia. While citrullination mediated by host PADs is generally considered a fundamental process (e.g apoptosis), it is also associated with inflammation in mammals [10].

When investigating potential common causal links between periodontitis and RA, the ability of *P. gingivalis* to citrullinate peptides is noteworthy as auto-antibodies against citrullinated peptides are highly specific and sensitive in RA diagnosis [11]. Post-translationally modified peptides and proteins containing citrulline can exhibit altered epitopes compared to those that are unmodified [12]. Accordingly, citrullination has been reported to trigger an auto-immune response [11,13] via modified self-proteins and peptides perceived as foreign by the immune system [14]. While citrullinated peptides may be involved in the pathogenesis of RA the nature of their role is unclear and the contributions of host or prokaryote PADs to citrullination is unknown.

It has been proposed that the increased levels of *P. gingivalis* in patients suffering from chronic periodontitis might influence the development of RA, via PPAD promotion of peptide citrullination, thus explaining the over representation of patients presenting with periodontitis suffering from RA [15–17].

Therefore the aims of this investigation were to construct a PAD-deficient *P. gingivalis* strain and compare the onset and severity of arthritis and periodontitis in a mouse model in the presence of either the wild type or PAD-negative strain.

Materials and Methods

Ethics

Approval for the use of BALB/c mice in this study was obtained from the University of Adelaide, Animal Ethics Committee (Project N° M-2012-183R). The animals were housed in the University of Adelaide PC2 Animal holding facility (OGTR certification No 2067/2008). Approval to culture and prepare inoculates of the genetically modified *P. gingivalis* strain ECR527 was granted by the Institutional Biosafety Committee of the University of Adelaide (Approval No: IBC Dealing ID 10890). The animals were assessed daily for a number of general health parameters including dull/ruffled coat, a change in temperament, reduced food/water intake or a reluctance to move and body weight recorded.

Bacterial Strains and Culture Conditions

P. gingivalis strain W50 (wild type) was obtained from the culture collection of the Oral Health CRC, Melbourne Dental School, University of Melbourne. A PAD-deficient strain (ECR527) was derived from W50 for this study. *P. gingivalis* strains were routinely maintained on Horse Blood Agar (HBA) plates and antibiotic selection of 10 µg/mL erythromycin when appropriate. *E. coli* alpha-select gold cells (Bioline, London, UK) were grown at 37°C in Luria Bertani (LB) Broth or maintained on LB agar with 100 µg/mL ampicillin when harbouring pGEM-TEasy plasmids (Promega, Madison, WI, USA).

DNA Analysis and Manipulations

Oligonucleotide primers used in this study are listed in Table 1. Genomic DNA from *P. gingivalis* strains was prepared using the DNeasy Blood and Tissue kit (Qiagen) and plasmid DNA was extracted from *E. coli* using the QIAprep spin miniprep kit (Qiagen, Venlo, Netherlands). DNA was sequenced by Applied Genetics Diagnostics, The University of Melbourne.

RT-PCR

RNA was isolated using a NucleoSpin RNA II Total RNA Isolation kit (Macherey-Nagel, Duren, Germany) and cDNA was generated using a SuperScrip III Reverse Transcriptase First-Strand Synthesis SuperMix for qRT-PCR kit with random hexamers (Life Technologies, California, USA), both according to the manufacturer's instructions. BIOTAQ Red DNA Polymerase (Bioline, London, UK) was then used to PCR from the following templates: 125 ng of cDNA, 125 ng RNA that was not reverse transcribed, milliQ H_2O and 13 ng W50 genomic DNA in 50 µL reactions with gene-specific primer pairs (Table 1) for 30 cycles in a G-Storm GS1 thermal cycler (Gene Works, Adelaide, Australia). The expected product size from each primer pair was 682 bp for PG1424-RT-Fwd and PG1423-RT-Rev; and 1181 bp from PG1424-RT-Fwd and PG1422-RT-Rev. DNA was electrophoresed at 80 V for 40 min using a 1.0% agarose gel prepared with tris-acetate buffer (40 mM tris-acetate, 1 mM EDTA, pH 8).

Construction of *P. gingivalis* PAD-deficient Strain ECR527

The recombination cassette for deletion of the *pad* gene consisted of 972 bp upstream of the *PG1424* (*pad*) ORF which encompassed *PG1426*, followed by the *ermF* gene encoding erythromycin resistance in *P. gingivalis*, followed by 741 bp downstream of the *PG1424* ORF which encompassed *PG1423*. This recombination cassette resulted in replacement of *PG1424* with *ermF* and was constructed from three separate PCR products that were spliced together using gene splicing by overlap extension PCRs (SOE PCR) to form the final cassette. SOE PCRs were performed essentially as previously described [18]. The PCR products that flanked the PG1424 ORF were amplified from W50 genomic DNA: *PG1426* (primers PG1426-Fwd and ErmF-PG1426-Rev) and *PG1423* (primers ErmF-PG1423-Fwd and PG1423-Rev). The *ermF* gene was amplified from pVA2198 [19] with primers PG1426-ErmF-Fwd and PG1423-ErmF-Rev. All PCRs were performed with Herculase II DNA Polymerase (Stratagene, La Jolla, Ca, USA) except for the final SOE PCR which was amplified with Platinum Taq DNA Polymerase High Fidelity (Life Technologies, California, USA). PCR products were purified using the NucleoSpin Extract II purification kit (Macherey Nagel, Duren, Germany) according to manufacturer's instructions. The final PCR product was ligated with pGEM-TEasy and transformed into *E. coli* alpha-select gold competent cells (Bioline) by heat shock according to manufacturer's instructions. The resulting plasmid was sequenced to confirm the fidelity of the recombination cassette then it was linearised and 200 ng electroporated into *P. gingivalis* W50 in a 0.1 cm gap cuvette at 1.8 kV, 200 Ohms resistance. The resulting PAD-deficient strain was named ECR527.

Measurement of PAD Activity

A colorimetric microtitre plate assay for the determination of enzymatic deimination of the substrate N-α-benzoyl-L-arginine ethyl ester (BAEE) was performed as previously described [20,21]. Briefly, cells from three biological replicate cultures each of *P. gingivalis* W50 and ECR527 (OD_{650} 1.1–1.3) were washed and

Table 1. Oligonucleotide primers used in this study.

Oligonucleotide Primer	Sequence (5′-3′)[a]	Purpose
PG1424-RT-Fwd	ATCGAAGCAGATGTCGTCTCAT	RT PCR
PG1423-RT-Rev	TACGAAACCAATGCTCAGATTTTG	RT PCR
PG1422-RT-Rev	ATAGTTGGATGCGAGAGAAGGA	RT PCR
PG1426-Fwd	GAAGCACGTAATAAGGACAATGAC	*pad* recombination cassette
ErmF-PG1426-Rev	ACGGGCAATTTCTTTTTTGTCATTGTTTGATATGTTTTATGATGTTATGAA	*pad* recombination cassette
PG1426-ErmF-Fwd	TTCATAACATCATAAAACATATCAAACAATGACAAAAAAGAAATTGCCCGT	*pad* recombination cassette
PG1423-ErmF-Rev	GTATTCTCAAATAAGGGGCCTTACGAAGGATGAAATTTTTCAGG	*pad* recombination cassette
ErmF-PG1423-Fwd	CCTGAAAAATTTCATCCTTCGTAAGGCCCCTTATTTGAGAATAC	*pad* recombination cassette
PG1423-Rev	CATCGACGATGATATCTCCTGT	*pad* recombination cassette

[a]Underlined sequence of SOE primers indicates the part of the primer that is not complementary to the target sequence, but provides complementarity with a second PCR product for splicing.

resuspended in 0.2 M Tris-HCl (pH 8), 1 mM EDTA, 1 μM flavin mononucleotide and 10 mM cysteine. A 10 μL aliquot of BAEE (30 mM) was added to 50 μL cells (1×10^8 cfu) and incubated at 37°C for 30 min before addition of 200 μL of detection reagent. The detection reagent was assembled daily from its two components with one part A (0.5% diacetyl monoximine and 0.01% thiosemicarbazide) added to two parts B (0.25 mg of $FeCl_3$/mL in 24.5% sulphuric acid and 17% phosphoric acid). The reaction plate was heated at 105°C for 25 min, then cooled and optically measured at 490 nm using a Bio-Tek Powerwave

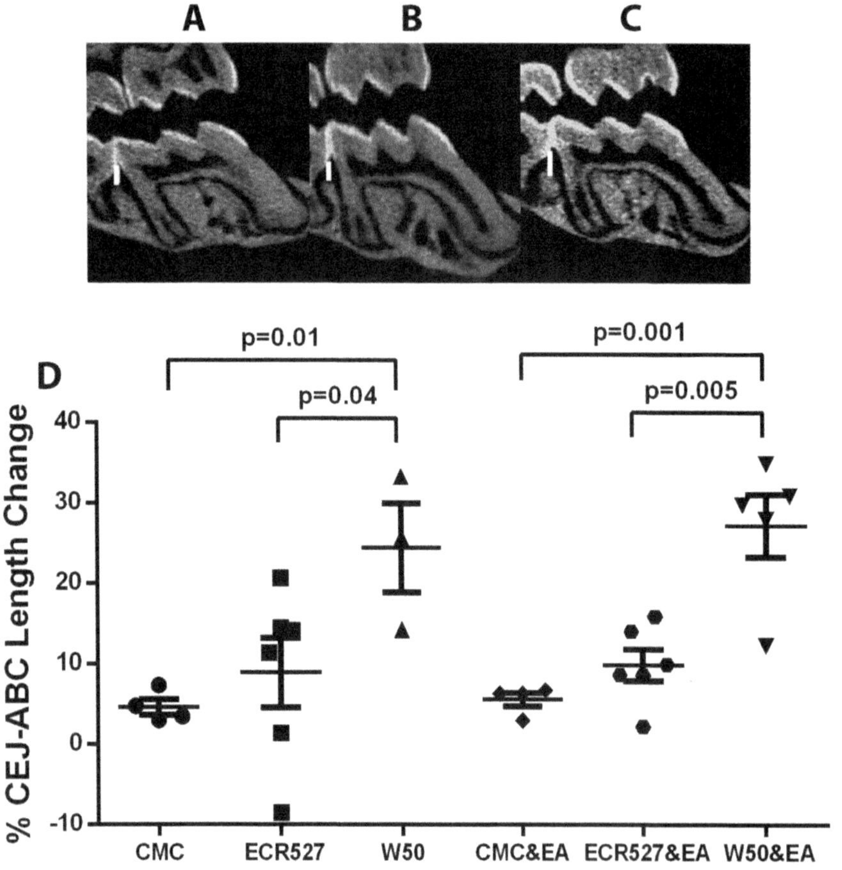

Figure 1. Micro CT appearance and analysis of periodontal bone loss. A. Micro CT of mouse jaw for CMC control group. B. Micro CT of mouse jaw for ECR527 & EA group. C. Micro CT of mouse jaw W50 & EA group. D. Measurements of bone changes in the jaw were calculated by measuring the cemento-enamel junction-alveolar bone crest on three slices for each mouse using CTAn sagital sections. Data represent mean (± SEM). The number of animals in each group was 6 and measurements were performed in triplicate. Statistical analysis was done by one way ANOVA and Tukey multiple comparisons. White bars represent CEJ/ABC distance measurements. *Abbreviations:* CMC = carboxymethyl cellulose; ECR527 = PAD-deficient *P. gingivalis*; W50 = wild type *P. Gingivalis*; EA = experimental arthritis

Table 2. Recovery of viable *P. gingivalis* from oral swabs after final inoculation.

Group	Recovery 0 hr	Recovery 6 hr	Recovery 24 hr	PPAD activity
Control	–	–	–	–
Wild-type (W50)	+	+	+	*
PAD-deficient (ECR527)	+	+	+	–

(+) Viable wild type (W50) and PAD-deficient (ECR527) *P. gingivalis strains* W50 and ECR527 were recovered from the gingiva of each group of mice inoculated separately with each strain at the three time points assayed. The colonies in both groups were black pigmented with gram negative staining organisms.
(−) No viable organisms were recovered from the control group receiving the vehicle (2% CMC).
(*) PPAD activity was only demonstrated in the group of mice where *P. gingivalis* W50 was recovered from gingival swabs.

spectrophotometer (Biotek Instruments, Winooski, VT, USA). A standard curve was generated using 0–400 µM L-citrulline using the same method to quantify citrulline in samples.

Animal Groupings

Thirty six female BALB/c mice between 6 and 8 weeks old were acquired from the Laboratory Animal Services (LAS) of the University of Adelaide. Six experimental groups each containing six mice were used. All groups received oral inoculations for the duration of the study and three groups in addition to the inoculations were induced with experimental arthritis (EA) using a mouse monoclonal antibody against type II collagen (Arthrogen-CIA Arthritogenic Monoclonal Antibody, Chondrex Inc., Redwood, WA, USA).

Group 1: Control: 2% Carboxylmethylcellulose (CMC) (Sigma, St Louis, MO, USA)

Group 2: PPAD$^-$: PAD-deficient *P. gingivalis* (ECR527)

Group 3: PPAD$^+$: Wild type *P. gingivalis* (W50)

Group 4: Control + EA: 2% CMC with induced EA

Group 5: PPAD$^-$ + EA: PAD-deficient *P. gingivalis* (ECR527) with induced EA

Group 6: PPAD$^+$ + EA: Wild type *P. gingivalis* (W50) with induced EA

Induction of Experimental Periodontitis by Oral Inoculation

The preparation of the inocula and the inoculation protocol to induce an experimental periodontitis in female BALB/c mice has been previously described [22]. All mice were inoculated with either wild type *P. gingivalis* (Groups 3 and 6) or PAD-deficient *P. gingivalis* (Groups 2 and 5). The control groups (Groups 1 and 4)

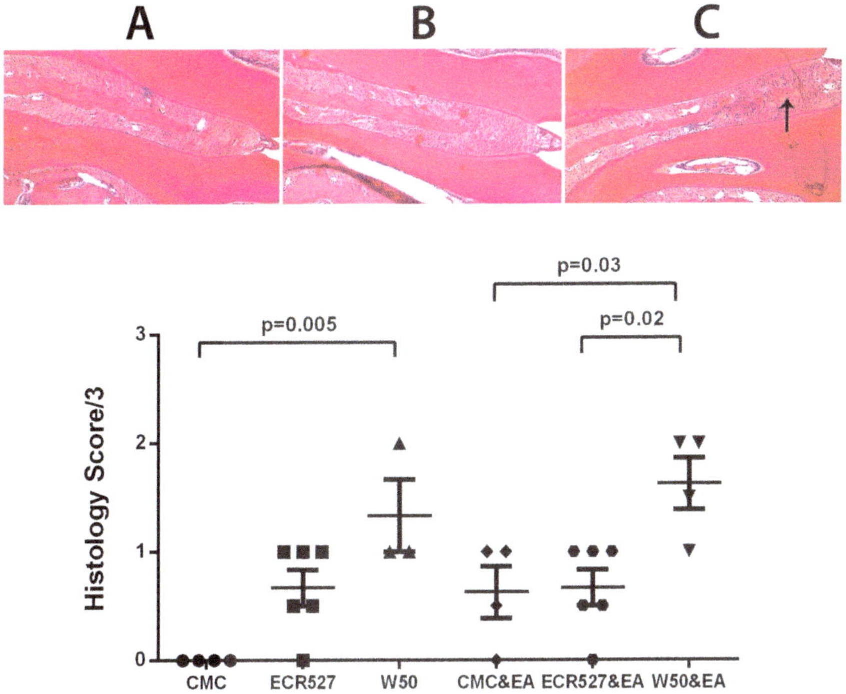

Figure 2. Histological analysis of maxillary periodontal tissues. A. Histology of mouse jaw for CMC control group at day 63. B. Histology of mouse jaw for ECR527 & EA group at day 63. C. Histology of mouse jaw for W50 & EA group at day 63. Arrow indicates increased inflammatory reaction in supra-crestal alveolar bone gingival tissue. D. Histological scores (mean ± SEM) for the presence of osteoclasts and evidence of bone erosion around the first and second upper molars for all groups in the study. Original magnification of A–C = 100X. The number of animals in each group was 6 and measurements were performed in triplicate. Statistical analysis was done by one way ANOVA and Tukey multiple comparisons. *Abbreviations:* CMC = carboxymethyl cellulose; ECR527 = PAD-deficient *P. gingivalis*; W50 = wild type *P. Gingivalis*; EA = experimental arthritis.

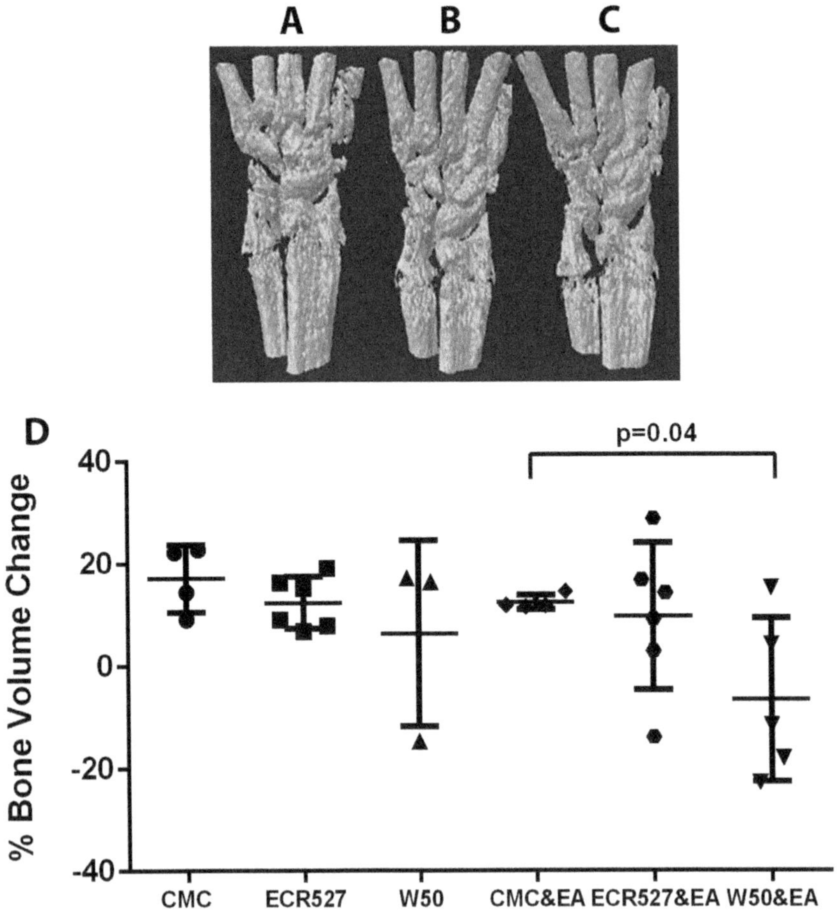

Figure 3. Micro CT appearance and analysis of bone erosion in front paw radio-carpal joint. A. Micro CT appearance of paw for CMC control group at day 63. B. Micro CT appearance of paw for ECR527 & EA group at day 63. C. Micro CT appearance of paw for W50 & EA group at day 63. D. The front paws (left and right combined), were processed to determine bone loss/growth between the two scanned time points in the radio-carpal joint. Data represent mean (± SEM). The number of animals in each group was 6 and measurements were performed in duplicate. Statistical analysis was done by one way ANOVA and Bonferroni multiple comparisons. *Abbreviations:* CMC = carboxymethyl cellulose; ECR527 = PAD-deficient *P. gingivalis*; W50 = wild type *P. Gingivalis*; EA = experimental arthritis

were inoculated with the suspension vehicle for *P. gingivalis* strains, 2% CMC. PPAD activity for both strains was assessed prior to the preparation of each inoculum using the colorimetric method described above. Animals were inoculated over two intensive sequences, each comprising four inoculations over an eight day period. The first sequence commenced two days after the mice had completed 7 days of antibiotic treatment of 1 mg/mL kanamycin (Sigma, St. Louis, MO, USA) in deionised water *ad libitum*. The inoculation sequences were separated by a period of two weeks and during this period mice were inoculated twice a week. Following the second intensive inoculation sequence all mice continued to be inoculated twice a week for the remainder of the experimental period. All animal inoculations were performed by experienced professional staff within a Class II Biological safety cabinet and PC2 animal holding facility.

Induction of Collagen Antibody-induced Arthritis - Experimental Arthritis

Experimental arthritis (EA) was induced in Groups 4–6 by intravenous tail vein injection with 1.5 mg of a mouse monoclonal antibody against type II collagen (Arthrogen-CIA Arthritogenic Monoclonal Antibody, Chondrex Inc., Redwood, WA, USA). This procedure was performed two days after completion of the second intensive inoculation sequence (day 44). To aid in the induction of EA a dose of 5 μg of lipopolysaccharide (LPS) was intraperitoneally administered three days after the antibody exposure, as described previously [23].

Visual Scoring of Paw Swelling

Front and rear paws were visually assessed and scored each day by two experienced observers to assess swelling and inflammation. Two different scales were used to assess paw changes throughout the experiment. Firstly each inflamed toe or knuckle received a score of 1 and a fully inflamed swollen wrist/ankle a score of 5. Each assessed paw received a score between 0–15 and the total score per mouse was 0–60 [24]. The second system employed a scoring system whereby each paw was allocated a score from zero to four according to the level of inflammation and swelling to make a total score of 16 for each animal. 0 = normal paw, 1 = mild but definite redness and swelling of the wrist/ankle, 2 = moderate swelling and redness of the wrist/ankle with digit involvement, 3 = severe swelling and redness of the paw with digit involvement and 4 = maximum inflammation the entire paw, with multiple digit involvement.

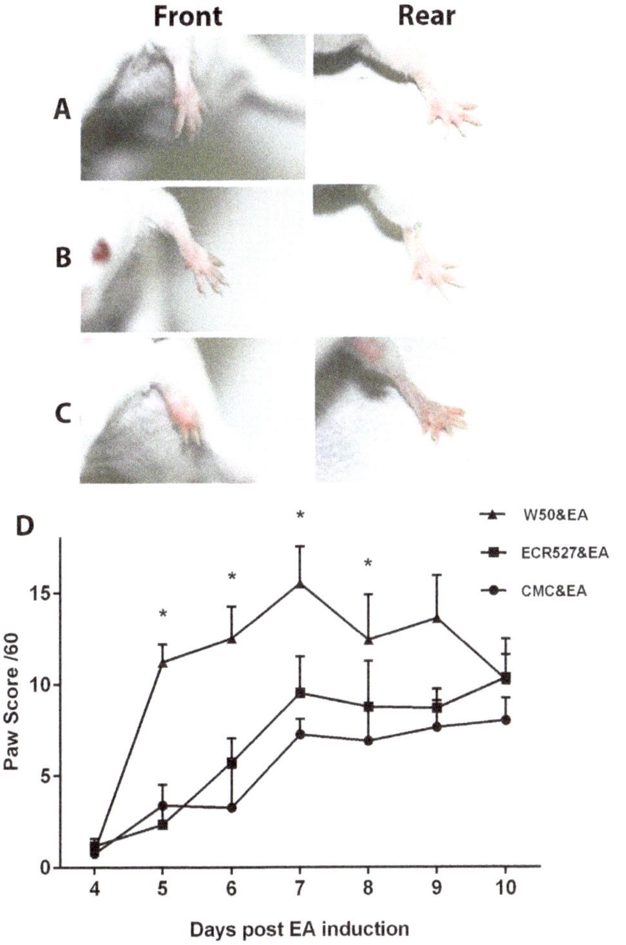

Figure 4. Visual appearance and scoring of paw swelling. A. Appearance of front and rear paws for CMC control group at day 7 post EA induction. B. Appearance of front and rear paws for ECR527 & EA group at day 7 post EA induction. C. Appearance of front and rear paws for W50 & EA group at day 7 post EA induction. D. Total paw score grade out of a 60 including front and back paws. Data represent mean (± SEM). The number of animals in each group was 6 and measurements were performed once daily per animal Statistical analysis was done by two way ANOVA and Tukey multiple comparisons. Raw data for data points are shown in Figure S1. *Abbreviations:* CMC = carboxymethyl cellulose; ECR527 = PAD-deficient *P. gingivalis*; W50 = wild type *P. Gingivalis*; EA = experimental arthritis

Live Animal Micro-computed Tomography

Mice were scanned using the Skyscan 1076 High Resolution live animal computed tomography (micro CT) (SkyScan, Bruker, Belgium) to determine changes in bone volume in the radio-carpal joint and cemento-enamel junction to the alveolar bone crest (CEJ-ABC) length in the jaws. The scanning width was set to 35 mm with a resolution of 9 μm. Detailed specifications for micro CT imaging have previously been published [22]. Animals were anaesthetised prior to scanning with a mixture of ketamine and xylazine and positioned on a polystyrene foam holder then placed within an enclosed container with a HEPA filter at the ends. The container was placed in the 3 cm carbon fibre bed of the micro CT scanner. Mice were scanned before the induction of experimental inflammatory disease to obtain baseline measurements and again at the completion of the study (10 days post experimental arthritis induction).

Micro-CT Data Processing

Scans were reconstructed using Skyscan NRECON software (Version 1.6.6.0). Settings used; smoothing = 1, ring artefact = 15, beam hardening = 30% and misalignment compensation was adjusted manually using the DataViewer program (Skyscan, Bruker, Belgium). The BMP files created were opened in CT Analyser (Version 1.12.0.0+) to create a volume of interest. To realign images and save the appropriate plane for either the radio-carpal joint or determining the CEJ-ABC distance, DataViewer (Version 1.4.4 64-bit) was used. Transaxial images were saved for the bone volume determinations in the radio-carpal joint, and sagittal images for the CEJ-ABC distance. The images were then opened in CTAnalyser to measure bone volume or CEJ-ABC distance. The histogram settings were set at 100 and 255 to measure both the bone volume in the radio-carpal joint and CEJ-ABC junction distance. The bone volume was calculated in a set number (200) 9 μm slices above and below a standard reference point set within the radiocarpal joint. The CEJ-ABC distance was measured between the second and third molars on three slices for each mouse [22,25].

Serum Collection

Approximately 100 μL of blood was collected from cheek puncture bleeds at the commencement of the study (Time = 0) and at 6 weeks. Cardiac puncture was used at the conclusion of the study (week 9). Blood was allowed to clot for 1 hour at room temperature, centrifuged at 1000 *g* for 20 min at room temperature and the serum removed and dispensed into aliquots and stored prior to analysis at −80°C.

ELISA Assays

An anti-CCP kit (AXIS-Shield, Dundee, Scotland) was modified and used to assess levels of anti-CCP antibodies in mouse sera. Week 9 serum was diluted 1:200 and analysed according to the manufacturer's instructions by substitution of an anti-mouse horseradish peroxidase-conjugated secondary to detect mouse IgG (Cell Signalling Technology, Boston, MA, USA).

Antibodies to wild type *P. gingivalis* were detected by coating Costar Maxisorp 96 well plates (Corning, Tewksbury, MA, USA) with 1×10^8 formalin fixed cells in 50 mM bicarbonate buffer, pH 9.4, overnight at 4°C. Wells were washed 3 times in PBS/0.05% Tween-20 (PBS-T) and blocked with 5% skim milk in PBS-T for 1 hr at room temperature followed by three washes of PBS-T. An antibody against *P. gingivalis* purchased from the Developmental Studies Hybridoma Bank (Iowa City, IA, USA) was used as a control and to produce a standard curve. Mouse serum samples from time (day 0, 6 weeks and 9 weeks) were diluted 1:100, added to wells in duplicate and incubated at room temperature for 2 hrs. Wells were washed three times and incubated with a mouse horseradish peroxidase-conjugated secondary antibody (1:10000) (Cell Signalling Technology, Boston, MA, USA) for 45 minutes at room temperature. After the final washes the substrate reagent was prepared (R&D, Minneapolis, MN, USA) and added to wells. The colour reaction was stopped with 2 M H_2SO_4 and the plate read at 450 nm on the Power-wave plate reader using dedicated KC4 microplate data analysis software (Biotek Instruments, Winooski, VT, USA).

Histological Evaluation

At the conclusion of the study (day 63) mice were euthanized by CO_2 inhalation. All paws and heads were retrieved from each mouse and placed into 10% buffered formalin for two days. Following fixation, the specimens were rinsed thoroughly in

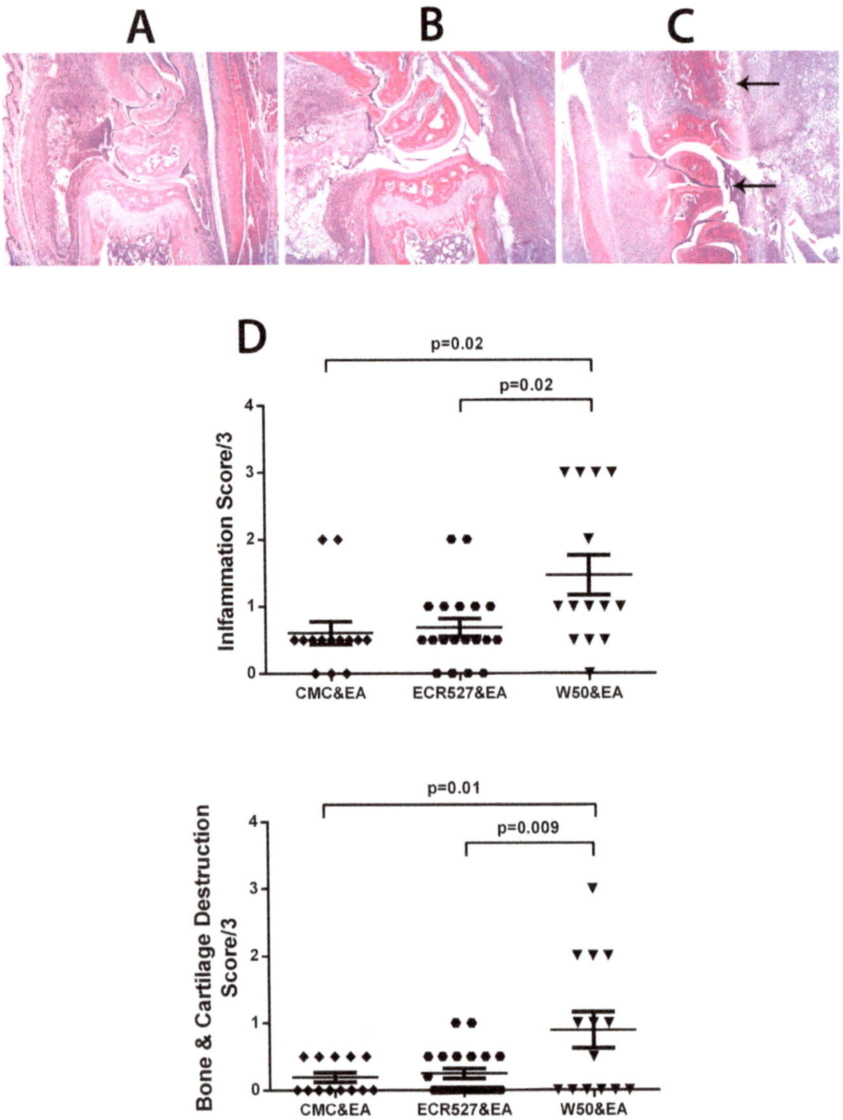

Figure 5. Histological assessment of joint inflammation. A. Histology of the radio-carpal joint for CMC control group at day 63. B. Histology of the radio-carpal joint for ECR527 & EA group at day 63. C. Histology of the radio-carpal joint for W50 & EA group at day 63. Arows indicate increased inflamaotry reaction in joint. D. Histological scores (mean ± SEM) for (a) inflammation and (b) bone and cartilage destruction for both front and rear paws combined. Original magnification of A–C = 100X. The number of animals in each group was 6 and measurements were performed in triplicate. Statistical analysis was done by One way ANOVA and Bonferroni multiple comparisons. *Abbreviations:* CMC = carboxymethyl cellulose; ECR527 = PAD-deficient *P. gingivalis*; W50 = wild type *P. Gingivalis*; EA = experimental arthritis

physiological buffered saline (PBS) and then decalcified in 10% EDTA for 14 days with regular replacement of the solution over this period. Complete decalcification was confirmed by digital radiography and specimens paraffin embedded and sectioned at a thickness of 7 μm. Sections were stained with haematoxylin and eosin for histological analysis. Slides were viewed using a Leica DM1000 microscope and imaged with a connected Leica DFC450 Camera system (Leica Microsystems, Wetzlar, Germany). The front and rear paws were assessed for inflammatory changes, bone and cartilage destruction and pannus formation. A point scale (0–3) was used to score the severity of inflammatory changes based on the number and type of inflammatory cells, (0 = normal tissue, 0–5% inflammatory cells; 1 = mild inflammation 5–25% inflammatory cells; 2 = moderate inflammation 25–50% inflammatory cells; 3 = severe inflammation >50% inflammatory cells). Bone and cartilage destruction was assessed in a similar fashion (0 = normal, 1 = mild cartilage destruction, 2 = evidence of bone and cartilage destruction, 3 = severe bone and cartilage destruction. Pannus formation in the joint was also noted. The periodontium of the maxillary molars was assessed for inflammation with interdental papilla reduction, and presence of osteoclasts with bone erosion particularly between the first and second molars. The severity of each parameter was scored separately on a scale from 0 to 3 (0 = normal, 1 = mild effect, 2 = moderate effect, 3 = severe effect). The sections assessed and selected for each mouse were all at the level where the distal root of the first molar and proximal root of the second molar was clearly visible [23].

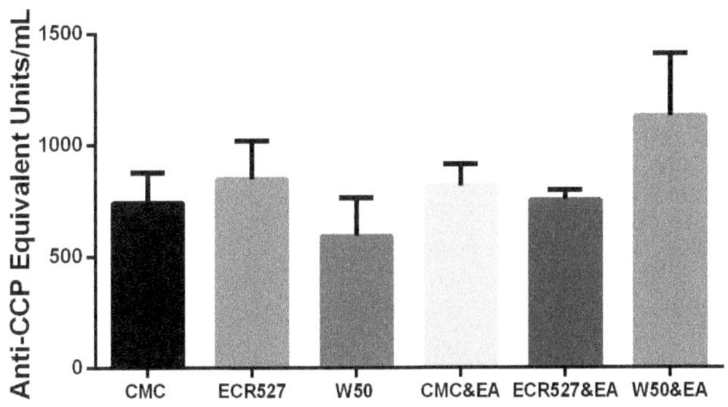

Figure 6. Serum anti-CCP antibody levels. The mean (± SEM) titre of anti-CCP antibodies detected in the sera of mice at week 9 from each of the 6 treatment groups. Raw data for data points are shown in Figure S2. The number in each group was 6 and measurements were performed in duplicate. Statistical analysis was done by one way ANOVA and Tukey multiple comparisons. *Abbreviations:* CMC = carboxymethyl cellulose; ECR527 = PAD-deficient *P. gingivalis;* W50 = wild type *P. Gingivalis;* EA = experimental arthritis

Recovery of *P. gingivalis* from the Oral Cavity

Three groups of six mice were inoculated with either 2% CMC (vehicle control), wild type *P. gingivalis* or PAD-deficient *P. gingivalis*. The inoculation sequence employed was identical to that of Groups 1–3 described previously. At 0, 6 and 24 hrs after the final inoculation sequence the animals gingivae were swabbed using periodontal strips and these were used to inoculate Brain Heart Infusion Broth. Broth cultures were gown under anaerobic conditions for seven days and an inoculum from each culture spread onto anaerobic blood agar plates. Following seven days of anaerobic incubation a typical black-pigmented colony from each group was Gram stained and assayed for PPAD activity.

Statistical Analysis

The data collected from all surviving mice in this study was analysed by one-way ANOVA. When the global test was statistically significant ($p<0.05$), post hoc comparisons were performed using the Tukey or Bonferroni's Multiple Comparison, 95% confidence level. Unpaired t-tests were also used for 2 group comparisons. All testing was carried out with Graph Pad Prism 6 as the statistical analysis package. Significance levels were set at $p<0.05$ for all tests.

Results

Construction of PAD-deficient *P. gingivalis* Strain (ECR527)

Peptidylarginine deiminase is encoded on the wild type *P. gingivalis* genome at locus PG1424. It is predicted by MicrobesOnline [26] to be the first gene in a 3 gene operon with PG1423 and PG1422, which we have confirmed in *P. gingivalis* W50 using reverse transcription PCR. The RT-PCR products corresponded to the predicted sizes of 682 bp for the primer pair specific for PG1424/PG1423 and 1181 bp for the primer pair specific for PG1424/PG1422 (data not shown). A recombination cassette was constructed using gene splicing by Overlap Extension PCRs where the open reading frame of the *ermF* gene, which confers erythromycin resistance was inserted in place of the PG1424 ORF, so that *ermF* would be expressed from the PG1424 promoter. Replacement of the PG1424 ORF with the *ermF* ORF was successfully achieved in *P. gingivalis* strain W50 with the resulting mutant (ECR527) noticeably slower to pigment than wild type W50. Loss of PPAD activity by the PAD-deficient *P. gingivalis*

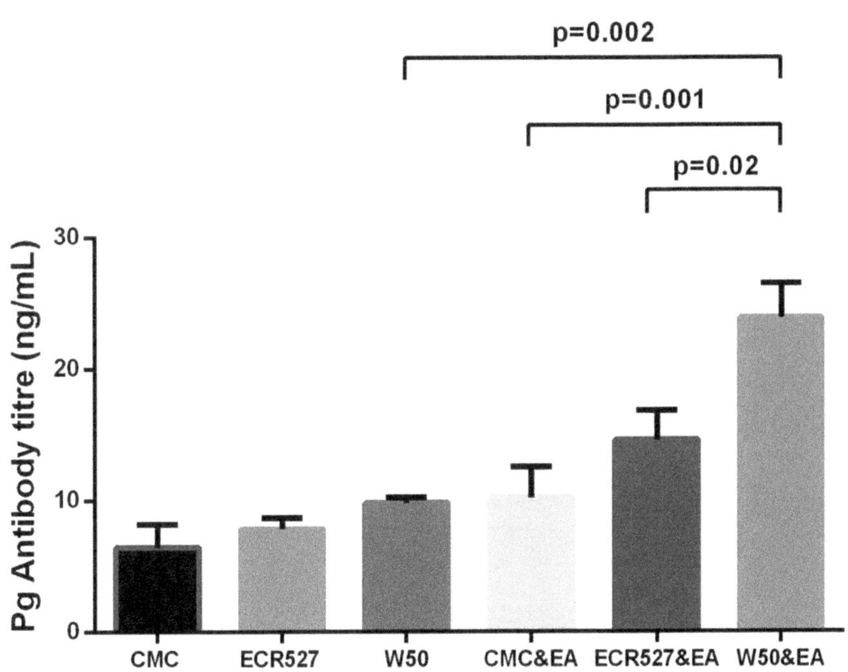

Figure 7. Serum anti-*P. gingivalis* levels. The mean (± SEM) titre of anti-*P.gingivalis* detected in the sera of mice over 9 week time course. Raw data for data points are shown in Figure S3. The number in each group was 6 and measurements were performed in duplicate. Statistical analysis was done by one way ANOVA and Tukey multiple comparisons. *Abbreviations:* CMC = carboxymethyl cellulose; ECR527 = PAD-deficient *P. gingivalis;* W50 = wild type *P. Gingivalis;* EA = experimental arthritis

was confirmed biologically by loss of the ability of ECR527 cultures to deiminate the substrate BAEE whereas 1×10^8 cfu of wild type *P. gingivalis* produced 20.4±0.8 nmol N-α-benzoylcitrulline ethyl ester in 30 min from 300 nmol BAEE.

Post Inoculation Recovery of *P. gingivalis* from Gingiva

Following incubation, black-pigmented colonies of Gram negative bacteria were observed on blood agar plates from the swabs obtained at 0, 6 and 24 hours post final inoculation with wild type *P. gingivalis* W50 and PAD-deficient *P. gingivalis*. However no growth was observed from swabs of animals inoculated with 2% CMC vehicle control. PPAD activity was positive only for bacteria recovered from animals exposed to W50 (Table 2).

Micro-CT Analysis of Periodontal Bone Loss

To determine the effect of PPAD on the periodontium, bone loss in the jaws of the mice, the cemento-enamel junction to alveolar bone crest (CEJ-ABC) length was measured in all 6 groups (Figure 1). No significant difference between PAD-deficient *P. gingivalis* and the CMC vehicle control was observed. However a significant increase in CEJ-ABC distance reflecting increased bone loss was observed between wild type P. *gingivalis* and CMC vehicle control ($p = 0.01$) and wild type *P. gingivalis* with experimental arthritis and CMC vehicle control with experimental arthritis ($p = 0.001$). Furthermore, there was significantly higher bone loss between wild type *P. gingivalis* W50 and PAD-deficient *P. gingivalis* ($p = 0.04$) over wild type *P. gingivalis* with experimental arthritis and PAD-deficient *P. gingivalis* with experimental arthritis ($p = 0.005$).

Histological Analysis of Maxillary Periodontal Tissues

Histological assessment of the periodontal tissue around the first and second maxillary molars demonstrated a statistically significant number of osteoclasts and evidence of bone resorption in the experimental arthritis groups where the difference between the PAD-deficient *P. gingivalis* and the CMC groups were also significantly different to the wild type *P. gingivalis* group ($p = 0.03$ and $p = 0.02$ respectively; Figure 2). There was no statistical difference seen between the non-experimental arthritis groups and the experimental arthritis group which had CMC or PAD-deficient *P. gingivalis* inoculations. Interestingly, the control group with induced experimental arthritis showed evidence of bone resorption which was not seen in the CMC group where there was no induced experimental arthritis.

Micro-CT Analysis of Bone Erosion in Front Paw Radio-carpal Joint

Animals were micro-CTscanned and the radio-carpal joints of both paws (combined) were analysed for changes in bone volume over time. The W50 group with EA showed significantly lower bone volume change reflecting increased bone loss, than the CMC with experimental arthritis group in the radio-carpal joint ($p < 0.04$) (Figure 3). Other group comparisons were not significant.

Visual Scoring of Paw Swelling

Front and rear paws of all mice induced with experimental arthritis were scored daily for swelling and inflammation. There was no significant difference between the control (CMC inoculated group) and the group inoculated with PAD-deficient *P. gingivalis* for the onset of disease and maximum paw score at the height of the disease (day 6–7). However this was not the case for the group that received wild type *P. gingivalis*. There was a rapid onset with swelling and inflammation evident at day 4 and continued for the next 3 days with paw scores significantly higher ($p < 0.0001$) than those of the CMC and PAD-deficient *P. gingivalis* groups (Figure 4).

Histological Assessment of Joint Inflammation

Histological assessment of the sections of inflamed paws in the experimental arthritis group of animals confirmed the observations from the clinical paw scores that the level of inflammation and cartilage and bone destruction was significantly higher in the group inoculated with wild type control groups ($p = 0.02$ and 0.01 respectively). A significant difference was also noted between the wild type *P. gingivalis* and PAD-deficient strain for inflammation and bone/cartilage destruction ($p = 0.02$ and $p = 0.009$ respectively). No differences were observed between the PAD-deficient strain and the CMC control groups (Figure 5). There was no paw inflammation observed in groups that did not undergo experimental arthritis induction.

Serum anti-CCP Antibody Levels

Control mice (inoculated with CMC) demonstrated a background level of anti-CCP antibodies (ACPA). Similar levels were demonstrated in the groups inoculated with wild type *P. gingivalis* and PAD-deficient *P. gingivalis* strains. There was no significant increases in anti-CCP titre in the CMC and *P. gingivalis* ECR527 inoculated groups compared to the groups with no EA. Only mice induced with EA and with pre-existing periodontitis induced by *P. gingivalis* W50 demonstrated a trend towards an increase in anti-CCP antibodies, but this was not significant (Figure 6).

Serum anti-*P. gingivalis* Levels

Mice developed antibodies to *P. gingivalis* over the course of the experiment. Antibody titres increased significantly following induction of experimental arthritis at week 9 in all groups. However those inoculated with wild type *P. gingivalis* produced a higher titre than experimental arthritis alone ($p = 0.001$) and experimental arthritis plus PAD-deficient *P. gingivalis*. ($p = 0.02$) (Figure 7)

Discussion

Of the many hypotheses proposed for a linking mechanism between periodontal disease and RA, the role of citrullination and production of anti-cyclic citrullinated antibodies is of particular interest [15,27]. Citrullination is a common post-translational modification based on the conversion of arginine into citrulline. It occurs frequently in various tissues of the body, particularly at sites of inflammation, and is initiated by peptidylarginine deiminases (PADs). A key concept in the pathogenesis of RA is the preclinical phase which precedes the clinical manifestation of RA [28]. This concept is predicated on the identification of serum autoantibodies years before the development of RA. Indeed there is good evidence to suggest that the immunological conflict often predates the onset of RA by several years. A key component in this process is the production of anti-citrullinated protein antibodies [10]. The production of citrullinated proteins and anti-citrullinated protein antibodies at extra-articular sites prior to the development of RA is well documented [10]. It has been proposed that the inflamed periodontal tissues may be one such site [29].

A number of animal models of experimental arthritis have been studied, each presenting certain advantages and disadvantages [30]. The model chosen for this study, collagen antibody induced arthritis, is characterized by macrophage and polymorphonuclear leukocyte infiltrate within the joints. In this model the anti-collagen antibody is adoptively transferred and therefore it does not rely on specific B- and T-cell responses for disease to ensue.

Nonetheless the development of arthritis in the CAIA model is similar to other models with regards to the inflammatory cytokine response and pannus formation within the affected joints [31,32].

While the role of anti-citrullinated protein antibodies in the pathogenesis of rheumatoid arthritis has been controversial, there is good evidence to support a pathogenic role for these antibodies in the development of both experimental arthritis and human rheumatoid arthritis. [33,34]. While not studied in as much detail as other experimental arthritis models, anti-citrullinated protein antibodies have been suggested to play a role in the severity of disease in the collagen antibody induced arthritis model of experimental arthritis [35,36]. To date there have been no reports concerning an anti-citrullinated protein antibody response in experimental periodontitis. In this regard the present study is significant since it reports that mice with experimental periodontitis and subsequent induction of experimental arthritis demonstrated a trend (not significant) towards an increase in anti-citrullinated protein antibody titre. The precise role that anti-citrullinated protein antibodies play in this process await further investigation.

Shortly after *P. gingivalis* was shown to be the only prokaryote to produce a peptidylarginine deiminase (PPAD) a hypothesis was presented in which the ability of this organism to citrullinate proteins through secretion of PPAD could be one mechanism whereby anti-citrullinated protein antibodies could develop and result in an exaggerated antibody response with subsequent joint inflammation and development of rheumatoid arthritis [9,15].

To explore this concept further we constructed a knock-out *P. gingivalis* strain deficient in PPAD expression (ECR527) with view to examining the role of PPAD in the development of both experimental periodontitis and arthritis. We have recently completed sequencing of the PAD-deficient *P. gingivalis* on our in-house ion torrent and found no secondary mutations, indicating that the experimental results were solely due to the deletion of *pad* from *P. gingivalis* (unpublished data).

There is only one other report in the literature that has used a PAD-deficient *P. gingivalis* strain in a experimental arthritis model [37]. However, our study complements and extends this earlier study [37] by investigating experimental periodontitis in addition to experimental arthritis and a combination of both. This is an important extension of the earlier study [37] which investigated the effect of subcutaneous inoculation of *P. gingivalis* on experimental arthritis only. Furthermore we demonstrated that both the wild type and PAD-deficient strain of *P. gingivalis* survived in the oral cavity after oral inoculation. Recent observations indicate that experimental periodontitis can only progress in the presence of a biofilm containing viable *P. gingivalis* [38]. In this study we used *P. gingivalis* W50 as it is highly virulent in murine periodontitis models [39–45].

With regards to the induction of experimental periodontitis it was noteworthy that oral inoculation with the PAD-deficient strain resulted in a significantly reduced amount of periodontal bone loss compared to oral inoculation with the wild type *P. gingivalis*. The reasons for this response are as yet unclear and require further investigation but this finding does implicate a role for PAD in the pathogenesis of periodontitis.

When periodontitis was first induced followed by induction of experimental arthritis studies it was noted that inoculation with the PAD-deficient *P. gingivalis* strain resulted in reduced severity and onset of arthritis. This is in agreement with a previous study in which it was noted that inoculation with PAD-deficient strain of *P. gingivalis* resulted in reduced severity of collagen-induced experimental arthritis [37].

In recent years the concepts of molecular mimicry and posttranslational modification of proteins in auto-immune reactions such as RA have been actively debated [28,46]. Interestingly, *P. gingivalis* appears as a likely agent involved in these processes. For example, cross reactivity of antibodies to *P. gingivalis* heat shock protein (HSP 60) and host-derived heat shock protein in the pathogenesis of RA has been documented [47]. Another case for molecular mimicry involving *P. gingivalis* has been made whereby antibodies against citrullinated human α-enolase cross react with citrullinated *P. gingivalis* enolase [27]. Similarly, the ability of *P. gingivalis* to produce PPAD which can citrullinate host proteins and lead to an early anti-citrullinated protein antibody response has also implicated this bacterium in the pathogenesis of RA [37]. While antibodies to PPAD have been detected in the sera of mice injected with *P. gingivalis*, the titre is very low and this reaction probably does not contribute to the process of *P. gingivalis*-induced exacerbation of experimental arthritis [37]. In the present study, when periodontitis was induced the anti-citrullinated protein antibody serum levels for control and PAD-deficient strains were similar. However, following induction of experimental arthritis the anti-citrullinated protein antibody titres were elevated only for the wild type strain and not for the controls or PAD-deficient strains. This implies a synergistic role for PPAD in the development of experimental arthritis. This observation is in line with those from a study using a different model of collagen-induced experimental arthritis [37].

The emerging data now significantly implicate local citrullination within inflamed periodontal tissues as having the potential to be an extra-articular source of citrullination and production of anti-citrullinated protein antibodies. To date, smoking has been considered a major risk factor in the pathogenesis of RA whereby smoking leads to citrullination within the lung and a priming anti-citrullinated protein antibody response which leads to exacerbation of the anti-citrullinated protein antibody response and associated tissue destruction within inflamed joints. In light of recent observations of the presence of inflammation-associated citrullination, presence of PAD-2 and PAD-4 in gingival tissues [28,48] as well as PPAD in serum [49] now provides good evidence for another important extra-articular source for citrullination and anti-citrullinated protein antibody production to occur years in advance of the development of the clinical signs and symptoms of RA. In this regard it is significant that individuals with untreated RA who are non-smokers but presenting with chronic periodontitis have a significantly high level of anti-citrullinated protein antibody titres [50].

In conclusion this study has demonstrated that PPAD appears to be a significant factor in the development of experimental periodontitis and exacerbation of experimental arthritis. Interpretation of these findings must be made in the context that the animal models used do not completely reflect the complexities of human dises for both periodontitis and rheumatoid arthrits.

Nonetheless these findings adds further evidence for a potentail role of *P. gingivalis* in the pathogenesis and exacerbation of arthritis. Further studies are now needed to elucidate the mechanisms which drive these processes.

Supporting Information

Figure S1 Raw data used for determination of data points in Figure 4.

Figure S2 Raw data used for determination of data points in Figure 6.

Figure S3 Raw data used for determination of data points in Figure 7.

Data S1

Acknowledgments

The authors wish to thank Ruth Williams from Adelaide Microscopy for her expert assistance with the Skyscan1076 live animal microCT scanner and Associate Professor Renato Morona from the School of Molecular and Biomedical Science for the use of his PC2 laboratory facilities to grow and maintain the genetically modified *P. gingivalis* strain ECR527.

Author Contributions

Conceived and designed the experiments: NG RB VM CM MC DRH CAB SD ECR PMB. Performed the experiments: NG RB VM CM MC CAB SD. Analyzed the data: NG RB VM CM MC DRH CAB SD ECR PMB. Contributed reagents/materials/analysis tools: NG RB VM CM MC DRH CAB SD ECR PMB. Wrote the paper: NG RB VM CM MC DRH CAB SD ECR PMB. Research Funding: NG DRH CAB PMB. Manuscript revision and submission: NG RB VM CM MC DRH CAB SD ECR PMB.

References

1. Page RC, Offenbacher S, Schroeder HE, Seymour GJ, Kornman KS (1997) Advances in the pathogenesis of periodontitis: summary of developments, clinical implications and future directions. Periodontol 2000 14: 216–48.
2. Linden GJ, Lyons A, Scannapieco FA (2013) Periodontal systemic associations: review of the evidence. J Clin Periodontol 40 Suppl 14: S8–19.
3. Kornman KS (2009) A Call to Action. J Periodontol 80: 1019–1020.
4. de Pablo P, Chapple IL, Buckley CD, Dietrich T (2009) Periodontitis in systemic rheumatic diseases. Nat Rev Rheumatol 5: 218–224.
5. Bartold PM, Marshall RI, Haynes DR (2005) Periodontitis and rheumatoid arthritis: a review. J Periodontol 76 (11 Suppl): 2066–2074.
6. Byrne SJ, Dashper SG, Darby IB, Adams GG, Hoffmann B, et al. (2009) Progression of chronic periodontitis can be predicted by the levels of *Porphyromonas gingivalis* and *Treponema denticola* in subgingival plaque. Oral Microbiol Immunol 24: 469–477.
7. Shiloah J, Patters MR, Waring MB (2000) The prevalence of pathogenic periodontal microflora in healthy young adult smokers. J Periodontol 71: 562–567.
8. van Winkelhoff AJ, Loos BG, van der Reijden WA, van der Velden U (2002) *Porphyromonas gingivalis, Bacteroides forsythus* and other putative periodontal pathogens in subjects with and without periodontal destruction. J Clin Periodontol 29: 1023–1028.
9. McGraw WT, Potempa J, Farley D, Travis J (1999) Purification, characterization, and sequence analysis of a potential virulence factor from *Porphyromonas gingivalis*, peptidylarginine deiminase. Infect Immun 67: 3248–3256.
10. Holers VM (2013) Autoimmunity to citrullinated proteins and the initiation of rheumatoid arthritis. Curr Op Immunol 25: 728–735.
11. Schellekens GA, de Jong BA, van den Hoogen FH, van de Putte LB, van Venrooij WJ (1998) Citrulline is an essential constituent of antigenic determinants recognized by rheumatoid arthritis-specific autoantibodies. J Clin Invest 101: 273–281.
12. Masson-Bessiere C, Sebbag M, Girbal-Neuhauser E, Nogueira L, Vincent C, et al. (2001) The major synovial targets of the rheumatoid arthritis-specific antifilaggrin autoantibodies are deiminated forms of the alpha- and beta-chains of fibrin. J Immunol 166: 4177–4184.
13. Girbal-Neuhauser E, Durieux JJ, Arnaud M, Dalbon P, Sebbag M, et al. (1999) The epitopes targeted by the rheumatoid arthritis-associated antifilaggrin autoantibodies are posttranslationally generated on various sites of (pro)filaggrin by deimination of arginine residues. J Immunol 162: 585–594.
14. Doyle HA, Mamula MJ (2002) Posttranslational protein modifications: new flavors in the menu of autoantigens. Curr Opin Rheumatol 14: 244–249.
15. Rosenstein ED, Greenwald RA, Kushner LJ, Weissmann G (2004) Hypothesis: the humoral immune response to oral bacteria provides a stimulus for the development of rheumatoid arthritis. Inflammation 28: 311–318.
16. Wegner N, Lundberg K, Kinloch A, Fisher B, Malmström V, et al. (2010) Autoimmunity to specific citrullinated proteins gives the first clues to the etiology of rheumatoid arthritis. Immunol Rev 233: 34–54.
17. Wegner N, Wait R, Sroka A, Eick S, Nguyen KA, et al. (2010) Peptidylarginine deiminase from *Porphyromonas gingivalis* citrullinates human fibrinogen and alpha-enolase: implications for autoimmunity in rheumatoid arthritis. Arthritis Rheum 62: 2662–2672.
18. Horton RM (1995) PCR-mediated recombination and mutagenesis. SOEing together tailor-made genes. Mol Biotechnol 3: 93–99.
19. Fletcher HM, Schenkein HA, Morgan RM, Bailey KA, Berry CR, et al. (1995) Virulence of a *Porphyromonas gingivalis* W83 mutant defective in the *prtH* gene. Infect Immun 63: 1521–1528.
20. Knipp M, Vasak M (2000) A colorimetric 96-well microtiter plate assay for the determination of enzymatically formed citrulline. Anal Biochem 286: 257–264.
21. Abdullah SN, Farmer EA, Spargo L, Logan R, Gully N (2013) *Porphyromonas gingivalis* peptidylarginine deiminase substrate specificity. Anaerobe 23: 102–108.
22. Cantley MD, Bartold PM, Marino V, Reid RC, Fairlie DP, et al. (2009) The use of live-animal micro-computed tomography to determine the effect of a novel phospholipase A2 inhibitor on alveolar bone loss in an in vivo mouse model of periodontitis. J Periodontal Res 44: 317–322.
23. Cantley MD, Haynes DR, Marino V, Bartold PM (2011) Pre-existing periodontitis exacerbates experimental arthritis in a mouse model. J Clin Periodontol. 38: 532–541.
24. Nandakumar KS, Andrén M, Martinsson P, Bajtner E, Hellström S, et al. (2003) Induction of arthritis by single monoclonal IgG anti-collagen type II antibodies and enhancement of arthritis in mice lacking inhibitory FcgammaRIIB. Eur J Immunol 33: 2269–2277.
25. Park CH, Abramson ZR, Taba M Jr, Jin Q, Chang J, et al. (2007) Three-dimensional micro-computed tomographic imaging of alveolar bone in experimental bone loss or repair. J Periodontol 78: 273–281.
26. Dehal PS, Joachimiak MP, Price MN, Bates JT, Baumohl JK, et al. (2010) MicrobesOnline: an integrated portal for comparative and functional genomics. Nucleic Acids Res 38 (Database issue): D396–400.
27. Lundberg K, Wegner N, Yucel-Lindberg T, Venables PJ (2010) Periodontitis in RA-the citrullinated enolase connection. Nat Rev Rheumatol 6: 727–730.
28. Demoruelle MK, Deane KD, Holers VM (2014) When and where does inflammation begin in rheumatoid arthritis. Curr Opin Rheumatol 26: 64–71.
29. Harvey GP, Fitzsimmons TR, Dhamarpatni AA, Marchant C, Haynes DR, et al. (2013) Expression of peptidylarginine deiminase-2 and -4, citrullinated proteins and anti-citrullinated protein antibodies in human gingiva. J Periodontal Res 48: 252–261.
30. Asquith DL, Miller AM, McInnes IB, Liew FY (2009) Animal models of rheumatoid arthritis. Eur J Immunol. 39: 2040–2044.
31. Nandakumar KS, Svensson L, Holmdahl R (2003) Collagen type II-specific monoclonal antibody-induced arthritis in mice: description of the disease and the influence of age, sex, and genes. Am J Pathol 163: 1827–1837.
32. Nandakumar KS, Holmdahl R (2006) Antibody-induced arthritis: disease mechanisms and genes involved at the effector phase of arthritis. Arthritis Res Ther 2006; 8: 223–234.
33. Klareskog L, Rönnelid J, Lundberg K, Padyukov L, Alfredsson L (2008) Immunity to citrullinated proteins in rheumatoid arthritis. Annu Rev Immunol 26: 651–675.
34. Thiele GM, Duryee MJ, Dusad A, Hunter CD, Lacy JP, et al. (2012) Citrullinated mouse collagen administered to DBA/1J mice in the absence of adjuvant initiates arthritis. Int Immunopharmacol 13: 424–431.
35. Kuhn KA, Kulik L, Tomooka B, Braschler KJ, Arend WP, et al. (2006) Antibodies against citrullinated proteins enhance tissue injury in experimental autoimmune arthritis. J Clin Invest 116: 961–973.
36. Willis VC, Gizinski AM, Banda NK, Causey CP, Knuckley B, et al. (2011) N-α-benzoyl-N5-(2-chloro-1-iminoethyl)-L-ornithine amide, a protein arginine deiminase inhibitor, reduces the severity of murine collagen-induced arthritis. J Immunol 186: 4396–4404.
37. Maresz KJ, Hellvard A, Sroka A, Adamowicz K, Bielecka E, et al. (2013) *Porphyromonas gingivalis* facilitates the development and progression of destructive arthritis through its unique bacterial peptidylarginine deiminase (PAD). PLoS Pathog 9: e1003627.
38. Dashper S, O'Brien-Simpson N, Liu SW, Paolini R, Mitchell H, et al. (2014) Oxantel disrupts polymicrobial biofilm development of periodontal pathogens. Antimicrob Agents Chemother. 58: 378–85. doi:10.1128/AAC.01375-13. Epub 2013 Oct 28.
39. Bird PS, Gemmell E, Polak B, Paton RG, Sosroseno W, et al. (1995). Protective immunity to *Porphyromonas gingivalis* infection in a murine model. J. Periodontol 66: 351–362.
40. Kesavalu L, Holt SC, Ebersole JL (1998) Virulence of a polymicrobic complex, *Treponema denticola* and *Porphyromonas gingivalis*, in a murine model. Oral Microbiol Immunol 13: 373–377.
41. O'Brien-Simpson NM, Paolini RA, Hoffmann B, Slakeski N, Dashper SG, et al. (2001) Role of RgpA, RgpB, and Kgp proteinases in virulence of *Porphyromonas gingivalis* W50 in a murine lesion model. Infect. Immun 69: 7527–7534.
42. Pathirana RD, O'Brien-Simpson NM, Veith PD, Riley PF, Reynolds EC(2006) Characterization of proteinase-adhesin complexes of *Porphyromonas gingivalis*. Microbiology 152: 2381–2394.
43. O'Brien-Simpson NM, Pathirana RD, Paolini RA, Chen YY, Veith PD, et al. (2005) An immune response directed to proteinase and adhesin functional epitopes protects against Porphyromonas gingivalis-induced periodontal bone loss. J Immunol 175: 3980–3989.
44. Orth RK, O'Brien-Simpson NM, Dashper SG, Reynolds EC (2011) Synergistic virulence of *Treponema denticola* and *Porphyromonas gingivalis* in a murine periodontitis model. Molecular Oral Microbiology 26: 229–240.

45. Rajapakse PS, O'Brien-Simpson NM, Slakeski N, Hoffmann B, Reynolds EC (2002) Immunization with the RgpA-Kgp proteinase-adhesin complexes of Porphyromonas gingivalis protects against periodontal bone loss in the rat periodontitis model. Infect Immun 70: 2480–2424
46. Wegner N, Wait R, Venables PJ (2009) Evolutionarily conserved antigens in autoimmune disease: implications for an infective aetiology. Int J Biochem Cell Biol 41: 390–397.
47. Jeong E, Lee J-Y, Kim S-J, Choi J (2012) Predominant immunoreactivity of *Porphyromonas gingivalis* heat shock protein in autoimmune disease. J Periodont Res 47: 811–816.
48. Nesse W, Westra J, van der Wal JE, Abbas F, Nicholas AP, et al. (2012) The periodontium of periodontitis patients contains citrullinated proteins which may play a role in ACPA (anti-citrullinated protein antibody) formation. J Clin Periodontol 39: 599–607.
49. Quirke AM, Lugli EB, Wegner N, Hamilton BC, Charles P, et al. (2014) Heightened immune response to autocitrullinated *Porphyromonas gingivalis* peptidylarginine deiminase: a potential mechanism for breaching immunologic tolerance in rheumatoid arthritis. Ann Rheum Dis 73: 263–269.
50. Potikuri D, Dannana KC, Kanchinadam S, Agrawal S, Kancharla A, et al. (2012) Periodontal disease is significantly higher in non-smoking treatment-naïve rheumatoid arthritis patients: results from a case-control study. Ann Rheum Dis 71: 1541–1544.

16

Global Metabolite Profiling of Synovial Fluid for the Specific Diagnosis of Rheumatoid Arthritis from Other Inflammatory Arthritis

Sooah Kim[1], Jiwon Hwang[2], Jinhua Xuan[1], Young Hoon Jung[1], Hoon-Suk Cha[2]*, Kyoung Heon Kim[1]*

1 Department of Biotechnology, Korea University Graduate School, Seoul, Republic of Korea, 2 Samsung Medical Center, Sungkyunkwan University School of Medicine, Seoul, Republic of Korea

Abstract

Currently, reliable biomarkers that can be used to distinguish rheumatoid arthritis (RA) from other inflammatory diseases are unavailable. To find possible distinctive metabolic patterns and biomarker candidates for RA, we performed global metabolite profiling of synovial fluid samples. Synovial fluid samples from 38 patients with RA, ankylosing spondylitis, Behçet's disease, and gout were analyzed by gas chromatography/time-of-flight mass spectrometry (GC/TOF MS). Orthogonal partial least-squares discriminant and hierarchical clustering analyses were performed for the discrimination of RA and non-RA groups. Variable importance for projection values were determined, and the Wilcoxon-Mann-Whitney test and the breakdown and one-way analysis of variance were conducted to identify potential biomarkers for RA. A total of 105 metabolites were identified from synovial fluid samples. The score plot of orthogonal partial least squares discriminant analysis showed significant discrimination between the RA and non-RA groups. The 20 metabolites, including citrulline, succinate, glutamine, octadecanol, isopalmitic acid, and glycerol, were identified as potential biomarkers for RA. These metabolites were found to be associated with the urea and TCA cycles as well as fatty acid and amino acid metabolism. The metabolomic analysis results demonstrated that global metabolite profiling by GC/TOF MS might be a useful tool for the effective diagnosis and further understanding of RA.

Editor: Yong-Sun Bahn, Yonsei University, Republic of Korea

Funding: This work was supported by the Advanced Biomass R&D Center of Korea (2011-0031353) and the National Foundation of Research (2013059103), both funded by the Korean Government. Experiments were performed by using the facilities of the Institute of Biomedical Science and Food Safety at the Korea University Food Safety Hall. The funders had no role in study design, data collection and analysis, decision to publish, or preparation of the manuscript.

Competing Interests: The authors have declared that no competing interests exist.

* E-mail: hoonsuk.cha@samsung.com (HSC); khekim@korea.ac.kr (KHK)

These authors contributed equally to this work.

Introduction

Rheumatoid arthritis (RA) is a chronic autoimmune disease characterized by synovial proliferation and damage of the affected joints. In spite of current treatment advances including the use of tumor necrosis factor-α (TNF-α) inhibitors, early diagnosis of RA using reliable biomarkers is important for early intervention. Rheumatoid factor (RF), a well-known biomarker for RA, is not useful for specific diagnosis of RA because RF is also detected in various other rheumatic (other than RA) and nonrheumatic disorders such as infection and malignancy, and even in normal individuals [1,2]. Anti-citrullinated protein antibodies (ACPA) have recently received much attention as a valuable tool to differentiate RA from other kinds of arthritis in the 2010 American College of Rheumatology/European League Against Rheumatism (ACR/EULAR) classification criteria [3,4]. However, not all RA patients are seropositive for ACPA, and the 2010 ACR/EULAR classification criteria does not satisfactorily rule in RA for patients with seronegative arthritis, especially involving only one joint. Therefore, more reliable biomarkers with diagnostic capabilities are still needed for RA.

Recently, omics technologies such as genomics, transcriptomics, proteomics, and metabolomics have been increasingly exploited for the discovery of disease biomarkers, including those for RA. Genomics has clearly revealed differences between ACPA-positive and ACPA-negative diseases [5]. In addition, transcriptomics has been used to discover immunity and defense-related genes in RA patients and to predict the efficacy of the anti-TNF-α biologic agent, infliximab, in RA patients [6,7]. Metabolomics, which is a non-targeted analysis of global changes of the complete set of metabolites in organisms [8], has shown its potential in the discovery in disease biomarkers [9–12]. Because metabolite profile changes can be indicative of a disease state [13–15], metabolomics may be a powerful tool for discovering new biomarkers for diseases. Recently, the application of metabolomics to plasma samples was successful in finding metabolic discrimination and potential biomarkers for RA by using nuclear magnetic resonance spectroscopy (NMR) [16], gas chromatography/mass spectrometry (GC/MS), and liquid chromatography/mass spectrometry (LC/MS) [17]. However, to date, reliable biomarkers of RA that discriminate RA from other inflammatory arthritis have not been identified using metabolomics.

Synovial fluid is a body fluid that provides nutrition and lubrication to the articular cartilage. In the pathological joint, the amount of synovial fluid is higher than normal, and a high number of inflammatory cytokines and immune cells are present in the synovial fluid [7]. Thus far, although synovial fluid is the direct medium for the pathological products of RA, no study has examined the changes in metabolism of RA synovial fluid, and biomarkers for RA have not been discovered using synovial fluid. In the present study, in order to find potential biomarkers for RA, discriminating from other kinds of inflammatory arthritis except for septic arthritis (i.e., ankylosing spondylitis (AS), Behçet's disease (BD), and gout), metabolite profiling of synovial fluid from the patients with inflammatory arthritis was performed using gas chromatography/time-of-flight mass spectrometry (GC/TOF MS). These biomarker candidates were verified by multivariate statistical analyses in comparison with other kinds of inflammatory arthritis.

Materials and Methods

Human synovial fluid collection and patients

Among patients visiting the rheumatology clinic at the Samsung Medical Center in Seoul, Korea between July 2000 and September 2007, 77 patients who received arthrocentesis were retrospectively screened. Patients with osteoarthritis or a septic condition were excluded from the screening, and thus 38 patients who were diagnosed with RA, ankylosing spondylitis (AS), Behçet's disease (BD), and gout were enrolled in our study. Medical records of the 38 patients were reviewed for age, gender, duration of disease, and laboratory data along with the disease category such as RF, ACPA, fluorescent anti-nuclear antibody, and human leukocyte antigen B27 (HLA-B27). Fulfillment of the above criteria was assessed following the 1987 ACR and 2010 ACR/EULAR classification criteria for RA, the 1984 modified New York criteria, the Assessment of SpondyloArthritis international Society (ASAS) classification criteria for axial spondyloarthritis, and the criteria of the 1990 International Study Group for BD. For gout, the presence of monosodium urate (MSU) crystals was examined in joint fluid. Radiographic findings for the involvement of sacroiliac joints in AS and BD were evaluated, and bony erosion with overhanging edges was checked for gout patients. Following disease categorization, treatment data were obtained for previous uses of non-steroidal anti-inflammatory drugs (NSAIDs) and disease-modifying anti-rheumatic drugs (DMARDs) or uric acid lowering treatment (ULT). In addition, the history of intraarticular steroid injection was investigated.

Synovial fluid samples were obtained from arthrocentesis for the sake of the clinical diagnosis of arthritis. This aspirated synovial fluid was routinely analyzed by examining the white blood cell count, polarizing microscopy, the Gram staining and culture, fungus culture, and acid-fast bacteria staining and culture. The final diagnosis was made by experienced rheumatologists. Synovial fluid samples were collected and stored at -80°C. To identify presumed biomarkers for RA, samples were divided into 2 groups: RA versus non-RA including AS, BD, and gout. The study was carried out in accordance with the Helsinki Declaration and approved by the Institutional Review Board of Samsung Medical Center, Seoul, Korea. All subjects were provided with written informed consent prior to study enrollment.

Patient characteristics

Synovial fluid samples from 38 patients with inflammatory arthritis were analyzed as RA (13 samples), AS (7 samples), BD (5 samples), and gout (13 samples), and their baseline characteristics are summarized in Table 1. The ages of patients with RA (44.2 ± 10.7) and non-RA (42.1 ± 10.3) did not significantly differ at a significance level of 0.05. Among them, 10 samples were obtained through diagnostic arthrocentesis, whereas other samples were obtained for therapeutic purposes. None of the diagnostic samples were positive for microbial culture. Sacroiliac joints were affected in all AS patients. Five patients with gout had typical erosive lesions as determined from the radiographs, and MSU crystals were confirmed in synovial fluid samples of 7 patients. All RA patients had a history of receiving DMARDs except one patient who was enrolled during the initial presentation of RA. Five of 7 AS patients and 2 of 5 BD patients were prescribed DMARDs before arthrocentesis. Of the 13 patients with gout, 9 had ULT and 10 had received colchicines before enrollment.

Metabolite sample preparation

Metabolite extraction from synovial fluid was conducted using 80% (v/v) methanol at -20°C according to a previously described procedure with a slight modification [18]. Synovial fluid samples were thawed on ice for 3 min and then centrifuged at $500 \times g$ at 4°C for 5 min to remove cells and debris. The supernatant from the centrifuged synovial fluid was mixed with 80% (v/v) methanol at -20°C for metabolite extraction, and this mixture was vortexed for 3 min and then centrifuged at $16100 \times g$ for 5 min at 4°C. The supernatant was then completely dried in a vacuum concentrator (Labconco, Kansas City, MO). To eliminate lipids and waxes, the metabolite extract was re-extracted with 500 μL of an aqueous acetonitrile solution (acetonitrile:water = 1:1, v/v) at 0°C. After centrifugation at $16100 \times g$ for 5 min, the supernatant was collected and concentrated to dryness. The dried metabolite was derivatized with 5 μL of methoxyamine hydrochloride in pyridine (40 mg/mL; Pierce, Rockford, IL) for 90 min at 30°C and 45 μL of *N*-methyl-*N*-(trimethylsilyl) trifluoroacetamide (Fluka, Buchs, Switzerland) was added for 30 min and 37°C. Subsequently, a mixture of fatty acid methyl esters as retention index markers was added to the derivatized sample.

Metabolite analysis

An Agilent 7890A GC (Hewlett-Packard, Atlanta, GA) coupled to a Pegasus HT TOF MS (Leco, St. Joseph, MI) was used for the analysis of derivatized metabolite samples. The derivatized extract (1 μL) was injected into the GC in splitless mode. An RTX-5Sil MS capillary column (30 m length, 25 mm inner diameter, and 0.25 mm film thickness; Restek, Bellefonte, PA) and an additional 10-m long integrated guard column were used for GC separation. The sample was initially held at a constant temperature of 50°C for 1 min, after which it was ramped to 330°C at 20°C/min and then finally held for 5 min. The transfer line temperature was set at 280°C. Mass spectra were acquired in a scanning range of 85–500 m/z at an acquisition rate of 10 spectra/sec. The ionization mode was subjected to electron impact at 70 eV with an ion source temperature set at 250°C. GC/TOF MS data were preprocessed by Leco ChromaTOF software (version 3.34; Leco) by using automated peak detection and mass spectral deconvolution. Preprocessed MS data were processed using BinBase, an in-house programmed database for the identification of metabolites, as described previously [19,20]. The abundance of each identified metabolite was obtained by normalizing the peak intensity of each metabolite using the median of sums of peak intensities of all the identified metabolites in each sample [21,22].

Table 1. Baseline characteristics of RA and non-RA groups.

	RA (n = 13)	Non-RA (n = 25)		
		AS (n = 7)	BD (n = 5)	Gout (n = 13)
Age, mean ± SD years	44.2±10.7	35.4±10.7	41.6±12.5	45.9±7.9
Female, no. (%)	13 (100)	3 (42.9)	2 (40.0)	0 (0.0)
Disease duration, years	6.5±6.3	3.1±3.3	6.3±7.9	7.9±2.7
RF, no. of positive/tested (%)	13 (100)	0/5 (0.0)	1/3 (33.3)	0/7 (0.0)
ACPA, no. of positive/tested (%)	3/3 (100)	n.a.	n.a.	n.a.
FANA, no. of positive/tested (%)	n.a.	0/3 (0.0)	0/2 (0.0)	0/2 (0.0)
HLA-B27, no. of positive/tested (%)	n.a.	6/6 (100.0)	n.a.	n.a.
Fulfillment of criteria, no. of positive/tested (%)				
1987 ACR	12/13 (92.3)	n.a.	n.a.	n.a.
1984 modified NY	n.a.	7/7 (100.0)	1/5 (20.0)	n.a.
2010 ACR/EULAR	13/13 (100.0)	n.a.	n.a.	n.a.
ASAS axial	n.a.	7/7 (100.0)	n.a.	n.a.
Previous NSAID, no. of positive/tested (%)	12/13 (92.3)	22/25 (88.0)	2/5 (40.0)	13/13 (100.0)
Previous intraarticular steroid injection, no. or no. of positive/tested (%)	10/13 (76.9)	4/7 (57.1)	3/5 (60.0)	3/13 (23.1)

ACPA, anti-CCP antibody; ACR, The American College of Rheumatology classification criteria of RA; ACR/EULAR, The American College of Rheumatology/European League Against Rheumatism classification criteria for RA; AS, ankylosing spondylitis; ASAS axial, Assessment of SpondyloArthritis international Society classification criteria for axial spondyloarthritis; BD, Behçet's disease; FANA, fluorescent anti-nuclear antibody; HLA-B27, human leukocyte antigen B27; modified NY, Modified New York criteria for the diagnosis of AS; n.a, not applicable; non-RA, non-rheumatoid arthritis including ankylosing spondylitis, Behçet's disease, and gout; Previous NSAID, previously use of non-steroidal anti-inflammatory drug; RA, rheumatoid arthritis; RF, rheumatoid factor.

Statistical analyses and validation

As the statistical analyses of metabolite profiles of synovial fluid from the RA and non-RA (AS, BD, and gout) groups, univariate analysis [19,20,23], orthogonal partial least squares discriminant analysis (OPLS-DA), hierarchical clustering analysis (HCA) [24], and receiver operating characteristic (ROC) curve analysis were performed. To obtain maximal covariance between the measured data and the response variable, OPLS-DA was performed using SIMCA-P+ (version 12.0; Umetric AB, Umea, Sweden). Seven-fold internal cross validation and external validation were also conducted using SIMCA-P+. For the external validation, RA patients and non-RA patients were randomly collected from another cohort. The mean age of 6 RA patients (five female and one male) was 66.5 years, and that of 11 non-RA patients (one female and ten male) consisting of 4 AS patients, 4 BD patients and 3 gout patients was 32.5 years. Hierarchical clustering analysis (HCA) was performed using MultiExperiment Viewer for visualization and organization of metabolite profiles [24]. Statistica (version 7.1; StatSoft, Tulsa, OK) was used for univariate analysis [19,20,23]. A further diagnostic property was deduced by receiver operating characteristic (ROC) curve analysis using MedCalc software (Broekstraat, Mariakerke, Belgium).

Results

Metabolite profiles of RA and non-RA groups

A total of 38 synovial fluid samples of inflammatory arthritis including RA, AS, BD, and gout were analyzed by GC/TOF MS. After deconvolution, 105 metabolites were identified across the synovial fluid samples of 38 patients, which were classified into the following chemical classes: sugars and sugar alcohols (25%), amino acids (21%), fatty acids (16%), organic acids (16%), amines (9%), phosphates (8%), and miscellaneous (Table S1).

Since principal component analysis (PCA) showed only slight discrimination between RA and non-RA groups ($R^2X = 0.34$, $Q^2 = 0.20$) in a preliminary study (data not shown), OPLS-DA was employed in this study. OPLS-DA successfully minimized the possible contribution of intergroup variability and further increased the discrimination between the RA and non-RA groups compared to the results obtained by the PCA. As shown in Figure 1a, metabolite profiles of the RA and non-RA groups were distinctively separated on the score plot of OPLS-DA. The OPLS-DA model established with one predictive component and two orthogonal components generated the explained variation values: 0.36 of R^2X and 0.99 of R^2Y and the predictive capability: Q^2 of 0.97. These high value parameters indicated the excellence in modeling and prediction with good discrimination between the RA and non-RA groups since OPLS-DA models with the parameters higher than 0.5 are considered to be satisfactory in explanatory and predictive capabilities [25]. To validate the OPLS-DA model, the PLS-DA model with the same number of components was used. All permuted R^2 values to the left were lower than the original point to the right, and the Q^2 regression line had a negative intercept (Figure S1-a). These results strongly indicated that the OPLS-DA models were statistically validated without overfitting of the original model since the intercept of Q^2 was less than 0.05. In addition, 6 RA patients and 11 non-RA patients collected from another cohort were predicted to be in correct classes (Figure S1-b).

A total of 105 identified metabolites were clustered and visualized by the HCA using the Euclidean distance and the average linkage method to determine possible variations in the metabolite profiling of the RA and non-RA groups. The normalized peak intensity of each metabolite was transformed by unit variance scaling and loaded into a clustered heat map (Figure 2). The higher the abundance of the metabolites, the more

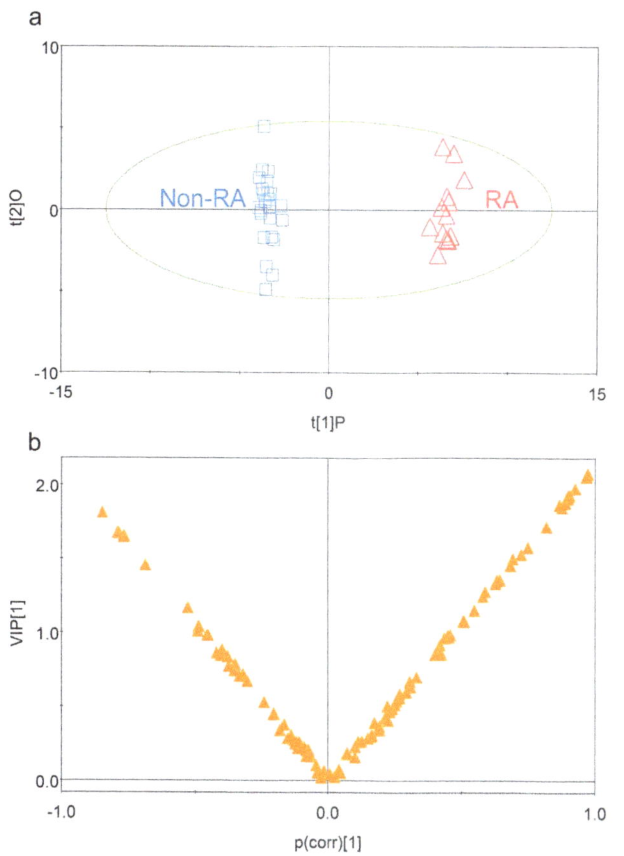

Figure 1. OPLS-DA of the metabolite profiles of RA and non-RA groups. (a) Score plot of the OPLS-DA model for RA and non-RA groups (t[1]P, score of the non-orthogonal component; t[2]O, score of the orthogonal component). (b) V-plot with p(corr) and VIP values of 105 metabolites. The metabolites with p(corr) <0 were those decreased in RA groups while the metabolites with p(corr) >0 were those increased in RA groups.

yellow in the heat map, and the lower the abundance of the metabolites, the more blue in the heat map. Clustering of the metabolites led to good separation between the RA and non-RA groups. The discrimination of metabolite profiles between the two groups was mainly caused by certain metabolites as shown in Figure 2.

Identification of biomarkers for RA

Identification of potential biomarker candidates that account for the differentiation of diseases is a necessary step not only for diagnosis but also for better understanding of the functional metabolism in clinical diseases. To screen putative biomarkers for RA, the variable importance for projection (VIP) values from the OPLS-DA model were obtained. Then, the nonparametric Wilcoxon-Mann-Whitney test and the breakdown and one-way analysis of variance (ANOVA) with post hoc Tukey's honestly significant difference (HSD) test led to further testing of the selected metabolites with high VIP values as biomarker candidates for RA.

VIP values were used to rank the contribution of metabolites to the discrimination between the RA and non-RA groups, which are based on weighted coefficients of the OPLS-DA model [25]. Using the p(corr) and VIP values of the 105 metabolites in synovial fluid, a V-plot was constructed (Figure 1b). VIP values and correlation coefficients (i.e., p(corr)) of each metabolites were shown in the V-plot. Metabolites in both terminals of V represented a high contribution to the discrimination of the RA and non-RA groups. In a VIP analysis, VIP values above 1 are considered important since the influence of variables with a VIP >1.0 on the explanation of the Y matrix is above average [25]. In this study, 33 metabolites were found to have VIP values higher than 1, of which 23 metabolites were higher in the RA group, whereas 10 metabolites were higher in the non-RA group.

Next, the Wilcoxon-Mann-Whitney test was employed to evaluate significant differences ($p<0.01$) of metabolite candidates and to eliminate variables without significant differences between the two groups. Because the abundance of ornithine between the RA and non-RA groups was not significantly different at the 99% significance level, ornithine was ruled out from the 33 biomarker candidates. Among the 32 metabolites that passed the Wilcoxon-Mann-Whitney test, the abundances of 22 metabolites, including succinate, octadecanol, asparagine, and terephthalate, were higher in the RA group than in the non-RA group. Meanwhile, the abundances of 10 metabolites, including isopalmitic acid, glycerol, myristic acid, and palmitoleic acid, were lower in the RA group than in the non-RA group.

One-way ANOVA was conducted to select putative biomarkers for the RA group only in comparison with the non-RA group representing other inflammatory arthritis including AS, BD, and gout. A post-hoc Tukey's HSD test at the 99% significance level was then performed to compare the mean values between groups. The following metabolites did not significantly differ in abundance between the RA group and each disease group of AS, BD, and gout in ANOVA and HSD tests: adipate, asparagine dehydrated, 2,5-dihydroxypyrazine NIST, lanosterol, lignoceric acid, *N*-methylalanine, palmitic acid, phosphoric acid, proline, pyrophosphate, serine, and stearic acid. All of these metabolites were eliminated from the putative biomarkers for RA.

The fold changes of the 20 metabolites selected as potential biomarkers to discriminate RA from non-RA are shown in Figure S2. The abundances of succinate, octadecanol, asparagine, terephthalate, salicylaldehyde, glutamine, citrulline, tyrosine, uracil, lysine, ribitol, tryptophan, xylose, and ribose were higher in the RA group than those in the non-RA group. However, the abundances of isopalmitic acid, glycerol, myristic acid, palmitoleic acid, hydroxylamine, and ethanolamine were lower in the RA group than those in the non-RA group. Notably, the fold change of succinate was highest in the RA group, and the fold changes of salicylaldehyde and glutamine were much higher than those of other metabolites in the RA group. The fold changes of the metabolite abundances increased in the RA group ranged from 1.7 to 73.6.

ROC analysis

Twenty putative biomarkers of the RA group were selected after employing multiple statistical analyses as described earlier. Prior to clinical utility of the 20 putative biomarkers, validation of the biomarkers is needed. For disease diagnosis, the ROC curve and the area under the ROC curve (AUC) provide a numerical value of the relationship between the specificity and sensitivity of a biomarker. These sensitivity and specificity indicate the probably tests for correctly identifying patients with the disease and without the disease, respectively [26]. An AUC value of 0.5 or less for a biomarker indicates no information and discrimination within the test, thus implying no diagnostic utility of the biomarker, whereas an AUC value of 1.0 indicates perfect prediction of the diagnostic test [27-29]. Figure 3 shows the ROC curve analysis for the predictive power of the 20

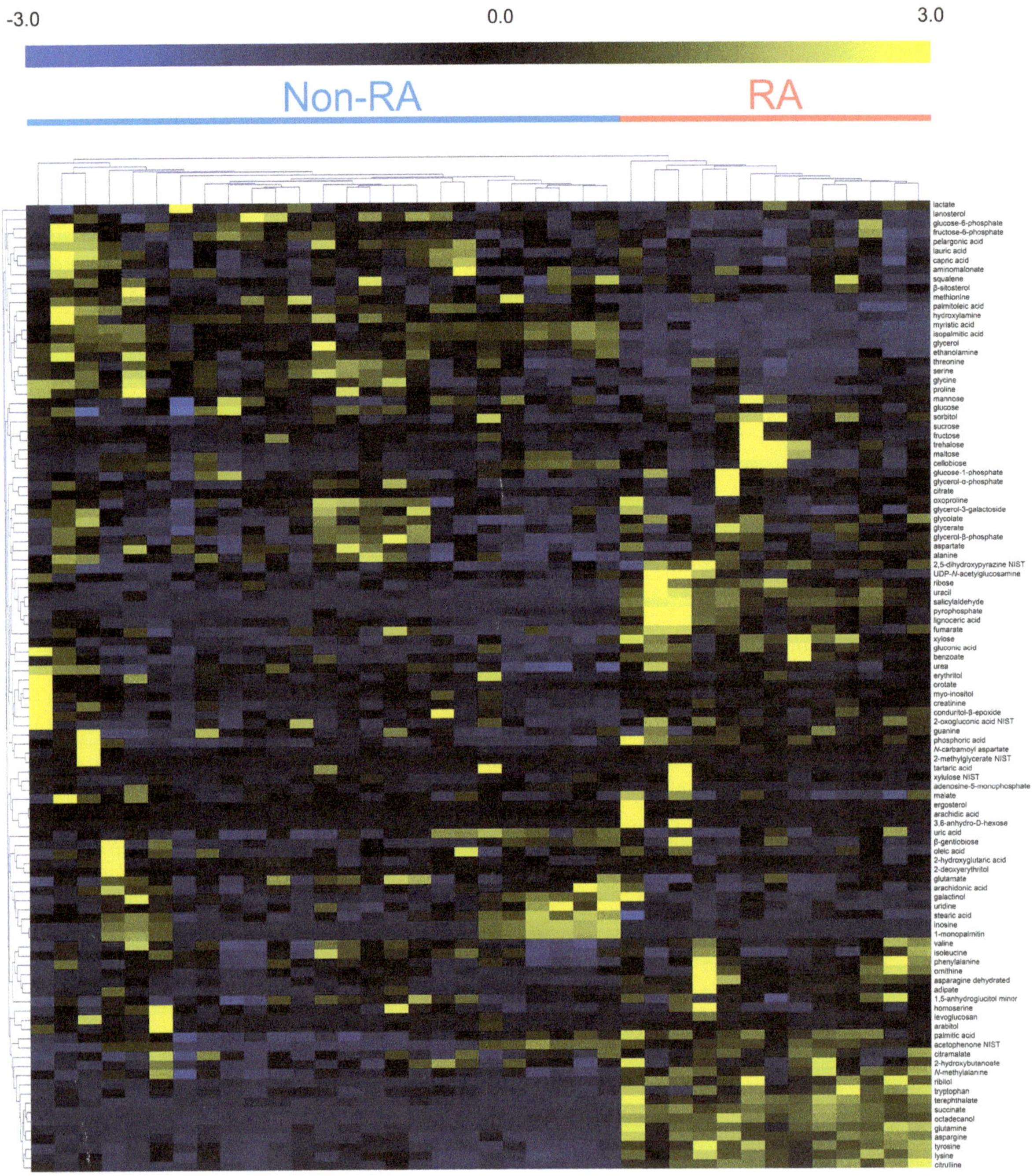

Figure 2. HCA of 105 metabolites from synovial fluid samples of RA and non-RA patients. Each column and row represents a disease and an individual metabolite, respectively.

combined biomarkers of the RA group to discriminate RA from non-RA. A sensitivity of 92.3% and a specificity of 68.0% were obtained from the ROC curve, and the value of AUC was 0.812. Since the 20 putative biomarkers showed the AUC value of greater than 0.8, they were selected as biomarkers of RA (Table 2).

Discussion

Recently, the importance of metabolomics for the study of disease biomarkers and metabolism is rapidly increasing [30–32]. Zahi et al. reported the branched-chain amino acids to histidine ratio as a novel serum biomarker of osteoarthritis using a metabolomics approach [33]. However, only a few studies have performed non-targeted metabolite profiling of RA on a global scale by using plasma or synovial fluid [16,17,34]. Especially, reliable biomarkers of RA distinguished from other inflammatory arthritis such as AS, BD, and gout have not been identified using metabolite profiling in synovial fluids, which is the direct medium showing the state of disease. For example, in a previous study of metabolite profiling of synovial fluid from RA, AS, and gout patients using ^{1}H-NMR identifying 35 metabolites, no differences

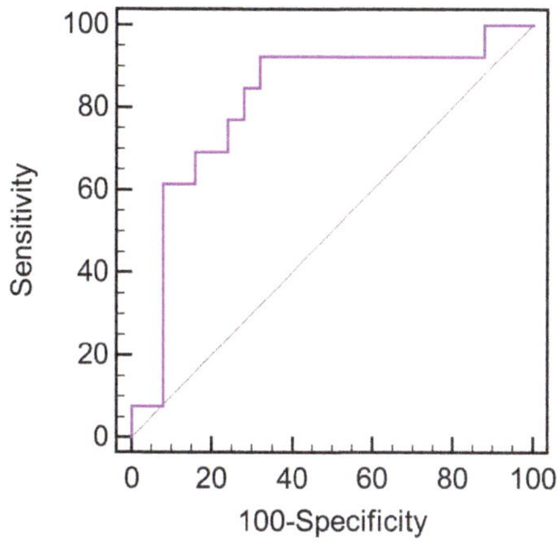

Figure 3. ROC analysis of the predictive power of the 20 combined biomarkers for distinguishing RA and non-RA groups. A sensitivity and specificity were 92.3% and 68.0%, respectively, and the value of AUC was 0.812.

in metabolite profiles were shown between those diseases [34]. In this study, GC/TOF MS was used to find possible biomarkers among metabolites in the synovial fluid of patients with inflammatory arthritis in order to differentiate RA from other inflammatory arthritis such as AS, BD, and gout by using metabolomics. The metabolite profiles of synovial fluid obtained from RA patients were distinguishable from those of other inflammatory arthritis, in which 20 metabolites were selected and validated as potential biomarkers with the capability of discriminating RA from the non-RA diseases like AS, BD, and gout with 92.3% sensitivity and 68.0% specificity. This is the first report of the discovery of potential biomarkers for RA, which discriminate RA from other inflammatory arthritis, by GC/TOF MS-based metabolomic analysis of synovial fluid.

In the present study, 105 metabolites classified into various chemical classes such as amines, amino acids, fatty acids, organic acids, phosphates, and sugars and sugar alcohols were identified by an in-house library. These metabolites are major intermediates of various metabolic pathways, including glycolysis, the TCA cycle, as well as pathways involving amino acid and fatty acid metabolism. The number of metabolites identified from synovial fluid of RA in this study was much higher than that in previous studies [34]. In this study, the metabolite profiles of synovial fluid from RA and non-RA groups were considerably discriminated by OPLS-DA. Following various statistical analyses, 20 metabolites of synovial fluid, including succinate, octadecanol, asparagine, terephthalate, salicylaldehyde, glutamine, citrulline, tyrosine, uracil, lysine, ribitol, tryptophan, xylose, ribose, isopalmitic acid, glycerol, myristic acid, palmitoleic acid, hydroxylamine, and ethanolamine were selected and validated as putative biomarkers for RA, which discriminated from non-RA diseases such as AS, BD, and gout.

Table 2. VIP and AUC values of the metabolites that significantly contribute to the discrimination between the RA and non-RA groups.

Metabolite	VIP value (rank)	*p*-value[a]	AUC[b]
Metabolites with higher abundances in the RA group than in the non-RA group			
succinate	2.09 (1)	<0.0001	1.000
octadecanol	2.07 (2)	<0.0001	1.000
asparagine	1.98 (3)	<0.0001	1.000
terephthalate	1.94 (4)	<0.0001	1.000
salicylaldehyde	1.93 (5)	<0.0001	1.000
glutamine	1.92 (6)	<0.0001	0.997
citrulline	1.91 (7)	<0.0001	1.000
tyrosine	1.89 (8)	<0.0001	1.000
uracil	1.87 (9)	<0.0001	0.997
lysine	1.86 (10)	<0.0001	0.994
ribitol	1.72 (12)	<0.0001	0.985
tryptophan	1.59 (17)	<0.0001	0.883
xylose	1.54 (18)	<0.0001	0.92
ribose	1.51 (19)	<0.0001	0.969
Metabolites with lower abundances in the RA group than in the non-RA group			
isopalmitic acid	1.82 (11)	<0.0001	0.994
glycerol	1.68 (13)	<0.0001	1.000
myristic acid	1.68 (14)	<0.0001	0.985
palmitoleic acid	1.66 (15)	<0.0001	1.000
hydroxylamine	1.65 (16)	<0.0001	1.000
ethanolamine	1.46 (20)	<0.0001	0.963

[a] *p*-values were determined using the Wilcoxon-Mann-Whitney test.
[b] Area under the receiver operator characteristics curve.

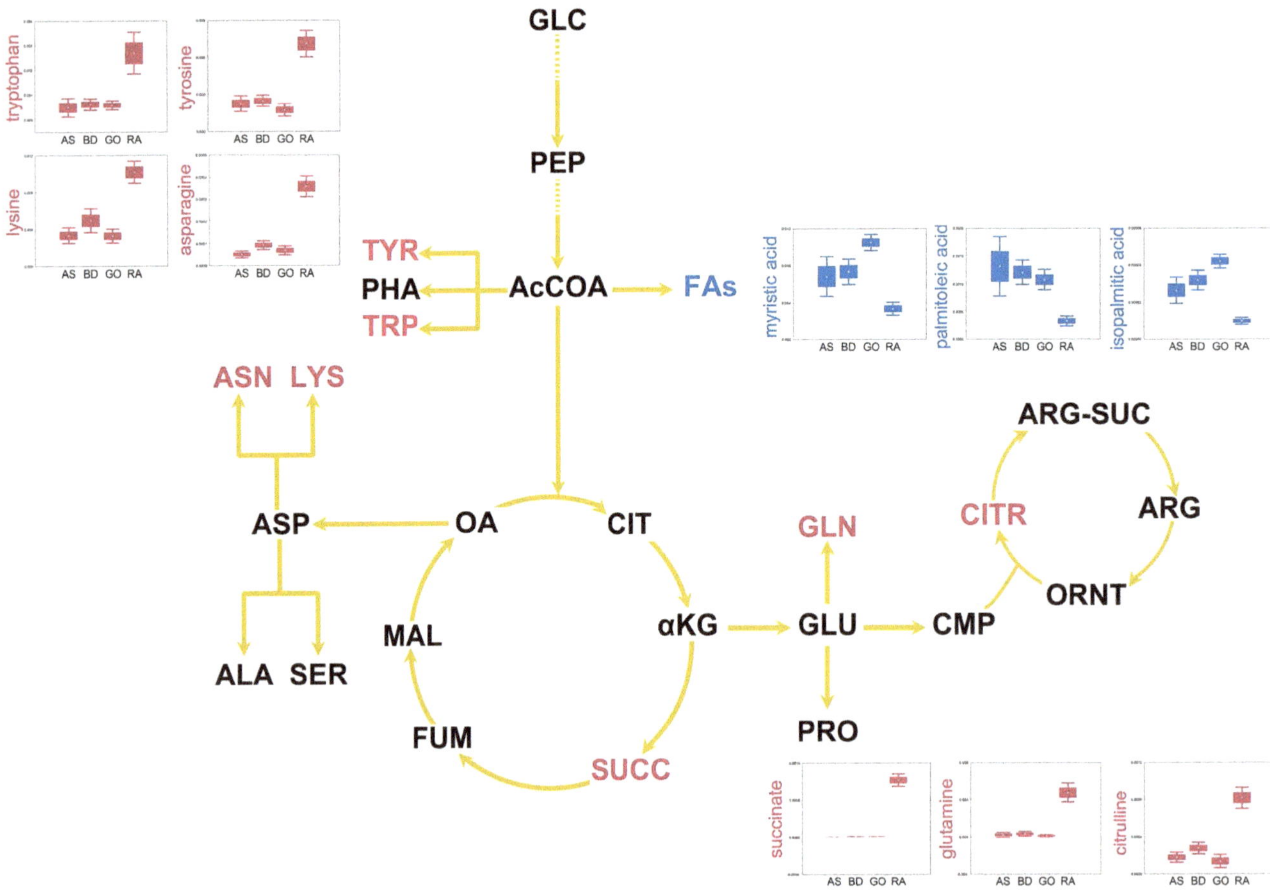

Figure 4. Schematic comparison of the primary metabolisms of RA vs. non-RA groups (AS, BD, and GO). The box and whisker plots indicate the intracellular metabolite levels for each disease group (red, increased in RA; green, increased in non-RA). *AcCOA*, acetyl-CoA; *ALA*, alanine; *ARG*, arginine; *ARG-SUC*, arginine-succinate; *ASN*, asparagine; *ASP*, aspartate; *CIT*, citrate; *CITR*, citrulline; *CMP*, carbamoyl phosphate; *FAs*, fatty acids; *FUM*, fumarate; *GLC*, glucose; *GLN*, glutamine; *GLU*, glutamate; *αKG*, α-ketoglutarate; *LYS*, lysine; *MAL*, malate; *OA*, oxalate; *ORNT*, ornithine; *PEP*, phosphoenolpyruvate; *PHA*, phenylalanine; *PRO*, proline; *SER*, serine; *SUCC*, succinate; *TRP*, tryptophan; *TYR*, tyrosine.

These metabolites are the major intermediates of the TCA cycle, urea cycle, and fatty acid and amino acid metabolism (Figure 4).

In particular, citrulline synthesized from ornithine and carbamoyl phosphate is a key intermediate of the urea cycle. It is also generated by posttranslational modification of arginine residues by peptidylarginine deiminase [35]. Because citrulline is a major antigenic determinant recognized by RA, ACPAs have been used for the diagnosis of RA and have been established as a useful tool to discriminate RA from other arthritic diseases [36]. Moreover, in this study, the abundances of citrulline and ornithine were significantly higher in the RA group than those in the non-RA group. In the TCA cycle, α-ketoglutarate is a precursor to such amino acids as glutamate, glutamine, proline, and arginine. Oxaloacetate, which is converted from succinate, fumarate, and malate, is also a precursor to such amino acids as asparagine, methionine, threonine, isoleucine, and lysine [37]. The abundances of asparagine, glutamine, tyrosine, lysine, and tryptophan were higher in the RA group than those in non-RA group. Although α-ketoglutarate and oxaloacetate from the TCA cycle were not identified as metabolites in the present study, the abundances of succinate and fumarate in the TCA cycle were higher in the RA group, as were their derivative amino acids asparagine, lysine, and glutamine. These results indicate that the urea and TCA cycles as well as amino acid metabolism were highly activated in the RA group compared with the non-RA group consisting of AS, BD, and gout patients. In addition to citrulline, succinate, asparagine, glutamine, and lysine can be considered as major biomarkers for RA diagnosis.

Fatty acids are synthesized from acetyl-CoA and play important roles in cellular metabolism. RA is known to be affected by n-3 and n-6 fatty acids. For example, n-3 fatty acids suppress inflammation by reducing TNF-α and interleukin-1β levels in RA patients by competitively inhibiting the production of leukotriene B4 from arachidonic acid [38]. In our study, arachidonic acid (an n-6 fatty acid) was identified, but the level of arachidonic acid between the RA and non-RA groups did not significantly differ at the 99% significance level. Other than arachidonic acid, major fatty acids such as isopalmitic acid, myristic acid, and palmitoleic acid were identified as the significant metabolites in the RA group because their levels were markedly lower in the RA group. These results indicate that the fatty acid metabolism was more activated in the non-RA group than in the RA group.

This study has some limitations in the sample size and gender ratio. Although the sample size was relatively small here, the OPLS-DA model was well validated by the permutation test (Figure S1-a), and the potential biomarkers of RA were also verified by external validation (Figure S1-b) and AUC (Table 2). The gender ratio was not controlled in each group in this study, but among the 20 biomarkers of RA found from 13 RA and 25 non-RA patients without gender ratio control, 14 metabolites reappeared as the biomarkers of RA from 13 RA and 5 non-RA patients with gender ratio control (Table S2). These results agreed with previous reports that the metabolic profiles of RA did not significantly affected by gender [16,39].

In conclusion, this is the first report on the identification of potential biomarkers for RA using human synovial fluid of RA and non-RA patients by metabolomics for the diagnosis of RA distinguished from other inflammatory arthritis such as AS, BD, and gout. We also demonstrated that metabolic profiling may be a useful tool to discover biomarkers, and envision a holistic view of metabolism for diseases.

Supporting Information

Figure S1 OPLS model of the metabolite profiles of RA and non-RA groups. (a) Validation of the OPLS-DA model using 100 permutation test. Y-axis intercept of R2 and Q2 were 0.514 and −0.231, respectively. (b) Y-predicted scatter plot of the OPLS-DA model validated with RA and non-RA patients from another cohort. Red, RA patients; Blue, non-RA patients; Orange, RA and non-RA patients from another cohort.

Figure S2 Fold changes of abundances of 20 metabolites in synovial fluid selected as potential biomarkers for RA. Positive values indicate the increased fold changes in the RA group and negative values the increased fold changes in the non-RA group.

Table S1 Metabolites identified from GC/TOF MS and BinBase analyses of synovial fluid.

Table S2 The potential biomarkers of RA found from metabolite analysis of synovial fluid with and without controlling gender ratios of RA and non-RA patients.

Author Contributions

Conceived and designed the experiments: HSC KHK. Performed the experiments: SK JH JX YHJ. Analyzed the data: SK JH HSC KHK. Contributed reagents/materials/analysis tools: SK JH HSC KHK. Wrote the paper: SK JH HSC KHK.

References

1. Cammarata RJ, Rodnan GP, Fennell RH (1967) Serum anti-γ-globulin and antinuclear factors in the aged. JAMA-J Am Med Assoc 199: 455–458.
2. Litwin SD, Singer JM (1965) Studies of the incidence and significance of anti-gamma globulin factors in the aging. Arthritis Rheum 8: 538–550.
3. Rantapaa-Dahlqvist S, de Jong BAW, Berglin E, Hallmans G, Wadell G, et al. (2003) Antibodies against cyclic citrullinated peptide and IgA rheumatoid factor predict the development of rheumatoid arthritis. Arthritis Rheum 48: 2741–2749.
4. Humphreys JH, Symmons DP (2012) Postpublication validation of the 2010 American College of Rheumatology/European League Against Rheumatism classification criteria for rheumatoid arthritis: where do we stand? Curr Opin Rheumatol 25(2): 157–163.
5. Kallberg H, Padyukov L, Plenge RM, Ronnelid J, Gregersen PK, et al. (2007) Gene-gene and gene-environment interactions involving HLA-DRB1, PTPN22, and smoking in two subsets of rheumatoid arthritis. Am J Hum Genet 80: 867–875.
6. Teixeira VH, Olaso R, Martin-Magniette ML, Lasbleiz S, Jacq L, et al. (2009) Transcriptome analysis describing new immunity and defense genes in peripheral blood mononuclear cells of rheumatoid arthritis patients. PLOS ONE 4(8): e6803.
7. Tanino M, Matoba R, Nakamura S, Kameda H, Amano K, et al. (2009) Prediction of efficacy of anti-TNF biologic agent, infliximab, for rheumatoid arthritis patients using a comprehensive transcriptome analysis of white blood cells. Biochem Biophys Res Commun 387: 261–265.
8. Villas-Boas SG, Roessner-Tunali U, Hansen MAE, Smedsgaard J, Nielsen J (2007) Metabolome Analysis: An Introduction. Hoboken, NJ: John Wiley and Sons, Inc.
9. Bogdanov M, Matson WR, Wang L, Matson T, Saunders-Pullman R, et al. (2008) Metabolomic profiling to develop blood biomarkers for Parkinson's disease. Brain 131: 389–396.
10. Zhang J, Bowers J, Liu LY, Wei SW, Gowda GAN, et al. (2012) Esophageal cancer metabolite biomarkers detected by LC-MS and NMR methods. PLOS ONE 7(1): e30181.
11. Chen TL, Xie GX, Wang XY, Fan J, Qiu YP, et al. (2011) Serum and urine metabolite profiling reveals potential biomarkers of human hepatocellular carcinoma. Mol Cell Proteomics 10(7): M110.004945.
12. Huang ZZ, Lin L, Gao Y, Chen YJ, Yan XM, et al. (2011) Bladder cancer determination via two urinary metabolites: A biomarker pattern approach. Mol Cell Proteomics 10(10): M111.007922.
13. Bell JD, Sadler PJ, Morris VC, Levander OA (1991) Effect of aging and diet on proton NMR spectra of rat urine. Magn Reson Med 17: 414–422.
14. Connor SC, Hansen MK, Corner A, Smith RF, Ryan TE (2010) Integration of metabolomics and transcriptomics data to aid biomarker discovery in type 2 diabetes. Mol Biosyst 6: 909–921.
15. Holmes E, Wilson ID, Nicholson JK (2008) Metabolic phenotyping in health and disease. Cell 134: 714–717.
16. Lauridsen MB, Bliddal H, Christensen R, Danneskiold-Samsoe B, Bennett R, et al. (2010) ^{1}H NMR Spectroscopy-based interventional metabolic phenotyping: A cohort study of rheumatoid arthritis patients. J Proteome Res 9: 4545–4553.
17. Madsen RK, Lundstedt T, Gabrielsson J, Sennbro CJ, Alenius GM, et al. (2011) Diagnostic properties of metabolic perturbations in rheumatoid arthritis. Arthritis Res Ther 13.
18. Borenstein DG, Gibbs CA, Jacobs RP (1982) Gas-liquid chromatographic analysis of synovial fluid. Arthritis Rheum 25: 947–953.
19. Lee DY, Fiehn O (2008) High quality metabolomic data for *Chlamydomonas reinhardtii*. Plant Methods 4: 7.
20. Fiehn O, Wohlgemuth G, Scholz M, Kind T, Lee DY, et al. (2008) Quality control for plant metabolomics: reporting MSI-compliant studies. Plant J 53: 691–704.
21. Hutschenreuther A, Kiontke A, Birkenmeier G, Birkemeyer C (2012) Comparison of extraction conditions and normalization approaches for cellular metabolomics of adherent growing cells with GC-MS. Anal Methods 4: 1953–1963.
22. Lee DY, Park JJ, Barupal DK, Fiehn O (2012) System Response of Metabolic Networks in *Chlamydomonas reinhardtii* to Total Available Ammonium. Mol Cell Proteomics 11: 973–988.
23. Denkert C, Budczies J, Kind T, Weichert W, Tablack P, et al. (2006) Mass spectrometry-based metabolic profiling reveals different metabolite patterns in invasive ovarian carcinomas and ovarian borderline tumors. Cancer Res 66: 10795–10804.
24. Saeed AI, Bhagabati NK, Braisted JC, Liang W, Sharov V, et al. (2006) TM4 microarray software suite. Methods Enzymol 411: 134–193.
25. Umetrics AB (2005) User's Guide to SIMCA-P, SIMCA-P+ version 11.0. Umeå, Sweden: Umetrics AB.
26. Lalkhen AG, McCluskey A (2008) Clinical tests: sensitivity and specificity. Contin Educ Anaesth Crit Care Pain 8: 221–223.
27. Swets JA (1988) Measuring the accuracy of diagnostic systems. Science 240: 1285–1293.
28. Lasko TA, Bhagwat JG, Zou KH, Ohno-Machado L (2005) The use of receiver operating characteristic curves in biomedical informatics. J Biomed Inform 38: 404–415.
29. Greiner M, Pfeiffer D, Smith RD (2000) Principles and practical application of the receiver-operating characteristic analysis for diagnostic tests. Prev Vet Med 45: 23–41.
30. Mamas M, Dunn WB, Neyses L, Goodacre R (2011) The role of metabolites and metabolomics in clinically applicable biomarkers of disease. Arch Toxicol 85: 5–17.
31. Madsen R, Lundstedt T, Trygg J (2010) Chemometrics in metabolomics-A review in human disease diagnosis. Anal Chim Acta 659: 23–33.
32. Vinayavekhin N, Homan EA, Saghatelian A (2010) Exploring Disease through Metabolomics. ACS Chem Biol 5: 91–103.
33. Zhai G, Wang-Sattler R, Hart DJ, Arden NK, Hakim AJ, et al. (2010) Serum branched-chain amino acid to histidine ratio: a novel metabolomic biomarker of knee osteoarthritis. Ann Rheum Dis 69: 1227–1231.
34. Hugle T, Kovacs H, Heijnen I, Daikeler T, Baisch U, et al. (2012) Synovial fluid metabolomics in different forms of arthritis assessed by nuclear magnetic resonance spectroscopy. Clin Exp Rheumatol 30: 240–245.
35. Tarcsa E, Marekov LN, Mei G, Melino G, Lee SC, et al. (1996) Protein unfolding by peptidylarginine deiminase – Substrate specificity and structural

relationships of the natural substrates trichohyalin and filaggrin. J Biol Chem 271: 30709–30716.
36. Bas S, Perneger TV, Seitz M, Tiercy JM, Roux-Lombard P, et al. (2002) Diagnostic tests for rheumatoid arthritis: comparison of anti-cyclic citrullinated peptide antibodies, anti-keratin antibodies and IgM rheumatoid factors. Rheumatology 41: 809–814.
37. Jetten MSM, Pitoc GA, Follettie MT, Sinskey AJ (1994) Regulation of phospho(enol)-pyruvate-and oxaloacetate-converting enzymes in *Corynebacterium glutamicum*. Appl Microbiol Biotechnol 41: 47–52.
38. Kremer JM, Lawrence DA, Jubiz W, Digiacomo R, Rynes R, et al. (1990) Dietary fish oil and olive oil supplementation in patients with rheumatoid arthritis. Arthritis Rheum 33: 810–820.
39. Xie GX, Chen TL, Qiu YP, Shi P, Zheng XJ, et al. (2012) Urine metabolite profiling offers potential early diagnosis of oral cancer. Metabolomics 8: 220–231.

17

Circulating Protein Fragments of Cartilage and Connective Tissue Degradation Are Diagnostic and Prognostic Markers of Rheumatoid Arthritis and Ankylosing Spondylitis

Anne C. Bay-Jensen[1]*, Stephanie Wichuk[2], Inger Byrjalsen[1], Diana J. Leeming[1], Nathalie Morency[2], Claus Christiansen[1], Morten A. Karsdal[1], Walter P. Maksymowych[2]

1 Rheumatology, Nordic Bioscience, Herlev, Denmark, **2** Division of Rheumatology, University of Alberta, Edmonton, Alberta, Canada

Abstract

Inflammation driven connective tissue turnover is key in rheumatic diseases, such as ankylosing spondylitis (AS). Few biomarkers are available for measuring disease prognosis or the efficacy of interventions applied in these tissue-related conditions. Type II collagen is the primary structural protein of cartilage and type III collagen of connective tissues, and obvious targets for the collagenalytic, which increase during tissue inflammation. The objective of the study was to investigate the diagnostic and prognostic utility of cartilage, C2M, and synovial, C3M, turnover biomarkers in AS. Serum samples were retrieved from patients suffering from AS (n = 103), RA (n = 47) and healthy controls (n = 56). AS progressors were defined as having new vertebral syndesmophytes or more that 3 unit change in mSASSS over a two-year period. Type II collagen degradation markers in serum were measured by the C2M ELISA, and type III collagen degradation by the C3M ELISA. Logistic regression and dichotomized decision tree were used to analyze the prognostic value of the markers individually or in combination. Both C2M and C3M levels were significantly higher in RA patients than in healthy controls (*p*<*0.0001*). Diagnostic utility was analyzed by ROC and areas under the curve (AUCs) were 72% and 89% for C2M and C3M, respectively. Both C2M and C3M, were significantly higher in serum samples from AS patient than from healthy controls (*p*<*0.0001*). The AUCs of C2M and C3M, respectively, were 70% and 81% for AS. A combination of C2M and C3M, dichotomized according to best cut-offs for individual markers, could correctly identify 80% of the progressors and 61% of the non-progressors. The present study is the first to show that specific biomarkers of cartilage and connective tissue degradation facilitate both diagnosis and prediction of progression of RA and AS.

Editor: Masataka Kuwana, Keio University School of Medicine, Japan

Funding: The study was partly supported by the Danish Research Foundation and partly by the research budgets of the departments of ACBJ and WP at Nordic Bioscience and University of Alberta, respectively. The funders had no role in study design, data collection and analysis, decision to publish, or preparation of the manuscript.

Competing Interests: ACBJ, IB, DJL and MK are full time employees at, and CC and MK hold stocks in, Nordic Bioscience. This study was partly funded by Nordic Bioscience. Nordic Bioscience is a privately-owned; small-medium size enterprise partly focused the development of biomarkers for rheumatic and fibrotic diseases. The two biomarkers described in the manuscript are patented by Nordic Bioscience (C2M, "ASSAY FOR A TYPE II COLLAGEN BIOMARKER" Patent Application WO/2012/038331; C3M, "FIBROSIS BIOMARKER ASSAY" Patent Application WO/2010/115749 & United States Patent Application 20100209940). Further research on the markers will be conducted which may lead to commercialization. There are no further patents, products in development or marketed products to declare. This does not alter the authors' adherence to all the PLOS ONE policies on sharing data and materials. None of the authors received fees, bonuses or other benefits for the work described in the manuscript. WP, SW and NM have no financial or competing interest to declare. WP is a Medical Scientist of the Alberta Heritage Foundation for Medical Research.

* E-mail: acbj@nordicbioscience.com

Introduction

Ankylosing spondylitis (AS) and rheumatoid arthritis (RA) are both chronic inflammatory arthropathies that are associated with excessive turnover of connective tissues, such as cartilage and ligaments, in and surrounding the affected joint [1]. RA is a systemic autoimmune disease that primarily attacks synovial joints leading to deterioration and loss of mobility. Moreover synovial inflammation and fibrosis are key events in the pathogenesis of RA [1]. Bone changes such as erosions, bone marrow lesions, and osteitis are also common pathological features of RA [2]. AS is also a systemic disease characterized by chronic inflammation of the sacroiliac joints, entheses, bone marrow, and structural lesions such as, syndesmophytes and joint ankylosis [3–5]. Accordingly, a common denominator of RA and AS is an elevated, inflammation-dependent turnover of connective tissue, specifically the extracellular matrix (ECM), in cartilage and synovium. ECM composition varies between connective tissues. The major ECM protein of cartilage is type II collagen, while type III collagen is the key protein of soft tissue (such as the synovium and entheses). Monitoring the turnover of these collagens may aid the understanding of the pathogenesis of RA and AS.

In pathological situations, such as RA and AS, inflammation disturbs the normal repair response leading to excessive remodeling and tissue turnover. The consequence of this heightened ECM remodeling is the release of a range of protein-degradation products generated by the proteases expressed locally in the pathologically affected area. The degradation fragments result in the exposure of *de novo* sites in the proteins, referred to as neo-epitopes. These protein degradation fragments may be specific for the tissue of origin and for the involved enzymes, and may consequently be used for the identification of molecular biochemical markers [6]. Recently, neo-epitope-based biochemical markers measured in serum have received increased attention for their diagnostic and prognostic potential in rheumatic diseases [7]. In slowly progressing diseases, such as osteoporosis and osteoarthritis (OA), bone resorption and cartilage degradation markers have been studied extensively [8].

It has been shown that cartilage degradation is highly elevated in RA patients, as measured by C-terminal telopeptide of type II collagen (CTX-II) in urine and *in situ* histological assessments [9]. These specific activities are precisely coordinated under physiological situations, with a specified sequence of events resulting in controlled tissue turnover.

Only a few serological biomarkers with diagnostic and prognostic properties are available for rheumatic diseases [10]. Most available biomarkers measure systemic and inflammatory factors, which do not reflect pathogenesis in the affected tissue. There is also a lack of sensitive biomarkers that can be used to predict those patients who will progress and those who will respond to treatment. One of the few examples of a prognostic biomarker is MMP3 measured in serum [11], which was elevated in patients who had an mSASSS change of more than 3 over a 3-year period. We recently developed two neo-epitope biomarkers C2M [12] and C3M [13], which directly measure tissue remodeling, and ultimately might be used to predict progression in inflammatory diseases. C2M is a serum biomarker that measures a matrix metalloproteinase (MMP)-generated neo-epitope of type II collagen and correlates with the severity of knee OA. C2M therefore reflects cartilage degradation [14]. C3M is a biomarker of soft tissue turnover associated with inflammation [15–17], which has been shown to be elevated in liver, skin and lung fibrosis. We recently reported that both biomarkers were highly elevated in AS and that the diagnostic utility for the combination of these two biomarkers was high (AUC 0.87, $p<0.0001$) [14]. The primary aims of the present study were to (i) to compare the diagnostic utility of these markers in AS versus RA and (ii) to investigate the prognostic potential of these novel connective tissue turnover markers in patients with AS.

Methods

Serum samples from healthy individuals and patients

Serum samples from controls were retrieved from two separate studies [12,14]. Subjects were all lean (BMI<25 kg/m2), between 21 and 72 years of age, had no history of rheumatic or arthritic disease or treatment for such. All subjects felt healthy and had no reported pain or symptoms of any disease. All patients signed an informed consent. Baseline characteristics are shown in Table 1.

Serum samples were collected from patients suffering from AS (n = 106). Of the 106 patients, 94 had 2-year radiographic follow-up. All patients had an established diagnosis of AS according to the modified New York Criteria [18]. Patients had received standard care, including physical therapy and treatment with a non-steroidal anti-inflammatory drug (NSAID), but were naïve to biologics at baseline. For progression analysis, patients were separated into two groups based on the presence (Yes/No) of a new syndesmophyte at 2-year follow-up. Bath AS Disease Activity Index (BASDAI) [19] and modified Stoke AS Spinal Score (mSASSS)[20] were recorded for each AS patient. Baseline characteristics are shown in Table 1.

Serum samples from RA patients (n = 47) were retrieved prior to the start of treatment with biologics. Patients are eligible for biologics in the Province of Alberta, Canada, if they had active disease despite treatment with methotrexate, a methotrexate combination with a second disease-modifying agent, or leflunomide. Baseline characteristics are shown in Table 1.

The retrieval of serum samples from healthy subjects and patients was approved by the Danish national Committee on Biomedical Research ethics (approval no KA 2006–0054), and by the Ethical board of University of Alberta, Edmonton, Canada. The study was conducted in the countries of residence of the authors, Denmark and Canada respectively.

Biomarker assays

Cartilage degradation and connective tissue inflammation were measured in all serum samples, whether from controls or patients with AS or RA, using competitive enzyme-linked immune sorbent assays (ELISAs) for C2M [12] and C3M [15], respectively. The C2M ELISA measures type II collagen fragments generated by MMPs in cartilage. Briefly, a streptavidin-coated microtiter plate was coated with 4 ng/mL biotinylated peptide. Unbound peptide was washed off and 20 µL 1:2 prediluted serum samples were added, followed by 100 µL of 60 ng/mL peroxidase-labeled monoclonal antibody (MAb-C2M-3C1). The plate was incubated at 4C for 18 hours, washed and developed using 3,3',5,5'-Tetramethylbenzidine (TMB) and stopped with sulfuric acid. The plate was read on a standard plate reader at 450 nm. The C3M ELISA measures type III collagen fragments generated by MMPs in connective tissue. Briefly, a streptavidin-coated microtiter plate was coated with 1.25 ng/mL biotinylated peptide. Unbound peptide was washed off and 20 µL 1:4 prediluted serum samples were added, followed by 100 µL 25 ng/mL peroxidase-labeled monoclonal antibody (MAb-C3M-610T1). The plate was incubated at 20°C for 1 hour, washed and developed using the TMB and stopped with sulfuric acid. The plate was read on a standard plate reader at 450 nm. Technical performances of the assays were assessed according to in-house standard operating procedures and final inspections included tests on detection range, sample stability and linearity, a sample and assay stress test, matrix and interference test, prolonged storage of the assays and normal range tests. In addition, analyte stability was investigated in terms of freeze-thaw, ambient temperatures, prolonged storage, etc. Serum C-reactive protein (CRP) levels were assessed by standard measures. The final inspection results concerning serum testing are summarized in Table 2.

Statistics

Statistical analyses of correlations and logistic regression were performed using MedCalc® version 12 and GraphPad Prism® version 5. The primary objectives were to investigate: i) the serum levels of the two novel biomarkers, C2M and C3M, in RA and AS patients as compared to controls, and ii) whether there was an association between the biomarkers and progression of AS over a 2-year period. Comparison between the log transformed mean levels of the markers was performed using the Student's t-test (fig. 1, 2). Data was shown as the geometric mean with 95% confidence intervals (95%-CI), which depicts the principal distribution of the biomarker levels. The diagnostic power were investigated by area under the receiver-operator curve (AUROC) giving the AUC with 95%-CI (fig. 1, 2). Using the principle of Z-score normalization, cut-off values for the diagnostic test were set

Table 1. Baseline demographics and clinical assessment scores for the healthy controls, RA and AS patients.

	Controls Mean (SD)	RA patients Mean (SD)	AS patients Mean (SD)
N	56	47	103
Mean age (SD), years	42.8 (10.5)	55.3 (12.4)	42.0 (13.6)
Number of Female/male	21/35	12/35	30/94
NSAID users, %	0	17	84
Disease duration, years	–	14.4 (10.7)	18.0 (11.9)
RF positive, %	–	86	0
Mean ESR (SD), mm/hour	–	40 (29)	22 (20)
CRP (mg/L)	–	33.5 (45.1)	14.2 (22.2)
BASDAI	–	–	5.6 (2.2)
mSASSS	–	–	14.2 (18.5)
DAS28	–	6.6 (1.2)	–
HAQ	–	1.9 (0.8)	–
TJC	–	18.2 (7.9)	–
SJC	–	13.5 (5.9)	–

as 1 standard deviation (SD) above the mean of the controls which will include 84% below this cut-off assuming a normal distribution. Using these cut-off values the number of patients below and above the cut-off was counted and put into a 2×2 contingency table. From this the odds ratios (ORs), sensitivity, specificity and likelihood ratios were calculated by Fisher's exact test (fig. 1, 2).

Table 2. ELISA technical performance.

	C2M	C3M
Assay specifications		
Slope of Standard curve (CV %)	1.10 (6.6)	1.03 (10.8)
IC50, nmol/L (CV %)	0.45 (3.8)	5.22 (11.9)
Intra-assay variation, CV%	6.2	6.7
Inter-assay variation, CV%	7.3	12.1
Lower limit of detection, nmol/L	0.037	0.28
Quantifiable range, nmol/L	0.274–4.36	0.54–42.1
Analyte recovery		
Serum dilution linearity (analyte recovery)	Neat to 1:4; >82%	1:4 to 1:64; >88%
Freeze-thaw	> 7 cycles	> 10 cycles
On-table stability	>48hours	>48hours
Interference		
Hemoglobin	<11%	<7%
Lipidimia	<6%	<2%
Biotin	<0.1%	<0.1%
Rheumatoid factor	<0.1%	<0.1%
HAMA	<0.1%	<0.1%
Biological variation		
Correlation to age, R, *p-value*	0.083, *ns*	0.13, *ns*
Gender difference, Difference, *p-value*	0.055, *ns*	3.12, *ns*

Univariate correlation analyses between the biomarkers and clinical scores, or between the individual biomarkers, were analyzed by non-parametric Spearman's test (table 3, 4).

The prognostic utility was investigated by a decision tree approach by asking following questions: how many AS progressors were we able to select and how many patients were we able to deselect by measuring the two biomarkers in question. The biomarkers for disease progression (NewSynd) was calculated using dichotomized values for the markers by discriminating high biomarker levels by Classification and Regression Tree Analysis (using the 2×2 diagnostic contingency table). Sensitivity (fraction progressors) and specificity (fraction non-progressors) values were produced. Data were considered significant when the P-value was below 0.05.

Results

Technical performance of the C2M and C3M ELISAs

The technical performance of the C2M and the C3M ELISAs was assessed before serum levels were measured in patients with RA, AS and healthy controls. Table 2 describes the basic technical characteristics of the two assays, both of which had good technical performance. Intra- and inter-assay coefficients of variation were less than 7% and 13%, respectively. The data analyte recovery, interference (hemoglobin, lipidimia, and biotin, rheumatoid factor (RF) and human anti-mouse antibody (HAMA)) and biological variation are shown in Table 2. None of the markers were significantly correlated to age. There was no gender difference for either marker investigated by Mann-Whitney test.

The level of cartilage and connective tissue degradation fragments in serum of RA patients

Both serum C2M and C3M levels were significantly higher in RA patients than in healthy controls ($p<0.0001$, fig. 1). Diagnostic utility, as analyzed by ROC and the AUCs, was 72% and 89% for C2M and C3M, respectively (fig. 1C). The odds ratio (OR) for identifying RA patients were 6.3 and 16 for C2M and C3M respectively (fig. 1C). Serum C2M levels were not associated with age, disease duration or any of the clinical outcome scores (Table 3). In contrast, serum C3M levels were highly correlated

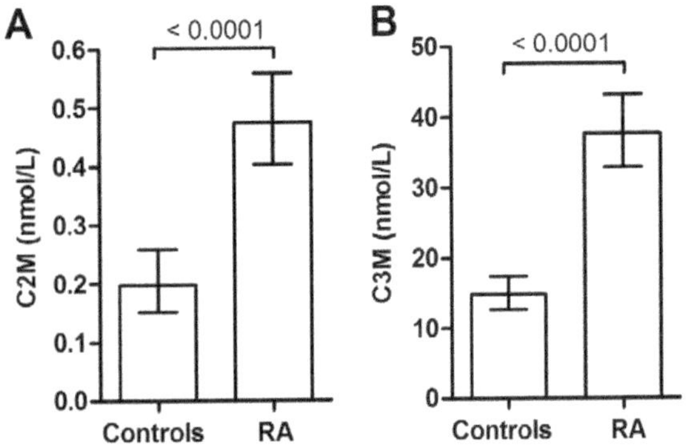

C

	C2M	C3M
n, controls / RA	56 / 47	56 / 47
AUC (95%-CI)	0.72 (0.62 - 0.82)	0.89 (0.83 - 0.95)
p -value	0.0001	<0.0001
OR (95%-CI)	6.33 (2.13 - 18.9)	15.5 (5.88 - 40.7)
Sensitivity	0.64 (0.52 - 0.74)	0.83 (0.70 - 0.92)
Specificity	0.78 (0.56 - 0.93)	0.76 (0.62 - 0.87)
LR+ / LR-	2.93 / 0.46	3.46 / 0.22
Cut-off (nmol/L)	0.538	27.3

Figure 1. The level of the cartilage degradation and connective tissue inflammation in RA patients (n = 47) and healthy controls (n = 56). A) Cartilage degradation measured by C2M in serum. B) Connective tissue degradation measured by C3M in serum. C) The diagnostic utility depicted as area under the curve (AUC), odds ratio (OR), sensitivity, specificity and likelihood ratio (LR). Cut-off values were set as 1 SD above the mean of the healthy controls. Comparison of RA patients and controls was performed on log transformed data with student's t-test. Results are shown as geometric mean with 95% CI. Diagnostic utility was calculated by a contingency table applying Fisher's exact test.

with disease activity score (DAS), health assessment questionnaire (HAQ), erythrocyte sedimentation rate (ESR), C-reactive protein (CRP), swollen (SJC) and tender joint count (TJC). There was no correlation (table 3) between serum C2M and C3M.

The level of cartilage and connective tissue degradation in serum of AS patients

Both C2M and C3M levels were significantly higher in AS patients than in healthy controls (fig. 1A and 1B). The diagnostic utility of C2M in discriminating between controls and AS patients was 70% ($p<0.0001$) (Fig. 2C) and thereby similar to that in the RA analysis (Fig. 1C). A high C2M level could correctly identify 40% of the AS patients and 80% of the healthy controls. A high C3M value could correctly identify 46% of the AS patients and 82% of the healthy controls. Thus the sensitivity was markedly lower for AS than for RA. The diagnostic utility of C3M was 81% ($p<0.0001$, Fig. 2C), which was 10% lower than the utility in RA patients (Fig. 1C). The ORs for AS were 3.4 ($p = 0.003$) and 4.7 ($p<0.0001$) for C2M and C3M, respectively (Fig. 2C).

The evaluation of all patients collectively showed C2M correlated with neither of the disease scores; Disease duration, ESR, CRP, mSASSS or BASDAI (table 4). Serum C3M was significantly correlated with ESR ($p<0.0001$) and CRP ($p<0.0001$), as well as with mSASSS ($p = 0.0006$), but was of only borderline significant correlation ($p = 0.054$) with BASDAI (table 4). No correlation was observed between the two biomarkers C2M and C3M when measured in either AS patients, or RA patients (data not shown).

Clinical predictive utility of measuring serum C2M and C3M

An abnormally high serum C2M level, defined as one SD above the mean of that found in healthy controls, could positively predict 44% of the progressors of AS and exclude 70% of the non-progressors (table 5). High serum C3M levels could positively predict 59% of the progressors and excluded 55% of the non-progressors. A high serum level of both C2M and C3M could predict 80% of the progressors and 61% of the non-progressors.

Discussion

In the current study we firstly validated the diagnostic utility of the two novel markers, C2M and C3M, in RA and found that the serum levels of the markers were elevated in patients compared

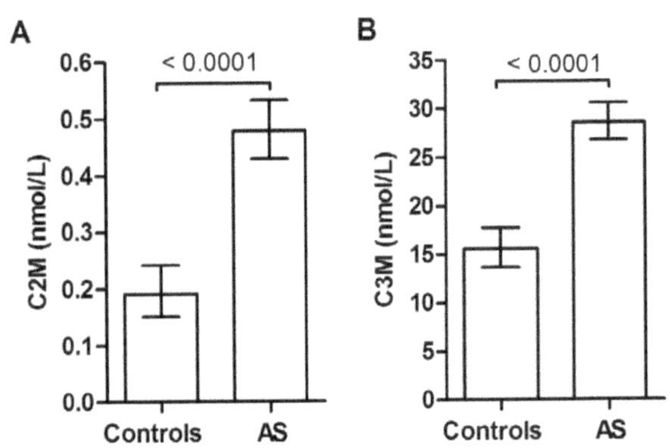

C

	C2M	C3M
n, controls / AS	56 / 106	56 / 106
AUC (95%-CI)	0.70 (0.61 - 0.79)	0.81 (0.73 - 0.88)
p -value	<0.0001	<0.0001
OR (95%-CI)	4.05 (1.48 - 11.1)	4.02 (1.92 - 8.43)
Sensitivity	0.40 (0.31 - 0.49)	0.46 (0.36 - 0.56)
Specificity	0.86 (0.71 - 0.95)	0.82 (0.72 - 0.91)
LR+ / LR-	2.85 / 0.70	2.64 / 0.66
Cut-off (nmol/L)	0.538	27.3

Figure 2. The level of the cartilage degradation and connective tissue inflammation in AS patients (n = 103) and controls (n = 56). A) Cartilage degradation measured by C2M in serum. B) Connective tissue degradation measured by C3M in serum C) The diagnostic utility depicted as area under the curve (AUC), odds ratio (OR), sensitivity, specificity and likelihood ratio (LR). Cut-off values were set as 1 SD above the mean of the healthy controls. Comparison of AS patients and controls was performed on log transformed data with student's t-test. Results are shown as geometric mean with 95% CI. Diagnostic utility was calculated by a contingency table applying Fisher's exact test.

Table 3. Univariate analysis for C2M and C3M associations with age, disease duration and RA clinical characteristics; Disease activity score (DAS), health assessment questionnaire (HAQ), erythrocyte sedimentation rate (ESR), high sensitive C-reactive protein (CRP), tender joint count (TJC) and swollen joint count (SJC).

	C2M	C3M
Age	−0.12, *ns*	0.13, *ns*
Disease Duration	0.16, *ns*	0.18, *ns*
DAS	0.09, *ns*	0.54, *p<0.001*
HAQ	0.01, *ns*	0.52, *p<0.001*
ESR	0.05, *ns*	0.60, *p<0.0001*
CRP	−0.06, *ns*	0.59, *p<0.0001*
TJC	−0.02, ns	0.34, *p<0.05*
SJC	−0.10, *ns*	0.18, *ns*
C2M		−0.10, *ns*

Data are shown as Spearman's correlation coefficient R and *p-value*.

Table 4. Univariate analysis for C2M and C3M associations with age, disease duration and AS clinical characteristics; erythrocyte sedimentation rate (ESR), high sensitive C-reactive protein (CRP), mSASSS and BASDAI.

	C2M	C3M
Age	0.06, *ns*	0.17, *ns*
Disease duration	0.01, *ns*	0.14, *ns*
ESR	0.03, *ns*	0.40, *p<0.0001*
CRP	0.06, *ns*	0.55, *p<0.001*
mSASSS	0.02, *ns*	0.32, *p<0.001*
BASDAI	−0.04, *ns*	0.19, *ns*
C2M		0.12, *ns*

Data are shown as Spearman's correlation coefficient R and p-value.

with controls with an OR of more than 6. This is expected since RA is characterized by massive joint turnover, which includes cartilage degradation and connective tissue turnover, such as occurs during synovial inflammation. While elevated serum C2M did not seem to be correlated with any disease characteristics in RA, high serum C3M was highly correlated with DAS, HAQ and ESR, as well as TJC. These results support the concept that connective tissue degradation is indeed related to the inflammatory component of RA, whereas cartilage degradation seemed to be partly uncoupled from this component. This suggests that the two biomarkers contribute independent and additive information about the disease pathogenesis and maybe supplementary diagnostic tools for clinical diagnosis. These markers can not compete with diagnostic markers such as RF and CRP, however in stead they can provide additional information on tissue integrity, which may aid in the understanding of disease severity.

Secondly, we investigated whether these joint turnover markers could be used for AS. In contrast to RA, RF and CRP are not applicable diagnostic markers in AS. The present study supports a role of C2M and C3M as potential diagnostic biomarkers in AS. We also saw a strong correlation between connective tissue degradation as measured by serum C3M and the radiographic score, mSASSS. Cartilage degradation as measured by serum C2M levels was likewise elevated in AS patients compared with controls. But C2M did not correlate with the mSASSS. These results are interesting because they indicate that cartilage degradation and soft tissue turnover may provide independent information also in AS.

The first part of the study validated and supports the importance of monitoring connective tissue remodeling in the pathogenesis of rheumatic diseases. The second part of the study evaluated the prognostic potential of the markers. We demonstrated that a combination of these novel markers could identify 80% of the progressors in AS. This combination could be used to select only the likely progressors for clinical trials, and thus reduce the number of patients exposed to treatment in such studies. Furthermore, by identifying likely progressors in an AS population, one could test strategies aimed at early intervention to prevent deterioration of structural damage using anti-inflammatory therapies [21,22]. Our data also shows that the combination of biomarkers may possess higher prognostic utility than individual biomarkers. We showed that cartilage and soft tissue turnover is indeed increased in AS patients, and that the level of increase is predictive of those who will progress–a potential which CRP does not possess [23].

There are considerable limitations to the information provided by standard clinical and laboratory parameters to guide treatment decisions. Consequently, there has been a particular interest in evaluating biomarkers in AS that reflect disease activity and predict structural progression [5,24,25]. Although CRP and ESR are sensitive detectors of disease activity in RA, they are not so in AS, probably because these markers are elevated in only about 50% of AS patients [23]. Unlike in RA, they also correlate poorly with clinical measures of AS, although good correlations have been noted with MRI assessment of inflammation in the spine [26–28]. In contrast to RA, CRP and ESR do not appear to predict progression of structural damage in AS although CRP does predict clinical response to anti-TNF therapy in both RA and AS [29,30].

Cartilage degradation and connective tissue turnover are hallmarks of most arthropathies. We have developed two new serological biomarkers of cartilage degradation (C2M) [12] and soft tissue turnover (C3M) [13,16]. Both biomarkers are MMP-mediated collagen fragments, which are also called collagen neo-epitopes. Assays for these two biomarkers are specific for the cleavage site in the respective collagens. Hence the assays do not measure full-size collagens, but only the pathogenic fingerprint of that collagen. We have previously demonstrated that serum C2M was associated with increased Kellgreen-Lawrence score in knee osteoarthritis [12], indicating a correlation with cartilage loss and joint deterioration. C3M is derived by degradation of type III collagen, which is a central component of most connective tissues. The turnover of both types II and III collagens is high [31]. There was a strong correlation between CRP and C3M in both RA and AS, which supports the concept that inflammation accelerates the turnover of connective tissue and thereby the release of C3M [14]. This may contribute to the increased levels of these biomarkers in AS which could arise from excessive remodeling of the joint. However, additional contributions may be derived from multiple organs of the body affected by inflammation.

A previous report showed that other markers of extracellular remodeling had limited association with baseline BASDAI and mSASSS [11]. Cartilage oligomeric protein and YKL-40 were both correlated with baseline mSASSS ($p<0.05$), but they were not associated with 2-year change in mSASSS. Interestingly that

Table 5. Clinical predictive utility of the serum markers.

	High C2M (n = 94)	High C3M (n = 94)	High C2M & high C3M (n = 33)
Cut-offs	>0.538 nmol/L	>27.3 nmol/L	
Sensitivity (%)	44.1 (28.6–61.7)	58.8 (40.7–75.6)	80.0 (51.9–95.7)
Specificity (%)	70.0 (56.8–81.2)	55.0 (41.6–67.9)	61.1 (35.8–82.7)
Positive/Negative Likelihood ratio	1.46/0.80	1.31/0.75	2.06/0.33
Proportion of progressors with a positive test	15/34	20/34	12/15
Proportion of non-progressors with a negative test	42/60	33/60	11/18

Progressors were defined as NewSynd Yes/No over at a two year period.

study showed a clear association between elevated MMP-3 and radiographic progression. MMP-3 is widely up-regulated by inflammation in the connective tissue surrounding the joints (e.g. synovial tissue). Thus MMP-3 might very well be one of the MMPs responsible for the degradation of type II and type III collagens. It would interesting to investigate the relationship between MMP-3 and type II and type III collagen turnover and potentially combine the markers in an algorithm for predicting inflammatory disease. This kind of investigation will increase our understanding of the role of MMPs in AS and the proteolytical products resulting from MMP activity.

Conclusions

This is the first study to show the prognostic value of two novel biomarkers of MMP-mediated degradation of types II and III collagen. These two biomarkers, C2M and C3M, might be the best diagnostic [14] and prognostic markers available to date for AS. Further longitudinal study is needed to confirm these preliminary data. We speculate that markers measuring joint tissue turnover and deterioration may assist better understanding of disease pathogenesis and eventually disease severity. In the era of personalized medicine markers that are direct measures of disease status and severity may aid in designing the best treatment for the individual patients.

Acknowledgments

We would like to acknowledge our skilled technicians Kathrine Mikkelsen, Sedi Tavallaee, Maibritt Andersen and Trine Overgaard whom all contributed in the development of the ELISAs. Furthermore we would like to thank *Den Danske Forskningsfond*.

Author Contributions

Conceived and designed the experiments: ACBJ SW MK WPM CC. Performed the experiments: ACBJ DJL SW NM. Analyzed the data: ACBJ SW MK WPM CC. Contributed reagents/materials/analysis tools: ACBJ SW IB DJL NM CC MK WPM. Wrote the paper: ACBJ SW MK WPM CC.

References

1. Lories RJ, Baeten DL (2009) Differences in pathophysiology between rheumatoid arthritis and ankylosing spondylitis. Clin Exp Rheumatol 27: S10–S14.
2. Goldring SR (2003) Pathogenesis of bone and cartilage destruction in rheumatoid arthritis. Rheumatology (Oxford) 42: ii11–ii16.
3. Braun J, Pincus T (2002) Mortality, course of disease and prognosis of patients with ankylosing spondylitis. Clin Exp Rheumatol 20: S16–S22.
4. Tam LS, Gu J, Yu D (2010) Pathogenesis of ankylosing spondylitis. Nat Rev Rheumatol 6: 399–405.
5. Colbert RA, Deodhar AA, Fox D, Gravallese EM, Khan MA, et al. (2009) Entheses and bones in spondyloarthritis: 2008 Annual Research and Education Meeting of the Spondyloarthritis Research and Therapy Network (SPARTAN). J Rheumatol 36: 1527–1531.
6. Karsdal MA, Henriksen K, Leeming DJ, Mitchell P, Duffin K, et al. (2009) Biochemical markers and the FDA Critical Path: how biomarkers may contribute to the understanding of pathophysiology and provide unique and necessary tools for drug development. Biomarkers 14: 181–202.
7. Segovia-Silvestre T, Bonnefond C, Sondergaard BC, Christensen ST, Karsdal MA, et al. (2011) Identification of the Calcitonin receptor in osteoarthritic chondrocytes. BMC Res Notes 4: 407.
8. Schaller S, Henriksen K, Hoegh-Andersen P, Sondergaard BC, Sumer EU, et al. (2005) In vitro, ex vivo, and in vivo methodological approaches for studying therapeutic targets of osteoporosis and degenerative joint diseases: how biomarkers can assist? Assay Drug Dev Technol 3: 553–580.
9. Garnero P, Desmarais S, Charni N, Percival MD (2005) The CII fragments Helix-II and CTX-II reveal distinct enzymatic pathways of cartilage collagen degradation: diagnostic and therapeutic implications in rheumatoid arthritis and osteoarthritis. Arthritis Rheum 52: P51.
10. de VK (2010) Soluble and tissue biomarkers in ankylosing spondylitis. Best Pract Res Clin Rheumatol 24: 671–682.
11. Maksymowych WP, Landewe R, Conner-Spady B, Dougados M, Mielants H, et al. (2007) Serum matrix metalloproteinase 3 is an independent predictor of structural damage progression in patients with ankylosing spondylitis. Arthritis Rheum 56: 1846–1853.
12. Bay-Jensen AC, Liu Q, Byrjalsen I, Li Y, Wang J, et al. (2011) Enzyme-linked immunosorbent assay (ELISAs) for metalloproteinase derived type II collagen neoepitope, CIIM--increased serum CIIM in subjects with severe radiographic osteoarthritis. Clin Biochem 44: 423–429.
13. Barascuk N, Veidal SS, Larsen L, Larsen DV, Larsen MR, et al. (2010) A novel assay for extracellular matrix remodeling associated with liver fibrosis: An enzyme-linked immunosorbent assay (ELISA) for a MMP-9 proteolytically revealed neo-epitope of type III collagen. Clin Biochem *In press*.
14. Bay-Jensen AC, Leeming DJ, Kleyer A, Veidal SS, Schett G, et al. (2011) Ankylosing spondylitis is characterized by an increased turnover of several different metalloproteinase-derived collagen species: a cross-sectional study. Rheumatol Int.
15. Veidal SS, Vassiliadis E, Barascuk N, Zhang C, Segovia-Silvestre T, et al. (2010) Matrix metalloproteinase-9-mediated type III collagen degradation as a novel serological biochemical marker for liver fibrogenesis. Liver Int 30: 1293–1304.
16. Vassiliadis E, Larsen DV, Clausen RE, Veidal SS, Barascuk N, et al. (2011) Measurement of CO3-610, a Potential Liver Biomarker Derived from Matrix Metalloproteinase-9 Degradation of Collagen Type III, in a Rat Model of Reversible Carbon-Tetrachloride-Induced Fibrosis. Biomark Insights 6: 49–58.
17. Vassiliadis E, Veidal SS, Simonsen H, Larsen DV, Vainer B, et al. (2011) Immunological detection of the type V collagen propeptide fragment, PVCP-1230, in connective tissue remodeling associated with liver fibrosis. Biomarkers .
18. van der LS, Valkenburg HA, Cats A (1984) Evaluation of diagnostic criteria for ankylosing spondylitis. A proposal for modification of the New York criteria. Arthritis Rheum 27: 361–368.
19. Garrett S, Jenkinson T, Kennedy LG, Whitelock H, Gaisford P, et al. (1994) A new approach to defining disease status in ankylosing spondylitis: the Bath Ankylosing Spondylitis Disease Activity Index. J Rheumatol 21: 2286–2291.
20. Creemers MC, Franssen MJ, van't Hof MA, Gribnau FW, van de Putte LB, et al. (2005) Assessment of outcome in ankylosing spondylitis: an extended radiographic scoring system. Ann Rheum Dis 64: 127–129.

21. Maksymowych WP, Landewe R, Tak PP, Ritchlin CJ, Ostergaard M, et al. (2009) Reappraisal of OMERACT 8 draft validation criteria for a soluble biomarker reflecting structural damage endpoints in rheumatoid arthritis, psoriatic arthritis, and spondyloarthritis: the OMERACT 9 v2 criteria. J Rheumatol 36: 1785–1791.
22. Maksymowych WP, FitzGerald O, Wells GA, Gladman DD, Landewe R, et al. (2009) Proposal for levels of evidence schema for validation of a soluble biomarker reflecting damage endpoints in rheumatoid arthritis, psoriatic arthritis, and ankylosing spondylitis, and recommendations for study design. J Rheumatol 36: 1792–1799.
23. Ruof J, Stucki G (1999) Validity aspects of erythrocyte sedimentation rate and C-reactive protein in ankylosing spondylitis: a literature review. J Rheumatol 26: 966–970.
24. Schett G (2007) Joint remodelling in inflammatory disease. Ann Rheum Dis 66 Suppl 3: iii42–iii44.
25. Schett G, Sieper J (2009) Inflammation and repair mechanisms. Clin Exp Rheumatol 27: S33–S35.
26. Spoorenberg A, van der HD, de KE, Dougados M, de VK, et al. (1999) Relative value of erythrocyte sedimentation rate and C-reactive protein in assessment of disease activity in ankylosing spondylitis. J Rheumatol 26: 980–984.
27. Lukas C, Braun J, van der HD, Hermann KG, Rudwaleit M, et al. (2007) Scoring inflammatory activity of the spine by magnetic resonance imaging in ankylosing spondylitis: a multireader experiment. J Rheumatol 34: 862–870.
28. Maksymowych WP, Dhillon SS, Park R, Salonen D, Inman RD, et al. (2007) Validation of the spondyloarthritis research consortium of Canada magnetic resonance imaging spinal inflammation index: is it necessary to score the entire spine? Arthritis Rheum 57: 501–507.
29. Wanders AJ, Gorman JD, Davis JC, Landewe RB, van der Heijde DM (2004) Responsiveness and discriminative capacity of the assessments in ankylosing spondylitis disease-controlling antirheumatic therapy core set and other outcome measures in a trial of etanercept in ankylosing spondylitis. Arthritis Rheum 51: 1–8.
30. de Vries MK, van E, I, van der Horst-Bruinsma IE, Peters MJ, Nurmohamed MT, et al. (2009) Erythrocyte sedimentation rate, C-reactive protein level, and serum amyloid a protein for patient selection and monitoring of anti-tumor necrosis factor treatment in ankylosing spondylitis. Arthritis Rheum 61: 1484–1490.
31. Gelse K, Poschl E, Aigner T (2003) Collagens--structure, function, and biosynthesis. Advanced Drug Delivery Reviews 55: 1531–1546.

18

Optimising Use of Electronic Health Records to Describe the Presentation of Rheumatoid Arthritis in Primary Care: A Strategy for Developing Code Lists

Amanda Nicholson[1¤], Elizabeth Ford[1*], Kevin A. Davies[1], Helen E. Smith[1], Greta Rait[2], A. Rosemary Tate[3], Irene Petersen[2], Jackie Cassell[1]

1 Division of Primary Care and Public Health, Brighton and Sussex Medical School, Brighton, United Kingdom, **2** Research Department of Primary Care and Population Health, University College London, London, United Kingdom, **3** Department of Informatics, University of Sussex, Brighton, United Kingdom

Abstract

Background: Research using electronic health records (EHRs) relies heavily on coded clinical data. Due to variation in coding practices, it can be difficult to aggregate the codes for a condition in order to define cases. This paper describes a methodology to develop 'indicator markers' found in patients with early rheumatoid arthritis (RA); these are a broader range of codes which may allow a probabilistic case definition to use in cases where no diagnostic code is yet recorded.

Methods: We examined EHRs of 5,843 patients in the General Practice Research Database, aged ≥30y, with a first coded diagnosis of RA between 2005 and 2008. Lists of indicator markers for RA were developed initially by panels of clinicians drawing up code-lists and then modified based on scrutiny of available data. The prevalence of indicator markers, and their temporal relationship to RA codes, was examined in patients from 3y before to 14d after recorded RA diagnosis.

Findings: Indicator markers were common throughout EHRs of RA patients, with 83.5% having 2 or more markers. 34% of patients received a disease-specific prescription before RA was coded; 42% had a referral to rheumatology, and 63% had a test for rheumatoid factor. 65% had at least one joint symptom or sign recorded and in 44% this was at least 6-months before recorded RA diagnosis.

Conclusion: Indicator markers of RA may be valuable for case definition in cases which do not yet have a diagnostic code. The clinical diagnosis of RA is likely to occur some months before it is coded, shown by markers frequently occurring ≥6 months before recorded diagnosis. It is difficult to differentiate delay in diagnosis from delay in recording. Information concealed in free text may be required for the accurate identification of patients and to assess the quality of care in general practice.

Editor: Christian Lovis, University Hospitals of Geneva, Switzerland

Funding: The study was funded by the Wellcome Trust (http://www.wellcome.ac.uk/), grant number 086105/Z/08/Z – the PREP (Patient Record Enhancement Project) study. The funders had no role in study design, data collection and analysis, decision to publish, or preparation of the manuscript.

Competing Interests: The authors have declared that no competing interests exist.

* E-mail: e.m.ford@bsms.ac.uk

¤ Current address: Faculty of Health and Medicine, Lancaster University, Lancaster, United Kingdom

Introduction

Electronic health records and their potential for research and clinical audit

Electronic health records (EHR) are a key data source for health-related research [1,2]. EHR systems are developing rapidly in the US in response to government directives and incentives [3,4]. EHRs in the UK are most advanced in primary care where they provide complete electronic data about primary care consultations, as well as a summary of care received elsewhere and reported to the practice. EHRs are now seen as valuable resources for research such as healthcare provision audits, disease registries, and epidemiological studies [5,6]. Traditional epidemiological studies have either used data collected within the study in purpose-built datasets [7,8,9] or used routine hospital data which have gone through a separate coding stage (e.g. Hospital Episode Statistics). These can be considered as "static" data, by contrast with "live" electronic health data, produced and coded in the context of clinical consultation and shaped by the context of recording. Many factors influence recording, from financial incentives to the desire to protect a patient from stigma – and these can often change rapidly over time [10]. This means that defining and finding all cases of the disease of interest can be problematic. This paper describes a methodology to maximise the probability of finding cases in EHRs by developing "indicator markers" which are codes that may be combined to make a probabilistic or logical definition of a case in conjunction with, or in the absence of, a diagnostic code. We describe the development of these markers for cases of rheumatoid arthritis (RA) and explore the utility of these markers for case definition in the early presentation of RA.

The use of indicator markers instead of solely diagnostic codes

When general practitioners (GPs) code the results of clinical consultations, they may not apply a diagnostic code on the first suspicion of a diagnosis, especially of a complex or chronic disease. Instead they may code symptoms, tests or referrals for a specialist opinion. The first firm diagnosis may be found in the text of a specialist's letter to the GP which is attached to the record but coded under an administrative code such as "letter from specialist". The diagnostic code may only be recorded in the EHR when, for example, a specialised drug prescription is issued. The date of recording of the diagnostic code may therefore bear little relationship to the date of actual diagnosis.

When using EHRs to examine the presentation and diagnosis of a specific condition, it is therefore not sufficient to rely upon the diagnostic codes alone for case definition. Such practice will miss cases for which a diagnostic code has not yet been recorded, and may also misrepresent the date of diagnosis and result in the loss of valuable information about presentation and diagnosis which comes before the code. Two systematic reviews of EHR data quality in the UK [11,12] found the recording of diagnostic codes for diseases varied, from 40% agreement with other sources for angina, up to 100% for myocardial infarction and diabetes, both of which have clear diagnostic criteria or their recording incentivised in the UK's national health service. Several studies suggest that cancer, for example, is not recorded systematically. Pascoe and colleagues [13] found that when comparing GP records to a cancer registry, 19.3% of patients had no code for a malignancy in their GP records, but that by combining codes for malignancy, abnormal test results and prescriptions they could identify 96.3% of cancer patients in their sample. Tate and colleagues [14] found evidence that a cancer code was recorded late in the diagnostic process, with relevant investigations found in almost three quarters (71%) of patients in the year before the date of recorded diagnosis and 87% having relevant recorded symptoms. In addition, 7.5% had evidence of cancer treatment or oncology referral before any specific mention of cancer as a diagnosis in the EHR.

In order to define cases of the disease of interest in an EHR, it is therefore not sufficient to rely solely on diagnostic codes [15]. Instead it is necessary to draw up lists of a range of related codes, such as symptom, referral, test or treatment codes, which are strongly associated with, and indicative of, the disease of interest. We term these codes "indicator markers". Indicator markers may be used singly or in combination to indicate the suspicion of, or presumptive presence of, the clinical entity.

The methodology of drawing up code-lists

Even for studies using only diagnostic codes, the methodology of drawing up code lists for any given clinical entity is poorly described in the literature. Preparing lists for all the various entities that need to be considered within a study – case definition, endpoints, covariates – is a major undertaking. Researchers working on similar diseases in different settings may replicate effort in drawing up code-lists as there is rarely standardisation or transparency to the process. This lack of collaboration means that code-lists and case definitions may vary across studies. Variations in code lists may lead to cases being missed or identified cases differing between studies, and create biased, inaccurate or non-replicable results [15,16]. Similarly, incidence estimates may be affected leading to inaccurate assessment of the health need, which in turn may have major implications for commissioning and the distribution of resources.

Code lists for studies using primary care EHRs are normally prepared through an *a priori* process of consultation between researchers, GPs and disease specialists [17,18]. A dictionary of Read codes (the hierarchical system for coding diagnoses, symptoms and procedures used in UK primary care) is consulted, and relevant codes selected, which are then operationalised in a case definition. Cases of a disease or "clinical entity" are often defined by the first occurrence of a diagnostic Read code considered as sufficient to define a case (e.g. cancer of the colon). We propose that cases can also be identified by combinations of Read codes and other categories of coded data (e.g. migraine could be ascertained by the occurrence of general terms for headache, together with multiple prescriptions of a migraine specific drug). The multiplicity of potentially relevant data types is shown in Figure 1. A range of these may be combined to form a probabilistic or logical definition. The data types which contribute to case definition of a clinical entity may vary from diagnosis, through symptoms, to consultations and recording of correspondence and may not be confined to the health data of individuals, but may include social, demographic and lifestyle factors. In addition to coded data in the record, much information may be hidden in free text portions of the EHR and this concealed information has very rarely been used to classify cases [19]. Computer based methodologies for reliably extracting written clinical information are still in their early stages [20]. Several authors have shown that including data from free text increases case ascertainment for both acute conditions such as respiratory infections and chronic diseases such as angina [21,22,23] as well as RA [19] and can enhance estimates of symptoms in cancer presentation by 40% [24]. Indicators of a disease can be drawn from both coded data and the free text in the record. This study focuses on the use of coded data for this purpose.

Rheumatoid arthritis as an exemplar

Using descriptions of the early presentation and management of rheumatoid arthritis (RA) in primary care as an exemplar, we aimed to demonstrate the potential impact of supplementing existing approaches to case definition using an *a posteriori*, data driven approach. We hypothesised that if a broad range of indicator markers are to be used to identify cases of RA, they could not be exclusively drawn up using an *a priori* method. Instead, to form a truly comprehensive list of these codes, some scrutiny of data within RA patients' records would be needed. The consequent list of codes developed was then examined for its ability to augment our ability to (i) identify recently incident cases of RA, and (ii) provide information about the diagnostic process in primary care.

Rheumatoid arthritis was selected because robust data on the diagnosis and management of RA in primary care setting is lacking and referral practices are highly variable across the NHS in the UK. However, there is increasing evidence that early intervention with disease modifying anti-rheumatic drugs (DMARD) improves prognosis [25]. Such early intervention requires early recognition and referral to specialist services. Reliable case definition would enable better estimation of presentation and service use as well as facilitate research on this disease. It was hypothesised that there would be significant activity in the record indicative of RA presentation before an RA code was found in the record. RA is not an incentivised condition in UK primary care and there are no universally used codes so identification is problematic. This fact, however, also gave us the opportunity to explore coding in a

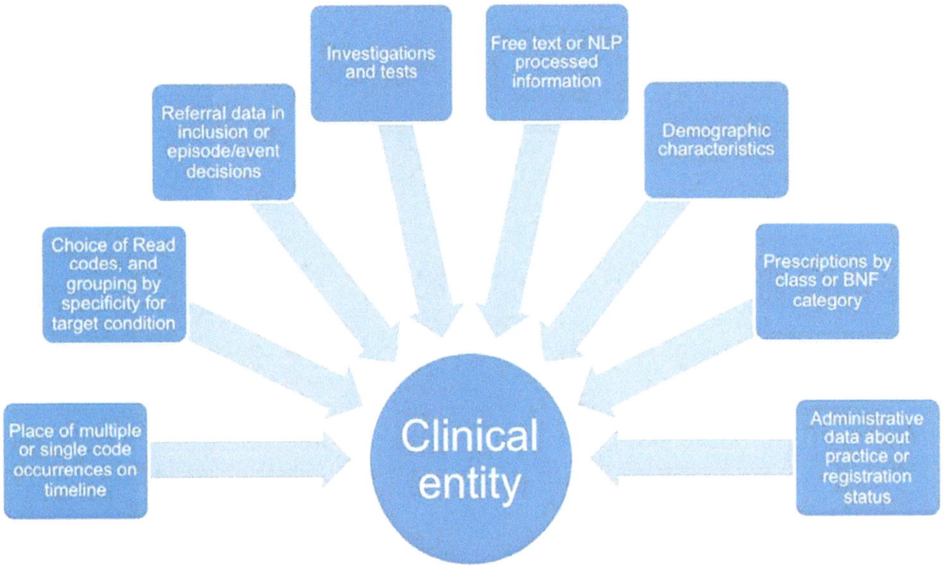

Figure 1. Data types contributing to characterisation of a clinical entity.

disease for which there are no agreed coding standards and in which coding practices may vary widely.

Objectives

Our objectives were to:

1. Draw up a comprehensive list of indicator markers for the early presentation and diagnostic process of rheumatoid arthritis.
2. Describe how much additional information is acquired by supplementing the *a priori* code lists with the *a posteriori* approach.
3. Explore the extent to which the indicator markers could a) be used to identify cases of rheumatoid arthritis prior to an RA diagnostic code and b) describe the diagnostic process of RA in primary care.
4. Explore differences in the recording of indicator markers between genders to confirm that there were no systematic differences between genders which would affect case definition.

Methods

Ethics Statement

The study was approved by the MHRA Independent Scientific Advisory Committee (protocol number 09_033R).

Population and participants

The General Practice Research Database (GPRD) is an electronic database of anonymised longitudinal patient records from general practice [1]. Established in 1987, it is a nationwide dataset currently covering 8.5% of the population, with data from over 600 practices, broadly representative of the UK population. There are 5.25 million currently active patients (in January 2012). Records are derived from a widely used GP software system (VISION) and contain complete prescribing and coded diagnostic and clinical information as well as information on tests requested, laboratory results and referrals made at or following on from each consultation. The structure of the data is shown in Figure 2, with different elements of data held in separate record tables. Each clinical event has a code assigned by the GP using the Read coding system, version 2. General practitioners enter medical diagnoses and symptoms using these Read codes. Read codes are a hierarchical recording system used to record clinical summary information. The codes are not limited to diagnostic and procedural codes, but also include codes for symptoms, test results, screening, history and other areas.

Our target population was permanently registered patients in the GPRD within the study period (1/1/2005 to 31/12/2008). From this group we identified patients with a first diagnostic code for RA between 1/1/2005 and 31/12/2008 who were aged 30 years and over at the time of diagnosis.

Development of indicator markers

Figure 3 provides an overview of the preparation of the lists of indicator markers. Lists of diagnostic codes for rheumatoid arthritis, used to define the cases used in this study, were also drawn up using the *a priori* methods described here. The methods used two complementary approaches:

1. **a priori** development using clinical opinion, code hierarchy and dictionaries.
2. **a posteriori** modification examining the records of identified RA cases to supplement lists with codes actually used in these records in the period leading up to RA diagnosis.

A priori development of indicator markers

We were seeking to capture events and consultations involved in the presentation and early management of inflammatory arthritis and which would be recorded in the electronic health record. The lead researcher (AN) met with two rheumatologists (KAD and one other), as well as two GPs (HS, GR) to discuss how patients with early inflammatory arthritis might present and how this might be recorded by the GP in codes in the primary care record. The following domains were considered: diagnoses; symptoms; signs; tests; referrals; treatment. Within each domain, this group of four clinicians identified possible markers of RA presentation along with key terms that might be used to record this presentation

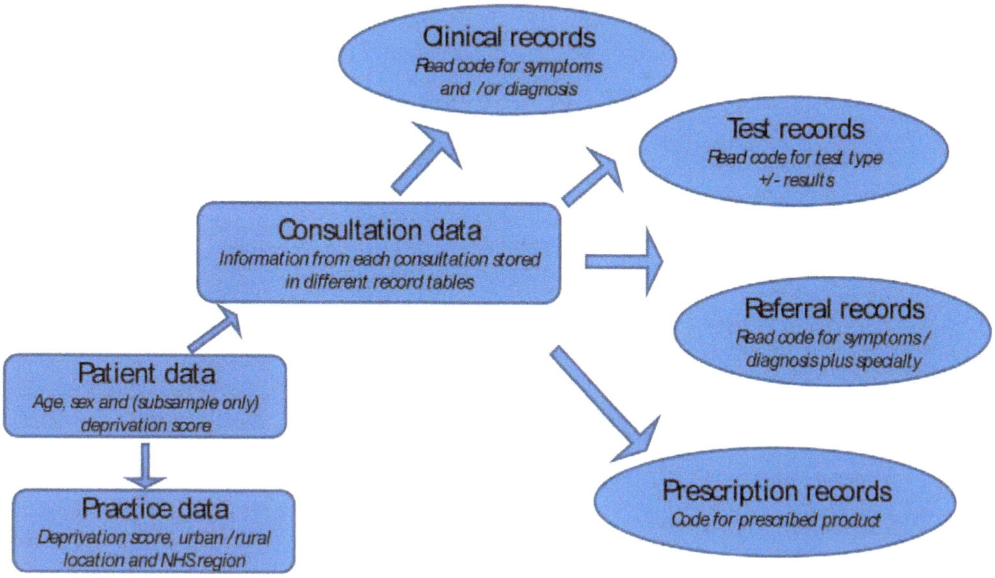

Figure 2. Schematic model of the GPRD database.

(Table 1). Those marked with asterisks were felt to be most specific and were selected as the initial markers.

We then undertook searches for Read codes used to represent these markers of RA presentation. This was designed to be an inclusive, sensitive search strategy leading to the production of lists of potential codes to be considered. The following combination of techniques was used, often in an iterative fashion.

1. Text searching. This was carried out in the medical browser supplied by the GPRD which lists the codes available to GPs to use in the records. Using the list of keywords that might be used for each marker we searched in as many fields (primarily the Read-Oxmis-Code table) as possible to find suitable codes.

2. Using the code hierarchy. By examining the Read codes obtained from text searches, the main Read code groups involved were identified. Using the NHS Browser, which lists Read codes in hierarchies, related areas in the hierarchy were identified and searches were then repeated including these terms and code-groups.

Figure 4 summarises the marker groups which underpinned the searches that were undertaken. Full details are available in Appendix S1. The search process was complicated by the structure of the Read code hierarchy because the codes for diagnoses and presenting symptoms of musculoskeletal disorders are not clearly differentiated. In order to maintain a complete record of the methods, all codes returned by each search were saved. Code-lists used for studies of RA available from other researchers were reviewed and this led to 15 extra codes being included [15]. Search results were then collated and ten duplicates removed, resulting in a total of 1248 codes relating to markers indicating some aspect of RA presentation. A classification system was prepared so that codes were classified to correspond to provisional indicator marker groups and those that were not relevant to these groups were discarded, with documentation of the process. All codes identified in the searches were examined for relevance and to assign them to marker groups, separately by two clinically trained investigators, AN and either GR or HS. Disagreements were discussed by the coders and if not agreed referred to third party (KD, GR or HS).

A posteriori modification of indicator markers

We used data from previously identified RA cases in three ways to confirm or modify the *a priori* marker lists drawn up during the first process.

1. Commonly-used codes. The complete records of an initial random sample of 1,743 RA cases defined using the rheumatoid arthritis or juvenile inflammatory arthritis codes in the *a priori* provisional code list were examined. All the codes that related to RA presentation in the year preceding diagnosis were totalled. Any codes that had been used in more than 50 cases but had not been included in the *a priori* marker code lists were reviewed. These codes included a group that described *non-specific investigations* such as C-reactive protein levels, anti-nuclear antibody or other auto-antibody tests. These were added as new marker group. Additional symptom codes for knee pain and neck pain were added to the *other symptoms* marker and polymyalgia rheumatica was added to the *other named inflammatory arthritis diagnosis* marker.

2. Patient histories. For selected time periods all the codes used in 30 randomly selected RA patients from the sample above were reviewed. The time periods selected were 30 days either side of first *referral* code, first *Disease Modifying Anti-Rheumatic Drug (DMARD)* prescription (especially if more than six months before diagnosis), and 30 days either side of the first one out of *inflammatory diagnosis*, *rheumatoid factor test*, and *non – specific investigation* code (especially if these were more than six months before diagnosis). This review revealed that one code for *psoriatic arthropathy* had been missed. It additionally suggested that many oral steroid prescriptions were unrelated to arthritis, so the codes for DMARD were revised to remove *steroids*. It also revealed use of codes for *monitoring DMARD usage*. New searches were undertaken for codes related to *drug monitoring*, the results were classified by two coders and the agreed codes added to the DMARD code-list.

3. Pre-anonymised text. We had access to 10,000 entries of pre-anonymised text from the GPRD unrelated to this study dataset. These had been used in a variety of other studies, including an investigation into the use of non-steroidal anti-inflammatory drugs. The free text entered in association with 1307 codes which were one of the assigned *a priori* codes or had the term

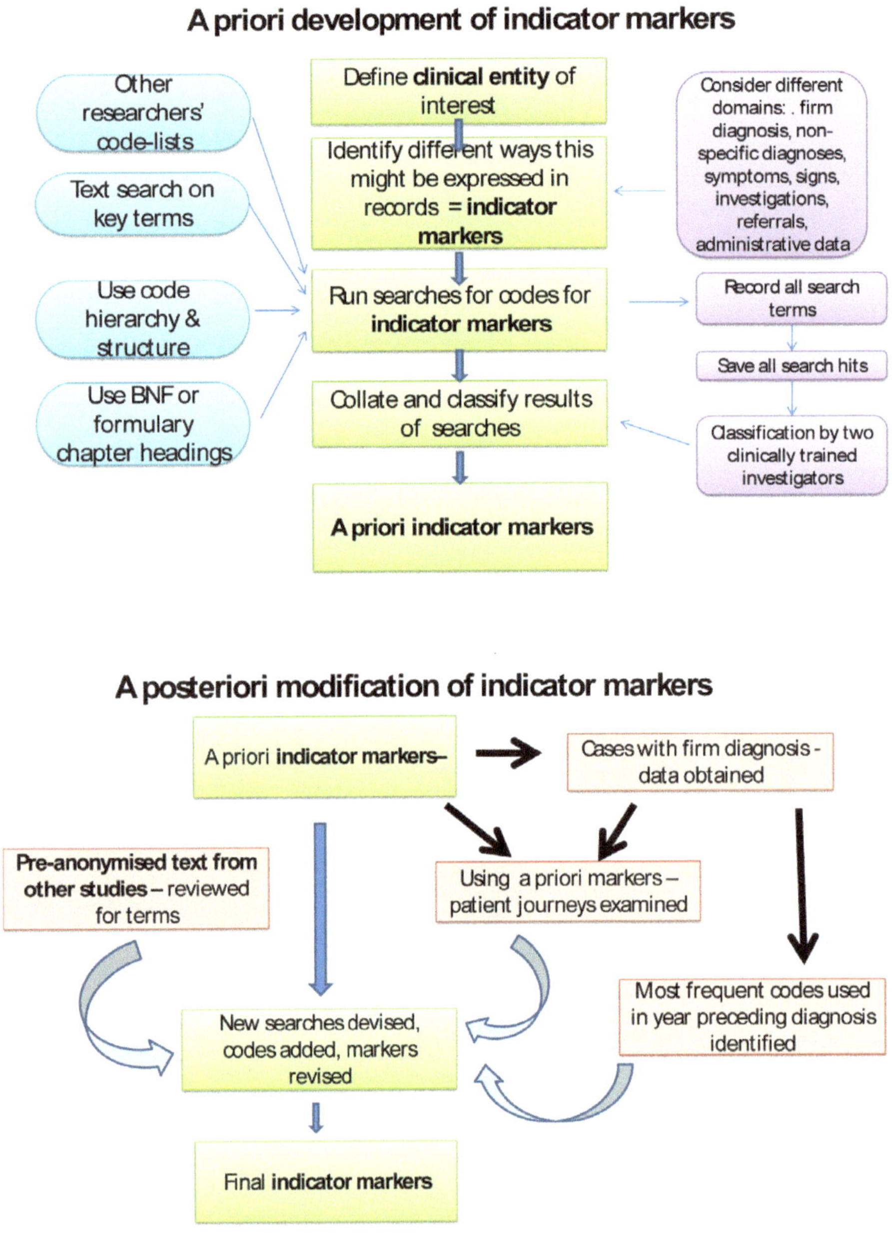

Figure 3. ***A priori* and *a posteriori* strategies for developing code lists.**

arthritis in the text was reviewed. Terms in text that might be useful in identifying cases were added and new searches performed (as in the *a priori* code – searching process) and classified using methods described above. This led to a marker of *synovitis* being created (Figure 4).

Final code-lists for the indicator markers are in Appendix S2. Markers were separated into *specific markers* of rheumatoid arthritis (inflammatory arthritis, other inflammatory condition, referral to rheumatology, rheumatoid factor test, synovitis or DMARD prescription) and *non-specific markers* (non-specific or other arthritis diagnosis, non-specific inflammatory or auto-immune investigations, joint signs and symptoms and NSAID prescriptions). No changes were made to the diagnostic codes for Rheumatoid Arthritis or Juvenile Inflammatory Arthritis in this *a posteriori* modification process.

Identification of cases

All patients with a first coded diagnosis of RA (from an *a priori* list of diagnostic codes) and aged 30 years or more at the time of diagnosis were identified in the study period (2005–2008). Patients who had an RA code anywhere in their record before the study period were not included. GPRD allows for a date to be entered for an event, in case this differs from the date the event was recorded. However, if an event date had not been entered into the GP system, the date that the record was created was used (10,986 events (0.1%) were imputed). Events were discarded if they occurred before the start date (the later of the patient's registration date or the date that the practice's records were considered up-to-standard by the GPRD) or after the end date (the earlier of the date of the patient leaving the practice or the last date records were received from the practice). The indicator markers (asterisked

Table 1. Initial list of indicator markers for early inflammatory arthritis across different clinical domains, based on round-table clinical discussions.

Diagnosis	Symptoms	Signs	Investigations	Therapy
***Rheumatoid arthritis**	*Stiffness especially morning	*Polyarthritis	*Rheumatoid factor	*NSAID
*Inflammatory arthritis	*Painful joints *especially hands/ feet/wrists*	*Joint effusion *(not knee)*	C-reactive protein	*DMARD
*Arthritis NOS	Pyrexia of Unknown Origin	Synovitis	ESR (erythrocyte sedimentation rate)	Steroid (non-oral)
*Palindromic RA	Night sweats		Anaemia	Cox II inhibitors
*Reactive arthritis	Fever		X-rays *hand & feet (not knee)*	
Reiter's syndrome			Auto-antibodies	
Fibromyalgia			Thyroid function tests	
Lupus				
Sicca syndrome				

*these markers were selected for initial searches.

in Table 1) were identified in the records within one year of RA diagnosis. Having established the markers, we then sought these codes throughout the records of RA patients. To standardise follow up times, analyses were restricted to RA cases who had records for at least three years before through to 14 days after the first coded RA diagnosis. All records were cut off at three years prior to diagnosis. The first diagnostic code had to be within the study period (2005–2008) but indicator marker events occurring before the study period were included in analyses.

Statistical analysis

The data were prepared using Stata version 11 (Statacorp LP, Texas). For each indicator marker, any relevant code from any GPRD entry resulted in a positive marker. Within a marker group, the date of the earliest code was taken as the first example of an indicator for that patient and the date intervals were calculated from this earliest code. For medication markers (DMARD and NSAID) we looked for the presence of a prescription of these medications. The prevalence of different indicator markers was compared using chi-squared tests. The time interval between the first indicator marker within a group and the first coded diagnosis of RA was calculated. Since the time-intervals were skewed, medians and non-parametric tests were used to compare groups (Mann Whitney U). Survival analysis was performed constructing survival time from 14 days after diagnosis backwards to three years, with the earliest code in any indicator marker group as a failure event.

Results

Results describe the value of the addition of indicator markers to diagnostic code case definitions and how their exploration changes the view of RA management in primary care.

Cases defined by diagnostic codes

Cases were defined by a first occurrence of an RA diagnostic code during the study period (and no code prior to this in their entire record). The study sample comprised 5,843 cases of RA, of which 1,831 were men and 4,012 were women. Men were older (median age 63 years; inter-quartile range, (IQR) 51–73) than women at the time of diagnosis (median age 60 years; IQR 50–71, $p<0.001$).

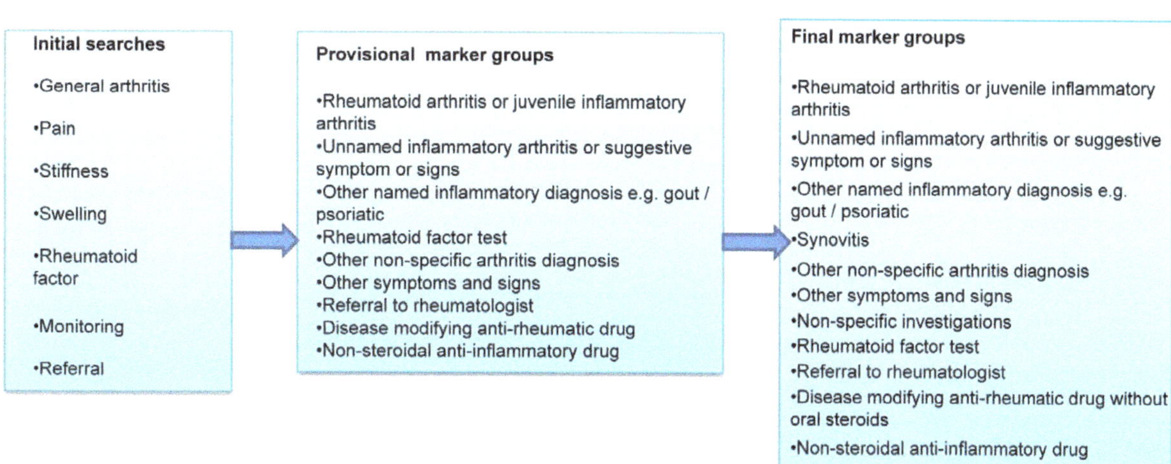

Figure 4. Indicator marker groups.

Prevalence of Indicator Markers

Table 2 summarises the prevalence of the indicator marker groups both in the whole study period and within particular time periods. The most common **specific marker** was a rheumatoid factor test, for which 62.9% patients had a code. There were codes for referral to rheumatology services in 42.4% of patients. Codes for clinical findings related to any inflammatory arthritis were uncommon, present in only 14.8% of patients. Likewise synovitis codes were present in only 4.1%. A third (33.6%) of patients had a prescription for a DMARD and in 14% of patients this had occurred *at least six months before* the diagnosis of RA was coded. Overall, 86.0% of patients had one or more specific indicator markers including DMARD prescriptions, with 34.2% having one marker, 30.5% having two markers and 21.3% having three or more specific markers.

Non-specific markers. were more common in the records but these may reflect activity relating to events other than RA. The most common indicator marker was a prescription for a non-steroidal anti-inflammatory drug (NSAID) which was present in over three-quarters of patients (79.3%). Two-thirds of patients (66.1%) had evidence of a non-specific investigation, such as CRP or autoantibody level and two-thirds (65.4%) had evidence of other joint signs and symptoms. Non-specific arthritis diagnoses were found in 18.0% of patients. Overall 94.5% of patients had one or more non-specific indicator markers. When NSAIDs were excluded from this analysis, as they may have been prescribed for many conditions other than RA, 86.0% of patients had at least one non-specific marker, with 32.8% having one, 42.8% having two, and 10.4% having three non-specific markers.

In this sample, only 4.9% of patients (288) had no indicator markers whether specific or non-specific. Only 11.5% (674) patients had a single indicator marker, whereas 18.3% had two markers, 23.6% had three markers, 21.1% had four markers and 20.5% of patients had five or more indicator markers in their record before the RA diagnostic code was recorded.

Combinations of Markers

The combinations of specific indicator markers were examined to assess their utility in presumptive case definition. These are shown in Table 3. The most common specific indicator markers (DMARD prescription, referral to rheumatology and rheumatoid factor test) were assessed in combination with each other, as well as with joint signs & symptoms from the non-specific markers.

DMARD prescription. This was commonly found in combination with other markers: 1175 patients (20.1%) had both a DMARD prescription and a referral to rheumatology services before their RA code, 1032 (17.7%) had both DMARD and a rheumatoid factor test and 1263 (21.6%) of patients had DMARD and a non-specific joint sign or symptom.

Referral. 1640 patients (28.1%) had both a referral to rheumatology services and a rheumatoid factor test coded in their file before the RA code was recorded and a similar number (1764; 30.2%) had both a referral and a joint sign or symptom.

Rheumatoid factor test. Nearly half of patients (2670; 45.7%) had codes for both a rheumatoid factor test and a joint sign or symptom.

When the three most common specific markers were investigated (DMARD prescription, referral and rheumatoid factor test), it was found that 1846 patients (31.6%) had two of these markers and 667 patients (11.4%) had all three of these markers in their file before an RA code was recorded. When joint signs & symptoms was added to this list, 2080 patients (35.6%) had two of these markers, 1426 patients (24.4%) had three markers and 531 (9.1%) had all four of these common markers.

Prevalence of Markers by Gender

The prevalence of markers was similar in men and women as shown in Table 4. Only two marker groups showed statistically significant gender differences in prevalence. Diagnosis of a named inflammatory arthritis was more common in men, 8.3% compared to 6.5% in women (chi square $=6.18$, DF $=1$; $p=0.01$) (not shown in table). A DMARD prescription was also more frequent in men, 35.7% compared to 32.6% in women, (chi square $=5.47$, DF $=1$; $p=0.02$), although when a Bonferroni correction was applied for multiple comparisons, these differences were no longer significant.

Timing of Markers

The timings of the first occurrence of the indicator markers in relation to RA diagnostic code are shown in Table 2 and Table 4. Referral to rheumatology services, rheumatoid factor tests and DMARD prescriptions were coded closest in time to diagnosis, whereas non-specific markers such as general investigations or symptoms were frequently present more than a year before diagnosis. It was found that 20.6% of patients had a rheumatoid factor test coded more than six months before a specific diagnostic code was recorded, 16.8% had a referral to rheumatology and 14.4% had a DMARD prescription. Overall, 44.7% of patients had a specific marker occurring more than six months before a diagnostic code was recorded. Intervals between markers and RA diagnostic code were longer in women than men for non-specific auto-immune type investigations (men 147 days (median), women 189 days; $p=0.006$), for presentation of joint signs and symptoms (men 323 days (median), women 448 days; $p<0.001$), and for first evidence of referral (men 88 days (median), women 109 days; $p=0.02$).

Figure 5 shows "survival" curves for selected indicator markers, with time reversed, from 15 days after diagnosis to three years before diagnosis with a "failure event" being the earliest marker in that indicator category. The curves show that rheumatoid factor tests, referral and DMARD most often occur close to diagnosis with a more gradual occurrence more than one year previously.

Discussion

This study described in detail a two stage, iterative process for drawing up code lists and looked at the utility of indicator markers prior to the definitive diagnostic code in a) the description of early care, and b) the case definition, of rheumatoid arthritis patients, with a view to defining uncoded cases (false negatives). Following a panel of clinicians drawing up a first list of codes, data from RA patients was scrutinised to see if additions to the lists should be made. The second stage of this process resulted in considerable modification of the lists, suggesting this is a valuable addition to traditional methods of approaching code list design. The indicator markers chosen were found to exist in the file well before the RA diagnostic code and to give important information on the diagnostic process of RA. Indicator markers were wide-spread in the records of RA patients with 83.5% of patients having at least two markers in their file before the RA diagnostic code was recorded.

This strategy of drawing up code lists, with the combination of *a priori* and *a posteriori* data-driven stages, will be applicable to other conditions and coding systems. Using the second stage, *a posteriori* approach allowed us to make significant modifications to code lists. For example, synovitis and non-specific auto-immune investigations had been raised by the expert group at the initial stages but not included in the *a priori* searches as they were considered too non-specific. However, they were discovered, during the data-

Table 2. Prevalence of indicator markers during study period.

Marker present		Timing of first marker within study period (in relation to RA diagnosis)			
		14 days after to <1 month before	1–3 months before	3–6 months before	6 months - 3 yrs before
Non-specific inflammatory arthritis diagnosis or signs					
n	867	209	143	124	391
%	14.8	3.6	2.5	2.1	6.7
Other named inflammatory condition					
n	410	32	32	49	297
%	7.0	0.6	0.6	0.8	5.1
Referral to rheumatology services					
n	2,480	725	467	306	982
%	42.4	12.4	8.0	5.2	16.8
RhF test - regardless of result					
n	3,674	1326	657	488	1,203
%	62.9	22.7	11.2	8.4	20.6
Synovitis					
n	241	46	44	33	118
%	4.1	0.8	0.8	0.6	2
DMARD prescription - excluding oral steroids					
n	1,962	842	154	123	843
%	33.6	14.4	2.6	2.1	14.4
Any specific marker (date of earliest marker used)					
n	2057	1395	771	607	2243
%	86.0	27.8	15.4	12.1	44.7
Non-specific arthritis diagnosis					
n	1,053	200	224	151	478
%	18.0	3.4	3.8	2.6	8.2
Joint signs & symptoms					
n	3,823	363	440	421	2,599
%	65.4	6.2	7.5	7.2	44.5
Non-specific investigations e.g. CRP, auto-antibodies					
n	3,861	844	611	519	1,887
%	66.1	14.4	10.5	8.9	32.3
NSAID prescription					
n	4,631	385	390	373	3,483
%	79.3	6.6	6.7	6.4	59.6
Any non-specific Markers (date of earliest marker used)					
n	5524	404	370	400	4318
%	94.5	7.4	6.7	7.3	78.6

driven stage, to be found with some regularity in the records of RA patients. The data-driven stage then revealed codes that had been missed and some errors in classification and so served as a form of triangulation. The finding that this data-driven modification stage is of such importance poses a challenge to researchers and data providers, as this additional stage of code searching may not be possible in the design stage of all research studies, due to difficulties with advance access to data.

Secondly, our study looked at the value of using indicator markers to understand the diagnostic process of early RA as presenting in primary care. Using these markers, we aimed to indicate locations in the EHR where the diagnosis of RA was being considered and to describe the early course of disease presentation in these patients, as shown by coded symptoms of the disease, referrals to appropriate services or because of tests being ordered or results recorded. Indicator markers were widespread within the RA patient records, in many cases a long time before the RA diagnostic code was found on the file. These results suggest, as was hypothesised, that the diagnosis of RA may have been known about for some time before a diagnostic code was added, with specific markers frequently found more than six months before recorded diagnosis. This discrepancy between dates may indicate diagnostic uncertainty or delay in coding a known or presumptive diagnosis. Further field work would be needed to

Table 3. Frequency of combinations of indicator markers.

Code 1	Code 2	N (5843)	%
DMARD	Referral	1175	20.1
	RhF Test	1032	17.7
	Joint Symptom	1263	21.6
Referral	RhF Test	1640	28.1
	Joint Symptom	1764	30.2
RhF Test	Joint Symptom	2670	45.7
DMARD, referral and RhF Test			
- any two		1846	31.6
- all three		667	11.4
DMARD, referral, RhF Test and Joint symptom			
- any two		2080	35.6
- any three		1426	24.4
- all four		531	9.1

determine which of these two processes has most influence in these data. UK guidance from NICE [25] suggests that RA should only be diagnosed after it has been in evidence for 6 months. However, these data precede this guidance and this is unlikely to be a full explanation for the delay in diagnostic coding.

We were also able to explore gender differences in indicator markers, to check for systematic differences in recording by gender, but found no evidence of gender differences in the prevalence of most, except for named inflammatory arthritis and DMARD prescriptions both of which were more common in men. The prevalence of referral and investigation markers was similar in men and women although there was some evidence that the gap between referral, non-specific symptoms, non-specific investigations and coding of diagnosis was longer in women than in men.

Thirdly, this study explored indicator markers as a way of broadening case definitions in this disease, thereby potentially identifying individuals with the disease who do not yet have a diagnostic code. The majority of patients (83.5%) had two or more indicator markers, and therefore combinations of codes may help to describe the early presentation and diagnostic process of these patients. One finding, however, was that the most common symptom codes found in our study were the non-specific ones, and these could relate to conditions other than RA. Despite this, 86% of patients had at least one specific marker. When a combination of the four most indicative markers were examined, it was found that 36% had two of these markers, 24.4% had three markers and 9.1% had all four of these common markers. This suggests that using these markers in combination may facilitate the identification of RA cases, both in the early stages before an RA code is recorded and in cases where no code has been recorded and the cases would ordinarily slip "under the radar", leading to false negatives and biasing a subsequent study.

However, these findings suggest that while coded indicator markers do give a good indication of the presentation of RA, in 16.5% of patients there was no marker or only one marker before the RA diagnostic code. With coded information alone it may not be possible to reliably identify the early presentation of every case. Extra information may be available in unstructured free text, and may include both notes made by the GP during a consultation and the content of referral letters and correspondence from specialists. Information governance requirements mean that free text must be anonymised before release to researchers. It is not currently possible to do this reliably automatically and therefore manual, expensive labour is required to ensure that datasets are anonymised. Research projects using EHRs have therefore relied almost exclusively on coded structured data rather than accessing free text [12]. Text data is also difficult to analyse in large numbers of patients and requires some form of processing or structuring to

Table 4. Intervals between first indicator marker and diagnosis in RA cases (days).

	n	%	Mean	Median	25% quartile	75%% quartile	n	%	Mean	Median	25% quartile	75%% quartile	p for gender difference*
Inflammatory arthritis diagnosis	273	14.9	278	126	34	454	594	14.8	307	159	34	511	0.31
Rheumatoid factor test	1,142	62.4	193	74	13	250	2,532	63.1	212	75	9	303	0.94
Referral	801	43.7	233	88	16	326	1,679	41.8	269	109	22	445	0.02
DMARD prescription	654	35.7	321	51	0	693	1,308	32.6	351	103	0	749	0.23
Non-specific arthritis diagnosis	351	19.2	258	141	44	370	702	17.5	304	154	45	508	0.19
Non-specific auto-immune test	1,198	65.4	295	147	38	478	2,663	66.4	336	189	42	588	0.006
Joint signs and symptoms	1,186	64.8	424	323	94	747	2,637	65.7	481	448	129	813	<0.001
NSAID prescription	1,455	79.5	577	595	160	1010	3,176	79.2	614	689	194	1021	0.02

*non-parametric Mann-Whitney U test.

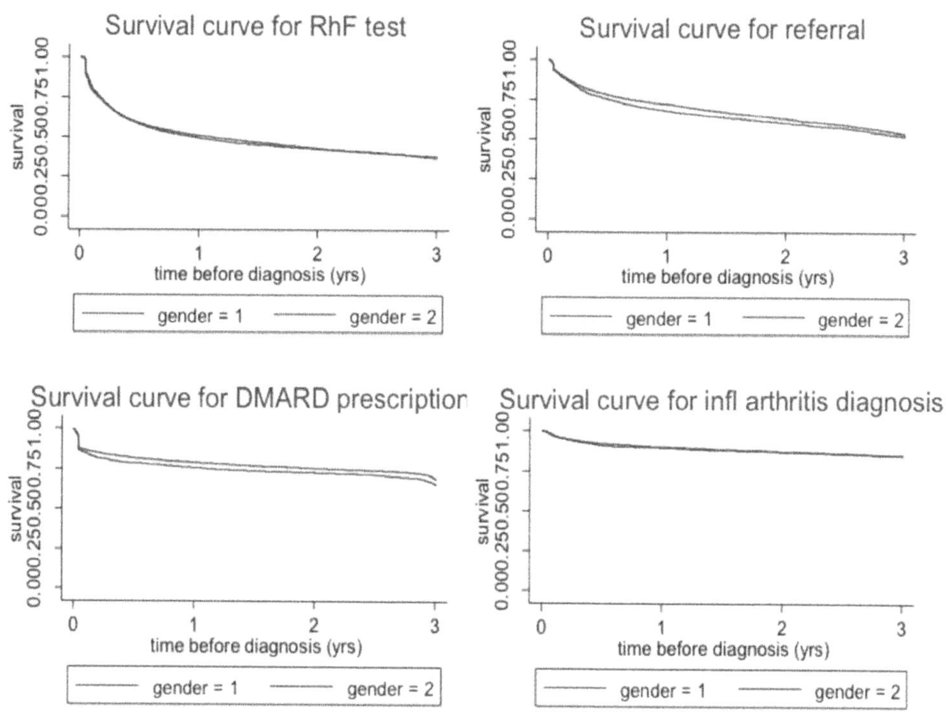

Figure 5. Survival curves for selected indicator markers in the 3 years preceding RA diagnosis, by gender.

allow quantitative analysis [13]. The supplementation of coded information with free text would significantly strengthen findings in studies using EHRs, as has been found in previous studies of case definition of RA using EHRs [19,26].

In order to identify a "case" for a study using EHRs we therefore propose that there are three levels of classification for sources of variation in recording, each level posing an increasing challenge to the researcher. **Level 1** consists of diagnostic codes from within the same domain, such as different diagnostic codes for rheumatoid arthritis. Because these are diagnostic codes, it is probable that patients with these codes have the condition of interest. However, the sole use of these codes may miss cases where diagnostic coding is delayed or incomplete. At **level 2**, codes from different domains are used, such as symptoms or test results rather than a diagnosis e.g. "joint stiffness", "referral to rheumatology clinic" or "rheumatoid factor positive". A combination of these codes would result in a probabilistic definition of the condition, but these coding patterns result in less certainty in the diagnosis for the researcher and may also result in the inclusion of cases which do not have the disease of interest. The final level, **level 3**, is where additional disease specific information is found in free text – either along with a more general diagnostic code or a code for a symptom or a more general code such as "had a chat to patient". Free text may supply additional information to allow a diagnosis to be made with more certainty than if coded data alone were used.

How findings fit with previous literature

Literature on the methodology of drawing up code-lists for the identification of cases, treatment or outcomes for health research is sparse, despite its pivotal importance in such research. Some work been published on the operationalisation of code-lists into statistical programmes [27]. There are techniques available to address the proliferation of diagnostic codes such as ancestor/descendant tracing within SNOMED ("Systematised Nomenclature of Medicine Clinical Terms" – an international comprehensive terminology system being adopted by the NHS), hierarchies within Read codes and query building within clinical trial systems. However, high-level search strategies, and how to address variations in lists of codes below Level 1 variation (outlined above) have not been discussed in the literature.

A lack of standardisation in methodology means that code-lists, and hence case definitions, may vary across studies in a variety of research contexts. Very little is known about how this variation in code-lists affects study results, although there are implications that it may be important, such as high rates of false negatives or positives introducing biases in the estimation of uptake of certain tests or treatments within disease populations [16,28]. An additional concern is that the use and type of coding structures may be individual to software systems so that the codes used to describe, for example a polyarthritis, may differ across different primary care software systems. Such system-specific coding reinforces the need for a data-driven stage in any case-finding process and the need to explore the data before finalizing code selections.

Other authors have also highlighted the deficits from coded data [29]. Jordan and colleagues showed that the number of consultations related to knee pain were underestimated without the use of text from primary care databases [21], and as mentioned Tate and colleagues have shown that the diagnosis date of ovarian cancer recorded in primary care records is later than other evidence in the record [14]. This is consistent with our results indicating that the diagnosis may have been known for some time before it was formally coded. In addition two studies have found that using free text within algorithms for case definition significantly improves the positive predictive value of subject classification in RA when using EHRs [19,26].

Previous studies looking at the presentation and management of early RA have been situated in secondary care and are therefore prone to substantial referral bias [30,31,32]. The existing work suggests that delay in seeking medical attention is a more important factor than delay in recognition and referral to specialist services [33]. Data from primary care describing the care process from the first presentation are needed, but our results suggest that this cannot be achieved within routine primary care electronic databases using codes alone as much information, particularly that which occurs outside primary care, may be recorded in free text.

Limitations

The indicator markers have not been validated by a review of the associated text in the record and therefore it is possible that non-specific codes, for example for a painful ankle, were unrelated to the subsequent RA diagnosis. Similarly prescriptions for DMARD such as methotrexate, and especially NSAIDs, may be unrelated to RA. This will lead to an over-estimation of the presenting symptoms and treatment in RA patients. The risk of under-estimation is perhaps greater. This will occur if events or consultations relating to RA diagnosis and management are missed because general codes have been used and the important information recorded in text, which we have described as level 3 variation. The next stage in the project is to extract text around the time of indicator markers, and perform keyword searches on extracted text.

Although we used a panel of four experts for generating the *a priori* lists of indicator markers, a larger panel or a more in depth process, such as a Delphi process, might have generated a different or fuller list. However, other studies in this field have used similar size panels of experts [15] to scrutinise possible codes. Indeed, some studies have not drawn up lists but used a single diagnostic Read code to identify RA patients [34,35]. We are not aware of any studies which have reported the details of a data-driven stage for modifying their lists. Greater clarity of reporting for drawing up lists would result increased standardisation of case definition and increase the generalisability of EHR study results. Previous studies reporting validation of cases using EHRs have inadequately described the methods for this validation [36]. We believe that this documentation of the process is an important resource for researchers new in the field, and encourage other researchers to publish their code list strategies in a replicable way.

Furthermore we did not look at control data to compare the incidence of the indicator markers in patients with no RA diagnostic code. This comparison would be valuable to ascertain whether these markers do indeed occur in greater numbers just before an RA diagnostic code compared to at other times or in other patients. Further work will examine these markers in control data and also assess their utility in estimating the rates of false negatives which may result by only using diagnostic codes for case definition, thereby introducing bias into the study [28]. The use of control data will allow us to estimate the positive predictive value of clusters of indicator markers to ascertain which combinations are most predictive of a RA diagnostic code being added to the file. However, given the small proportions of patients with three or more of the chosen codes in their record (around 10%) prior to the RA code, there is likely to be more information concealed in the free text which would contribute to case definition. Therefore our plan is to extract this free text information to estimate its contribution to case definition before estimating the predictive value of clusters of indicators.

Implications for future research and practice

Preparing indicator markers and code-lists is time-consuming and requires input from clinical experts. Context and temporal relationships are often important in looking at markers and building up patterns. It is likely to be a rate-limiting step in future research projects – particularly if multiple clinical entities need to be included in any one study. The design of future EHR systems should consider the need for reporting and aggregation of cases and facilitate the recording of the code-selection process, including a data-driven stage and the ability to search within code-sets. Future research might also consider whether machine learning techniques could contribute to this process.

If EHRs are to be used appropriately in research we need to develop a wider understanding of the drivers of coding in the clinical environment. As work on different diseases develops, it may also be possible to develop a typology of what kind of clinical entities are liable to long gaps between the onset of clinical suspicion, referral and treatment, and where the two are reliably contemporaneous, in order to minimise wasted effort doing over-complex analyses. Our findings here may generalise to some other chronic diseases, but not all.

Sharing of resources between researchers is desirable, to avoid unnecessary duplication. The process of breaking up search strategies into different markers, with publication of precise search terms and results, may allow transparency and replicability in the preparation of code-lists and facilitate their sharing. For example codes relating to a certain presentation might be stored and available for use by another study. At present there is no standardisation of methods for preparing case definitions and code-lists which limits the possibilities of sharing results. No recognised repository to aid sharing exists. Any standardisation would require a common set of meta-data relating to case-finding – detailing what has been done, decisions that have been made and why. The format these meta-data should take is not obvious.

These findings emphasise the need for research using EHR to go beyond simple use of diagnostic codes and adopt more sophisticated strategies for case-finding, including the use of free text. Relying on coded diagnosis may not lead to accurate case definition thereby leading to inaccurate estimates for disease registries and assessments of service needs. The development of automated methods to allow access to information in text without anonymisation should be an urgent priority.

Acknowledgments

The authors wish to thank Sara Thomas at the London School of Hygiene and Tropical Medicine, who assisted in sharing code lists from previous RA studies, and Dr Karen Walker-Bone at Brighton & Sussex Medical School, who helped in the initial stages of the study to suggest indicator marker groups. We also wish to thank Elizabeth Morris for reading versions of the manuscript.

Author Contributions

Gave clinical expertise for drawing up code lists: JC KD HS GR. Gave advice on analysing data: ART IP. Conceived and designed the experiments: AN KD HS GR ART IP JC. Performed the experiments: AN. Analyzed the data: AN EF. Wrote the paper: AN EF.

References

1. Lawson DH, Sherman V, Hollowell J (1998) The General Practice Research Database. Q J Med 91: 445–452.
2. Hansell A, Hollowell J, Nichols T, McNiece R, Strachan D (1999) Use of the General Practice Research Database (GPRD) for respiratory epidemiology: a comparison with the 4th Morbidity Survey in General Practice (MSGP4). Thorax 54: 413–419.
3. Blumenthal D (2010) Launching HITECH. N Engl J Med 362: 382–385.
4. Blumenthal D, Tavenner M (2010) The "Meaningful Use" Regulation for Electronic Health Records. N Engl J Med 363: 501–504.
5. Linder JA, Haas JS, Iyer A, Labuzetta MA, Ibara M, et al. (2010) Secondary use of electronic health record data: spontaneous triggered adverse drug event reporting. Pharmacoepidemiol Drug Saf 19: 1211–1215.
6. Sharp J (2010) Beyond 'Meaningful Use': EHR data in Research. iHealthBeat. California, USA: California Healthcare Foundation.
7. Doll R, Hill AB (1950) Smoking and Carcinoma of the Lung. BMJ 1 1451–1455.
8. Marmot MG, Stansfeld S, Patel C, North F, Head J, et al. (1991) Health inequalities among British civil servants: the Whitehall II study. The Lancet 337: 1387–1393.
9. Hansen K, Joshi H, Dex S (2010) Children of the 21st Century: First Five Years v. 2 (UK Millennium Cohort Study Series). Bristol, UK: Policy Press.
10. Hippisley-Cox J, Vinogradova Y, Coupland C (2007) Time Series Analysis for selected clinical indicators from the Quality and Outcomes Framework 2001–2006. Leeds: The Information Centre for Health and Social Care.
11. Thiru K, Hassey A, Sullivan F (2003) Systematic review of scope and quality of electronic patient record data in primary care. BMJ 326: 1070.
12. Jordan K, Porcheret M, Croft P (2004) Quality of morbidity coding in general practice computerized medical records: a systematic review. Family Practice 21: 396–412.
13. Pascoe SW, Neal RD, Heywood PL, Allgar VL, Miles JN, et al. (2008) Identifying patients with a cancer diagnosis using general practice medical records and Cancer Registry data. Fam Pract 25: 215–220.
14. Tate AR, Martin AG, Murray-Thomas T, Anderson SR, Cassell JA (2009) Determining the date of diagnosis – is it a simple matter? The impact of different approaches to dating diagnosis on estimates of delayed care for ovarian cancer in UK primary care. BMC Med Res Methodol 9: 42.
15. Thomas SL, Edwards CJ, Smeeth L, Cooper C, Hall AJ (2008) How accurate are diagnoses for rheumatoid arthritis and juvenile idiopathic arthritis in the general practice research database? Arthritis Rheum 59: 1314–1321.
16. Gulliford MC, Charlton J, Ashworth M, Rudd A, Toschke AM, et al. (2009) Selection of Medical Diagnostic Codes for Analysis of Electronic Patient Records. Application to Stroke in a Primary Care Database. PLoS ONE 4: e7168.
17. Cassell JA, Mercer CH, Sutcliffe L, Petersen I, Islam A, et al. (2006) Trends in sexually transmitted infections in general practice 1990–2000: population based study using data from the UK general practice research database. BMJ 332: 332–334.
18. Tate AR, Nicholson A, Cassell JA (2010) Are GPs under-investigating older patients presenting with symptoms of ovarian cancer? Observational study using General Practice Research Database. Br J Cancer 102: 947–951.
19. Liao KP, Cai T, Gainer V, Goryachev S, Zeng-Treitler Q, et al. (2010) Electronic Medical Records for Discovery Research in Rheumatoid Arthritis. Arthritis Care Res (Hoboken) 62: 1120–1127.
20. Meystre SM, Savova GK, Kipper-Schuler KC, Hurdle JF (2008) Extracting information from textual documents in the electronic health record: a review of recent research. Yearb Med Inform: 128–144.
21. Jordan K, Jinks C, Croft P (2006) Health care utilisation: measurement using primary care records and patient recall both showed bias. J Clin Epidemiol 59: 791–797.
22. Pakhomov SS, Hemingway H, Weston SA, Jacobsen SJ, Rodeheffer R, et al. (2007) Epidemiology of angina pectoris: role of natural language processing of the medical record. Am Heart J 153: 666–673.
23. DeLisle S, South B, Anthony JA, Kalp E, Gundlapallli A, et al. (2010) Combining Free Text and Structured Electronic Medical Record Entries to Detect Acute Respiratory Infections. PLoS ONE 5: e13377.
24. Koeling R, Tate AR, Carroll JA. (2011) Automatically estimating the incidence of symptoms recording in GP free text notes. Proceedings of the first international workshop on Managing interoperability and complexity in health systems 43–50; Glasgow, Scotland, UK.
25. NICE (2009) Rheumatoid arthritis. The management of rheumatoid arthritis in adults. Clinical guideline 79. London, UK.
26. Carroll RJ, Eyler AE, Denny JC (2011) Naïve Electronic Health Record Phenotype Identification for Rheumatoid Arthritis. AMIA Annu Symp Proc 2011: 189–196.
27. Dave S, Petersen I (2009) Creating medical and drug code lists to identify cases in primary care databases. Pharmacoepidemiol Drug Saf 18: 704–7.
28. Manuel DG, Rosella LC, Stukel TA (2010) Importance of accurately identifying disease in studies using electronic health records. BMJ 341: c4226.
29. Jordan K, Porcheret M, Kadam UT, Croft P (2006) The use of general practice consultation databases in rheumatology research. Rheumatology (Oxford) 45: 126–128.
30. Arndt U, Behrens F, Ziswiler HR, Kaltwasser JP, Moller B (2007) Observational study of a patient and doctor directed pre-referral questionnaire for an early arthritis clinic. Rheumatol Int 28: 21–26.
31. Houssien DA, Scott DL (1998) Early referral and outcome in rheumatoid arthritis. Scand J Rheumatol 27: 300–302.
32. van der Horst-Bruinsma IE, Speyer I, Visser H, Breedveld FC, Hazes JM (1998) Diagnosis and course of early-onset arthritis: results of a special early arthritis clinic compared to routine patient care. Br J Rheumatol 37: 1084–1088.
33. Kumar K, Daley E, Carruthers DM, Situnayake D, Gordon C, et al. (2007) Delay in presentation to primary care physicians is the main reason why patients with rheumatoid arthritis are seen late by rheumatologists. Rheumatology (Oxford) 46: 1438–1440.
34. Edwards CJ, Arden NK, Fisher D, Saperia JC, Reading I, et al. (2005) The changing use of disease-modifying anti-rheumatic drugs in individuals with rheumatoid arthritis from the United Kingdom General Practice Research Database. Rheumatology (Oxford) 44: 1394–1398.
35. Edwards CJ, Cooper C, Fisher D, Field M, Van Staa TP, et al. (2007) The Important of the Disease Process and Disease-Modifying Antirheumatic Drug Treatment in the Development of Septic Arthritis in Patients with Rheumatoid Arthritis. Arthritis Rheum 57: 1151–1157.
36. Herrett E, Thomas SL, Schoonen WM, Smeeth L, Hall AJ (2010) Validation and validity of diagnoses in the General Practice Research Database: a systematic review. Br J Clin Pharmacol 69: 4–14.

TRAF5 and TRAF3IP2 Gene Polymorphisms Are Associated with Behçet's Disease and Vogt-Koyanagi-Harada Syndrome: A Case-Control Study

Qin Xiang[1]⁹, Lu Chen[1]⁹, Shengping Hou[1], Jing Fang[1], Yan Zhou[1], Lin Bai[1], Yunjia Liu[1], Aize Kijlstra[2], Peizeng Yang[1]*

1 Chongqing Key Laboratory of Ophthalmology and Chongqing Eye Institute; The First Affiliated Hospital of Chongqing Medical University, Chongqing, P. R. China, **2** University Eye Clinic Maastricht, Maastricht, The Netherlands

Abstract

Background: TRAF5 and TRAF3IP2 have been reported to be associated with several autoimmune diseases. Behçet's disease (BD) and Vogt-Koyanagi-Harada (VKH) syndrome are two autoimmune uveitis entities whereby both genetic and environmental factors are thought to be involved.

Objective: The role of TRAF5 and TRAF3IP2 in BD and VKH has not yet been reported and was therefore the subject of this study.

Methods: The study included 789 BD patients, 940 VKH patients and 1601 healthy unrelated individuals. Genotyping was performed by polymerase chain reaction-restriction fragment length polymorphism (PCR-RFLP) or TaqMan® SNP Genotyping Assay. Real-Time PCR was used to detect mRNA expression from PBMCs obtained from healthy controls with (n = 22) or without (n = 79) stimulation. Levels of TNF-α, IL-6 and IL-8 in culture supernatants were measured by ELISA (n = 22).

Results: Three SNPs (rs6540679, rs12569232, rs10863888) of TRAF5 and rs13210247 of TRAF3IP2 were significantly associated with Behçet's disease and VKH syndrome (corrected P values ranging from 9.45×10^{-12} to 0.027). TRAF3IP2 rs33980500 and rs13190932 were not polymorphic in Han Chinese. Following stimulation by lipopolysaccharide (LPS), carriers of the GG genotype of rs6540679/TRAF5 had a higher TRAF5 mRNA expression (p = 0.004) and an increased TNF-α (p = 0.0052) and IL-6 (p = 0.0014) level compared with AA and AG genotype carriers.

Conclusion: This study provides evidence that TRAF5 and TRAF3IP2 genes are involved in the development of BD and VKH syndrome. Functional research suggested that TRAF5 gene polymorphisms may regulate TRAF5 expression and downstream inflammatory cytokines such as TNF-α and IL-6.

Editor: Yong-Gang Yao, Kunming Institute of Zoology, Chinese Academy of Sciences, China

Funding: This work was supported by National Basic Research Program of China (973 Program) (2011CB510200), Key Project of Natural Science Foundation (81130019), Clinic Key Project of Ministry of Health, Basic Research Program of Chongqing, Research Fund for the Doctoral Program of Higher Education of China (20115503110002), Research Fund for the Doctoral Program of Higher Education of China (20115503110002), Chongqing Key Laboratory of Ophthalmology (CSTC,2008CA5003), Key Project of Health Bureau of Chongqing (2012-1-003) and Fund for PAR-EU Scholars Program. The funders had no role in study design, data collection and analysis, decision to publish, or preparation of the manuscript.

Competing Interests: The authors have declared that no competing interests exist.

* E-mail: peizengycmu@126.com

⁹ These authors contributed equally to this work.

Introduction

Uveitis is an intraocular inflammation that is caused by either infectious or noninfectious mechanisms and which can lead to serious visual impairment. To unravel the immunological mechanisms that cause uveitis we have focused on two commonly occurring uveitis entities in China, namely Behcet's disease (BD) and Vogt Koyanagi Harada (VKH) syndrome [1,2].

BD is an autoinflammatory disease characterized by a diverse spectrum of clinical manifestations including recurrent oral aphthae, uveitis, multiform skin lesions and genital ulceration [3,4]. It has a relatively high prevalence along the Silk Road countries such as Japan, China, Turkey, and the Mediterranean region [5]. The usual onset is between the age of twenty to forty. The cause of BD is still unknown but epidemiological studies have suggested that certain genetic factors play an important role in its development [6]. We and others have recently identified polymorphisms in multiple immunoregulatory genes as a risk factor for developing BD, such as CD40, STAT3, STAT4 and JAK2 [7,8,9]. These pathways are extremely complex and many other gene polymorphisms remain to be studied to unravel the exact genetic susceptibility to BD.

VKH syndrome is a multisystem autoimmune disorder directed against melanocytes and is characterized by bilateral granulomatous uveitis with meningeal irritation sign (MIS), dysacusis, vitiligo, poliosis and alopecia [10]. It is one of the most common uveitis entities in Chinese as well as in individuals of American-Indian descent. VKH has been shown to be associated with certain HLA genes [11,12]. However, this association cannot explain the whole genetic risk for VKH and further research is needed to identify potential non-HLA susceptibility genes. We have recently studied polymorphisms of various immune response genes in the pathogenesis of VKH syndrome and showed associations with several non HLA genes [13,14,15].

In our search for a possible role of as yet not identified polymorphisms in immunoregulatory genes in the pathogenesis of uveitis, we assessed factors that have been shown to play a role in autoimmune diseases that share features with uveitis. One of the polymorphic genes that were recently shown to be involved in autoimmune disease such as inflammatory bowel disease, rheumatoid arthritis and diabetes belong to the so called family of Tumor necrosis factor (TNF)-receptor-associated factors (TRAF).

TRAF5 is one of the factors belonging to the TRAF family and is significantly expressed in lung, thymus, spleen and kidney as well as in peripheral blood cells [16]. It is an adapter protein and signal transducer that links members of the tumor necrosis factor (TNF) receptor family to different signaling pathways and plays a critical role in the activation of NF-kappa-B leading to the expression of various inflammatory cytokines [17]. It has been demonstrated that TRAF5 polymorphisms are associated with susceptibility to rheumatoid arthritis (RA) [18].

TRAF3IP2 is another member of the TRAF family and encodes Act1 protein, which binds to TRAF5 thereby playing an important role in controlling inflammatory responses and autoimmunity through its effect on CD40L and IL-17 signaling [19,20,21]. Mutations of the TRAF3IP2 gene have been associated with susceptibility to several autoimmune diseases, such as psoriasis, psoriatic arthritis, chronic plaque psoriasis, inflammatory bowel disease and type 1 diabetes [22,23,24,25,26]. Of interest are the observations that IL-17 can induce Act1-TRAF2-TRAF5 complex formation leading to a downstream inflammatory response [20,27]. Earlier studies showed that Il-17 plays an important role in the pathogenesis of both BD and VKH [28,29] , providing support for a further study into a possible role of TRAF gene polymorphisms in uveitis.

Based on earlier reports in RA, psoriasis and psoriatic arthritis [18,23,24,25] and linkage disequilibrium patterns in Han Chinese, in combination with Japanese data in the Hap Map database, we selected three SNPs (rs6540679 Chr.1: 211491152, rs12569232 Chr.1: 211553064, rs10863888 Chr.1: 211502769) of TRAF5 and three SNPs (rs13210247 Chr.6: 111922720, rs33980500 Chr.6: 111913262, rs13190932 Chr.6: 111913070) of TRAF3IP2 as candidate SNPs for our study (Figure 1).

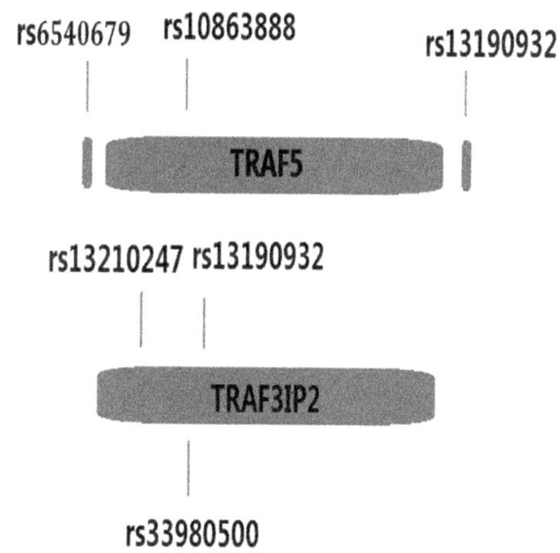

Figure 1. Schematic location of the chosen SNPs of TRAF5 and TRAF3IP2.

Methods

Patients and healthy controls study population

All subjects gave their written informed consent for this study, and the study protocol was approved by the Ethics Committee of the First Affiliated Hospital of Chongqing Medical University, Chongqing, China (Permit Number: 2009-201008). All procedures followed the tenets of the Declaration of Helsinki.

A case-control genetic study of two genes in individuals with or without uveitis was performed. 789 BD patients, 940 VKH patients and 1601 healthy unrelated individuals were included in this study. All subjects were of Han Chinese descent. Blood samples were obtained from the First Affiliated Hospital of Chongqing Medical University (Chongqing, China) and the Uveitis Study Center of the Sun Yat-sen University (Guangzhou, China) through 2005 until 2013.

The diagnosis of BD was based on the criteria of the International Study [30]. The clinical characteristics of the BD patients were assessed at the time of diagnosis and are summarized in Table S1. The diagnosis of VKH syndrome fulfilled the revised criteria for this disease [10]. The clinical characteristics of the patients are presented in Table S2.

DNA extraction and genotyping

Genomic DNA samples of BD, VKH patients and healthy controls were extracted by using the QIAamp DNA Blood Mini Kit (Qiagen, Valencia, CA). Rs6540679, rs33980500, rs13210247, rs13190932 were genotyped by polymerase chain reaction-restriction fragment length polymorphism (PCR-RFLP), the primers used to amplify the target DNA sequence by PCR are shown in Table S3. Digestion products were visualized on a 4% agarose gel and stained with GoldView^{TM} (SBS Genetech, Beijing, China). Rs12569232 (TagMan assay ID: C_26176827_20) and rs10863888 (TagMan assay ID: C_26176858_10) genotypes were investigated using the TaqMan® SNP Genotyping Assay (Applied Biosystems, Foster City, CA, USA) on the Applied Biosystems 7500 Real-Time PCR system. All the operations were performed according to manufacturers' instructions. The analysis was performed using TaqMan® Genotyper Software. Direct sequencing was also performed by the Beijing Biomed Co.,Ltd (Beijing, China) using randomly selected subjects (10% of all samples) to validate the accuracy of genotyping. The genotyping success rate of the various SNPs ranged between 93.6% and 100%.

Real-time PCR

Peripheral blood mononuclear cells (PBMCs) were prepared from heparinized blood by Ficoll-Hypaque density-gradient centrifugation. Isolated PBMCs were cultured in 24-well plates containing RPMI-1640 supplemented with 10% calf serum (Greiner, Wemmel, Belgium), 2 mM L-glutamine and 100 U/ml penicillin/streptomycin (Invitrogen, Carlsbad, CA). Cells were left unstimulated or were stimulated with a cocktail of anti-CD3 (5 µg/ml, eBioscience, San Diego, CA, USA) and anti-CD28 antibodies (5 µg/ml, eBioscience, San Diego, CA, USA) to mimic

Table 1. Polymorphisms of the TRAF5 and TRAF3IP2 genes in ocular Behçet's Disease.

Gene	SNPs	Genotype / Allele	BD n (%)	Control n (%)	P value	Pc value	OR (95%CI)
TRAF5	rs10863888	AA	74 (10)	170 (10.8)	0.566	5.094	0.919 (0.689–1.226)
		AG	359 (48.6)	650 (41.3)	0.001	0.009	1.343 (1.127–1.601)
		GG	306 (41.4)	754 (47.9)	0.003	0.027	0.769 (0.644–0.917)
		A	507 (34.3)	990 (31.4)	0.053	0.477	1.138 (0.998–1.298)
		G	971 (65.7)	2158(68.6)	0.053	0.477	0.879 (0.771–1.002)
	rs12569232	CC	9 (1.2)	20 (1.2)	0.893	8.037	0.947 (0.429–2.090)
		CG	96 (12.6)	304 (19.0)	1.20×10^{-4}	1.08×10^{-3}	0.617 (0.481–0.790)
		GG	655 (86.2)	1277(79.8)	1.56×10^{-4}	1.40×10^{-3}	1.583 (1.246–2.011)
		C	114 (7.5)	344 (10.7)	4.34×10^{-4}	1.30×10^{-3}	0.674 (0.540–0.840)
		G	1406(92.5)	2858(89.3)	4.34×10^{-4}	1.30×10^{-3}	1.484 (1.190–1.852)
	rs6540679	AA	58 (7.4)	81 (5.2)	0.036	0.324	1.449 (1.022–2.053)
		AG	355 (45.0)	497 (31.9)	4.00×10^{-10}	3.60×10^{-9}	1.750 (1.467–2.086)
		GG	376 (47.7)	982 (62.9)	1.35×10^{-12}	1.22×10^{-11}	0.536 (0.451–0.637)
		A	471 (29.8)	659 (21.1)	3.86×10^{-11}	1.16×10^{-10}	1.589 (1.384–1.824)
		G	1107(70.2)	2461(78.9)	3.86×10^{-11}	1.16×10^{-10}	0.629 (0.548–0.722)
TRAF3IP2	rs13210247	AA	539 (88.4)	1513(95.1)	1.79×10^{-8}	1.61×10^{-7}	0.391 (0.280–0.548)
		AG	71 (11.6)	76 (4.8)	7.83×10^{-9}	7.05×10^{-8}	2.626 (1.873–3.682)
		GG	0 (0.0)	2 (0.1)	0	0	
		A	1149(94.2)	3102(97.5)	6.91×10^{-8}	2.07×10^{-7}	0.417 (0.301–0.579)
		G	71 (5.8)	80 (2.5)	6.91×10^{-8}	2.07×10^{-7}	2.396 (1.728–3.322)

SNP, single-nucleotide polymorphism; VKH, Vogt-Koyanagi-Harada; BD, Behçet's disease; OR, odds ratio; CI, confidence interval; Pc, Bonferroni corrected p value which p_c equaled to a p value multiplied by 9 (for genotype) or 3 (for allele).

antigen presentation. Alternatively the cells were stimulated with LPS (1 ng/ml, Sigma-Aldrich Co. LLC), at 37°C in humidified 5% CO_2 for 72 hours at a density of 1×10^6 cells/ml. Total RNA was extracted from the cultured PBMCs using TRIzol (Invitrogen), followed by reverse transcription using a transcriptase kit (Takara Biotechnology Co. Ltd., Dalian, China.). Real-time quantitative PCR was performed to compare the mRNA expression of TRAF3IP2 and TRAF5 gene, using the Applied Biosystem 7500 Real-time PCR System and was determined using the SYBR Green I Assay kit (Applied Biosysterms) and normalized to β-actin mRNA. Relative expression levels were calculated using the $2^{-\Delta\Delta Ct}$ method. The sense and antisense primers used in this experiment are depicted in Table S4.

Cytokine Measurements

The concentration of IL-8, IL-6 and TNF-α in cell culture supernatants was measured with the human Duoset enzyme-linked immunosorbent assay (ELISA) Development kit (R&D System, Minneapolis, MN) according to the manufacturers' instructions.

Statistical analysis

Hardy-Weinberg equilibrium was tested using the $\chi2$ test for goodness of fit and a p-value<0.05 was considered as a significant disequilibrium. The patterns of linkage disequilibrium (LD) of the tested SNPs were compared using Haploview (version 4.0, Broad Institute of MIT and Harvard, Cambridge, MA). Allele and genotype frequencies were compared between patients and controls by the $\chi2$ test or two-sided Fisher' exact test using SPSS (version 13.0; SPSS Inc, Chicago, IL). The p values were corrected (p_c) with the Bonferroni correction by multiplying with the number of analyses performed. For Table 1 and Table 2, p_c equaled to a p value multiplied by 9 (for genotype analysis) or 3 (for allele analysis). A $p_c<0.05$ was considered significant.

Results

Six SNPs were successfully genotyped and confirmed to Hardy-Weinberg expectation in controls. A linkage disequilibrium analysis using Haploview software showed that the selected SNPs were not linked. Both rs33980500 and rs13190932 of the TRAF3IP2 gene were not polymorphic in Han Chinese and were therefore not analyzed further. Analysis of the clinical symptoms of our BD patients revealed six primary features, including oral ulcer (100.0%), skin lesions (78.0%), genital ulcer (57.9%), arthritis (39.1%), positive pathergy test (24.5%) and hypopyon (22.3%). The VKH patients could be subdivided according to seven clinical features, including nuchal rigidity (17.9%), headache (50.4%), scalp allergy (10.4%), tinnitus (40.5%), alopecia (39.8%), poliosis (36.6%) and vitiligo (21.5%).

Association of the TRAF5 and TRAF3IP2 gene polymorphisms with susceptibility to ocular Behçet's disease and VKH syndrome

Significant differences between BD patients and controls were observed for four SNPs. The frequencies of the rs12569232/TRAF5 CG genotype and C allele were significantly lower in BD patients ($p_c = 1.08\times10^{-3}$, OR = 0.617; $p_c = 1.30\times10^{-3}$, OR = 0.674, respectively), whereas a higher frequency of the GG genotype was observed ($p_c = 1.40\times10^{-3}$, OR = 1.583) com-

Table 2. Polymorphisms of the TRAF5 and TRAF3IP2 genes in VKH syndrome.

Gene	SNPs	Genotype	VKH	Control	P value	Pc value	OR (95%CI)
		Allele	n (%)	n (%)			
TRAF5	rs10863888	AA	94 (10.4)	170 (10.8)	0.734	6.606	0.955 (0.732–1.246)
		AG	416 (45.9)	650 (41.3)	0.027	0.243	1.204 (1.022–1.420)
		GG	397 (43.8)	754 (47.9)	0.047	0.423	0.847 (0.718–0.998)
		A	604 (33.3)	990 (31.4)	0.179	1.611	1.088 (0.962–1.231)
		G	1210 (66.7)	2158(68.6)	0.179	1.611	0.919 (0.812–1.040)
	rs12569232	CC	3 (0.3)	20 (1.2)	0.017	0.153	0.254 (0.075–0.857)
		CG	89 (9.5)	304 (19.0)	1.48×10^{-10}	1.33×10^{-9}	0.446 (0.347–0.574)
		GG	848 (90.2)	1277(79.8)	6.28×10^{-12}	5.65×10^{-11}	2.339 (1.826–2.995)
		C	95 (5.1)	344 (10.7)	3.15×10^{-12}	9.45×10^{-12}	0.442 (0.350–0.559)
		G	1785 (94.9)	2858(89.3)	3.15×10^{-12}	9.45×10^{-12}	2.262 (1.788–2.860)
	rs6540679	AA	20 (2.2)	81 (5.2)	2.90×10^{-4}	2.61×10^{-3}	0.411 (0.250–0.675)
		AG	284 (31.2)	497 (31.9)	0.751	6.759	0.972 (0.815–1.159)
		GG	605 (66.6)	982 (62.9)	0.071	0.639	1.171 (0.986–1.391)
		A	324 (17.8)	659 (21.1)	0.005	0.015	0.810 (0.699–0.939)
		G	1494 (82.2)	2461(78.9)	0.005	0.015	1.235 (1.065–1.431)
TRAF3IP2	rs13210247	AA	649 (90.0)	1513(95.1)	4.28×10^{-6}	3.85×10^{-5}	0.465 (0.333–0.648)
		AG	71 (9.8)	76 (4.8)	3.68×10^{-6}	3.31×10^{-5}	2.177 (1.556–3.048)
		GG	1 (0.1)	2 (0.1)	1.000	9.000	1.103 (0.100–12.189)
		A	1369 (94.9)	3102(97.5)	7.19×10^{-6}	2.16×10^{-5}	0.484 (0.350–0.668)
		G	73 (5.1)	80 (2.5)	7.19×10^{-6}	2.16×10^{-5}	2.068 (1.496–2.858)

pared with controls. As to rs10863888/TRAF5, an increased frequency of the AG genotype was observed in BD patients ($p_c = 0.009$, OR = 1.343), while a decreased GG frequency ($p_c = 0.027$, OR 0.769) was found. The frequency of the AG genotype and A allele of rs6540679/TRAF5 were remarkably increased ($p_c = 3.6\times10^{-9}$, OR = 1.750; $p_c = 1.16\times10^{-10}$, OR = 1.589 respectively), while the frequency of the homozygous GG genotype was markedly decreased ($p_c = 1.22\times10^{-11}$, OR = 0.536) in BD patients.

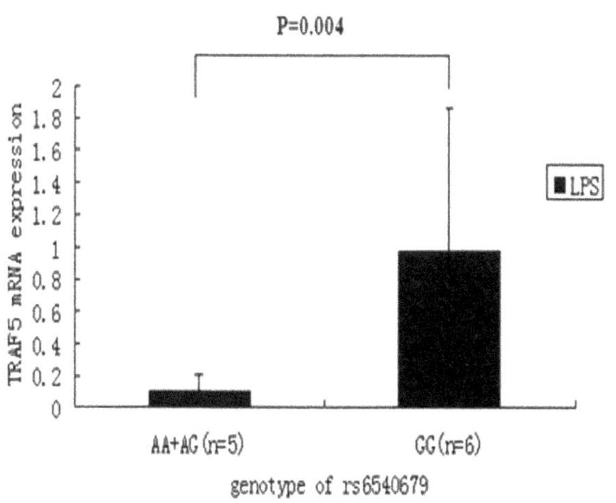

Figure 2. Effect of TRAF5 rs6540679 genotypes on mRNA expression by PBMCs stimulated with LPS (1 ng/ml). The mean ± SD is given for each genotype.

The frequencies of the AA genotype and A allele of rs13210247/TRAF3IP2 were significantly lower in BD patients ($p_c = 1.61\times10^{-7}$, OR = 0.391; $p_c = 2.07\times^{-7}$, OR = 0.417 respectively) while the frequency of the AG genotype and G allele was higher compared with controls ($p_c = 7.05\times10^{-8}$, OR = 2.626; $p_c = 2.07\times10^{-7}$, OR = 2.396 respectively) (Table 1).

Although obvious differences were found for the rs10863888 TRAF5 genotypes in VKH patients compared with healthy controls, they became non-significant after Bonferroni correction. The frequency of the CG genotype and C allele of rs12569232/TRAF5 was markedly lower in VKH patients as compared to controls. The frequency of the GG genotype was much higher ($p_c = 1.33\times10^{-9}$, OR = 0.446;. $p_c = 9.45\times10^{-12}$, OR = 0.442; $p_c = 5.65\times10^{-11}$, OR = 2.339), whereas the AA genotype and A allele of rs6540679/TRAF5 were both decreased in VKH patients ($p_c = 2.61\times10^{-3}$, OR = 0.411; $p_c = 0.015$, OR = 0.810).

As to rs13210247/TRAF3IP2, a decreased frequency of the AA genotype and A allele was observed ($p_c = 3.85\times10^{-5}$, OR = 0.465; $p_c = 2.16\times10^{-5}$, OR = 0.484) while the AG genotype was increased in VKH patients compared with normal controls ($p_c = 3.31\times10^{-5}$, OR = 2.177) (Table 2).

Relationship among genotypes, gene expression at the mRNA level and downstream inflammatory factors

Since the most significant association between TRAF gene polymorphisms and uveitis was found for TRAF5, we studied the effect of the different genotypes on the expression of TRAF5 under normal or inflammatory conditions. Real-Time PCR was performed to detect mRNA expression from PBMCs obtained from healthy controls. We genotyped 79 controls for the three SNPs of TRAF5 and then used Real-Time PCR to detect their

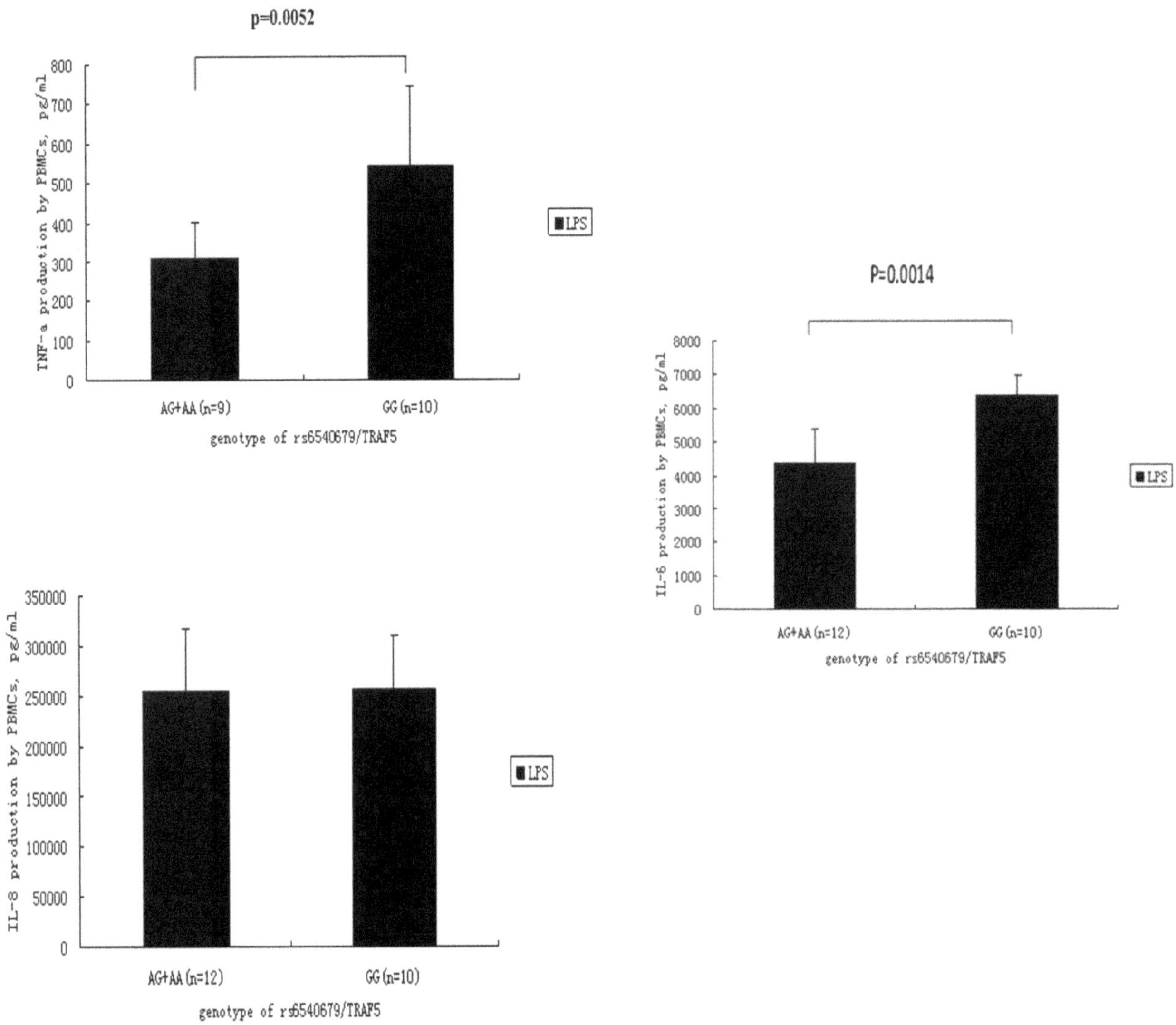

Figure 3. The effect of different genotypes of SNP rs6540679/TRAF5 on LPS-stimulated cytokine secretion by PBMCs obtained from healthy individuals. Supernatants of PBMCs co-cultured with 1 ng/mL LPS for 72 h were used to determine TRAF5 downstream cytokines (including TNF-α, IL-8, IL-6) levels by ELISA. Data are presented as means±SD.

TRAF5 expression at the mRNA level without stimulation. No difference could be detected under this condition (Figure S1). Following stimulation by LPS, carriers with the GG genotype in SNP rs6540679 had a higher TRAF5 mRNA expression compared with individuals carrying the AA and AG genotype ($p = 0.004$) (Figure 2). No effect on TRAF5 mRNA expression was observed for rs12569232 or rs10863888 (data not shown). Furthermore no effect on TRAF5 gene expression was observed when PBMCs were stimulated by a cocktail of anti-CD3/CD28 antibodies.

The aforementioned result showed that different genotypes of rs6540679/TRAF5 could affect TRAF5 expression and therefore a further study was designed to investigate if different genotypes of rs6540679/TRAF5 could also affect the cytokine response of PBMCs following LPS stimulation. We measured the level of TNF-α, IL-6 and IL-8 ($n = 22$), which are important TRAF5 downstream factors [31,32,33,34,35] in PBMC cultured supernatants by ELISA. Carriers of the GG genotype showed a higher TNF-α and IL-6 secretion, compared with AA and AG carriers ($p = 0.0052$, and $p = 0.0014$ respectively) (Figure 3). No effect of the various TRAF5 rs6540679 genotypes on IL-8 production could be detected.

Discussion

In this study, we show that TRAF5 and TRAF3IP2 gene polymorphisms are associated with VKH syndrome and ocular BD in a Han Chinese population. Highest p values were observed for the association between uveitis and TRAF5, and we therefore focused on this SNP to investigate a possible functional association. This approach revealed that carriers of the GG genotype in SNP rs6540679/TRAF5 had a higher TRAF5 mRNA expression level and enhanced TNF-α and IL-6 secretion, compared to AA and AG carriers. Expression was not altered for the other TRAF5 SNPs. We did not perform a haplotype analysis since the sample size was too small.

Our finding that the G allele of TRAF5 rs6540679 had a protective effect ($OR = 0.629$) in BD and a risk effect ($OR = 1.235$) in VKH suggests that the role of these factors depends on the

Table 3. TRAF family gene polymorphisms in autoimmune diseases.

Gene	SNP	Autoimmune Disease	Race	P value	OR (95%CI)
TRAF1 [51,52,53]	rs3761847	SLE	Japanese	0.016	1.36 (1.05–1.76)
		RA	North American & Swedish	4×10^{-14}	1.30 (1.23–1.42)
		RA	Japanese	0.031	1.18 (1.01–1.39)
	rs7021206	RA	Korean	0.0037	1.21 (1.06–1.38)
TRAF6 [54]	rs5030445	SLE	African American	0.00173	0.68 (0.53–0.87)
	rs5030437	SLE	African American	0.004456	0.70 (0.54–0.90)
	rs5030472	SLE	European	0.003342	0.65 (0.49–0.87)
	rs5030470	SLE	European	0.000179	0.55 (0.40–0.76)
TRAF3IP2 [23,24,55,56]	rs33980500	psoriasis	German	1.24×10^{-16}	*
		PsA	German	4.57×10^{-12}	1.95
		SLE	Italian	0.021	1.71
	rs13210247	psoriasis	German	$2..36\times10^{-10}$	*
		PsA	German	5.76×10^{-7}	2.08 (1.61–2.69)
		BD	Chinese	7.05×10^{-8}	2.63 (1.87–3.68)
		VKH	Chinese	3.31×10^{-5}	2.18 (1.56–3.05)
	rs13190932	PsA	German	9.19×10^{-7}	2.19 (1.66–2.88)
		UC	Italian	0.02	5.05 (1.12–2.83)
		CD	Italian	0.026	3.03 (1.1–8.3)
	rs13196377	PsA	German	9.36×10^{-7}	2.17 (1.66–2.88)
		SLE	Italian	0.002	2.59 (1.39–4.80)
		UC	Italian	0.049	4.1 (0.91–18.18)
TRAF5 [18]	rs10863888	RA	UK Caucasian	0.003	1.39 (1.11–1.75)
		BD	Chinese	0.009	1.34 (1.13–1.60)
	rs7514863	RA	UK Caucasian	0.005	1.2 (1.06–1.36)

*The data not stated in paper.
SLE, Systemic Lupus Erythematosus; RA, Rheumatoid Arthritis; PsA, Psoriatic Arthritis; UC, Ulcerative Colitis; CD, Crohn's Disease.

context whereby they are involved during the process of inflammation. Similarly TRAF rs12569232 is most significant in VKH while rs6540679 is the most significant in BD. The functional studies performed until now have only addressed the mRNA expression and as yet no studies have addressed the effect of the gene polymorphisms on the binding characteristics of the factors and their final effect on for instance NF-kappa-B activation. Both uveitis entities we investigated in this study differ markedly as to the causative mechanisms and the role of TRAF family members for each disease might be different. BD is considered to be caused by an aberrant inflammatory response towards certain environmental triggers whereas VKH is an autoimmune disease directed against melanocyte antigens [36,37]. How the members of the TRAF family exactly influence the inflammatory response in these two diseases remains to be elucidated.

Taken together, the results confirm earlier studies showing a role for TRAF5 in the control of inflammatory responses and the increased risk of certain polymorphisms of this gene for autoimmune or autoinflammatory diseases (Table 3) [17,18,32,33,34]. Of the TRAF5 polymorphisms included in our study, only rs10863888 was included in earlier studies on the association with RA. Associations with the TRAF5 SNPs rs6540679 and rs12569232 have not yet been reported earlier. On the other hand we did not include TRAF5 rs7514863, which showed an association with RA, because we designed six PCR primers of this SNP for PCR-RFLP, but none of their PCR product was satisfactory to be included in a following digestion step. In addition, no TaqMan® SNP Genotyping Assay is available for rs7514863.

VKH syndrome and BD are two of the most common uveitis entities in China [38,39]. Both diseases account for approximately one-third of the uveitis prevalence in our country [39]. The genetic background of both diseases is not yet completely clear. In recent years, we have reported on the association of various immune response related genes with the susceptibility to both BD and VKH including STAT4, STAT3, JAK2, CD40 [7,8,9,40]. In the present study, the selection of the candidate locus/gene was primarily based on GWAS data in patients with psoriasis, psoriatic arthritis (PsA) [24] and psoriasis vulgaris (PsV) [23], previously described associations for inflammatory diseases [17,25,41,42], as well as the involvement of the gene products in the control of the immune and inflammatory response [43,44,45].

TRAF5 and Act1, encoded by the TRAF3IP2 gene, have been implicated in the control of immune and inflammatory responses [44,45,46]. Both proteins act as regulators of NF-kappa-B activation. During recent years, evidence is mounting that they are involved in the pathogenesis of various autoimmune and autoinflammatory disorders [17,32,33,42,47]. In view of the fact that inflammation can induce Act1-TRAF2-TRAF5 complex formation, and in turn, can stimulate a downstream stress reaction, we aimed to assess whether these two genes were involved in the susceptibility to develop BD and VKH syndrome. The polymorphisms we used were based on earlier reports showing significant associations with RA, psoriatic arthritis, psoriasis and Inflammatory Bowel Disease [18,23,24,25] and included three SNPs (rs6540679, rs12569232, rs10863888) of TRAF5 and three SNPs (rs13210247, rs33980500, rs13190932) of TRAF3IP2 (Table 3).

To ensure the validity of our data we took the following measures. First, the sample sizes of VKH patients, BD patients and normal controls were large enough to ensure an association analysis, and our sample was larger than previous reports [7,8,18,25,32,48,49,50]. Second, the controls were strictly selected according to their birth origin to obtain a comparable immunogenetic background. Additionally, we randomly selected 10% of the samples to undergo direct sequencing to validate the results of genotyping by PCR-RFLP.

Although our results suggested that TRAF5 and TRAF3IP2 are associated with the development of BD and VKH syndrome, it is still unknown how these SNPs exert their roles in these two diseases. The complex and redundant function of the members of the TRAF family and the context they are involved in may dictate their possible divergent roles in immune mediated diseases.

Taken together, our study, for the first time, provides evidence for a role of TRAF5 and TRAF3IP2 polymorphisms in the development of BD and VKH syndrome.

Supporting Information

Table S1 Clinical features of the investigated BD patients.

Table S2 Clinical features of the investigated VKH patients.

Table S3 Primers and restriction enzymes used for RFLP analysis of the TRAF5 and TRAF3IP2 gene polymorphisms.

Table S4 RT-PCR primers for genes.

Figure S1 TRAF5 mRNA expression levels in PBMCs without stimulation, according to the genotypes of the three SNPs (rs6540679, rs10863888, rs12569232 respectively). Data are presented as means ± SD.

Acknowledgments

The authors would like to thank all donors enrolled in the present study.

Author Contributions

Conceived and designed the experiments: PY QX. Performed the experiments: QX LC SH JF YZ. Analyzed the data: QX LC SH. Contributed reagents/materials/analysis tools: YZ YL LB. Wrote the paper: QX PY AK.

References

1. Yang P, Fang W, Meng Q, Ren Y, Xing L, et al. (2008) Clinical features of Chinese patients with Behçet's disease. Ophthalmology 115: 312–318. e314.
2. Yang P, Ren Y, Li B, Fang W, Meng Q, et al. (2007) Clinical characteristics of Vogt–Koyanagi–Harada syndrome in Chinese patients. Ophthalmology 114: 606–614. e603.
3. Zhang Z, Peng J, Hou X, Dong Y (2006) Clinical manifestations of Behcet's disease in Chinese patients. APLAR Journal of Rheumatology 9: 244–247.
4. Ideguchi H, Suda A, Takeno M, Ueda A, Ohno S, et al. (2011) Behcet disease: evolution of clinical manifestations. Medicine (Baltimore) 90: 125–132.
5. Keino H, Okada AA (2007) Behcet's disease: global epidemiology of an Old Silk Road disease. Br J Ophthalmol 91: 1573–1574.
6. Meguro A, Inoko H, Ota M, Katsuyama Y, Oka A, et al. (2010) Genetics of Behçet disease inside and outside the MHC. Annals of the rheumatic diseases 69: 747–754.
7. Chen F, Hou S, Jiang Z, Chen Y, Kijlstra A, et al. (2012) CD40 gene polymorphisms confer risk of Behcet's disease but not of Vogt-Koyanagi-Harada syndrome in a Han Chinese population. Rheumatology (Oxford) 51: 47–51.
8. Hou S, Yang Z, Du L, Jiang Z, Shu Q, et al. (2012) Genome-wide association study identifies susceptible locus in STAT4 for Behcet's disease in Han Chinese. Arthritis Rheum.
9. Hu K, Hou S, Jiang Z, Kijlstra A, Yang P (2012) JAK2 and STAT3 polymorphisms in a Han Chinese population with Behcet's disease. Invest Ophthalmol Vis Sci 53: 538–541.
10. Read RW, Holland GN, Rao NA, Tabbara KF, Ohno S, et al. (2001) Revised diagnostic criteria for Vogt-Koyanagi-Harada disease: report of an international committee on nomenclature. American journal of ophthalmology 131: 647–652.
11. Davis J, Mittal K, Freidlin V, Mellow S, Optican D, et al. (1990) HLA associations and ancestry in Vogt-Koyanagi-Harada disease and sympathetic ophthalmia. Ophthalmology 97: 1137.
12. Zhao M, Jiang Y, Abrahams IW (1991) Association of HLA antigens with Vogt-Koyanagi-Harada syndrome in a Han Chinese population. Archives of ophthalmology 109: 368.
13. Jiang Z, Yang P, Hou S, Li F, Zhou H (2010) Polymorphisms of IL23R and Vogt–Koyanagi–Harada syndrome in a Chinese Han population. Human Immunology 71: 414–417.
14. Shu Q, Yang P, Hou S, Li F, Chen Y, et al. (2010) Interleukin-17 gene polymorphism is associated with Vogt–Koyanagi–Harada syndrome but not with Behçet's disease in a Chinese Han population. Human Immunology 71: 988–991.
15. Chu M, Yang P, Hu R, Hou S, Li F, et al. (2011) Elevated serum osteopontin levels and genetic polymorphisms of osteopontin are associated with Vogt-Koyanagi-Harada disease. Invest Ophthalmol Vis Sci 52: 7084–7089.
16. Au PY, Yeh WC (2007) Physiological roles and mechanisms of signaling by TRAF2 and TRAF5. Adv Exp Med Biol 597: 32–47.
17. Bulek K, Liu C, Swaidani S, Wang L, Page RC, et al. (2011) The inducible kinase IKKi is required for IL-17-dependent signaling associated with neutrophilia and pulmonary inflammation. Nat Immunol 12: 844–852.
18. Potter C, Eyre S, Cope A, Worthington J, Barton A (2007) Investigation of association between the TRAF family genes and RA susceptibility. Ann Rheum Dis 66: 1322–1326.
19. Ma AI (2012) The ubiquitous nature of IL-17. Nat Immunol 13: 1034–1035.
20. Doyle MS, Collins ES, Fitzgerald OM, Pennington SR (2012) New insight into the functions of the interleukin-17 receptor adaptor protein Act1 in psoriatic arthritis. Arthritis Res Ther 14: 226.
21. Sun D, Novotny M, Bulek K, Liu C, Li X, et al. (2011) Treatment with IL-17 prolongs the half-life of chemokine CXCL1 mRNA via the adaptor TRAF5 and the splicing-regulatory factor SF2 (ASF). Nature immunology 12: 853–860.
22. Rassi DM, Junta CM, Fachin AL, Sandrin-Garcia P, Mello S, et al. (2008) Gene expression profiles stratified according to type 1 diabetes mellitus susceptibility regions. Annals of the New York Academy of Sciences 1150: 282–289.
23. Ellinghaus E, Ellinghaus D, Stuart PE, Nair RP, Debrus S, et al. (2010) Genome-wide association study identifies a psoriasis susceptibility locus at TRAF3IP2. Nat Genet 42: 991–995.
24. Huffmeier U, Uebe S, Ekici AB, Bowes J, Giardina E, et al. (2010) Common variants at TRAF3IP2 are associated with susceptibility to psoriatic arthritis and psoriasis. Nat Genet 42: 996–999.
25. Ciccacci C, Biancone L, Di Fusco D, Ranieri M, Condino G, et al. (2012) TRAF3IP2 gene is associated with cutaneous extraintestinal manifestations in Inflammatory Bowel Disease. Journal of Crohn's and Colitis.
26. Bergholdt R, Brorsson C, Palleja A, Berchtold LA, Fløyel T, et al. (2012) Identification of novel type 1 diabetes candidate genes by integrating genome-wide association data, protein-protein interactions, and human pancreatic islet gene expression. Diabetes 61: 954–962.
27. O'Rielly DD, Rahman P (2011) Genetics of susceptibility and treatment response in psoriatic arthritis. Nat Rev Rheumatol 7: 718–732.
28. Chi W, Zhu X, Yang P, Liu X, Lin X, et al. (2008) Upregulated IL-23 and IL-17 in Behçet patients with active uveitis. Investigative ophthalmology & visual science 49: 3058–3064.

29. Chi W, Yang P, Li B, Wu C, Jin H, et al. (2007) IL-23 promotes CD4^{+} T cells to produce IL-17 in Vogt-Koyanagi-Harada disease. Journal of allergy and clinical immunology 119: 1218–1224.
30. International Study Group for Behcet's Disease (1990) Criteria for diagnosis of Behcet's disease. Lancet 335: 1078–1080.
31. Kraus ZJ, Nakano H, Bishop GA (2009) TRAF5 is a critical mediator of in vitro signals and in vivo functions of LMP1, the viral oncogenic mimic of CD40. Proceedings of the National Academy of Sciences 106: 17140–17145.
32. Cerhan JR, Liu-Mares W, Fredericksen ZS, Novak AJ, Cunningham JM, et al. (2008) Genetic variation in tumor necrosis factor and the nuclear factor-kappaB canonical pathway and risk of non-Hodgkin's lymphoma. Cancer Epidemiol Biomarkers Prev 17: 3161–3169.
33. Snell LM, Lin GH, McPherson AJ, Moraes TJ, Watts TH (2011) T-cell intrinsic effects of GITR and 4-1BB during viral infection and cancer immunotherapy. Immunol Rev 244: 197–217.
34. Zhang D, Gu T, Forsberg E, Efendic S, Brismar K, et al. (2011) Genetic and functional effects of membrane metalloendopeptidase on diabetic nephropathy development. Am J Nephrol 34: 483–490.
35. Zirlik A, Bavendiek U, Libby P, MacFarlane L, Gerdes N, et al. (2007) TRAF-1, -2, -3, -5, and -6 are induced in atherosclerotic plaques and differentially mediate proinflammatory functions of CD40L in endothelial cells. Arterioscler Thromb Vasc Biol 27: 1101–1107.
36. Sugita S, Takase H, Taguchi C, Imai Y, Kamoi K, et al. (2006) Ocular infiltrating CD4+ T cells from patients with Vogt-Koyanagi-Harada disease recognize human melanocyte antigens. Invest Ophthalmol Vis Sci 47: 2547–2554.
37. Ohno S (1981) Immunological aspects of Behçet's and Vogt-Koyanagi-Harada's diseases. Trans Ophthalmol Soc UK 101: 335–341.
38. Fang W, Yang P (2008) Vogt-koyanagi-harada syndrome. Curr Eye Res 33: 517–523.
39. Yang P, Zhang Z, Zhou H, Li B, Huang X, et al. (2005) Clinical patterns and characteristics of uveitis in a tertiary center for uveitis in China. Curr Eye Res 30: 943–948.
40. Hu K, Yang P, Jiang Z, Hou S, Du L, et al. (2010) STAT4 polymorphism in a Chinese Han population with Vogt–Koyanagi–Harada syndrome and Behçet's disease. Human Immunology 71: 723–726.
41. Jørgensen TN, Giltiay NV, Johnson A, Li X (2009) The role of Act1 in the control of autoimmunity. The Epigenetics of Autoimmune Diseases: 55–74.
42. Dolcino M, Cozzani E, Riva S, Parodi A, Tinazzi E, et al. (2012) Gene expression profiling in dermatitis herpetiformis skin lesions. Clin Dev Immunol 2012: 198956.
43. Kitamei H, Iwabuchi K, Namba K, Yoshida K, Yanagawa Y, et al. (2006) Amelioration of experimental autoimmune uveoretinitis (EAU) with an inhibitor of nuclear factor-κB (NF-κB), pyrrolidine dithiocarbamate. Journal of leukocyte biology 79: 1193–1201.
44. Niccoli L, Nannini C, Benucci M, Chindamo D, Cassara E, et al. (2007) Long-term efficacy of infliximab in refractory posterior uveitis of Behcet's disease: a 24-month follow-up study. Rheumatology (Oxford) 46: 1161–1164.
45. Okada AA, Goto H, Ohno S, Mochizuki M (2012) Multicenter study of infliximab for refractory uveoretinitis in Behçet disease. Arch Ophthalmol 130: 592–598.
46. Qian Y, Liu C, Hartupee J, Altuntas CZ, Gulen MF, et al. (2007) The adaptor Act1 is required for interleukin 17–dependent signaling associated with autoimmune and inflammatory disease. Nature immunology 8: 247–256.
47. Hunter CA (2007) Act1-ivating IL-17 inflammation. Nat Immunol 8: 232–234.
48. Li H, Liu Q, Hou S, Du L, Zhou Q, et al. (2013) TNFAIP3 gene polymorphisms confer risk for Behcet's disease in a Chinese Han population. Hum Genet 132: 293–300.
49. Zhou Q, Hou S, Liang L, Li X, Tan X, et al. (2012) MicroRNA-146a and Ets-1 gene polymorphisms in ocular Behcet's disease and Vogt-Koyanagi-Harada syndrome. Ann Rheum Dis.
50. Jiang Z, Yang P, Hou S, Du L, Xie L, et al. (2010) IL-23R gene confers susceptibility to Behcet's disease in a Chinese Han population. Ann Rheum Dis 69: 1325–1328.
51. Nishimoto K, Kochi Y, Ikari K, Yamamoto K, Suzuki A, et al. (2010) Association study of TRAF1-C5 polymorphisms with susceptibility to rheumatoid arthritis and systemic lupus erythematosus in Japanese. Annals of the rheumatic diseases 69: 368–373.
52. Plenge RM, Seielstad M, Padyukov L, Lee AT, Remmers EF, et al. (2007) TRAF1–C5 as a risk locus for rheumatoid arthritis—a genomewide study. New England Journal of Medicine 357: 1199–1209.
53. Han TU, Bang SY, Kang C, Bae SC (2009) TRAF1 polymorphisms associated with rheumatoid arthritis susceptibility in Asians and in Caucasians. Arthritis & Rheumatism 60: 2577–2584.
54. Namjou B, Choi CB, Harley IT, Alarcón-Riquelme ME, Kelly JA, et al. (2012) Evaluation of TRAF6 in a large multiancestral lupus cohort. Arthritis & Rheumatism 64: 1960–1969.
55. Perricone C, Ciccacci C, Ceccarelli F, Di Fusco D, Spinelli FR, et al. (2013) TRAF3IP2 gene and systemic lupus erythematosus: association with disease susceptibility and pericarditis development. Immunogenetics 65: 703–709.
56. Ciccacci C, Biancone L, Di Fusco D, Ranieri M, Condino G, et al. (2013) TRAF3IP2 gene is associated with cutaneous extraintestinal manifestations in Inflammatory Bowel Disease. Journal of Crohn's and Colitis 7: 44–52.

T Cell Post-Transcriptional miRNA-mRNA Interaction Networks Identify Targets Associated with Susceptibility/ Resistance to Collagen-induced Arthritis

Paula B. Donate[1,9], Thais A. Fornari[1,9], Claudia Macedo[1], Thiago M. Cunha[2], Daniele C. B. Nascimento[2], Elza T. Sakamoto-Hojo[3], Eduardo A. Donadi[4], Fernando Q. Cunha[2], Geraldo A. Passos[1,5*]

1 Molecular Immunogenetics Group, Department of Genetics, Faculty of Medicine of Ribeirão Preto, University of São Paulo, Ribeirão Preto, Brazil, **2** Inflammation and Pain Group, Department of Pharmacology, Faculty of Medicine of Ribeirão Preto, Ribeirão Preto, Brazil, **3** Department of Biology, Faculty of Philosophy, Sciences and Letters of Ribeirão Preto, Ribeirão Preto, Brazil, **4** Division of Clinical Immunology, Department of Medicine, Faculty of Medicine of Ribeirão Preto, Ribeirão Preto, Brazil, **5** Disciplines of Genetics and Molecular Biology, Department of Morphology, Faculty of Dentistry of Ribeirão Preto, Ribeirão Preto, Brazil

Abstract

Background: Due to recent studies indicating that the deregulation of microRNAs (miRNAs) in T cells contributes to increased severity of rheumatoid arthritis, we hypothesized that deregulated miRNAs may interact with key mRNA targets controlling the function or differentiation of these cells in this disease.

Methodology/Principal Findings: To test our hypothesis, we used microarrays to survey, for the first time, the expression of all known mouse miRNAs in parallel with genome-wide mRNAs in thymocytes and naïve and activated peripheral $CD3^+$ T cells from two mouse strains the DBA-1/J strain (MHC-H2q), which is susceptible to collagen induced arthritis (CIA), and the DBA-2/J strain (MHC-H2d), which is resistant. Hierarchical clustering of data showed the several T cell miRNAs and mRNAs differentially expressed between the mouse strains in different stages of immunization with collagen. Bayesian statistics using the $GenMir^{++}$ algorithm allowed reconstruction of post-transcriptional miRNA-mRNA interaction networks for target prediction. We revealed the participation of **miR-500, miR-202-3p** and **miR-30b***, which established interactions with at least one of the following mRNAs: Rorc, Fas, Fasl, Il-10 and Foxo3. Among the interactions that were validated by calculating the minimal free-energy of base pairing between the miRNA and the 3′UTR of the mRNA target and luciferase assay, we highlight the interaction of miR-30b*-Rorc mRNA because the mRNA encodes a protein implicated in pro-inflammatory Th17 cell differentiation (Rorγt). FACS analysis revealed that Rorγt protein levels and Th17 cell counts were comparatively reduced in the DBA-2/J strain.

Conclusions/Significance: This result showed that the miRNAs and mRNAs identified in this study represent new candidates regulating T cell function and controlling susceptibility and resistance to CIA.

Editor: Eric Jan, University of British Columbia, Canada

Funding: This study was supported by grants from Fundação de Amparo a Pesquisa do Estado de São Paulo (FAPESP) (grant number 08/56594-8), Conselho Nacional de Desenvolvimento Científico e Tecnológico (CNPq) and Coordenação de Aperfeiçoamento de Pessoal de Nível Superior (CAPES). The funders had no role in study design, data collection and analysis, decision to publish, or preparation of the manuscript.

Competing Interests: The authors declare that no competing interests exist.

* E-mail: passos@usp.br

9 These authors contributed equally to this work.

Introduction

Rheumatoid arthritis (RA) is a systemic autoimmune disorder characterized by inflammation of the synovial tissue that can lead to destruction of bone and cartilage, eventually leading to disability [1,2]. The mechanisms involved in disease initiation and progression are still incompletely understood, as RA has a complex component controlled by several genes that interact together with environmental and stochastic factors [2].

A hallmark feature of RA pathology is the infiltration and accumulation of T cells in the synovial tissue [3]. The T cells isolated from the synovial and joint tissue show an activated and memory phenotype. These cells appear to respond poorly to stimulation with mitogen or antigens in vitro and fail to undergo apoptosis [4]. The mechanisms underlying the impaired apoptosis of T cells in RA remain largely unclear. Inhibition of apoptosis causes these cells to accumulate in both the synovia and the periphery. Due to the inherent difficulty in studying these questions in humans, researchers use collagen-induced arthritis (CIA) in mice as an animal model of autoimmune inflammatory polyarthritis reproducing many of the clinical and pathological features of human RA [5]. Similar to RA, susceptibility to CIA has a genetic basis that is associated with certain MHC-II alleles (H2-Aq and H2-Ar) that make certain mouse strains susceptible [6].

The molecular genetics of RA and CIA is an emerging field with contributions from our group [7–10] and from others [11,12] that have demonstrated an association between transcriptional expression profiles of mRNAs and RA. Recent data suggest that certain microRNAs (miRNAs) in T cells might play a role in the onset of this disease [13], and several groups have focused their attention on the role played by miRNAs in the pathogenesis of RA, as well as their potential use as biomarkers to monitor the disease [14,15].

MiRNAs have emerged as post-transcriptional regulators of gene expression in a variety of biological processes [16–19]. They regulate protein expression via complementary sequence recognition of the 3′ untranslated region (3′UTR) of the target mRNA, triggering the degradation of the target transcript if miRNA-mRNA hybridization is faultless [20–22]. A recent paper indicated that the major effect of miRNAs is to decrease mRNA levels [23]. MiRNAs can potentially regulate hundreds of proteins [24] and modulate the concentration of proteins over a narrow range in a dose-dependent manner [25].

These molecules are involved in hematopoietic cell function and development, and a few miRNAs have been linked to specific T lymphocyte mechanisms. For example, miR-181a [26], miR-181c [27], miR-155 [28], miR-150 [29], miR-146 [13], and miR-142 [30] regulate T cell sensitivity to antigen stimulation, transcription factors, and activation-induced cell death.

Different miRNA expression patterns in RA patients and healthy controls or patients affected by osteoarthritis [14,31] have been the focus of many studies. Most studies have examined miRNA expression in plasma and serum, while others focused mainly on tissue analysis [15]. Several miRNAs were identified in the T cells of RA patients. MiR-223 is upregulated in $CD4^+$ naïve T lymphocytes [32]. As T lymphocytes are considered to play a role in the pathogenesis of RA, these results suggest that this miRNA could influence the T cell response and therefore contribute to disease onset. A recent study showed that miR-363 and miR-498 are downregulated in the $CD4^+$ T cells of RA patients, while miR-146a expression is significantly upregulated [13].

In this study, we used a multidimensional approach to integrate genome-wide miRNA and mRNA expression. We surveyed, for the first time, the expression of mouse miRNA sequences in thymocytes, naïve and activated T cells in two mouse strains, the DBA-1/J strain, which is susceptible to CIA, and the DBA-2/J refractory strain. In parallel, we profiled global mRNA levels, including the entire mouse genome (transcriptome profiling). Using the $GenMiR^{++}$ program, which is a Bayesian statistics-based data analysis algorithm and designed to reconstruct miRNA-mRNA networks interactions, important mRNAs related to the immune system, T cell function and differentiation were found as potential targets.

The majority of miRNA-mRNA interactions were validated by calculations of the minimal Gibbs free-energy using the RNA-Hybrid algorithm [33,34] and two of them (miR30b*-Rorγt mRNA and miR196b-CD8a mRNA) were confirmed to occurs within the cellular milieu by the luciferase assay. We highlighted miR-30b* interacting with RORγt mRNA because the encoded protein (RORγt) plays a role as a transcription factor involved in Th17 cell differentiation [35]. We observed that both RORγt mRNA and protein were down-regulated in the DBA-2/J strain, which is refractory to CIA. Moreover, the proportion of Th17 cells in this strain is lower than that found in the DBA-1/J strain.

In this study we identified novel miRNAs involved in T cell function in the context of autoimmunity of CIA model-system and provided evidence for their role in post-transcriptional networks involving key mRNAs. Evidence was taken that modulation of which might control the susceptibility/resistance to CIA in mice.

Materials and Methods

Animals

Male DBA/1J and DBA-2/J mice (4 and 12 weeks old) weighing 18–22 g each were housed in temperature-controlled rooms (22°C) in the animal facility of the School of Medicine of Ribeirão Preto, University of São Paulo, Ribeirão Preto, Brazil, and received water and food *ad libitum*. All experimental protocols were approved by the local Ethical Committee on Animal Experimentation of the Faculty of Medicine of Ribeirão Preto (Permit Number: 119/2008).

Induction and Assessment of Collagen-induced Arthritis

Male DBA/1J and DBA-2/J mice received 200 μg of a chicken type II collagen (Sigma-Aldrich St. Louis, MO, USA) emulsion in complete Freund's adjuvant (CFA) by intradermal injection (day 0). A second injection of collagen (200 μg dissolved in sterile apyrogenic pH 7.2 phosphate buffered saline, (PBS) was given on day 21 by intradermal injection [36]. Mice were monitored daily for signs of arthritis for which severity scores were derived as follows: 0 = normal paw, 1 = paw with erythema, 2 = paw with erythema plus swelling, and 3 = paw with extension/loss function. The total score indicated the sum of the individual scores for all four limbs. Disease onset characterized by erythema and/or paw swelling was observed between days 25 and 35. The control group corresponded to the sham-immunized mice, which only received an injection of CFA.

Thymocytes and $CD3^+$ T cell Isolation

The thymi from five 4-week-old male DBA-1/J and DBA-2/J mice were dissected and trimmed of fat and connective tissue in DMEM/F10 medium, and thymocytes were obtained by 2–3 passages of the thymic fragments throughout a 10-μm mesh nylon membrane (Sefar Inc. Depew, NY, USA). Pelleted thymocytes were suspended in PBS. Fluorescent-activated cell sorting (FACS) analysis in a BD-FACScalibur flow cytometer with a phycoerythrin (PE)-labeled anti-CD3 antibody indicated that this procedure yielded approximately 93% purity of the thymocyte population. These cells were then used for total RNA preparation. The peripheral $CD3^+$ T lymphocytes from five 4-week-old non-immunized mice (here, considered as naïve) and five 12-week-old control and collagen immunized male mice of both strains were isolated from the inguinal lymph nodes and spleens using magnetic beads for negative selection (Pan T-cell isolation kit, mouse, Miltenyi Biotec), according to the manufacturer's instructions. The FACS analysis with PE-labeled anti-CD3 antibody indicated that this procedure yielded a $CD3^+$ T lymphocyte population of approximately 88% purity. These cells were then used for total RNA preparation. All hybridizations of RNA pools were performed in triplicate for mRNA or in duplicate for miRNA microarrays.

Total RNA Extraction

The total RNA was extracted from approximately 1×10^7 thymocytes or peripheral T CD3+ lymphocytes using the mirVana total RNA isolation kit (Ambion, NY, USA), according to the manufacturer's instructions. RNA preparations were confirmed to be free of proteins and phenol by UV spectrophotometry. RNA degradation was assessed by microfluidic electrophoresis using Agilent 6000 RNA Nano chips and an Agilent 2100 Bioanalyzer (Agilent Technologies, Santa Clara, CA, USA). Only RNA samples that were free of proteins and phenol and featured an RNA Integrity Number (RIN) ≥9.0 were used.

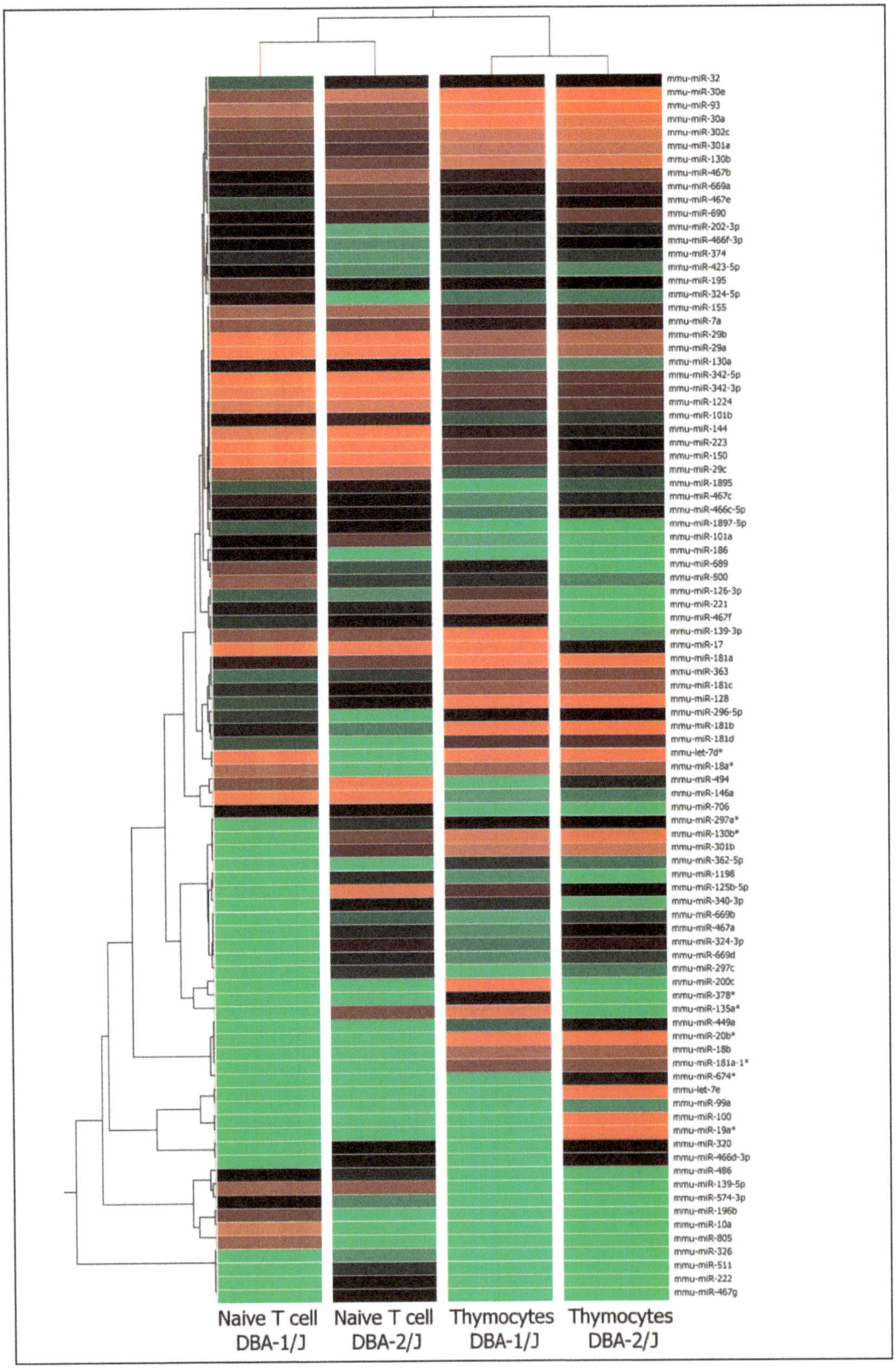

Figure 1. Modulation of miRNAs as evaluated by microarrays. Hierarchical clustering and color heat-map of miRNome (miRNAs) of thymocytes isolated from 4-week-old DBA-1/J and DBA-2/J mice and $CD3^+$ T cells from the spleen and lymph nodes of 4-week-old mice from both strains based on microarray expression profiling. The dendrogram and heat-map were obtained using cluster and tree-view algorithms through Agilent GeneSpring platform. Heat map legend: Red = up regulation, green = down regulation, black = unmodulated (Pearson correlation metrics).

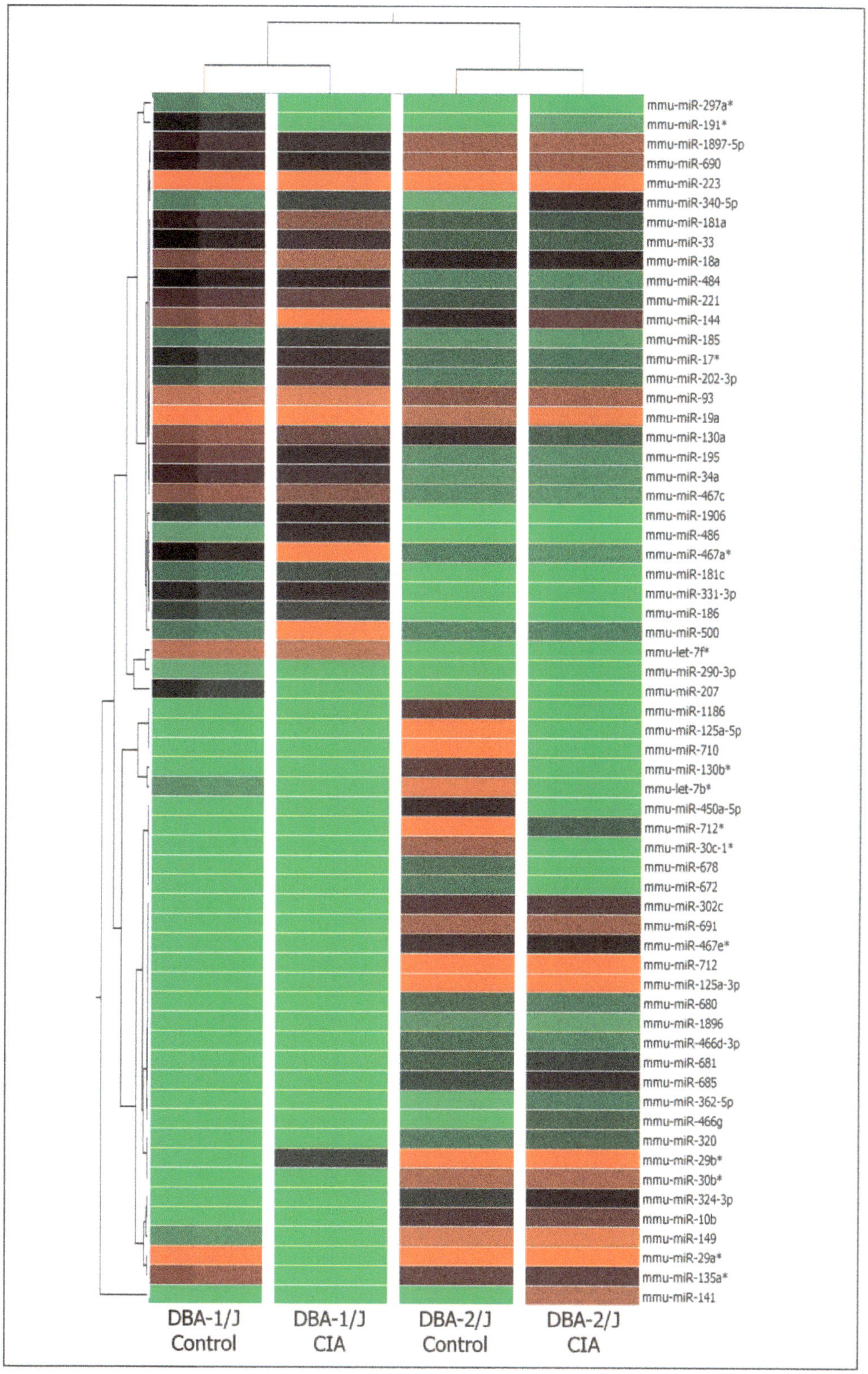

Figure 2. Modulation of miRNAs as evaluated by microarrays during collagen induced arthritis (CIA). Hierarchical clustering and color heat-map of miRNome (miRNAs) of CD3$^+$ T cells from the spleen and lymph nodes of 12-week-old mice from the resistant DBA-2/J and the susceptible DBA-1/J strain, both immunized with chicken type II collagen, based on microarray expression profiling. The control mice were immunized just with complete Freund's adjuvant (CFA) without any collagen. The dendrogram and heat-map were obtained using cluster and tree-view algorithms through Agilent GeneSpring platform. Heat map legend: Red = up regulation, green = down regulation, black = unmodulated (Pearson correlation metrics).

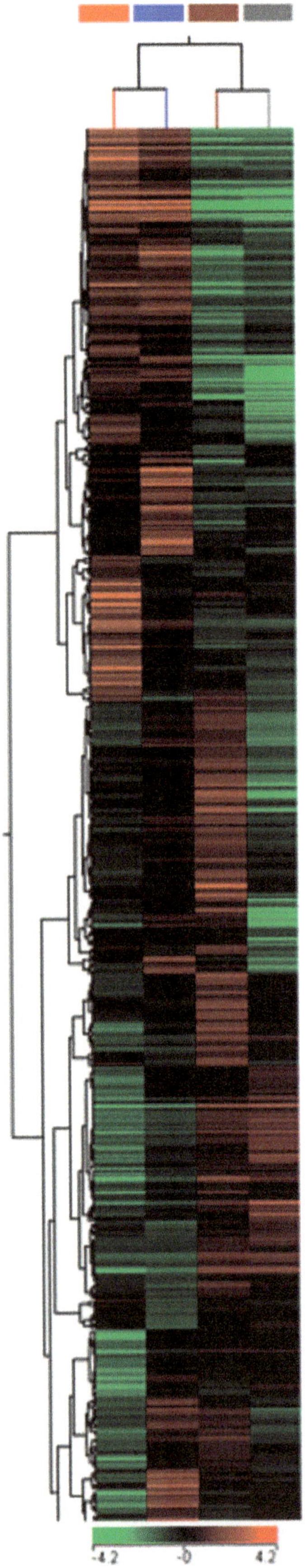

Figure 3. Modulation of mRNAs as evaluated by microarrays. Hierarchical clustering and color heat-map of the transcriptome (mRNAs) of thymocytes isolated from 28-day-old DBA-1/J and DBA-2/J mice and $CD3^+$ T cells from the spleen and lymph nodes of 4-week-old mice from both strains based on microarray expression profiling. The dendrogram and heat-map were obtained using cluster and tree-view algorithms through Agilent GeneSpring platform. This figure shows the modulation of genes related to immune system based on Gene Ontology (GO terms). Heat map legend: Red = up regulation, green = -down regulation, black = unmodulated (Pearson correlation metrics). Sample dendrogram legend: red-line = Naïve T cell DBA-1/J; blue-line = Naïve T cell DBA-2/J; brown-line = Thymocytes DBA-1/J; gray-line = Thymocytes DBA-2/J.

Microarray Hybridizations

mRNA expression profiling using agilent 4×44 K mouse oligo arrays. Individual 500 ng total RNA were used to synthesize double-stranded cDNA and cyanine 3 (Cy3)-CTP-labeled complementary amplified RNA (cRNA) using the Agilent Linear Amplification Kit (Agilent Technologies, Santa Clara, CA, USA), according to the manufacturer's instructions. Cyanine-labeled complementary RNA was hybridized to microarrays in SureHyb chambers (Agilent) in a rotator oven using Agilent mouse 4×44 K oligonucleotide microarrays (Agilent Technologies) for 18 h at 60°C. Each array contained 44,000 oligonucleotide probes covering the entire mouse functional genome plus internal control probes. The arrays were washed according to the manufacturer's instructions and scanned using an Agilent DNA Microarray scanner.

miRNA Expression Profiling using Agilent 8×15 K Mouse Oligo Arrays

The total RNA samples were Cy-3-labeled using the Agilent miRNA Complete Labeling and Hybridization Kit (Agilent Tech, Mississauga, ON, Canada). Briefly, 100 ng of total RNA was dephosphorylated by incubation with calf intestinal phosphatase at 37°C for 30 min, denatured in 100% DMSO at 100°C for 5 minutes and labeled with perCp-Cy3 using T4 ligase at 16°C for 1 h. Each labeled RNA sample was hybridized to an individual array on an 8×15 K format Agilent mouse miRNA array slides. Each array contained probes for 567 mouse miRNAs and 10 mouse gamma herpes virus miRNAs. Hybridizations were performed in SureHyb chambers (Agilent) for 20 h at 55°C, washed according to the manufacturer's instructions and scanned.

Microarray Data Analysis

The oligo-mRNA and oligo-miRNA array slides were scanned using a DNA microarray scanner (Agilent Technologies), and the hybridization signals were extracted using the Agilent Feature Extraction software version 10.5. Gene expression profiles from independent preparations of thymocytes (from 4-week-old DBA-1/J and DBA-2/J mice) or $CD3^+$ peripheral lymphocytes (from 4 and 12-week-old DBA-1/J and DBA-2/J mice) were analyzed by comparing the microarray hybridizations of the respective samples. Figure S1 depicts the experimental design for further comparison of the gene profiling. The microarray numerical quantitative data were normalized to the 75th percentile and were analyzed using the GeneSpring GX bioinformatics platform (http://www.agilent.com/chem/genespring) according to default instructions allowing for hierarchical clustering of samples of mice or genes based on an ANOVA statistical analysis ($P<0.05$), fold change ≥2.0 and uncentered Pearson correlation metrics [37].

The similarities and dissimilarities in gene expression (mRNA and miRNA) are presented as dendrograms in which the pattern and length of the branches reflect the relatedness of the samples or

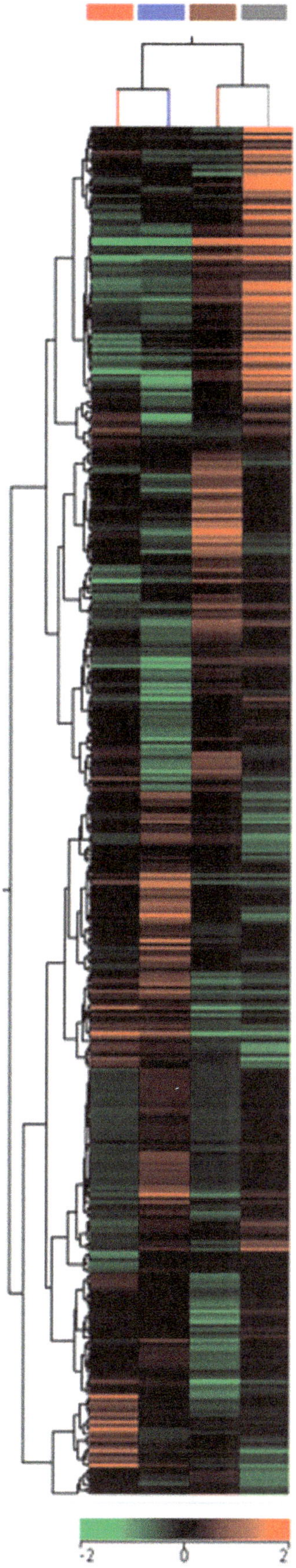

Figure 4. Modulation of mRNAs as evaluated by microarrays during collagen induced arthritis (CIA). Hierarchical clustering and color heat-map of the transcriptome (mRNAs) of CD3+ T cells from the spleen and lymph nodes of 12-week-old mice from the resistant DBA-2/J strain and the susceptible DBA-1/J strain immunized with chicken type II collagen, based on microarray expression profiling. The control mice were immunized just with complete Freund's adjuvant (CFA) without any collagen. The dendrogram and heat-map were obtained using cluster and tree-view algorithms through Agilent GeneSpring platform. This figure shows the expression of genes related to immune system function based on Gene Ontology (GO terms). Heat map legend: Red = up regulation, green = down regulation, black = unmodulated (Pearson correlation metrics). Sample dendrogram legend: red-line = -DBA-1/J control; blue-line = DBA-1/J CIA; brown-line = DBA-2/J control; gray-line = DBA-2/J CIA.

genes and heat maps. Gene ontology annotations were retrieved from the GeneSpring platform and were used to assess the biological functions of mRNAs based on a corrected p value <0.05 and cut-off = 0.1. Information about the miRNAs was retrieved from the miRBase data bank (www.mirbase.org).

A complete file that provides all of the mRNAs and miRNAs present in the arrays used in this study, as well as the experimental conditions, is available online at the MIAME public database (http://www.ebi.ac.uk/miamexpress), Array Express accession E-MEXP-3369 (for mRNA hybridizations) and E-MEXP-3370 (for miRNA hybridizations).

Reconstruction of miRNA-mRNA Post-transcriptional Interaction Networks

We used the GenMiR^{++} algorithm to reconstruct the miRNA-mRNA interaction networks, which use as a basis the respective miRNA and mRNA expression profiles from the same sets of tissues or cell types to identify candidate miRNA-mRNA target pairs that are best supported by the expression data, and a database of a potential set of mRNA targets for each miRNA identified [38]. In this study, we used the TargetScanS database (http://www.targetscan.org/) to select the target mRNA set.

For each mRNA differentially expressed, the candidate miRNA regulators were scored according to how much the miRNA expression profile contributed to explaining the down-regulation of the mRNA expression, given all other miRNA candidates.

GenMiR^{++} calculates the scores by attempting to reproduce an mRNA's profile by a weighted combination of the genome-wide average normalized expression profile and the negatively weighted profiles of a subset of the miRNA regulators. The miRNAs that often appear in subsets whose reproductions are good fits to the mRNA profile are assigned the highest scores. The scores are plotted and a reasonable threshold was determined to select no more than the top 20% of interactions predicted by GenMiR++. The graphical Cytoscape v 2.1 program (www.cytoscape.org) was used to design the networks.

Validations of miRNA-mRNA Interactions

Determination of hybridization minimum free energy. Observing the miRNA-mRNA interaction networks generated by the GenMiR^{++} algorithm, we selected pairs based on the biological function of the mRNA target. The RNA-hybrid algorithm [33,34], which is available at (http://bibiserv.techfak.uni-bielefeld.de/rnahybrid), was then used to validate the annealing. This method involves a dynamic programming algorithm that calculates the most favorable hybridization between a given miRNA and its mRNA target, calculating the minimum free energy (MFE) based on a thermodynamic state that postulates

Table 1. Up-regulated microRNAs in thymocytes and CD3+T lymphocytes in DBA-1/J and DBA-2/J mice strains and their potential targets related to immune system predicted by GenMiR++.

MicroRNAs	Potencial targets
miR-221	Add2, Ank1, Camp, Meis1, Pawr, S100a9, Sox6, Tlr3
miR-126-3p	Add2, Ank1, Camp, Epb4.2, Meis1, Pawr, Sox6, Spna1, Tlr3
miR-200c	Add2, Ahsp, Ank1, Bcl11a, Car2, Cd55, Cd59a, Cd59b, Cd83, Ctsg, Cxcl9, Enpp3, Epb4.2, Epor, Hspa1b, Igj, Il1rl1, Klf1, Lmo2, Meis1, Mpo, Ncf1, Pawr, Ptger3, Snca, Sox6, Sphk1, Spna1, Spon2, Tal1, Tlr3, Trim10, Zbtb32
miR-let-7e	Add2, Adora2b, Ahsp, Ank1, C4bp, Cd59a, Csf1r,Defb6, Enpp3, Epas1, Epb4.2, Fyb, Ghr, Gm5077, Gnas, Grin2b, H28, H2-Q10, Hoxa9, Klf1, Lifr, Lmo2, Mecom, Meis1, Mpl, Ms4a2, Pawr, Pbx1, Snca, Sox6, Sphk1, Spna1, Tal1, Tgfb2, Tlr3, Trim10
miR-100	Add2, Adora2b, Ahsp, Ank1, Cd59a, Csf1r, Ctsg, Defb6, Enpp3, Epas1, Epb4.2, Epor, Fyb, Ghr, Gm5077, Grin2b, H28, H2-Q10, Hdac9, Hoxa9, Il1rl1, Klf1, Lifr, Lmo2, Meis1, Mpl, Mpo, Ms4a2, Pawr, Smap1, Snca, Sox6, Sphk1,Spna1,Tal1, Tgfb2, Tlr3, Trim10, Zbtb7a
miR-19a*	Add2, Ahsp, Ank1, Cd59a, Csf1r, Defb6, Enpp3, Epas1, Epb4.2, Epor, Fyb, Gm5077, Grin2b, H28, H2-Q10, Hdac9, Hoxa9, Klf1, Lifr, Lmo2, Meis1,Mpl, Ms4a2,Pawr, Snca, Sox6, Sphk1, Spna1, Tal1, Tgfb2, Tlr3, Trim10
miR-195	Add2, Ank1, Camp, Enpp3, Epb4.2, Meis1, Ms4a2, Pawr, S100a9, Sox6, Spna1, Tlr3
miR-689	Add2, Ank1, Camp, Endou, Ly6d, Meis1, Pawr, Rag1, S100a9, Sox6, Tlr3
miR-500	Add2, Ank1, Camp, Meis1, Pawr, Rag1, S100a9, Sox6, Tlr3
miR-196b	Bcl11b, Camp, Ccl12, Cd247, Cd8a, Endou, Il5ra, Lig4, Ly6d, Mr1, Pax1, Rag1, Rag2, Rorc, S100a9, Sh2d1a, Themis, Thy1
miR-10a	Bcl11b, C1qc, Camp, Ccl12, Ccl24, Ccl8, Cd247, Cd4, Cd8a, Cfb,Endou, Esr2, Il5ra, Lig4, Ly6d, Mr1, P2rx1, Pax1, Rag1, Rag2, Rorc, Rtkn2, S100a9, Satb1, Sh2d1a, Sla2, Socs1, Sox4, Themis, Thy1
miR-805	Bcl11b, C1qc, Camp, Ccl12, Ccl24, Cd247, Cd8a, Endou, Esr2, Il5ra, Lifr, Lig4,Ly6d, Rag1, Rag2, Rorc, S100a9, Themis, Thy1
miR-125-5p	Add2, Adora2b, Ank1, Cd59a, Enpp3, Epas1, Epb4.2, H28, Hspa1b, Klf1, Lmo2, Meis1, Ms4a2, Pawr, Pbx1, Sox6, Sphk1, Spna1, Tlr3
miR-467e	Add2, Ank1, Camp, Enpp3, Epb4.2, H28, Meis1, Ms4a2, Pawr, Sox6, Spna1, Tlr3
miR-669a	Add2, Adora2b, Ank1, Camp, Enpp3, Epas1, Epb4.2, Meis1, Ms4a2, Pawr, Pbx1, S100a9, Sox6, Spna1, Tlr3
miR-101a	Add2, Ank1, Camp, Endou, Ly6d, Meis1,Pawr, Rag1, Rag2, S100a9, Sox6
miR-144	Aicda, Azgp1, Bank1, Btla, Cbfb, Cd1d2, Cd247, Cd38, Cd79b, Cx3cr1, Cxcr4, Cxcr5, Fcgr2b, Gimap5, Gnas, H2-Ab1, H2-DMb2, H2-Ea, H2-Eb1, H2-T3, Hdac9, Hspa1b, Icam1, Igh-6, Il1rap, Inhba, Klhl6, Ly6d, Lyn, Mll5, Ms4a1, Mx1, Mx2, Oas1b, Orm2, Pdcd1lg2, Pou2f2, Prkca, Prkcd, Ptprc, Ripk2, Rogdi, Sh2d1b1, Spib, Tlr1, Tlr7, Tnfrsf13c, Twsg1, Fas, Gzma, Gzmm, Il10
miR-17*	Bad, Btla, Cd28, Cd38, Csf1r, Cxcr4, Dock2, Gnas, Hdac9, Hspa1b, Kdr, Klhl6, Lyn, Mll5, Nfkb1, Orm2, Pdcd1lg2, Pecam1, Pou2f2, Ptprc, Rab27a, Rogdi, Rsad2, Sh2b3, Sh2d1b1, Slc11a1, Tlr1, Tlr2, Tlr7
miR-181a	Aicda, Bank1, Btla, Cbfb, Cd79b, Cx3cr1, Gnas, H2-Ab1, H2-DMb2, H2-Ea, H2-Eb1, H2-T3, Hdac9, Hspa1b, Icam1, Il1rap, Inhba, Klhl6, Lyn, Ms4a1, Mx1, Orm2, Pdcd1lg2, Prkcd, Ptprc, Ripk2, Sh2d1b1, Spib, Tnfrsf13c, Gzma, Gzmm, Il10
miR-202-3p	Aicda, Azgp1, Bank1, Btla, C3, Cbfb, Cd1d2, Cd247, Cd38, Cd79b, Cx3cr1, Cxcr4, Cxcr5, Ddx58, Fcgr2b, Gimap5, Gnas, H2-Aa, H2-Ab1, H2-DMa, H2-DMb2, H2-Ea, H2-Eb1, H2-T3, Hdac9, Hspa1b, Hspa1b, Icam1, Igh-6, Il1rap, Il2ra, Inhba, Klhl6, Ly6d, Lyn, Mll5, Ms4a1, Mx1, Mx2, Oas1b, Orm2, Pbx1, Pdcd1lg2, Pou2f2, Prkca, Prkcd, Ptprc, Ripk2, Rogdi, Sh2d1b1, Spib, Tlr1, Tlr7, Tnfrsf13c, Twsg1, Fas, Gzma, Gzmm, Il10
MicroRNAs	Potencial targets
miR-467a*	Aicda, Azgp1, Bad, Bank1, Blnk, Btla, C3, Cbfb, Cd1d2, Cd247, Cd28, Cd38, Cd55, Cd79b, Clcf1, Csf1r, Cx3cr1, Cxcr4, Cxcr5, Ddx58, Dock2, Fcgr2b, Gimap5, Gnas, H2-Aa, H2-Ab1, H2-DMa, H2-DMb1, H2-DMb2, H2-Ea, H2-Eb1, H2-T3, Hdac9, Hoxb3, Hspa1b, Icam1, Igh-6, Il1rap, Il2ra, Inhba, Kdr, Klhl6, Lat2, Ly6d, Lyn, Mll5, Ms4a1, Mx1, Mx2, Myo1e, Nfam1, Nfkb1, Oas1b, Orm2, Pbx1, Pdcd1lg2, Plcg2, Pou2f2, Prkca, Prkcd, Ptprc, Ripk2, Rogdi, Rsad2, Selp, Sfpi1, Sh2b3, Sh2d1b1, Slc11a1, Spib, Tapbp, Tlr1, Tlr7, Tnfrsf13c, Twsg1, Ywhaz, Fas, Fasl, Gzma, Gzmm
miR-500	Aicda, Azgp1, Bad, Bank1, Blnk, Btla, C3, Card11, Cbfb, Ccl1, Ccl5, Cd1d1, Cd1d2, Cd247, Cd28, Cd38, Cd40lg, Cd55, Cd79b, Cd80, Cebpg, Clcf1, Clec4a2, Clec4n, Csf1r, Csf1r, Cx3cr1, Cxcr4, Cxcr5, Ddx58, Dock2, Epas1, Fcer1g, Fcgr2b, Fkbp1b, G6pdx, Gapt, Gimap5, Gnas, H2-Aa, H2-Ab1, H2-DMa, H2-DMb1, H2-DMb2, H2-Ea, H2-Eb1, H2-T3, Hc, Hdac9, Hhex, Hoxb3, Hspa1b, Icam1, Igh-6, Ikbkg, Il16, Il1rap, Il2ra, Inhba, Irak1, Itgam, Kdr, Klhl6, Lat2, Lig4, Lst1, Ly6d, Lyn, Lyst, Mll5, Ms4a1, Mx1, Mx2, Myo1e, Myo1f, Nfam1, Nfkb1, Nlrx1, Oas1b, Orm2, Pbx1, Pdcd1lg2, Pecam1, Plcg1, Plcg2, Polm, Pou2f2, Prkca, Prkcd, Procr, Ptpn6, Ptprc, Rab27a, Rara, Rc3h1, Ripk2, Rogdi, Rsad2, S100a9, Selp, Sfpi1, Sh2b2, Sh2b3, Sh2d1a, Sh2d1b1, Slamf1, Slc11a1, Spib, Stap1, Stat6, Tac4, Tapbp, Tbk1, Tcfeb, Tgfbr2, Tinagl1, Tirap, Tlr1, Tlr2, Tlr4, Tlr7, Tnfaip8l2, Tnfrsf13b, Tnfrsf13c, Twsg1, Vnn1, Ywhaz, Fas, Fasl, Gzma, Gzmm
miR-10b	Ahsp, C3ar1, C4bp, Cd34, Cdk6, Cebpa, Crip2, Crkl, Ctla4, Cxcl9, Enpp3, Fyb, Gpam, H28, H2-Q1, H2-Q10,Hells, Hoxa9, Id2, Il12b, Il1r1, Il1rl1, Ilf2, Kit, Klf1, Masp2, Msh2, Pf4, Polr3h, Prg2, Prg3, Runx1, Serpinb9, Slc11a2, Sox6, Spna1, Tacc3, Tal1, Tap2, Tek, Tgtp1, Tlr3, Tnfsf9, Vpreb1, Cd28
miR-125a-3p	Ahsp, Alas2, Ank1, Bak1, Barx1,Bcl10, C3ar1, C4bp, C8a, Cd34, Cd47, Cdk6, Cebpa, Cplx2, Cr1l, Crip2, Crkl, Csf1, Ctla4, Ctse, Cxcl11, Cxcl13, Cxcl9, Daf2, Enpp2, Enpp3, Fech, Fyb, Gpam, H28, H2-Q1, H2-Q10, Hbb-b1, Hells, Heph, Hmgb1, Hoxa9, Icam1, Id2, Il12b, Il1r1, Il1rl1, Il2ra, Ilf2, Jarid2, Kcnj8, Kit, Klf1, Klf11, Klre1, Lrrc17, Masp1, Masp2, Mbl2, Mecom, Meis1, Msh2, Mx1, Nup85, Osm, Pf4, Pik3cd, Pml, Polr3h, Prg2, Prg3, Rag1, Runx1, Serpinb9, Serping1, Sfxn1, Sh2b2, Slc11a2, Sox6, Spna1, Tacc3, Tal1, Tap2, Tbx1, Tcf3, Tcfe3, Tek, Tgtp1, Tlr3, Tnfsf11, Tnfsf8, Tnfsf9, Traf3ip2, Txnrd2, Vegfa, Vpreb1, Cd28, Itgb6
miR-141	Ahsp, Alas2, Ank1, Bak1, Barx1, Bcl10, C3ar1, C4bp, C8a, Cd34, Cd47, Cdk6, Cebpa, Cplx2, Cr1l, Crip2, Crkl, Csf1, Ctla4, Ctse, Cxcl11, Cxcl13, Cxcl9, Daf2, Enpp2, Enpp3, Fech, Fyb, Gpam, H28, H2-Q1, H2-Q10, Hbb-b1, Hells, Heph, Hmgb1, Hoxa9, Icam1, Id2, Il12b, Il1r1, Il1rl1, Il2ra, Ilf2, Jarid2, Kit, Klf1, Klf11, Klre1, Lrrc17, Masp1, Masp2, Mbl2, Mecom, Meis1, Msh2, Mx1, Nup85, Osm, Pf4, Pik3cd, Pml, Polr3h, Prg2, Prg3, Rag1, Runx1, Serpinb9, Serping1, Sfxn1, Sh2b2, Slc11a2, Sox6, Spna1, Tacc3, Tal1, Tap2, Tbx1, Tcf3, Tcfe3, Tek, Tgtp1, Tlr3, Tnfsf11, Tnfsf8, Tnfsf9, Traf3ip2, Txnrd2, Vpreb1, Cd28
miR-149	Ahsp, Bak1, C3ar1, C4bp, C8a, Cd34, Cdk6, Cebp, Cplx2, Crip2, Crkl,Csf1, Ctla4, Ctse, Cxcl11, Cxcl13, Cxcl9, Enpp3, Fech, Fyb, Gpam, H28, H2-Q1, H2-Q10, Hbb-b1, Hells, Heph, Hoxa9, Icam1, Id2, Il12b, Il12b, Il1r1, Il1rl1, Il2ra, Ilf2, Kit, Klf1, Klf11, Lrrc17, Masp2, Meis1, Msh2, Mx1, Nup85, Osm, Pf4, Pik3cd, Pml,Polr3h, Prg2, Prg3, Rag1, Runx1, Serpinb9, Serping1, Sh2b2, Slc11a2, Sox6, Spna1, Tacc3, Tal1, Tap2, Tbx1, Tcf3, Tek, Tgtp1, Tlr3, Tnfsf8, Tnfsf9, Txnrd2, Vpreb1, Cd28

Table 1. Cont.

MicroRNAs	Potencial targets
miR-1897-5p	Cdk6, Cxcl9, Elf4, Fech, Foxo3, Fyb, Fyb, Gpam, H28, H2-Q1, H2-Q10, Hoxa9, Il12b, Il12b, Il1r1, Il1rl1, Klf1, Masp2, Masp2, Polr3h, Slc11a2, Slc11a2, Smap1, Tap2, Tek, Tgtp1
MicroRNAs	Potencial targets
miR-29b*	Add2, Ahsp, Ank1, Bak1, C3ar1, C4bp, C8a, Cd34, Cdk6, Cebpa, Cplx2, Crip2, Crkl, Csf1, Ctla4, Ctse, Cxcl11, Cxcl13, Cxcl9, Elf4, Enpp3, Fech, Fech, Fech, Foxo3, Fyb, Gpam, H28, H2-Q1, H2-Q10, Hbb-b1, Hells, Heph, Hoxa9, Icam1, Id2, Il12b, Il1r1, Il1rl1, Il2ra, Il6, Ilf2, Kit, Klf1, Klf11, Lrrc17, Masp2,Meis1, Msh2, Mx1, Nup85, Osm, Pf4, Pik3cd, Pml, Polr3h, Prg2, Prg3, Rag1, Rorc, Runx1, Serpinb9, Serping1, Sh2b2, Slc11a2, Smap1, Sox6, Spna1, Spon2, Tacc3, Tal1, Tap2, Tbx1, Tcf3, Tek, Tgtp1, Thy1, Tlr3, Tnfsf8, Tnfsf9, Txnrd2, Vpreb1, Cd28
miR-302c	Ahsp, Cdk6, Crkl, Ctla4, Cxcl9, Fyb, Gpam, H28, H2-Q1, H2-Q10, Hoxa9, Il12b, Il1r1, Il1rl1, Kit, Klf1, Masp2, Msh2, Polr3h, Prg2, Prg3, Runx1, Serpinb9, Slc11a2, Spna1, Tal1, Tap2, Tek, Tgtp1, Cd28
miR-30b*	Add2, Ahsp, Alas2, Ank1, Bak1, Barx1, Bcl10, C3ar1, C4bp, C8a, Cd34, Cd47, Cdk6, Cebpa, Cplx2, Cr1l, Crip2, Crkl, Csf1, Ctla4, Ctse, Cxcl11, Cxcl13, Cxcl9, Daf2, Elf4, Enpp2, Enpp3, Fech, Foxo3, Fyb, Gpam, H28, H2-Q1, H2-Q10, Hbb-b1, Hells, Heph, Hoxa9, Icam1, Id2, Il12b, Il1r1, Il1rl1, Il2ra, Il6, Ilf2, Jarid2, Kit, Klf1, Klf11, Klre1, Lrrc17, Masp1, Masp2, Mbl2, Mecom, Meis1, Msh2, Mx1, Nup85, Osm, Pf4, Pik3cd, Pml, Polr3h, Prg2, Prg3, Rag1, Rorc, Runx1, Serpinb9, Serping1, Sfxn1, Sh2b2, Slc11a2, Smap1, Sox6, Spna1, Tacc3, Tal1, Tap2, Tbx1, Tcf3, Tcfe3, Tek, Tgtp1, Thy1, Tlr3, Tnfsf8, Tnfsf9, Traf3ip2, Txnrd2, Vpreb1, Bcl2, Cd28
miR-690	Add2, Ahctf1, Ahsp, Alas2, Ank1, Bak1, Bcl10, C3ar1, C4bp, C8a, Cd34, Cdk6, Cebpa, Cplx2, Crip2, Crkl, Csf1, Ctla4, Ctse, Cxcl11, Cxcl13, Cxcl9, Daf2, Dyrk3, Elf4, Enpp3, Fech, Foxo3, Fyb, Gpam, H28, H2-Q1, H2-Q10, Hbb-b1, Hells, Heph, Hmgb3, Hoxa9, Icam1, Id2, Il12b, Il12b, Il18r1, Il1r1, Il1rl1, Il2ra, Il6, Ilf2, Kit, Klf1, Klf11, Lrrc17, Masp2, Meis1, Msh2, Mx1, Ncaph2, Nup85, Osm, Pf4, Pik3cd, Pml, Polr3h, Prdx2, Prg2, Prg3, Rag1, Rorc, Runx1, Serpinb9, Serping1, Sh2b2, Slc11a2, Slc11a2, Smap1, Sox6, Spna1, Spon2, Tacc3, Tal1, Tap2, Tbx1, Tcf3, Tcfe3, Tek, Tgtp1, Thy1, Tlr3, Tnfsf8, Tnfsf9, Traf3ip2, Txnrd2, Vpreb1, Bcl2, Cd28
miR-691	Ahsp, C3ar1, C4bp, Cd34, Cdk6, Cebpa, Crip2, Crkl,Ctla4, Ctse, Cxcl11, Cxcl9, Enpp3, Fyb, Gpam, H28, H2-Q1, H2-Q10, Hells, Hoxa9, Icam1, Id2, Il12b, Il1r1, Il1rl1, Il2ra, Ilf2, Kit, Klf1, Masp2, Msh2, Osm, Pf4, Polr3h, Prg2, Prg3, Runx1, Serpinb9, Slc11a2, Sox6, Spna1, Tacc3, Tal1, Tap2, Tek, Tgtp1, Tlr3, Tnfsf9, Vpreb1, Cd28
miR-712	Ahsp, C3ar1, C4bp, Cd34, Cdk6, Cebpa, Crip2, Crkl, Ctla4, Ctse, Cxcl11, Cxcl9, Enpp3, Fyb, Gpam, H28, H2-Q1, H2-Q10, Hells, Hoxa9, Icam1, Id2, Il12b, Il1r1, Il1rl1, Il2ra, Ilf2, Kit, Klf1, Masp2, Msh2, Osm, Pf4, Pml, Polr3h, Prg2, Prg3, Runx1, Serpinb9, Slc11a2, Sox6, Spna1, Tacc3, Tal1, Tap2, Tek, Tgtp1, Tlr3, Tnfsf9, Vpreb1, Cd28

that an RNA duplex is more stable and thermodynamically stronger when the free energy is low [39].

Luciferase reporter assay. The oligonucleotide pairs containing a portion of the Rorc or CD8a 3′UTR predicted binding site for miRNAs were synthetized by Sigma-Aldrich, St. Louis, MO, USA. The oligonucleotides were annealed and cloned into the pmirGLO Vector (Promega Corporation, USA) between the XhoI/XbaI restriction sites resulting in the miRNA target region in the correct 5′ to 3′ orientation, immediately 3′ downstream of the luciferase gene. For selected targets, we introduced point mutations into the 7-nt seed-binding sequence. These constructs, named "pMIR-Rorc" or "pMIR-CD8a" for the wild-type sequences and "pMIR-Rorc(m)" or "pMIR-CD8a(m)" for the mutant mismatch sequences were selected by colony-polymerase chain reaction (PCR) using the following pair of primers: forward 5′AGGTTA-CAACCGCCAAGAAG3′ and reverse 5′CAGCCAACT-CAGCTTCCTTT 3′, which flank the vector polycloning site.

For the luciferase reporter assay, 0.2 ug of each pmirGLO constructs was transfected together with 1.6 pmol of miR-30b*, miR-196b or scrambled miRNA (Thermo Scientific Dharmacon, Waltham, MA, USA) into HEK-293T cells (6×10^4 cells/well) in a 96-well plate. Transfections were done using Attractene Transfection Reagent (Qiagen, Hilden, Germany) according to the manufacturer's instructions. Transfected cells were incubated at 37°C in a 5% CO_2 incubator and 24 hours after transfections, cells were lysed in Passive Lysis Buffer and then firefly and renilla luciferase activities were measured in a Molecular Devices FlexStation 3 Luminometer with the Dual-Luciferase reporter system (Promega Corporation, USA) according to the manufacturer's instructions. Our laboratory has a CTNBio biosafety permission (Permit No. 0040/98).

Flow Cytometry

Spleen and lymph nodes were prepared as single-cell suspensions according to standard protocols, and the following monoclonal antibodies (BD Biosciences, New Jersey, USA) were used for staining: CD4 PerCP and CD8 FITC. For intracellular detection of RORγt, cells were first treated with anti-CD4 and then fixed, permeabilized, and stained with monoclonal RORγt PE. Flow cytometry was performed in a FACSCalibur instrument (Becton Dickinson, New Jersey, USA) and analyzed with FlowJo software (TreeStar, Ashland, USA).

Statistical Analysis

The real-time PCR and FACS results are presented as standard error of the mean (SEM). The differences were evaluated by one-way ANOVA followed by Student's t-test (two groups) or Bonferroni's test (three or more groups), $P<0.05$, $P<0.01$, and $P<0.001$ were considered statistically significant.

Results

Collagen-induced Arthritis (CIA)

Immunization with type II collagen induced CIA in male DBA-1/J mice, whose CIA scores reached a peak on day 35. Male DBA-2/J mice injected with the same schedule did not exhibit any features of arthritis development. Male mice from both strains immunized with only CFA were used as controls (data not shown).

miRNA Expression Profile in Thymocytes and Peripheral T Cells

We first compared miRNA expression in thymocytes and peripheral naïve $CD3^+$ total T cells from 4-week-old DBA-1/J and DBA-2/J non-immunized animals (Figure 1). We next compared miRNA expression in activated $CD3^+$ T cells from the spleen and

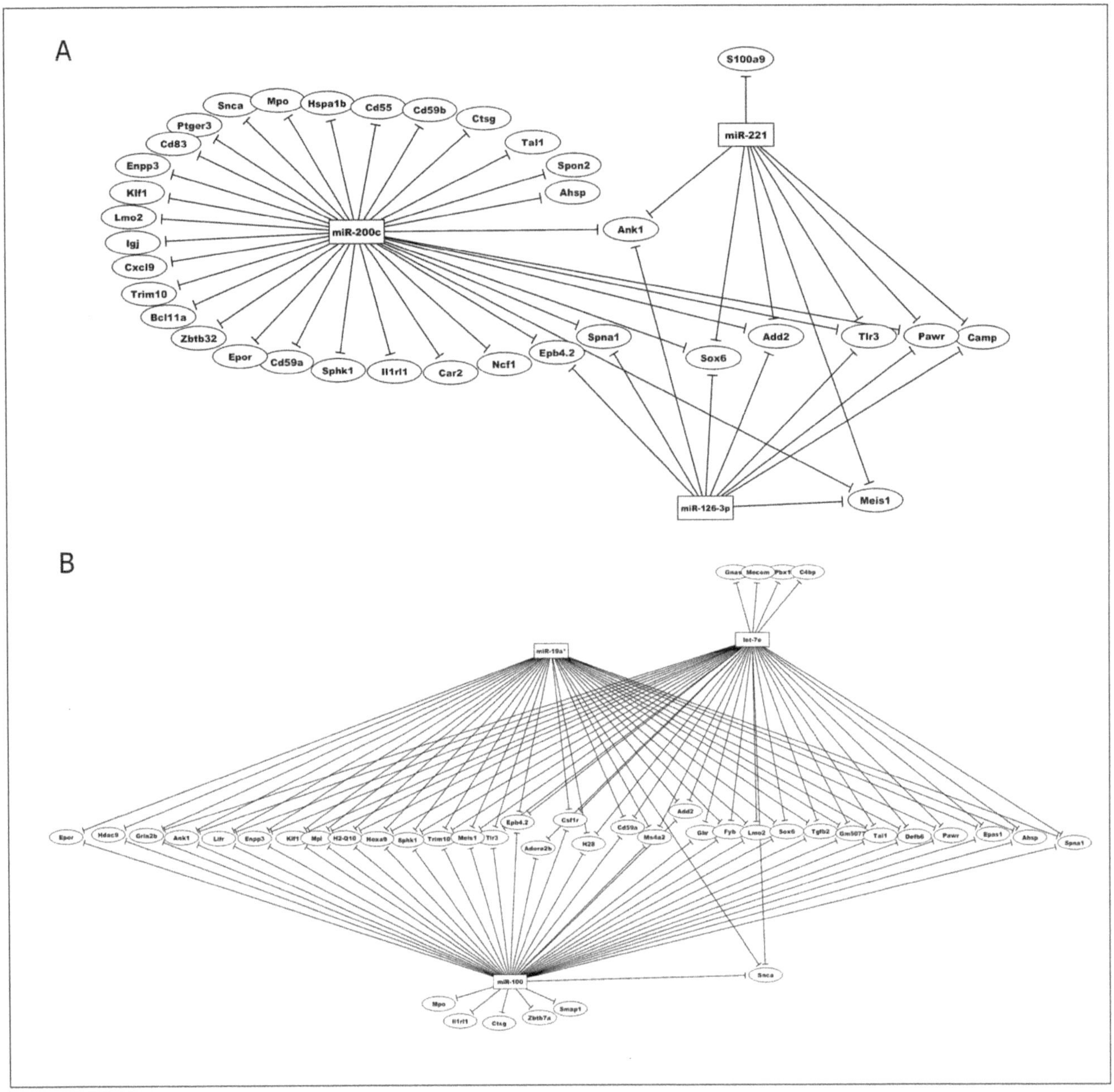

Figure 5. Post-transcriptional miRNA-mRNA interaction networks based on microarray expression data from thymocytes. The networks were obtained using the GenMir++ algorithm. This figure shows the participation of A) three miRNAs up-regulated in thymocytes of DBA-1/J strain and B) three miRNAs in up-regulated in thymocytes of DBA-2/J. These miRNAs interact with mRNAs related to immune system.

lymph nodes of 12-week-old mice that were immunized with collagen.

We identified 91 differentially expressed miRNAs ($p<0.05$, fold change ≥ 2.0) comparing thymocytes to naïve peripheral $CD3^+$ T cells from the DBA-1/J and DBA-2/J mouse strains (Figure 1), and 62 differentially expressed miRNAs ($p<0.05$, and fold change ≥ 2.0) comparing activated $CD3^+$ T cells during CIA development (Figure 2). We selected the specific up-regulated miRNAs from each group for subsequent of miRNA-mRNA interaction prediction. Three miRNAs (miR-126-3p, miR-221 and miR-200c) were exclusively up-regulated in thymocytes of DBA-1/J strain, and three others (miR-let-7e, miR-100 and miR-19a*) were exclusively up-regulated in the DBA-2/J strain.

In naïve peripheral $CD3^+$ T cells, we found six miRNAs exclusively up-regulated in DBA-1/J mice (miR-195, miR-689, miR-500, miR-196b, miR-10a and miR-805) and four exclusively up-regulated in DBA-2/J mice (miR-467e, miR-101a, miR-125-5p and miR-669a).

During the course of CIA, six miRNAs (miR-181a, miR-144, miR-17*, miR-202-3p, miR-467a* and miR-500) were up-regulated in peripheral $CD3^+$ T lymphocytes of DBA-1/J strain. In the peripheral $CD3^+$ T lymphocytes of DBA-2/J strain, we found 11 miRNAs (miR-302c, miR-691, miR-712, miR-125a-3p, miR-29b*, miR-30b*, miR-10b, miR-149, miR-141, miR-1897-5p and miR-690) that were up-regulated.

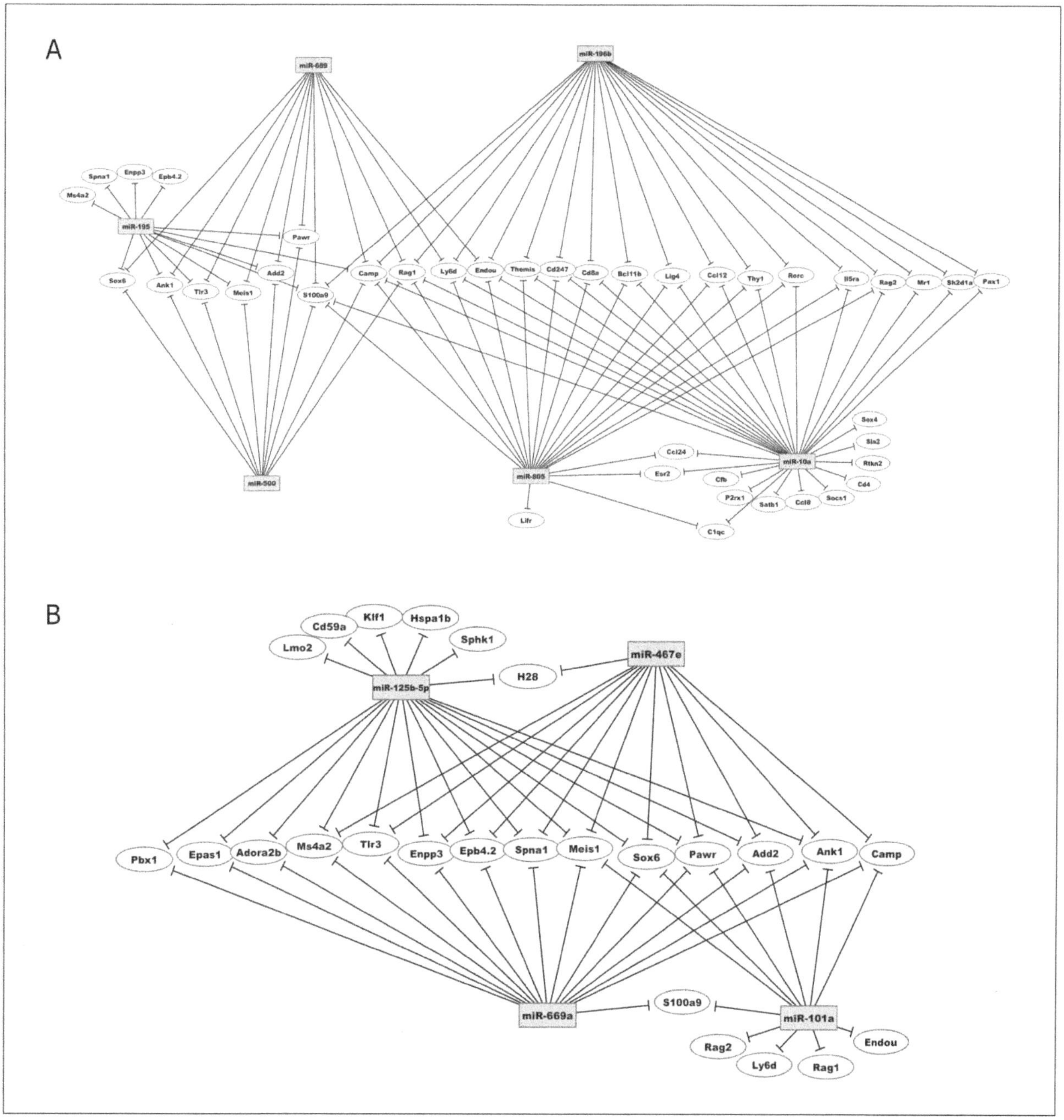

Figure 6. Post-transcriptional miRNA-mRNA interaction networks based on microarray expression data from peripheral CD3⁺ T cells. The networks were obtained using the GenMir++ algorithm. This figure shows the participation of A) six miRNAs up-regulated in CD3+ T cells of DBA-1/J strain and B) four miRNAs up-regulated in CD3+ T cells of DBA-2/J strain. These miRNAs interact with mRNAs related to immune system.

Messenger RNAs Differentially Expressed in Thymocytes and Peripheral T cells

Although the expression pattern remained unchanged during CIA development for the majority of the 44,000 sequences tested, 14,230 were differentially expressed in thymocytes compared to naïve T cells, and 3,155 were differentially expressed compared to activated $CD3^+$ T cells.

Functional annotation of the differentially expressed mRNAs using Gene Ontology (GO) (http://www.geneontology.org/) identified 1,813 immune system-related mRNAs among the 14,230 significantly expressed in thymocytes compared to naïve T cells (Figure 3) and 486 immune system-related mRNAs in $CD3^+$ T cells during CIA (Figure 4). Hierarchical clustering revealed that these sequences had distinct expression patterns. These sequences were then used to reconstruct miRNA-mRNA interaction networks to identify potential targets.

Reconstruction of miRNA-mRNA Interaction Networks

The miRNA-mRNA interaction networks predicting targeted immune system mRNAs in thymocytes and peripheral naïve and activated $CD3^+$ T cells from the DBA-1/J and DBA-2/J mouse

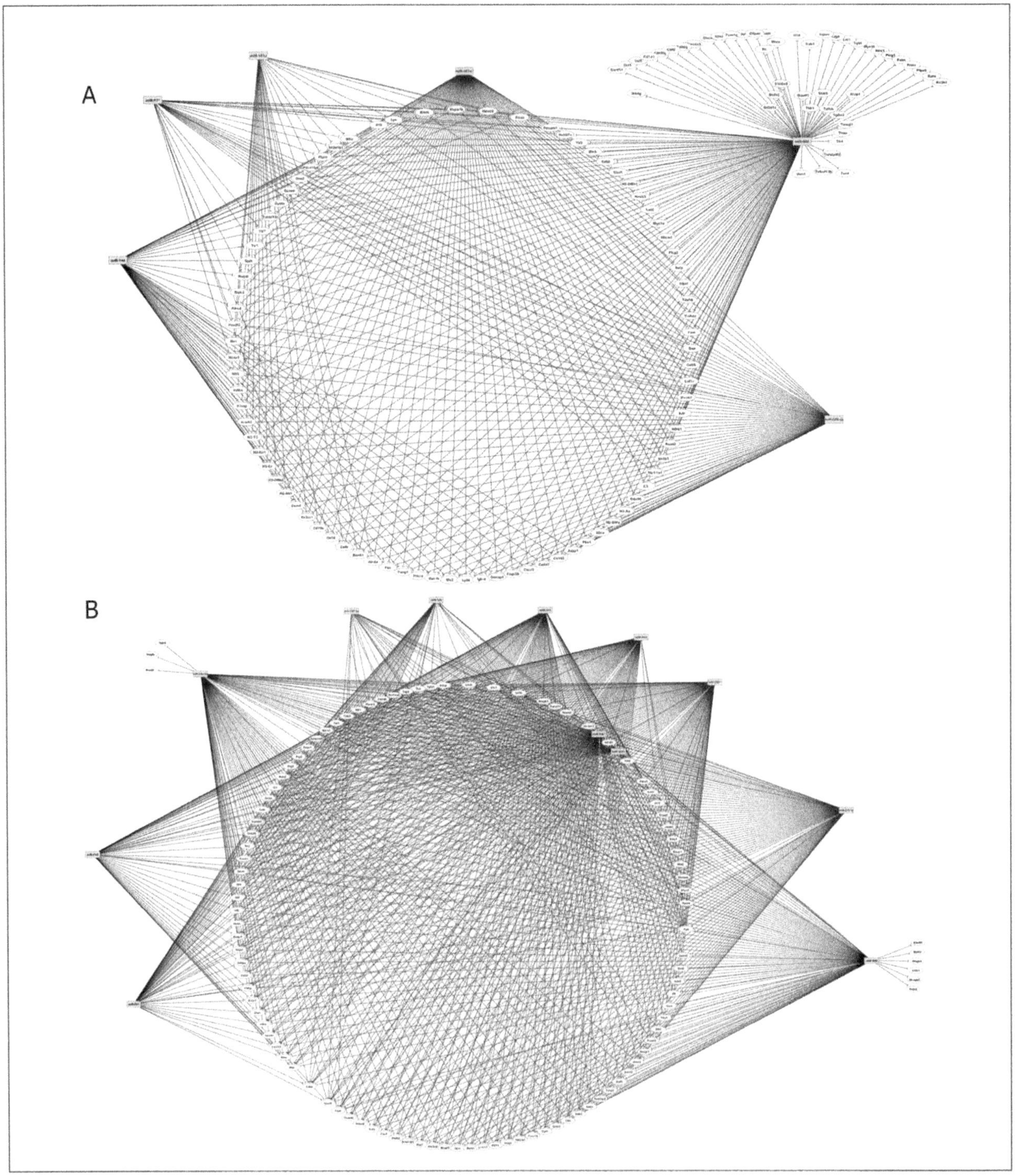

Figure 7. Reduced percentage of CD8^{+} T cells during collagen induced arthritis (CIA) in the DBA-1/J susceptible strain. The percentage of splenic or lymph nodes T cells of DBA-1/J and DBA-2/J mice expressing CD8a was evaluated by flow cytometry. Data from three independent experiments are shown. The results are presented as standard error of the mean (SEM). The differences were evaluated by Student's t-test. $^{**}P<0.01$ was considered statistically significant in DBA-2/J mice strain when compared to DBA-1/J.

strains were depicted and the selected miRNAs and their targets are shown in Table 1.

During the initial stage of T cell maturation in the thymus and their migration to the periphery, we found few potential targets related to immune functions when compared to activated T cells during immunization (Table 1). In general, the up-regulated miRNAs found in the DBA-2/J strain regulated higher numbers of targets (884 mRNA targets) than those found in the DBA-1/J strain (521 mRNA targets).

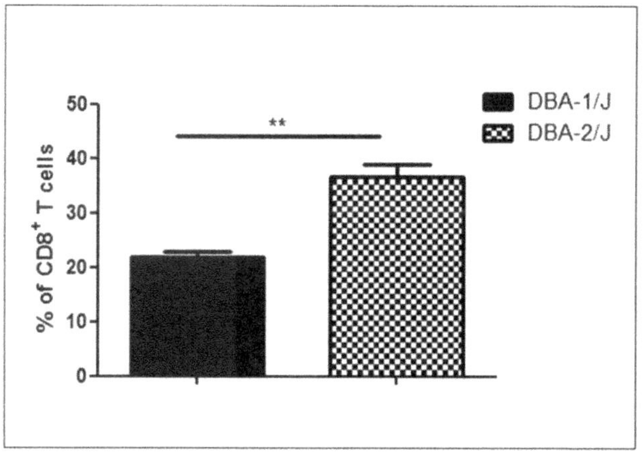

Figure 8. Post-transcriptional miRNA-mRNA interaction networks based on microarray expression data from peripheral CD3^{+} T cells during collagen induced arthritis (CIA). The networks were obtained using the GenMir++ algorithm. This figure shows the participation of A) six miRNAs up-regulated in peripheral CD3+ T cells of DBA-1/J mice and B) eleven miRNAs up-regulated in peripheral CD3+ T cells of DBA-2/J mice. These miRNAs interact with mRNAs related to immune system. The control mice were immunized just with complete Freund's adjuvant without any collagen.

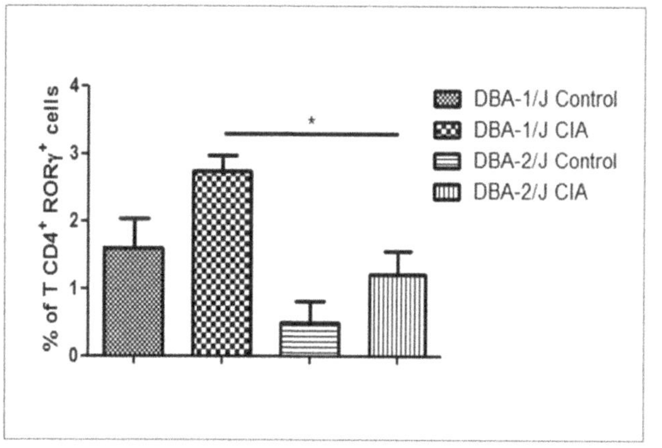

Figure 9. Reduced percentage of Rorγt^{+} T cells during collagen immunization of DBA-2/J strain. The percentage of splenic or lymph node expressing RORγt T cells of DBA-1/J and DBA-2/J mice during immunization with type II collagen was evaluated by flow cytometry. The control mice were immunized just with complete Freund's adjuvant without any collagen. Data from three independent experiments are shown. The results are presented as means standard error of mean (SEM). The differences were evaluated by a one-way ANOVA followed by Bonferroni's test. *$P<0.05$ was considered statistically significant in DBA-2/J mice strain when compared to DBA-1/J after CIA induction.

Interestingly, in thymocytes of both mouse strains, two different sets of miRNAs regulated a common set of targets, the Sox6, Tlr3 and Add2 mRNAs (Figure 5).

As expected, the peripheral mature T lymphocytes from these strains showed regulation of the Rag1, Rag2, and Themis mRNAs, which are associated with T cell differentiation and maturation (Figure 6).

Figure 6a shows that miRNAs miR-196b, miR-805 and miR-10a regulated CD8a mRNA in the peripheral T cells of the DBA-1/J strain. Flow cytometry analysis shows that the percentage of peripheral CD8^{+} T cells is lower in DBA-1/J mice than in DBA-2/J mice (Figure 7), which suggest the participation of these miRNAs as negative regulatory controllers.

During CIA development in DBA-1/J mice, the number of mRNA targets increased, which included important mRNAs such as Fas and FasL that encode apoptosis proteins, IL-10, Stat6, and granzymes Gzmm and Gzma (Figure 8a).

However, during collagen immunization of DBA-2/J mice, the mRNA targets Rorc, IL-6, Foxo3 and Bcl2 were found (Figure 8b). Because Th17 cells are strongly correlated with arthritis development, we highlighted the Rorc mRNA, which encodes the transcription factor Rorγt implicated in the differentiation of these cells. Rorc mRNA was regulated by miR-30b*, miR-690 and miR-29b* (Table 1). Our flow cytometry analysis showed that the percentage of CD4^{+} Rorγt^{+} T cells was lower in the DBA-2/J strain (Figure 9), and again the participation of these miRNAs as negative regulatory controllers is suggested.

As the most of the miRNA-mRNA interactions found in this study are new, we validated some of such using the RNAhybrid bioinformatic tool, which shows the most favorable hybridization between a given miRNA and its predicted mRNA target by calculating the minimum free energy (MFE). The miRNA-mRNA molecular interactions and respective MFEs are shown on Figure 10.

Moreover, the luciferase reporter assay was useful to confirm the occurrence of miRNA-mRNA interactions within the cellular milieu focusing on Rorc and CD8a mRNAs targets. We confirmed that miR-30b* interacts with Rorc mRNA and miR-196b interacts with CD8a mRNA by hybridization with their respective 3′UTR sequences containing the predicted binding sites for these miRNAs. Introduction of point mutations into the 3′UTR targeted sequences significantly abolished miRNA hybridization (Figure 11).

Discussion

Rheumatoid arthritis (RA) is an autoimmune disease that is characterized by an uncontrolled influx of inflammatory T cells to the joints, eventually leading to tissue damage. Pro- and anti-inflammatory cytokines and chemokines and/or their receptors, which are key mediators of the effector function of T cells, appear to be centrally involved in the pathogenesis of RA [1].

The role that T cells play in inflammation and joint damage has been elucidated through the usage of animal models, mainly mice [40]. The DBA-1/J and DBA-2/J strains of mouse, which are respectively susceptible and resistant to CIA [41], represent in these days a unique model-system for studying the mechanisms involved in arthritis susceptibility.

Although the main effector cells and proteins involved in human RA and experimental murine CIA have already been identified, efforts to better understand its molecular and genetic control are just beginning. In this regard, our group recently demonstrated that thymic stroma of the DBA-1/J and DBA-2/J strains differ in their transcriptional expression of joints, cartilage and bone peripheral tissue antigens (PTAs). Interestingly, in the DBA-1/J CIA-susceptible strain, the MHC-H2 gene represents a key regulator of downstream genes that code joints and bone PTAs [10]. We show that MHC-H2 at least partly control the expression of autoantigens in the thymus, a phenomenon known as promiscuous gene expression that is important for the negative selection of autoreactive thymocytes [42–44].

In the present study, we asked whether thymocytes, T cells in different phases of development and activation, naïve and

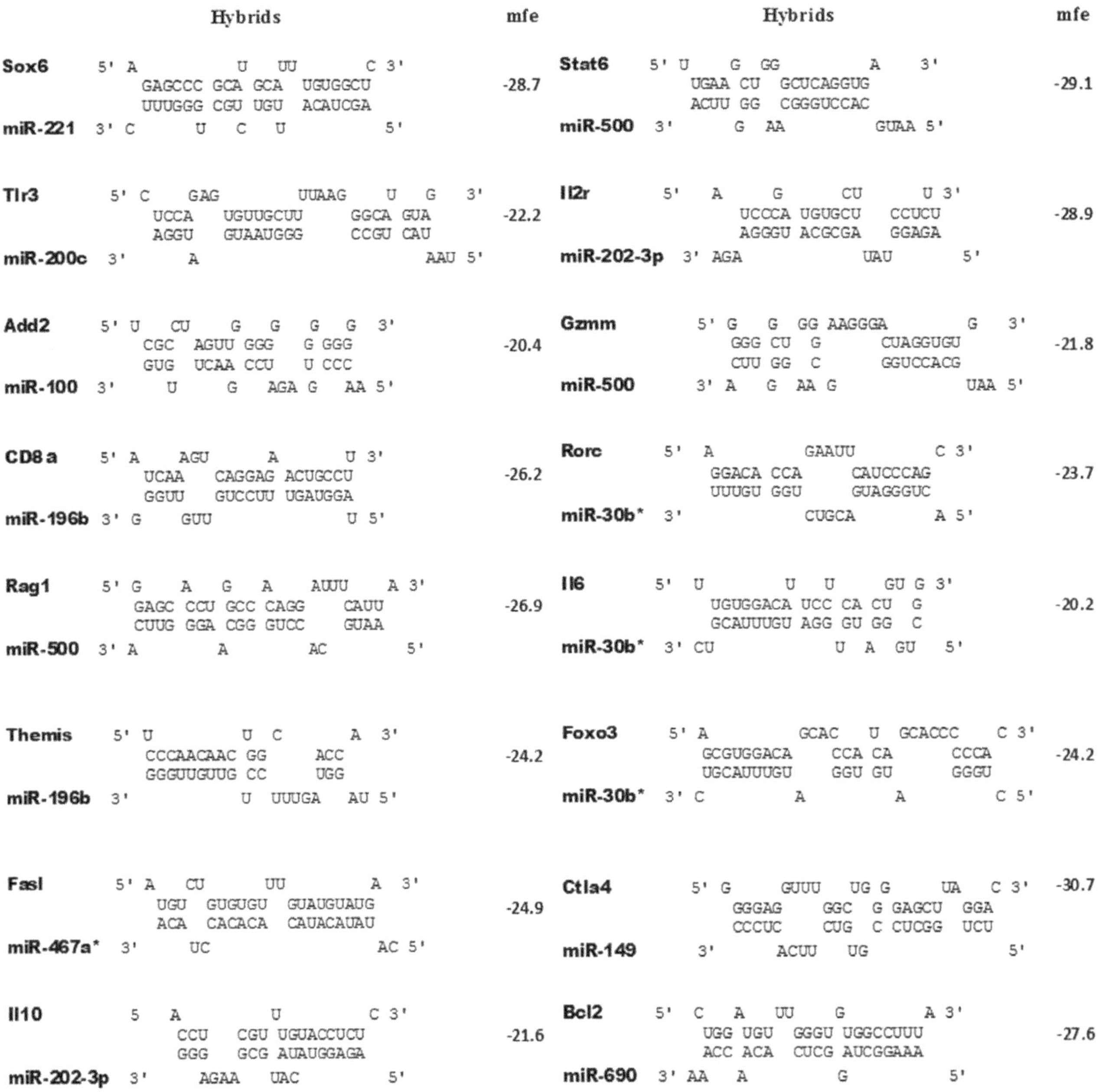

Figure 10. Validation of miRNA-mRNA interactions using RNAhybrid software. The miRNA:mRNA hybrid structures were calculated for selected examples of miRNA-mRNA interactions from GenMir++ predictions. Sixteen miRNA:mRNA hybrid structures are presented. The miRNA binding site of the target mRNA is shown at the top, the complementary miRNA is shown at the bottom strand, and the calculated minimum free energy (MFE) values are given to the right (kcal/mol). The gene names as well as the designation of the miRNA (miRBase) are shown to the left.

activated peripheral CD3$^+$ T lymphocytes in the context of CIA, also featured differences in their transcriptional expression of miRNAs and mRNAs.

Considering the role played by miRNAs in the post-transcriptional control of gene expression in immune cells [45], we also asked whether these molecules could differentially interact with mRNA targets. To test this, we used the microarray method and bioinformatics programs to trace gene expression signatures and miRNA-mRNA interactions (Figure S1).

Initially we conducted genome-wide transcriptional profiling of miRNAs and mRNAs, as depicted in Figures 1–4.

When thymocytes where compared to naïve T cells, we noticed that some miRNAs, including miR-30e, miR-363 and miR-130b, did not show altered expression. We also found T cell developmental stage-specific miRNAs with no difference between DBA-1/J and DBA-2/J mouse strains. This suggests that these miRNAs were related to common processes between the two strains. As our aim was to identify the miRNAs associated with susceptibility or resistance to CIA, then we focused our analysis on cell-type and strain-specific miRNAs.

We show the clustering of peripheral CD3$^+$ T lymphocyte miRNA profiles from the DBA-1/J and DBA-2/J strains after collagen immunization. Interestingly, most of the miRNAs differ

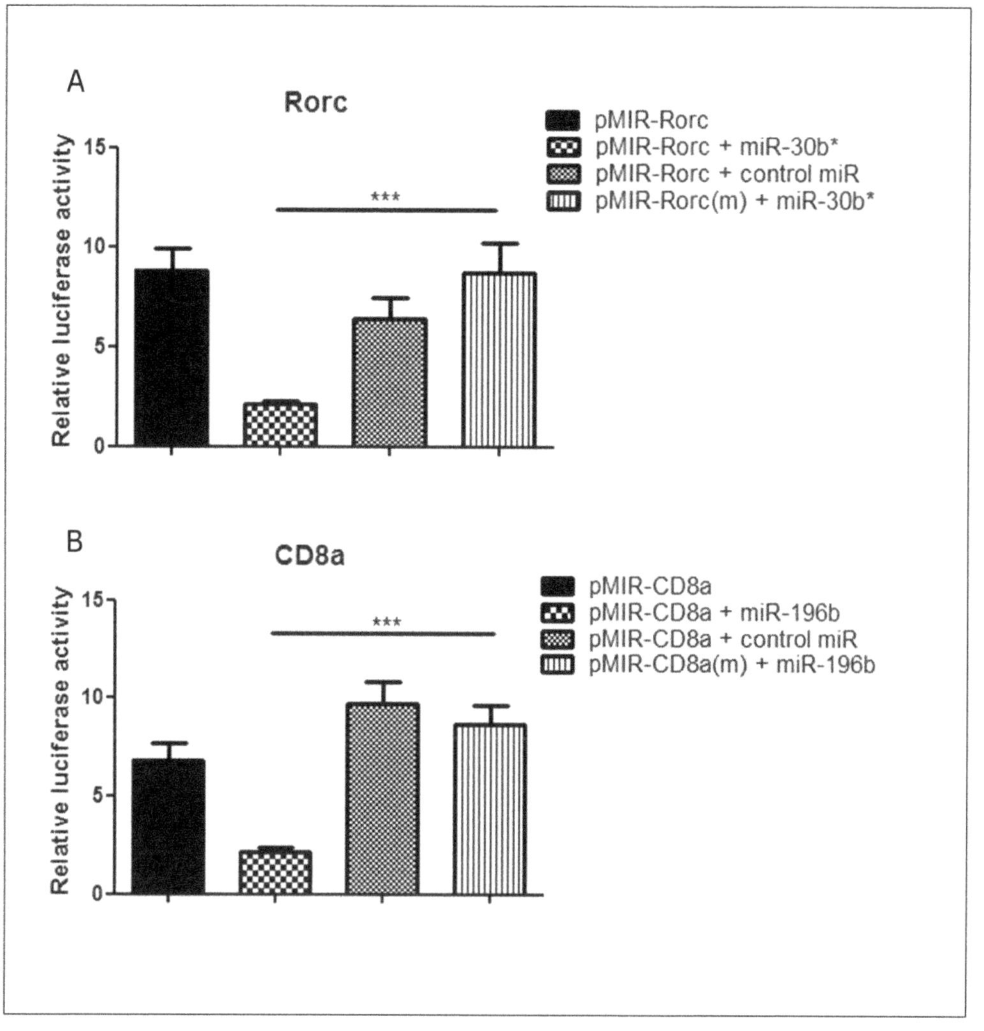

Figure 11. Luciferase reporter gene assay. pMIR-Rorc and pMIR-Rorc(m) 3′UTR luciferase plasmid were co-transfected with control or miR-30b* mimic (A), and pMIR-CD8a and pMIR-CD8a(m) with control or miR-196b (B) into HEK293 cells. Luciferase activity was evaluated at 24 h post transfections. Data are presented as means standard error of mean (SEM). The differences were evaluated by a one-way ANOVA followed by Bonferroni's test. ****P<0.001* was considered statistically significant when the wild-type pMIR was compared to the mutant mismatch sequence in the presence of the respective miRNA mimic.

in their expression profile between the mouse strains. The miR-223 among some other represents exception of miRNAs that were induced in both strains.

The mRNA expression profile of thymocytes and peripheral $CD3^+$ T lymphocytes from the DBA-1/J and DBA-2/J strains was also compared. Using Gene Ontology (GO), we identified those mRNAs that are related to the immune system due to their importance to arthritis. GO allowed identifying 1,813 immune system-related mRNAs in thymocytes and naïve T cells and 486 in $CD3^+$ T cells during collagen immunization of DBA-1/J and DBA-2/J mouse strains (Figures 3–5).

These results were important in demonstrating that the transcriptional programming of T cells is somewhat different between the mice strains studied, answering the first question of this study.

The hierarchical clustering of microarray data is very useful in grouping biological samples and represents the gold standard method. However, this does not address the possibility that the differentially expressed RNAs are somehow interacting with each other. As our second question addressed on the miRNA-mRNA interactions, we had to use a dedicated method for estimating this. Therefore, we choose the GenMir^{++} program [38], which establishes network interactions based on Bayesian statistics of opposite expression levels of miRNAs and mRNAs from actual microarray data. The set of miRNA and mRNA microarray data was then inputted to this program, which was used to identify potential targets through reconstruction of miRNA-mRNA interaction networks.

In general, miRNA-mRNA target pairs are penalized if both the miRNA and mRNA are highly expressed in the same sample and are rewarded if a given miRNA is highly expressed in a sample that a given mRNA has low expression in, especially if few of its other predicted miRNA regulators are highly expressed therein.

Each data set of differentially expressed RNAs (miRNAs and mRNAs) from the same sample was analyzed together to reconstruct interaction networks. The reconstructed networks show that one given miRNA can interact with several mRNA targets and that one mRNA can interact with several miRNAs at once. The interactions shown in these figures are clearly identified in Table 1.

During T cell maturation in the thymus of DBA-1/J and DBA-2/J mice, potential mRNA targets related to the immune system were found, including Sox6 Tlr3, and Add2. Despite the differential miRNA profiles of thymocytes from the two mouse strains studied, they do have common mRNA targets in addition to exclusive targets. Because of this, we next asked if transcriptional deregulation in the periphery could be associated with CIA.

Although the number of mRNA targets in naïve T cells was low, interesting differences were observed. For example, the Ragl, Rag2 and Themis mRNAs, which are involved in the differentiation and maturation of thymocytes, were regulated in both strains (Figure 6). Themis is expressed in a tightly regulated manner during T cell development in late double-negative (DN) and especially in double-positive (DP) thymocytes [46]. It is down-regulated after positive selection and is expressed at low levels in mature T cells. As expected, we found that genes involved with early T cell differentiation processes, Ragl, Rag2 and Themis, were regulated by miRNAs and consequently down-regulated in the periphery.

Another interesting mRNA target regulated in the DBA-1/J strain is the Cluster of differentiation 8 (CD8). $CD8^+$ T cells seem to be important in the effector phase of arthritis disease but are dispensable for its initiation [47]. However, the importance of the $CD8^+$ T cells in arthritis and their role in induction or protection are still controversial. Interestingly, we found that the DBA-1/J strain showed lower numbers of $CD8^+$ T cells in the periphery compared with the DBA-2/J strain (Figure 7).

Figure 8 shows the miRNA-mRNA interactions in the DBA-1/J and DBA-2/J strains during CIA development. Among the mRNAs differentially expressed and downregulated in peripheral $CD3^+$ T cells during collagen immunization and CIA development in DBA-1/J mice, we found genes that positively regulate inflammation, including Fas and FasL involved with apoptosis and IL-10 involved in suppressing Treg function.

Fas and FasL are part of the activation-induced cell death (AICD) pathway involved in the removal of activated T cells in vivo [48,49]. IL-10 production by Tregs is one of the mechanisms involved in inhibiting the production of inflammatory mediators and lymphocyte proliferation [50,51]. Our results suggest that the strong regulation of these genes in the CIA-susceptible DBA-1/J strain might contribute to the exacerbated T cell response observed in CIA.

Among the targets that are down-regulated during collagen immunization of the DBA-2/J strain, we found Rorc, which is involved in Th17 differentiation, and Foxo3, which is involved in cell cycle and survival, both of which are directly related to arthritis pathogenesis. In fact, Foxo3 has already been associated with RA. Foxo3 mRNA is increased in patients, and its overexpression may lead to the prolonged T cell survival in RA, thereby contributing to chronic inflammation [52].

Rorc mRNA encodes the transcription factor Rorγt, which is involved in the differentiation of $CD4^+$ T cells to Th17 pro-inflammatory cells. The role of IL-17 in the pathogenesis of arthritis is well known and was first confirmed in the CIA model [53]. In agreement with the FACS results of $CD8^+$ naïve T cells, we also found that the CIA-resistant DBA-2/J strain has diminished numbers of $Ror\gamma t^+$T cells in the periphery (Figure 9).

An intriguing result from this study was the finding that Rorc mRNA was regulated by miR-500 in naïve T cells in the DBA-1/J strain. However, during collagen immunization and CIA development in this strain, none miRNA regulation upon this mRNA was observed. In contrast, in DBA-2/J mice, Rorc mRNA expression was regulated by miR-29b*, miR-30b* and miR-690.

To the best of our knowledge, only miR-181a and miR-221, from the interaction networks showed in this study, have been previously identified as playing a role in T lymphocytes [26,54]. Moreover, we found new miRNAs that were up-regulated during the development and activation of T lymphocytes in the context of susceptibility or resistance to CIA.

Finally, we highlight the validation in this study of the miRNA-mRNA interactions that were not previously predicted in data bases such as TargetScan: miR-30b*-Rorc and miR-196b-CD8a. These interactions were initially validated by minimal free energy calculations of the respective RNA-RNA hybridizations. We used the RNAhybrid program for this purpose, which allowed us to know the specific miRNA-mRNA annealing sequence (Figure 10).

The portion of the mRNA 3′UTR sequences (annealing sequence) identified through RNAhybrid program was then synthesized, cloned in the pmirGlo vector, which was designed to assay the miRNA-mRNA interaction within the cell milieu (luciferase reporter assay). This assay allowed confirming the in vivo occurrence of the two new miRNA-mRNA interactions studied, which represent important pieces in the study of susceptibility/resistance to CIA. For each miRNA-mRNA interaction, the minimum free energy (MFE) was calculated based on the respective thermodynamic state (Figure 10). We used an MFE threshold of -20 kcal/mole based on the interaction between miRNAs with lengths of 22 nucleotides (nt) and a target with a length of 1,000 nt [33].

In this study, we identified a set of new miRNAs that regulate mRNA targets in different stages of T cell differentiation and activation in the context of murine CIA. These miRNAs differed in their expression profiling between DBA-1/J and DBA-2/J mice, which are susceptible and resistant to CIA, respectively. The modulation of miRNA expression allowed for the identification of miRNA-mRNA interactions, which were visualized through networks reconstructed based on actual microarray transcriptional profile and then validated through luciferase assay (Figure 11).

Important mRNA targets related to T cell differentiation and activation were predicted, including those related to inflammatory processes (Rorc), which were strongly regulated in the CIA-resistant DBA-2/J strain. The mRNAs involved in the control of an aggressive immune response, such as Fas and FasL, were found as miRNA targets in the CIA susceptible DBA-1/J strain.

The meaningful of these findings is reinforced since the mRNAs identified in this study encode proteins related to the pathogenesis of arthritis. Moreover, our results suggest a deregulation of miRNAs that could be associated with the control of molecules involved in inflammation development in the susceptible DBA-1/J strain following CIA induction.

These results contribute to a better understanding of the transcriptional and post-transcriptional modulation that might be contributing to the susceptibility/resistance to CIA in mice.

Supporting Information

Figure S1 Experimental design. Workflow for discriminating between the biological samples used (animal groups and cell types), total RNA extraction, hybridizations, microarray data analysis and miRNA-mRNA validation.

Acknowledgments

FACs experiments were carried out at the laboratory of Dr. João Santana da Silva (USP, Ribeirão Preto, Brazil). We thank Ieda Regina dos Santos and Denise Brufato Ferraz (USP, Ribeirão Preto, Brazil) and Ana Elisa C. S. Azzolini (USP, Ribeirão Preto, Brazil) by their technical assistance and

Dr. Yara M. Lucisano Valin (USP, Ribeirão Preto, Brazil) by make accessible the luminometer apparatus. Nicole Pezzi (FMRP USP) and Derek Gilchrist (University of Glasgow, UK) helped us with the cloning of microRNAs.

Author Contributions

Conceived and designed the experiments: PBD TMC ETSH FQC EAD GAP. Performed the experiments: PBD TAF CM. Analyzed the data: PBD DCBN. Contributed reagents/materials/analysis tools: ETSH EAD FQC GAP. Wrote the paper: PBD GAP.

References

1. Firestein GS (2003) Evolving concepts of rheumatoid arthritis. Nature 423: 356–361.
2. Klareskog L, Catrina AI, Paget S (2009) Rheumatoid arthritis. Lancet 373: 659–672.
3. Panayi GS, Lanchbury JS, Kingsley GH (1992) The importance of the T cell in initiatingand maintaining the chronic synovitis of rheumatoid arthritis. Arthritis Rheum 35: 729–735.
4. Ali M, Ponchel F, Wilson KE, Francis MJ, Wu X, et al. (2001) Rheumatoid arthritis synovial T cells regulate transcription of several genes associated with antigen-induced anergy. J Clin Invest 107: 519–528.
5. Trentham DE, Townes AS, Kang AH (1977) Autoimmunity to type II collagen an experimental model of arthritis. JExp Med 146: 857–868.
6. Griffiths MM, Nabozny GH, Hanson J, Harper DS, McCall S, et al. (1994) Collagen-induced arthritis and TCRs in SWR and B10Q mice expressing an Ek alpha transgene. J Immunol 153: 2758–2768.
7. Silva GL, Junta CM, Mello SS, Garcia PS, Rassi DM, et al. (2007) Profiling meta-analysis reveals primarily gene coexpression concordance between systemic lupus erythematosus and rheumatoid arthritis. Ann N Y Acad Sci 1110: 33–46.
8. Silva GL, Junta CM, Sakamoto-Hojo ET, Donadi EA, Louzada-Junior P, et al. (2009) Genetic susceptibility loci in rheumatoid arthritis establish transcriptional regulatory networks with other genes. Ann N Y Acad Sci 1173: 521–537.
9. Junta CM, Sandrin-Garcia P, Fachin-Saltoratto AL, Mello SS, Oliveira RD, et al. (2009) Differential gene expression of peripheral blood mononuclear cells from rheumatoid arthritis patients may discriminate immunogenetic, pathogenic and treatment features. Immunology 127: 365–372.
10. Donate PB, Fornari TA, Junta CM, Magalhães DA, Macedo C, et al. (2011) Collagen induced arthritis (CIA) in mice features regulatory transcriptional network connecting major histocompatibility complex (MHC H2) with autoantigen genes in the thymus. Immunobiology 216: 591–603.
11. Haeupl T, Witt H, Koczan D, Krenn V, Huber H, et al. (2010) Molecular signatures and new candidates to target the pathogenesis of rheumatoid arthritis. Physiol Genomics 29: 267–282.
12. Wu G, Zhu L, Dent JE, Nardini C (2010) A comprehensive molecular interaction map for rheumatoid arthritis. PLoS One 16: e10137.
13. Li J, Wan Y, Guo Q, Zou L, Zhang J, et al. (2010) Altered miRNA expression profile with miR-146a upregulation in CD4+ T cells from patients with rheumatoid arthritis. Arthritis ResTher 12: R81.
14. Pauley KM, Satoh M, Chan AL, Bubb MR, Reeves WH, et al. (2008) Upregulated miR-146a expression in peripheral blood mononuclear cells from rheumatoid arthritis patients. Arthritis Res Ther 10: R101.
15. Murata K, Yoshitomi H, Tanida S, Ishikawa M, Nishitani K, et al. (2010) Plasma and synovial fluid miRNAs as potential biomarkers of rheumatoid arthritis and osteoarthritis. Arthritis Res Ther 12: R86.
16. Ambros V (2004) The functions of animal miRNAs. Nature 431: 350–355.
17. Bartel DP (2004) MiRNAs: genomics, biogenesis, mechanism, and function. Cell 116: 281–297.
18. Chen CZ, Lodish HF (2005) MiRNAs as regulators of mammalian hematopoiesis. Semin.Immunol 17: 155–165.
19. Plasterk RH (2006) Micro RNAs in animal development. Cell 124: 877–881.
20. Engels BM, Hutvagner G (2006) Principles and effects of miRNA mediated posttranscriptional gene regulation. Oncogene 25: 6163–6169.
21. Behm-Ansmant I, Rehwinkel J, Izaurralde E (2006) MiRNAs silence gene expression by repressing protein expression and/or by promoting mRNA decay. Quant. Biol 71: 523–530.
22. Rajewsky N (2006) MiRNA target predictions in animals. Nat Genet 38: S8–S13.
23. Guo H, Ingolia NT, Weissman JS, Bartel DP (2010) Mammalian miRNAs predominantly act to decrease target mRNA levels. Nature 466: 835–840.
24. Grimson A, KFarh K, Johnston WK, Garrett-Engele P, Lim LP, et al. (2007) MiRNA targeting specificity in mammals: determinants beyond seed pairing Mol Cell 27: 91–105.
25. Selbach M, Schwanhausser B, Thierfelder N, Fang Z, Khanin R, et al. (2008) Widespread changes in protein synthesis induced bymiRNAs. Nature 455: 58–63.
26. Li QJ, Chau J, Ebert PJ, Sylvester G, Min H, et al. (2007) MiR-181a is an intrinsic modulator of T cell sensitivity and selection. Cell 129: 147–161.
27. Xue Q, Guo ZY, Li W, Wen WH, Meng YL, et al. (2010) Human activated CD4(+)T lymphocytes increase IL-2 expression by downregulating miRNA-181c. Mol Immunol 48: 592–599.
28. Thai TH, Calado DP, Casola S, Ansel KM, Xiao C, et al. (2007) Regulation of the germinal center response by miRNA-155. Science 316: 604–608.
29. Wu H, Neilson JR, Kumar P, Manocha M, Shankar P, et al. (2007) MiRNA profiling of naive, effector and memory CD8T cells. PLoS ONE 2: e1020.
30. Huang B, Zhao J, Lei Z, Shen S, Li D, et al. (2009) MiR-142–3p restricts cAMP production in CD4+CD25- T cells and CD4+CD25+ TREG cells by targeting AC9 mRNA. EMBO Rep 10: 180–185.
31. Stanczyk J, Pedrioli DM, Brentano F, Sanchez-Pernaute O, Kolling C, et al. (2008) Altered expression of miRNA in synovial fibroblasts and synovial tissue in rheumatoid arthritis. Arthritis Rheum 58: 1001–1009.
32. Fulci V, Scappucci G, Sebastiani GD, Giannitti C, Franceschini D, et al. (2010) MiR-223 is overexpressed in T-lymphocytes of patients affected by rheumatoid arthritis. Hum Immunol 71: 206–211.
33. Rehmsmeier M, Steffen P, Hochsmann M, Giegerich R (2004) Fast and effective prediction of microRNA/target duplexes. RNA 10: 1507–1517.
34. Kruger J, Rehmsmeier M (2006) RNAhybrid: microRNA target prediction easy, fast and flexible. Nucleic Acids Research 34: W451–W454.
35. Jetten AM (2009) Retinoid-related orphan receptors (RORs): critical roles in development, immunity, circadian rhythm, and cellular metabolism. Nuclear Receptor Signal 7: e003.
36. Leung BP, Sattar N, Crilly A, Prach M, McCarey DW, et al. (2003) A novel anti-inflammatory role for simvastatin in inflammatory arthritis. J Immunol 170: 1524–1530.
37. Eisen MB, Spellman PT, Brown PO, Botstein D (1998) Cluster analysis and display of genome-wide expression patterns. Proc Natl Acad Sci U S A 95: 14863–14868.
38. Huang JC, Morris QD, Frey BJ (2007) Bayesian inference of MiRNA targets from sequence and expression data. J Comput Biol 14: 550–563.
39. Lewis BP, Burge CB, Bartel DP (2005) Conserved seed pairing, often flanked by adenosines, indicates that thousands of human genes are microRNA targets. Cell 120: 15–20.
40. Alzabin S, Williams RO (2011) Effector T cells in rheumatoid arthritis: lessons from animal models. FEBS lett 585: 3649–3659.
41. Wooley PH, Luthra HS, Stuart JM, David CS (1981) Type II collagen induced arthritis in mice. I. Major histocompatibility complex (I-region) linkage and antibody correlates. J Exp Med 154: 688–700.
42. Magalhães DA, Silveira EL, Junta CM, Sandrin-Garcia P, Fachin AL, et al. (2006) Promiscuous gene expression in the thymus: the root of central tolerance. Clin and Develop.Immunol 13: 81–99.
43. Derbinski J, Kyewski B (2010) How thymic antigen presenting cells sample the body's self antigens. CurrOpinImmunol 22: 592–600.
44. Irla M, Hollander G, Reith W (2010) Control of central self-tolerance induction by autoreactive CD4+ thymocytes. Trends Immunol 31: 71–79.
45. Dai R, Ahmed SA (2011) MicroRNA, a new paradigm for understanding immunoregulation, inflammation and autoimmune diseases. Translational Research 157: 163–179.
46. Fu G, Vallee S, Rybakin V, McGuire MV, Ampudia J, et al. (2009) Themis controls thymocyte selection through regulation of T cell antigen receptor-mediated signaling. Nat Immunol 10: 848–856.
47. Ehinger M, Vestberg M, Johansson AC, Johannesson M, Svensson A et al. (2001) Influence of CD4 or CD8 deficiency on collagen-inducedarthritis. Immunology 103: 291–300.
48. Hughes PD, Belz GT, Fortner KA, Budd RC, Strasser A, et al. (2008) Apoptosis regulators Fas and Bim cooperate in shutdown of chronic immune responses and prevention of autoimmunity. Immunity 28: 197–205.
49. Weant AE, Michalek RD, Khan IU, Holbrook BC, Willingham MC, et al. (2008) Apoptosis regulators Bim and Fas function concurrently to control autoimmunity and CD8+ T cell contraction. Immunity 28: 218–230.
50. Bluestone JA, Abbas AK (2003) Natural versus adaptive regulatory T cells. Nat Rev 3: 253–257.
51. Roncarolo MG, Levings MK (2000) The role of different subsets of T regulatory cells in controlling autoimmunity.Curr.Opin.Immunol 12: 676–683.
52. Turrel-Davin F, Tournadre A, Pachot A, Arnaud B, Cazalis MA, et al. (2010) FoxO3a involved in neutrophil and T cell survival is overexpressed in rheumatoid blood and synovial tissue. Ann Rheum Dis 69: 755–760.
53. Yamaguchi Y, Fujio K, Shoda H, Okamoto A, Tsuno NH, et al. (2007) IL-17B and IL-17C are associated with TNF-alpha production and contribute to the exacerbation of inflammatory arthritis. J Immunol 179: 7128–7136.
54. Grigoryev YA, Kurian SM, Hart T, Nakorchevsky AA, Chen C, et al. (2011) MiRNA Regulation of Molecular Networks Mapped by Global MiRNA, mRNA, and Protein Expression in Activated T Lymphocytes. JImmunol 187: 2233–2243.

Serum Levels of Vasoactive Intestinal Peptide as a Prognostic Marker in Early Arthritis

Carmen Martínez[1]*, Ana M. Ortiz[2], Yasmina Juarranz[3], Amalia Lamana[2], Iria V. Seoane[3], Javier Leceta[3], Rosario García-Vicuña[2], Rosa P. Gomariz[3], Isidoro González-Álvaro[2]

1 Departamento de Biología Celular, Facultad de Medicina, Universidad Complutense de Madrid, Madrid, Spain, **2** Servicio de Reumatología, Hospital Universitario de la Princesa, Instituto de Investigación Sanitaria la Princesa, Madrid, Spain, **3** Departamento de Biología Celular, Facultad de Biología, Universidad Complutense de Madrid, Madrid, Spain

Abstract

Objective: Suitable biomarkers are essential for the design of therapeutic strategies in personalized medicine. Vasoactive intestinal peptide (VIP) has demonstrated immunomodulatory properties in autoimmune murine and ex vivo human models. Our aim was to study serum levels of VIP during the follow-up of an early arthritis (EA) cohort and to analyze its value as a biomarker predicting severity and therapeutic requirements.

Methods: Data from 91 patients on an EA register were analyzed (76% rheumatoid arthritis (RA), 24% undifferentiated arthritis, 73% women, and median age 54 years; median disease duration at entry, 5.4 months). We collected per protocol sociodemographic, clinical, and therapeutic data. VIP levels were determined by enzyme immunoassay in sera harvested from the 91 patients (353 visits; 3.9 visit/patient) and from 100 healthy controls. VIP values below the 25th percentile of those assessed in healthy population were considered low. To determine the effect of independent variables on VIP levels, we performed a longitudinal multivariate analysis nested by patient and visit. A multivariate ordered logistic regression was modeled to determine the effect of low VIP serum levels on disease activity at the end of follow-up.

Results: VIP concentrations varied considerably across EA patients. Those fulfilling the criteria for RA had the lowest values in the whole sample, although no significant differences were observed compared with healthy donors. Disease activity, which was assessed using DAS28, inversely correlated with VIP levels. After a two-year follow-up, those patients with low baseline levels of VIP displayed higher disease activity and received more intensive treatment.

Conclusion: Patients who are unable to up-regulate VIP seem to have a worse clinical course despite receiving more intense treatment. Therefore, measurement of VIP levels may be suitable as a prognostic biomarker.

Editor: Oliver Frey, University Hospital Jena, Germany

Funding: This work was supported by the Fondo de Investigación Sanitaria, Instituto de Salud Carlos III (PI08/0025, PI11/00195, PI11/00505, PI12/0758, RETICS RD08/0075, RD12/0009) and by FEDER funds from EU, S2010/BMD-2350 from Comunidad de Madrid. The funders had no role in study design, data collection and analysis, decision to publish, or preparation of the manuscript.

Competing Interests: A patent application (P201230827) for the use of VIP as a marker of prognostic in autoimmune diseases has been deposited by the Fundación de Investigación Biomédica del Hospital Universitario de la Princesa at the Oficina Española de Patentes y Marcas. The full name of the patent application is: VIP use as a prognostic marker of autoimmune diseases. This does not alter the authors' adherence to all the PLOS ONE policies.

* E-mail: cmmora@bio.ucm.es

These authors contributed equally to this work.

Introduction

Rheumatoid arthritis (RA) is a systemic autoimmune disease with a heterogeneous clinical spectrum. At present, our ability to predict this heterogeneity is poor, likely because of limitations in understanding its molecular complexity. Recent efforts to improve outcome in patients with RA have focused on the early stages of the disease [1], when aggressive treatment can slow progression and change long-term course. Currently, another crucial therapeutic goal is to delay/prevent progression of undifferentiated arthritis (UA) and one of the challenges faced by rheumatologists is the classification of these patients. Thus, many studies have attempted to identify prognostic markers in early RA or UA that correlate with disease progression in order to establish which patients are at risk for poor outcome or, conversely, which are destined to have a more benign disease so that overtreatment can be avoided [2]. However, criteria for this clustering of patients are scarce. To date, validated biomarkers of severity such as rheumatoid factor (RF) or anti-citrullinated peptide antibodies (ACPA) do not enable us to identify those patients who require more intensive treatment. Although challenging, identification of such predictive tools would help us tailor treatment.

Vasoactive intestinal peptide (VIP) is produced by neural, endocrine, and immune cells. It has anti-inflammatory and immunoregulatory effects [3], which are mediated by three G-protein–coupled receptors (VPAC1, VPAC2, and PAC1) [4,5]. First studies evaluating the endogenous role of VIP were performed in transgenic mice harboring a chimeric VIP gene

Table 1. Baseline characteristics of patients with early arthritis.

	Rheumatoid artritis (n = 69)	Undifferentiated arthritis (n = 22)	Total (n = 91)	P value
Age (years)	54 [45–66]	55 [44–69]	54 [45–66]	n.s.
Female gender (%)	78	54	73	0.004
Disease duration (months)	5 [3–8]	7 [3–11]	5.4 [3.2–8.4]	n.s.
GDAPa	46 [29–60]	46 [28–58]	46 [28–60]	n.s.
GDAPh	50 [30 - 72]	30 [14–50]	42 [25–66]	0.002
VAS Pain	52 [25–70]	48 [13–60]	50 [20–70]	n.s.
HAQ	1.125 [0.625–1.750]	0.875 [0.375–1.375]	1 [0.625–1.625]	n.s.
TJC	6 [2–12]	3 [0–10]	6 [1–12]	n.s.
SJC	7 [3–10]	3 [0–6]	5 [2–9]	0.004
ESR	32 [19–54]	17 [8–34]	30 [15–46]	0.006
CRP (mg/dl)	0.92 [0.2–1.96]	0.48 [0.1–0.82]	0.72 [0.16–1.7]	0.047
DAS28 (0–10)	5.0 [4.0–6.1]	3.6 [3.1–4.5]	4.8 [3.5–6.0]	0.002
RF (%)	54	18	45	0.004
ACPA+ (%)	60	14	49	<0.001
VIP (pg/ml)	342 [262–440]	375 [243–490]	352 [261–444]	n.s.

Data are shown as the median or percentage. GDAPa: global disease assessment by patient; GDAPh: global disease assessment by physician; VAS: visual analog scale; HAQ: health assessment questionnaire; TJC: tender joint count; SJC: swollen joint count; ESR: erythrocyte sedimentation rate; CRP: C-reactive protein; DAS28:28-joint count Disease Activity Score; RF: rheumatoid factor; ACPA: anti-citrullinated peptide antibodies; VIP: vasoactive intestinal peptide. n.s.: not significant.

which showed reduced brain VIP content and deficiencies in learning abilities supporting an important function for VIP in vivo [6]. Recently, it has been described that VIP-deficient mice display certain physiological abnormalities [7,8] and exhibit reduced mortality and impaired proinflammatory responses to lipopolysaccharide-induced endotoxemia [9], suggesting that defects in the innate arm of immunity may occurs in the chronic absence of VIP. Numerous reports have focused on the effects of VIP treatment. Thus, administration of VIP has demonstrated therapeutic effects in several murine models of inflammatory/autoimmune diseases [10–14]. In a murine model of collagen-induced arthritis, administration of VIP reduced joint inflammation and destruction, thus decreasing the inflammatory response and inducing a shift in the Th1/Th2 balance [10,15]. Research in human models has confirmed the modulatory effects of VIP in *ex vivo* assays with fibroblast-like synoviocytes and peripheral blood lymphocytes from patients with RA through down-regulation of proinflammatory mediators [16–18]. Decreased expression of VIP was recently reported in the synovial fluid of patients with osteoarthritis (OA) and poor radiological progression, indicating a protective role for VIP [19]. Moreover, patients with juvenile idiopathic arthritis have lower serum levels of VIP than healthy controls [20].

Consequently, the role of endogenous VIP in the pathophysiology of RA is becoming clearer. Our hypothesis is that VIP serum levels are correlated with disease severity. Therefore, the objective of this work was to assess VIP levels during the follow-up of patients with early arthritis (EA) and to explore its potential value as a biomarker in RA.

Methods

Ethics Statement

The register protocol was reviewed and approved by the Ethics Committee for Clinical Research at the Instituto de Investigación Sanitaria La Princesa. All patients were informed about the study and signed an informed consent form before inclusion in the EA register.

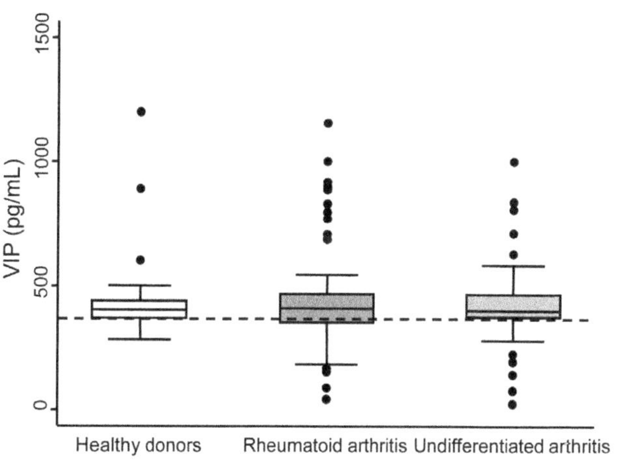

Figure 1. Variability of VIP levels in healthy controls (n = 100) and patients with early arthritis (Rheumatoid arthritis n = 69, Undifferentiated arthritis n = 22). Data are presented as the interquartile range (p75 upper edge of the box, p25 lower edge, p50 midline), p90 (line above the box), and p10 (line below the box) of the serum VIP levels. Dots represent outliers. Dashed lines show the 25th percentile of the healthy donor group.

Patients and Controls

The study sample comprised 91 patients enrolled on our EA register. The inclusion criteria included more than 1 swollen joint for at least 4 weeks and symptoms for less than a year. Only data from patients fulfilling the 1987 American College of Rheumatology criteria for RA [21] within the 5-year follow-up (n = 69) or with chronic undifferentiated arthritis (n = 22) were analyzed.

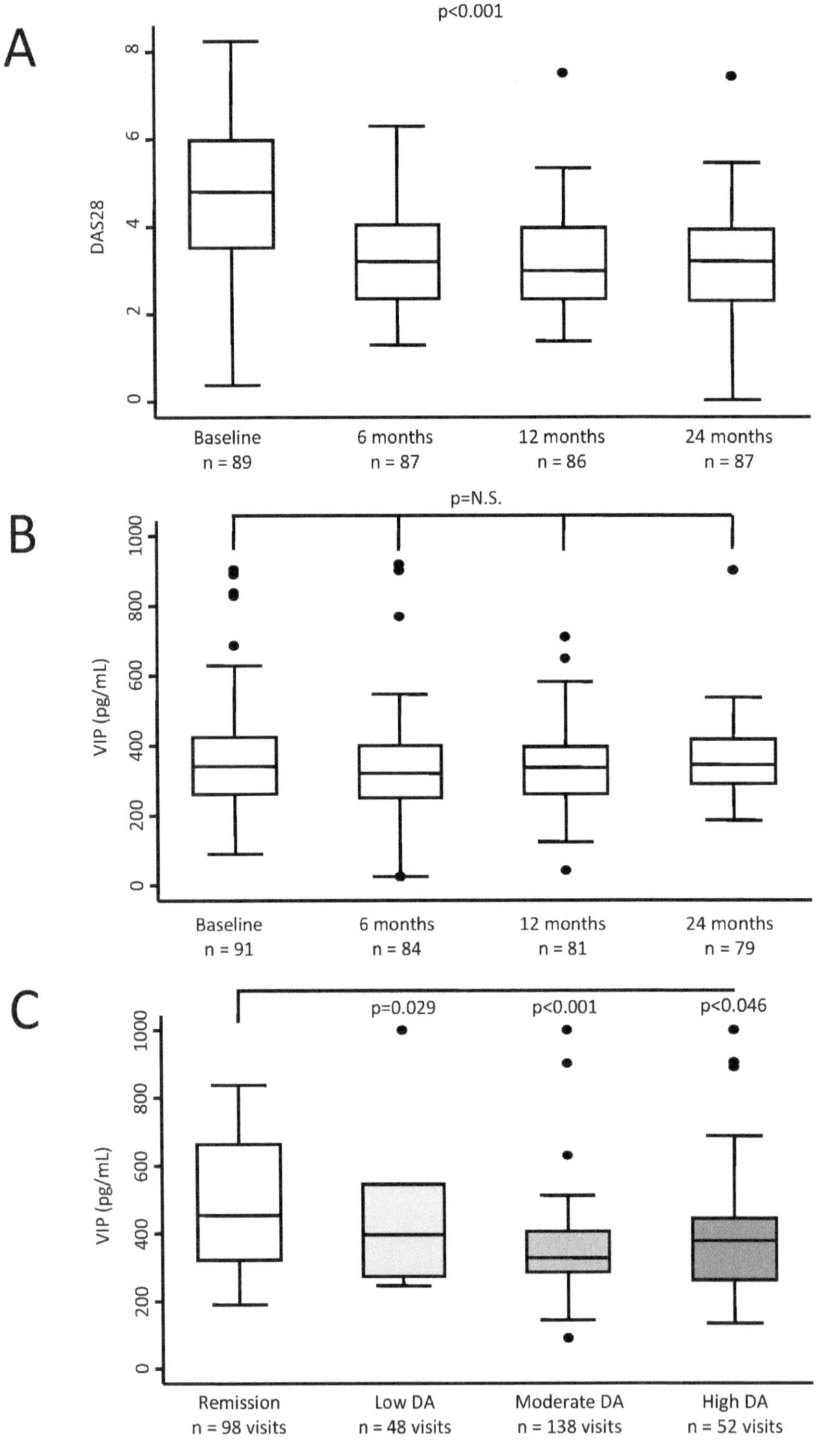

Figure 2. VIP serum levels correlate inversely with disease activity in patients with early arthritis. A) Progress of disease activity estimated by DAS28 at follow-up visits. **B)** Serum levels of VIP during the follow-up period. **C)** Serum VIP levels considering disease activity level. Data are presented as the interquartile range (p75 upper edge of the box, p25 lower edge, p50 midline), p90 (line above the box), and p10 (line below the box) of the serum VIP levels. Dots represent outliers. Statistical significance was established using the Kruskal-Wallis test in panels A and B. In panel C the significance level is that obtained in the multivariable analysis displayed in Table 2, model 2.

Patients with diagnosis of spondyloarthritis, connective tissue diseases or crystal induced arthritis, were excluded from the analysis. The register protocol included 5 visits (baseline, 6, 12, 24, and 60 months), and at each one we recorded the following data in

Table 2. Variables associated with VIP serum levels during follow-up of patients with early arthritis.

	Model 1		Model 2	
	β coeff ± SE	P	β coeff ± SE	P
Gender				
Male	Reference		Reference	
Female	0.108±0.067	0.106	0.105	0.086
Diagnosis				
RA	n.i.	n.s.	n.i.	n.s.
UA				
ACPA	n.i.	n.s.	n.i.	n.s.
Age (by 10 yr)	0.05±0.019	0.013	0.05±0.018	0.008
GDA Pat	n.i.	n.s.	n.i.	n.s.
GDA Phy	n.i.	n.s.	n.i.	n.s.
HAQ	n.i.	n.s.	n.i.	n.s.
SJC	n.i.	n.s.	n.i.	n.s.
MS	n.i.	n.s.	n.i.	n.s.
DAS28	−0.027±0.014	0.045	–	–
Disease activity				
Remission	–	–	Reference	
Low			−0.094±0.043	0.029
Moderate			−0.187±0.049	<0.001
High			−0.113±0.057	0.046
Leflunomide (mg/d)	n.i.	n.s.	n.i.	n.s.
TNF blockers	0.183±0.075	0.01	0.165±0.065	0.011

The longitudinal analysis was performed with data (logarithmic transformation of censored VIP levels; see figure S2) from 340 visits corresponding to the 88 patients with all information available in, at least, two visits. Model 1 was fitted using the continuous value of DAS28 as measure of disease activity while model 2 includes the categorical variable based in cut-off values of this index. The average number of visits by patient was 3.9. The table shows all the variables reaching p<0.15 at the bivariate analysis (see Methods section for further information on multivariable analysis modeling). Coeff: coefficient; CI: confidence interval; RA: rheumatoid arthritis; UA: undifferentiated arthritis; ACPA: anti-citrullinated peptide antibodies; yr, year; GDA: global disease assessment; Pat: patient; Phy: physician; HAQ: health assessment questionnaire; SJC: swollen joint count; MS: morning stiffness; DAS28, 28-joint Disease Activity Score; TNF: tumor necrosis factor; n.s.: not significant; n.i.: not included.

an electronic database: clinical and demographic information; disease duration at the beginning of follow-up; 28-joint Disease Activity Score (DAS28) [22]; global disease activity on a 100-mm visual analogue scale assessed by both the patient and the physician; Health Assessment Questionnaire score (HAQ; Spanish version) [23]; and the results of laboratory tests including erythrocyte sedimentation rate (ESR), C-reactive protein (CRP), rheumatoid factor (RF, assessed by nephelometry; positive >20 IU/ml), and anti-citrullinated peptide antibody (ACPA, measured by enzyme immunoassay [EIA]: Euro-Diagnostica Immunoscan RA; positive >50 IU/ml).

Healthy donors (n = 100) were recruited from the Centro de Transfusiones de la Comunidad de Madrid. Following the Spanish Personal Data Protection Law, their demographic information was confidential.

Measurement of Serum VIP

VIP levels were determined using a competitive EIA with a commercially available kit according to the manufacturer's instructions (Phoenix Pharmaceutical, Karlsruhe, Germany). We previously optimized sample preparation procedure to obtain optimal results. First, it was tested the extraction of peptides from serum using a SEP-COLUMN containing 200 mg of C18, according to the manufacturer's recommendations. Second, serum samples were concentrated by using a lyophilizer to assay different concentrations. Then, VIP levels were determined. The best results were obtained in reconstituted dried extract (2:1) without the use of columns. The assay was performed as follow, briefly, the samples were freeze-dried and dissolved in EIA buffer (2:1), added to an immunoplate pre-coated with a secondary antibody, and incubated with biotinylated VIP and a primary antibody whose Fab fragment competitively binds to the biotinylated peptide and targeted peptide in samples. After washes, the wells were incubated with streptavidin-horseradish peroxidase, which catalyzed the oxidation of the substrate solution. The reaction was stopped using the stop solution and absorbance measured at 450 nm. A standard curve of known concentration was established. The concentration in the samples was determined by extrapolation to this curve and by applying the corresponding dilution factor. Samples from each patient were assayed twice. The minimum detectable concentration was 0.12 ng/ml of sample, with an intra-assay and interassay variation of ≤5% and 15%, respectively.

Since serum samples were stored at −80°C for different periods of time until assay (range, 1 to 112 months), we first analyzed the effect of sample frozen-time on the ability of our assay to detect VIP. As shown in Figure S1, no significant correlation was observed between VIP serum level and frozen-time.

Statistical Analysis and New Variables

Normally distributed quantitative variables were expressed as the mean ± standard deviation, while non-normally distributed variables were expressed as the median and interquartile range (IQR). Qualitative variables were described using an estimation of the proportions. Variables with a normal distribution were analyzed using the *t* test, while the Mann-Whitney or Kruskal-Wallis tests were used for variables with a non-normal distribution. A χ^2 test or the Fisher exact test was used to compare categorical variables.

Considering that the raw data contained considerably left-shifted values (Figure S2A), we decided to censor values higher than 1000 pg/ml in this figure (Figure S2B) to avoid missing information if patients with very high VIP values were excluded. In addition, since the censored variable does not show a Gaussian distribution, data were normalized through logarithmic transformation (Figure S2C).

Additional variables were defined to further describe the role of VIP in the progress of arthritis. VIP levels were considered to be low when the concentration was below the 25th percentile of its concentration in the healthy population (370 pg/ml). The intensity of disease-modifying anti-rheumatic drugs (DMARDs) treatment (IDT) was assessed as the number of days of treatment with each DMARD during follow-up adjusted for weighted coefficients, as described elsewhere [24].

To identify factors that influenced VIP levels during follow-up (logarithmic transformation of the censored VIP levels as the dependent variable), we used data from 340 visits in the 88 patients with all information available in at least 2 visits to fit a population-averaged model by means of generalized linear models nested by patient and visit using the *xtgee* command of Stata 12 for

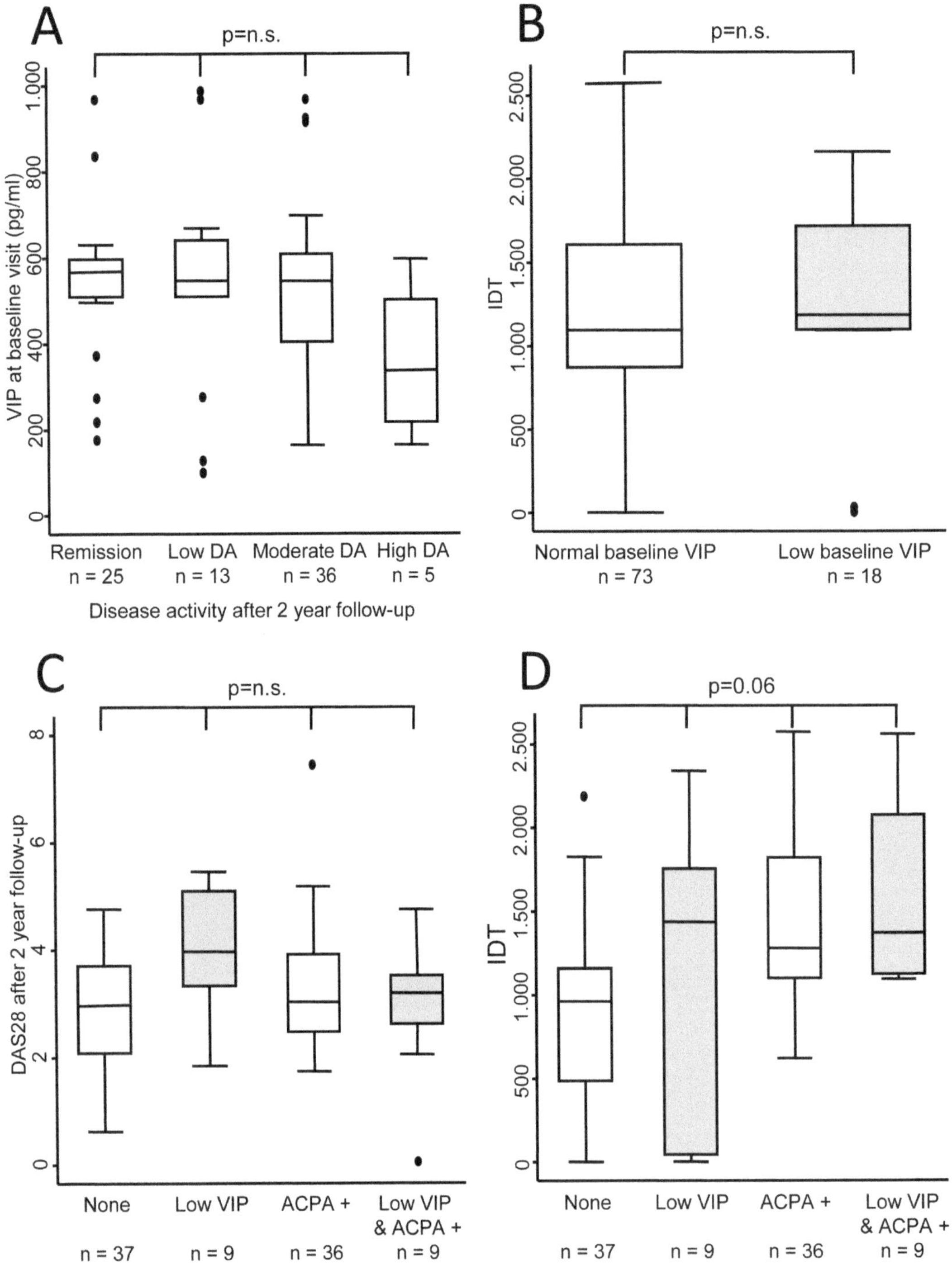

Figure 3. Serum VIP level as a prognostic marker. A) VIP levels at baseline according to the degree of disease activity after two years of follow-up. **B)** Intensity of treatment in two subpopulations of early arthritis patients clustered according to serum VIP level. Cumulative DMARD treatment during the follow-up period was estimated using the intensity of DMARD treatment (IDT) variable (see Methods). **C)** Disease activity estimated by DAS28 after two years of follow-up in a population of patients with early arthritis according to VIP levels and the presence of anti-citrullinated peptide antibody (ACPA+). **D)** Intensity of DMARD treatment in different subpopulations clustered by serum VIP levels and the presence of ACPA. Data are presented as the interquartile range (p75 upper edge of the box, p25 lower edge, p50 midline), p90 (line above the box), and p10 (line below the box). Dots represent outliers. Statistical significance was established using the Kruskal-Wallis test in panels A, C and D or Mann-Whitney test in panel B.

Windows (StataCorp LP, College Station, Texas, USA). The population-averaged generalized estimating equations were first modeled by adding all variables with a p value <0.15 in the bivariate analysis. The final models were constructed using a quasi-likelihood estimation based on the independence model

Table 3. Effect of low baseline VIP levels in serum on disease activity after a two-year follow-up.

	Odds ratio (95% CI)	P
Age (years)		
<45	Ref.	
45–65	–	n.s.
>65	–	n.s.
Gender		
Man	Ref.	
Woman	4.35 (1.46–12.99)	0.008
Diagnosis		
RA	Ref.	
UA	–	n.s.
Positive RF	–	n.s.
Interaction VIP, ACPA		
Normal VIP, ACPA-negative	Ref.	
Low VIP, ACPA-negative	6.11 (1.28–29.22)	0.023
Normal VIP, ACPA-positive	0.68 (0.24–1.9)	0.458
Low VIP, ACPA-positive	0.24 (0.03–1.85)	0.170
DMARD treatment		
None	Ref.	
Monotherapy	2.2 (0.30–12.96)	0.437
Combined therapy	6.62 (0.84–51.93)	0.071
Baseline DAS28	–	n.s.
Cutpoints	β coeff. (95% CI)	
Remission/Low disease activity	1.59 (–0.40 to 3.59)	–
Low/Moderate disease activity	2.46 (0.44–4.49)	–
Moderate/High disease activity	5.97 (3.57–8.38)	–

DAS28:28-joint Disease Activity Score; HAQ: Health Assessment Questionnaire; Coeff.: coefficient; Ref.: reference; RA: rheumatoid arthritis; UA: undifferentiated arthritis; ACPA: anti-citrullinated peptide antibody; n.s.: not significant.

information criterion [25] and Wald tests, after removing all variables with $p>0.15$.

To determine the usefulness of baseline VIP levels for predicting disease progress, we performed an ordered logistic model using the *ologit* command of Stata 12. The dependent variable was the disease activity level at the 2-year follow-up, using the cut-off points for DAS28 proposed by Prevoo et al. (<2.6, remission; 2.6 to 3.2, low disease activity; 3.2 to 5.1, moderate disease activity; >5.1 high disease activity) [22]. In this model, the dependent variable considered remission as 0 and low, moderate, and high disease activity as 1, 2, and 3. Thus, the ordered logistic analysis can also estimate cut-off points that aid the interpretation of the coefficients for each independent variable according to the levels of the dependent variable. The analysis was modeled as described above for *xtgee*.

The significance level was set at $p<0.05$.

Results

Characteristics of Patients with EA. VIP Levels in Patients and Healthy Donors

A total of 91 patients with RA (n = 69) or UA (n = 22) were included in the study. The main difference between these two subgroups was a higher frequency of female patients in the RA group, in which more severe disease at baseline and a higher prevalence of RF and ACPA positivity were also found (Table 1). No significant differences were detected between the groups in variables expressing a subjective component such as pain, global disease assessment by patient, tender joint count, and HAQ.

Considering serum levels of VIP at baseline, no significant differences were detected between the groups (Table 1) or between patients and healthy controls (Figure 1). Nevertheless, the distribution of the VIP serum concentration was considerably heterogeneous, especially among RA patients, and ranged from 100 to >1000 pg/ml. In addition, the lowest levels of VIP tended to be more frequent in RA and UA patients than in healthy donors (Figure 1).

Low VIP Levels are Associated with Higher Disease Activity in Patients with EA

Despite a significant decrease in disease activity during follow-up (Figure 2A), we could not detect a parallel down-regulation of serum VIP levels (Figure 2B). Therefore, we performed a multivariate analysis to achieve a more accurate appraisal of the potential relationship between VIP levels and disease activity in patients with EA. Our data showed that elderly patients expressed slightly but significantly higher serum levels of VIP during follow-up (Table 2 and Figure S3). In addition, VIP levels tended to be significantly higher in visits at which patients were treated with TNF blockers. Interestingly, after adjustment for these confounders, we observed a significant and negative correlation between disease activity, estimated through DAS28, and VIP serum levels (Table 2, model 1).

Next, we analyzed the concentration of VIP at the different visits after clustering the results in four groups: remission, low, moderate, and high disease activity. As shown in Figure 2C, we observed lower levels of VIP in those visits with moderate or high activity compared to visits at which patients were in remission and those differences reached statistically significance after adjusting by confounders (Table 2, model 2). However, this approach did not reveal whether inflammation induced low VIP levels or those patients with low VIP showed more intense disease activity.

Low Baseline VIP Serum Levels as a Biomarker of Disease Severity

Next, we studied whether having low VIP serum levels at baseline could predict long-term disease activity. As Figure 3A shows, those patients who continued to have high or moderate disease activity levels after a two-year follow-up had lower baseline VIP serum levels. This behaviour was detected despite the observed trend toward higher prescription of DMARDs in patients with low VIP serum levels (Figure 3B).

In view of the various confounding factors that could influence disease activity level after two years of follow-up, we performed a multivariate ordered logistic regression to determine which variables contribute to an increased level of disease activity. Female patients showed an odds ratio (OR) of 4.3 for poorer disease outcome than male patients (Table 3). In addition, patients requiring combined therapy displayed an OR of 6.6 for remaining at a higher disease activity level than those who did not require DMARDs. After adjustment for these confounders, having low baseline VIP levels was associated with a higher level of disease activity after two years of follow-up. However, marked interference with ACPA positivity was observed (Table 3). Thus, patients with low VIP serum levels but negative ACPA had an OR of 6.1 for being at a higher disease activity level than those with negative

ACPA levels and normal VIP serum levels (Table 3 and Figure 3C). By contrast, patients with positive ACPA levels showed a nonsignificant trend toward lower disease activity regardless of VIP levels (Table 3 and Figure 3C). In addition, the model revealed that the effect of gender, treatment, and baseline VIP level was more intense when the level of disease activity increased (β coefficients for cutpoints in Table 3).

In terms of treatment, ACPA positivity was associated with higher prescription of DMARDs, as occurred when low VIP levels were associated with ACPA positivity (Figure 3D). More heterogeneous regimens were found in patients with low VIP levels (treating physician blinded) and negativity for ACPA, but they undoubtedly received more intensive treatment than the population that met neither of these conditions (Figure 3B and 3D).

Discussion

Rheumatoid arthritis is a complex heterogeneous disease resulting from the interaction between genetic and environmental triggers and from the intervention of key molecules that modulate its severity. To date, there are no published data demonstrating an association between abnormal regulation of VIP and an increased risk for developing RA. However, growing evidence supports the ability of VIP to regulate the intensity of the inflammatory process and the immune response that contribute to the pathogenesis of rheumatic diseases [26]. In this work, we showed that the lowest values of serum VIP levels were clustered in the EA group, despite no significant differences compared with healthy donors. Furthermore, our results reveal an inverse correlation between disease activity and VIP concentration in serum. Thus, patients with lower VIP levels showed higher DAS28 scores, and, conversely, higher VIP levels were detected in the group of patients in remission and in those with significantly weaker disease activity.

Several experimental findings support this observation. Treatment with VIP reduced the incidence and severity of arthritis in murine models of RA by decreasing the production of proinflammatory cytokines and chemokines, and inducing a shift in the Th phenotype from a Th1-type toward a Th2-type response and generating efficient regulatory T cells [10,27]. In human fibroblast-like synoviocytes from RA patients, VIP downregulated the expression and production of proinflammatory cytokines, chemokines and COX2 as well as the production of IFNβ, CXCL8, and the matrix metalloproteinase-3 induced by TLR ligands [16,17,28].

Given the above evidence on the role of VIP, it seems reasonable that patients in whom production of this immunoregulatory peptide did not increase have more severe autoimmune and inflammatory responses and poor outcomes. In close correlation with our data, expression of VIP in synovial fluid and articular cartilage from patients with OA was negatively associated with progressive joint damage as a potential indicator of disease severity, thus suggesting that VIP could play a protective role in progression of OA [19]. Moreover, low serum levels of VIP have been described in patients with juvenile idiopathic arthritis who show clinical evidence of cardiac autonomic neuropathy associated with a parasympathetic dysfunction. In these patients, a significant positive association was found between cardiac autonomic neuropathy and major disease manifestations, including activity; therefore, the authors suggested that serum VIP should be assessed in these patients [20].

Although several parameters (eg, RF, ACPA, ESR, and CRP) have been proposed as predictors of long-term outcome of EA, they enable us to classify only 65% of patients [2,24,29–31]. Furthermore, as RF and ACPA largely overlap, identifying new prognostic markers would be essential for providing complementary information in order to improve the performance of a biomarker-guided strategy. In this setting, the association between VIP levels and disease activity reported here suggests that baseline serum VIP could be a feasible biomarker that enables EA patients to be stratified for therapeutic decision making. In fact, our data support that measurement of serum VIP levels at baseline enhances the predictive value of ACPA in determining long-term outcome in patients with EA. Thus, ACPA-negative patients with low VIP serum levels had a higher degree of disease activity than ACPA-negative patients with normal serum VIP levels and an even higher degree of disease activity than ACPA-positive patients. This finding likely reflects selection bias, since the presence of ACPA, a recognized marker of poor prognosis to which the attending rheumatologist was not blinded, was associated with more intense prescription of DMARDs. As a consequence, ACPA-positive patients with normal VIP showed similar disease activity to ACPA-negative patients with normal VIP. Interestingly, although the difference was not significant, ACPA-positive patients with low VIP serum levels had a slightly higher degree of disease activity and a greater requirement for DMARDs than ACPA-positive patients with normal VIP serum levels. On the other hand, ACPA-negative patients with low VIP levels received more heterogeneous treatment, probably because of the lack of a suitable marker, since physicians were entirely unaware of the value of this parameter.

An additional advantage of VIP as a prognostic marker is its scarce variation during follow-up, which indicates that VIP levels depend on the individual and do not change owing to external factors during follow-up. Thus, VIP concentrations could predict the outcome of arthritis independently of the treatment prescribed and the phase of the disease.

Our study is subject to a series of limitations. First, our data show that elderly patients have slightly but significantly higher serum levels of VIP. However, as demographic information in the healthy volunteers was confidential, we were unable to draw a comparison with the patients. In this regard, the correlation between VIP levels and gender and age has received little attention in the literature. The only study that does examine this correlation found no differences in VIP concentrations between men and women with secondary hyperparathyroidism undergoing dialysis [32]. Nevertheless, variation attributable to age in our study is lower than individual variability among EA patients (Figure S3). Second, the absence of a pre-established treatment strategy in our unit means that variations in the prescription of DMARDs by the rheumatologists involved in the study could interfere with the results. Third, considering the dispersion of VIP values owing to the variability of ELISA, we had to apply mathematical modifications to optimize the statistical analysis, thus hampering implementation in daily clinical practice.

Our study has the following strengths. First, exhaustive and rigorous collection of data on treatment with DMARDs goes some way to resolving the second limitation. VIP levels were measured retrospectively; therefore, the rheumatologists were blinded to serum VIP levels but not to ACPA reactivity when they selected therapy. Consequently, they were able to prescribe more intensive treatment to ACPA-positive patients. Second, we included a high number of samples and clinical data (about 4 visits per each of the 91 patients).

In conclusion, our study demonstrates that EA patients with low baseline VIP levels have worse disease outcome. Validation of the predictive value of serum VIP levels would enable earlier and more intensive treatment of patients with the most aggressive forms of RA.

Supporting Information

Figure S1 Frozen storage does not affect the measurement of serum VIP levels. VIP concentration at serum from samples stored from one month to 10 years is shown. The red line represents the linear prediction obtained with the command *lfit* of Stata 12.

Figure S2 Normalization of the VIP serum levels variable in order to obtain a distribution closer to Gaussian.

Figure S3 Correlation between age and VIP serum levels. Data are shown as dot plot and the exponential linear prediction with 95% confidence interval at ages 20, 30, 40, 50, 60, 70 and 80. These data were obtained using the command *marginsplot* of Stata 12 after performing the multivariable analysis displayed in Table 2 (dependent variable logarithmic transformation of censored VIP).

Acknowledgments

The authors are grateful to the patients of the EA Register and to the Centro de Transfusiones de la Comunidad de Madrid for recruiting healthy donors.

Author Contributions

Conceived and designed the experiments: CM AMO RPG IG-A. Performed the experiments: CM YJ AL IVS IG-A AMO JL. Analyzed the data: IG-A CM RPG AMO. Wrote the paper: CM IG-A RPG RG-V.

References

1. Schoels M, Knevel R, Aletaha D, Bijlsma JW, Breedveld FC, et al. (2010) Evidence for treating rheumatoid arthritis to target: results of a systematic literature search. Ann Rheum Dis 9: 638–643.
2. Smolen JS, Aletaha D, Grisar J, Redlich K, Steiner G, et al. (2008) The need for prognosticators in rheumatoid arthritis. Biological and clinical markers: where are we now? Arthritis Res Ther 10: 208–219.
3. Gomariz RP, Juarranz Y, Abad C, Arranz A, Leceta J, et al. (2006) VIP-PACAP system in immunity: new insights for multitarget therapy. Ann N Y Acad Sci 1070: 51–74.
4. Couvineau A, Laburthe M (2012) VPAC receptors: structure, molecular pharmacology and interaction with accessory proteins. Br J Pharmacol 166: 42–50.
5. Harmar AJ, Fahrenkrug J, Gozes I, Laburthe M, May V et al. (2012) Pharmacology and functions of receptors for vasoactive intestinal peptide and pituitary adenylate cyclase-activating polypeptide: IUPHAR Review 1. Br J Pharmacol 166: 4–17.
6. Gozes I, Glowa J, Brenneman DE, McCune SK, Lee E, et al. (1993) Learning and sexual deficiencies in transgenic mice carrying a chimeric vasoactive intestinal peptide gene. J Mol Neurosci 4: 185–193.
7. Szema AM, Hamidi SA, Lyubsky S, Dickman KG, Mathew S et al. (2006) Mice lacking the VIP gene show airway hyperresponsiveness and airway inflammation, partially reversible by VIP. Am J Physiol Lung Cell Mol Physiol 291: L880–886.
8. Colwell CS, Michel S, Itri J, Rodríguez W, Tam J et al. (2003) Disrupted circadian rhythms in VIP- and PHI-deficient mice. Am J Physiol Regul Integr Comp Physiol 285: R939–949.
9. Abad C, Tan YV, Cheung-Lau G, Nobuta H and Waschek JA (2012) VIP deficient mice exhibit resistance to lipopolysaccharide induced endotoxemia with an intrinsic defect in proinflammatory cellular responses. PLOS One 7: e36922.
10. Delgado M, Abad C, Martínez C, Leceta J, Gomariz RP (2001) Vasoactive intestinal peptide prevents experimental arthritis by downregulating both autoimmune and inflammatory components of the disease. Nat Med 7: 563–568.
11. Delgado M, Martínez C, Pozo D, Calvo JR, Leceta J, et al. (1999) Vasoactive intestinal peptide (VIP) and pituitary adenylate cyclase-activating polypeptide (PACAP) protect mice from lethal endotoxemia through the inhibition of TNF-α and IL-6. J Immunol 162: 1200–1205.
12. Abad C, Martínez C, Juarranz MG, Calvo JR, Leceta J, et al. (2003) Therapeutic effects of vasoactive intestinal peptide in the trinitrobenzene sulfonic acid mice model of Crohn's disease. Gastroenterology 124: 961–971.
13. Jimeno R, Gomariz RP, Gutiérrez-Cañas I, Martínez C, Juarranz Y, et al. (2010) New insights into the role of VIP on the ratio of T-cell subsets during the development of autoimmune diabetes. Immunol Cell Biol 88: 734–745.
14. Abad C, Waschek JA (2011) Immunomodulatory roles of VIP and PACAP in models of multiple sclerosis. Curr Pharm Des 17: 1025–1035.
15. Juarranz Y, Abad C, Martínez C, Arranz A, Gutierrez-Cañas I, et al. (2005) Protective effect of vasoactive intestinal peptide on bone destruction in the collagen-induced arthritis model of rheumatoid arthritis. Arthritis Res Ther 7: R1034–R1045.
16. Juarranz MG, Santiago B, Torroba M, Gutierrez-Cañas I, Palao G, et al. (2004) Vasoactive intestinal peptide modulates proinflammatory mediator synthesis in osteoarthritic and rheumatoid synovial cells. Rheumatology 43: 16–22.
17. Carrión M, Juarranz Y, Pérez-García S, Jimeno R, Pablos JL, et al. (2011) RNA sensors in human osteoarthritis and rheumatoid arthritis synovial fibroblasts: immune regulation by vasoactive intestinal peptide. Arthritis Rheum 63: 1626–1636.
18. Gutiérrez-Cañas I, Juarranz Y, Santiago B, Martínez C, Gomariz RP, et al. (2008) Immunoregulatory properties of vasoactive intestinal peptide in human T cell subsets: Implications for rheumatoid arthritis. Brain Behav Immun 22: 312–317.
19. Jiang W, Gao SG, Chen XG, Xu XC, Xu M, et al. (2012) Expression of synovial fluid and articular cartilage VIP in human osteoarthritic knee: A new indicator of disease severity? Clin Biochem 45: 1607–1612.
20. El-Sayed ZA, Mostafa GA, Aly GS, El-Shahed GS, El-Aziz MM, et al. (2009) Cardiovascular autonomic function assessed by autonomic function tests and serum autonomic neuropeptides in Egyptian children and adolescents with rheumatic diseases. Rheumatology 48: 843–848.
21. Arnett FC, Edworthy SM, Bloch DA, McShane DJ, Fries JF, et al. (1988) The American Rheumatism Association 1987 revised criteria for the classification of rheumatoid arthritis. Arthritis Rheum 31: 315–324.
22. Prevoo ML, van't Hof MA, Kuper HH, van Leeuwen MA, van de Putte LB, et al. (1995) Modified disease activity scores that include twenty-eight-joint counts. Development and validation in a prospective longitudinal study of patients with rheumatoid arthritis. Arthritis Rheum 38: 44–48.
23. Esteve-Vives J, Batlle-Gualda E, Reig A (1993) Spanish version of the Health Assessment Questionnaire: reliability, validity and transcultural equivalency. Grupo para la Adaptación del HAQ a la Población Española. J Rheumatol 20: 2116–2122.
24. González-Álvaro I, Ortiz AM, Álvaro-Gracia JM, Castañeda S, Díaz-Sánchez B, et al. (2011) Interleukin 15 levels in serum may predict a severe disease course in patients with early arthritis. PLOS One 6: e29492.
25. Pan W (2001) Model selection in estimating equations. Biometrics 57: 529–534.
26. Gonzalez-Rey E, Anderson P, Delgado M (2007) Emerging roles of vasoactive intestinal peptide: a new approach for autoimmune therapy. Ann Rheum Dis 66 Suppl 3: iii70–76.
27. Gonzalez-Rey E, Fernandez-Martin A, Chorny A, Delgado M (2006) Vasoactive intestinal peptide induces CD4+CD25+ T regulatory cells with therapeutic effect in collagen-induced arthritis. Arthritis Rheum 54: 864–876.
28. Pérez-García S, Juarranz Y, Carrión M, Gutiérrez-Cañas I, Margioris A, et al. (2011) Mapping the CRF-urocortins system in human osteoarthritic and rheumatoid synovial fibroblasts: effect of vasoactive intestinal peptide. J Cell Physiol 226: 3261–3269.
29. de Vries-Bouwstra JK, Goekoop-Ruiterman YP, Verpoort KN, Schreuder GM, Ewals JA, et al. (2008) Progression of joint damage in early rheumatoid arthritis: association with HLA-DRB1, rheumatoid factor, and anti-citrullinated protein antibodies in relation to different treatment strategies. Arthritis Rheum 58: 1293–1298.
30. Raza K, Filer A (2009) Predicting the development of RA in patients with early undifferentiated arthritis. Best Pract Res Clin Rheumatol 23: 25–36.
31. Szodoray P, Szabo Z, Kapitany A, Gyetvai A, Lakos G, et al. (2010) Anticitrullinated protein/peptide autoantibodies in association with genetic and environmental factors as indicators of disease outcome in rheumatoid arthritis. Autoimmun Rev 9: 140–143.
32. Díez JJ, Miguel JL, Codoceo R, Iglesias P, Bajo MA, et al. (2008) Effects of cinacalcet on gastrointestinal hormone release in patients with secondary hyperparathyroidism undergoing dialysis. Nephrol Dial Transplant 23: 1387–1395.

Increased HEV Seroprevalence in Patients with Autoimmune Hepatitis

Sven Pischke[1], Anett Gisa[1], Pothakamuri Venkata Suneetha[1], Steffen Björn Wiegand[1], Richard Taubert[1], Jerome Schlue[2], Karsten Wursthorn[1], Heike Bantel[1], Regina Raupach[1], Birgit Bremer[1], Behrend Johann Zacher[1], Reinhold Ernst Schmidt[3], Michael Peter Manns[1], Kinan Rifai[1], Torsten Witte[3], Heiner Wedemeyer[1]*

1 Department of Gastroenterology, Hepatology and Endocrinology, Hannover Medical School, Hannover, Germany, **2** Institute for Pathology, Hannover Medical School, Hannover, Germany, **3** Department of Clinical Immunology, Hannover Medical School, Hannover, Germany

Abstract

Background: Hepatitis E virus (HEV) infection takes a clinically silent, self-limited course in the far majority of cases. Chronic hepatitis E has been reported in some cohorts of immunocompromised individuals. The role of HEV infections in patients with autoimmune hepatitis (AIH) is unknown.

Methods: 969 individuals were tested for anti-HEV antibodies (MP-diagnostics) including 208 patients with AIH, 537 healthy controls, 114 patients with another autoimmune disease, rheumatoid arthritis (RA), and 109 patients with chronic HCV- or HBV-infection (HBV/HCV). Patients with AIH, RA and HBV/HCV were tested for HEV RNA. HEV-specific proliferative T cell responses were investigated using CFSE staining and in vitro stimulation of PBMC with overlapping HEV peptides.

Results: HEV-antibodies tested more frequently positive in patients with AIH ($n = 16$; 7.7%) than in healthy controls ($n = 11$; 2.0%; $p = 0.0002$), patients with RA ($n = 4$; 3.5%; $p = 0.13$) or patients with HBV/HCV infection ($n = 2$; 2.8%; $p = 0.03$). HEV-specific T cell responses could be detected in all anti-HEV-positive AIH patients. One AIH patient receiving immunosuppression with cyclosporin and prednisolone and elevated ALT levels had acute hepatitis E but HEV viremia resolved after reducing immunosuppressive medication. None of the RA or HBV/HCV patients tested HEV RNA positive.

Conclusions: Patients with autoimmune hepatitis but not RA or HBV/HCV patients are more likely to test anti-HEV positive. HEV infection should been ruled out before the diagnosis of AIH is made. Testing for HEV RNA is also recommended in AIH patients not responding to immunosuppressive therapy.

Editor: Ashok Chauhan, University of South Carolina School of Medicine, United States of America

Funding: This work was supported by a grant from the German Federal Ministry of Education and Research (reference number: 01EO0802), a grant from the Robert Koch Institute on hepatitis E to Sven Pischke and Heiner Wedemeyer (reference number 1362-1097), and by a grant to Torsten Witte and Reinhold E. Schmidt: KFO 250 TP 03. The funders had no role in study design, data collection and analysis, decision to publish, or preparation of the manuscript.

Competing Interests: The authors have declared that no competing interests exist.

* E-mail: Wedemeyer.Heiner@mh-hannover.de

Introduction

Autoimmune hepatitis (AIH) is an immune mediated liver disease more often affecting women than men. AIH is characterised by elevated serum IgG levels, the presence of certain autoantibodies and distinct histological features in the absence of other causes of liver disease [1]. The underlying pathomechanisms leading to autoimmune hepatitis are not well defined. One possibility is that viral infections trigger break of immunotolerance. Already 20 years ago an association between herpes simplex virus 1 (HSV 1) infection and autoimmune hepatitis has been described [2,3]. Other infectious agents including hepatitis C virus (HCV), cytomegalovirus, human T lymphotropic viruses 1 and 2 or salmonella typhimurum have been suggested to induce autoimmune liver disease [4]. If infections with the hepatitis E virus (HEV) are associated with AIH is unknown.

HEV infection takes a clinically silent course in the far majority of patients [5]. Few subjects may develop acute liver disease which can take a more severe course in particular in pregnant women or patients with underlying chronic liver diseases [6]. In recent years it became evident that HEV infection is not necessarily self limiting in all cases but may progress to chronic infection in immuno-compromised individuals [5,7]. Chronic hepatitis E has been described in liver and kidney transplant recipients [8] and also in some HIV-infected patients [9]. In Northern Germany, chronic hepatitis E was identified as the cause of graft hepatitis in 3% of liver transplant recipients with elevated liver enzymes [10]. Importantly persistent HEV infections have been associated with progressive liver disease [7,8,10,11]. To what extend HEV infections may lead to chronic hepatitis E in other patient groups receiving immunosuppressive medications including patients with autoimmune liver disease and rheumatoid arthritis is currently unknown.

The aims of this study were therefore, (i) to investigate the prevalence of antibodies to HEV in patients with autoimmune hepatitis and (ii) to determine if AIH patients receiving standard immunosuppressive medications are at risk for chronic hepatitis E in a low endemic Central European country and (iii) to rule out that rare cases of immunocompetent patients with chronic HEV infection had been misdiagnosed as autoimmune hepatitis.

Methods

From October 2009 until March 2010 all consecutive patients with AIH (n = 127) presenting our outpatient clinic were tested prospectively for presence of HEV RNA and anti HEV IgG. In addition, a control group of patients with viral hepatitis B or C (n = 109) was recruited. The diagnosis of autoimmune hepatitis was based on internationally accepted criteria [12]. Patients after liver transplantation were excluded. To compare the results with a cohort of patients with another autoimmune disease 114 consecutive patients receiving immunosuppressive medications followed by our Rheumatology outpatient clinic were studied between January 2012 and March 2012.

To enlarge the overall study cohort of patients with AIH, 81 additional patients were studied retrospectively. All retrospectively investigated patients were recruited at Hannover Medical School between 1998 and 2008. Furthermore 537 healthy subjects (employees of Hannover Medical School (n = 167) and blood donors (n = 370)) were studied for anti-HEV as already described as part of another project [10].

All AIH, HBV/HCV and RA patients were tested for the presence of HEV IgG antibodies by the MP assay (MP Biomedicals, formerly Genelabs Diagnostics, Singapore) according to the manufacture's instruction. Details of the primers used in the nested HEV RNA PCR were reported previously (11). Healthy subjects were only tested for anti-HEV-IgG.

Most AIH-patients received standard immunosuppressive regiments according to current guidelines [13] including mainly corticosteroids and partially azathioprine. Overall 70% of the AIH patients were female (n = 145). Age, gender and ALT levels of the overall study cohort are shown in table 1.

A subset of AIH patients (n = 123) was tested in addition with the Wantai anti-HEV assay (Wantai, Bejing). The frequency of anti-HEV in this subset was compared to 90 additional immunocompetent patients with chronic hepatitis B or C. Borderline test results were considered as positive for further statistical analysis.

Analysis of HEV-specific T cell responses

Cellular immune responses against HEV were studied in 1 AIH-patient with acute hepatitis E who tested HEV RNA and anti-HEV positive. Additional samples could be investigated from this subject 2 years after recovery. Furthermore, 4 anti-HEV-positive patients were tested for HEV-specific T cell responses. PBMC were stimulated with HEV overlapping peptide pools (spanning ORF2 and ORF3) as described previously [14,15]. T-cell proliferation was measured after 7 days by CFSE (5, 6-carboxyfluorescein diacetate succinimidyl ester) assay [14,15].

Statistics

Data for the different patient groups are presented as means and standard deviations. A comparison of continuous and categorical data between groups was performed using the chi-square test. Comparison of quantitative data between groups was performed using the Mann-Whitney test. A *p*-value<0.05 was considered significant.

Ethics

This study (including the analysis of HEV specific T-cell responses) was approved by the local research Ethics Committee (Ethics Committee of Hannover Medical School, Hannover, Germany). No research was conducted outside of our country. Patients agreed to hepatitis E testing as part of routine clinical work-up and thus no written informed consent was required. Retrospective testing of 81 samples from AIH patients was performed as part of the approved protocol and data were analysed anonymously according to the institutional and national ethics rules.

The need for written informed consent of participants of this study has been waived by the institutional review board according to our guidelines.

Results

Prevalence of HEV antibodies in patients with autoimmune hepatitis or persistent HBV- or HCV-infections

Anti HEV antibodies were detected in 16 out of 208 patients with autoimmune hepatitis (7.7%; 95% confidence interval 4.8–12). In contrast, anti HEV antibodies were detected in only 2/109 of control subjects with HCV or HBV infection (1.8%; CI 0.6–6.4). RA patients and healthy controls tested anti-HEV positive in 3.5% (4/115; CI 1.4–8.6) and 2.0% (11/537; CI 1.2–3.6), respectively (figure 1). Thus, anti HEV antibodies were more

Table 1. Prevalence of HEV antibodies and HEV-RNA in different patient groups.

	Patients with AIH (n = 208)	Patients with HBV or HCV infections (n = 109)	Patients with RA (n = 114)
Male	63 (30%)	59 (54%)**	29 (25%)
Age in years, mean (range, SD)	51 (18–84, 15)	49 (18–79, 13)	59 (19–85, 14)**
AST in U/ml	71 (15–684, 103)	69 (15–369, 59%)*	26 (13–63, 9)**
ALT in U/ml	94 (8–1422, 181)	82 (12–419, 78), p = 0.003**	26 (8–340, 32)**
HEV RNA positive	1 (0.5%)	0 (0%)	0 (0%)
Anti HEV IgG positive	16 (7.7%)	2 (1.8%)*	4 (3.5%)

p-values for comparison with AIH patients:
*p<0.05;
**p-values<0.01.

frequent in AIH patients than subjects with chronic viral hepatitis B or C (p = 0.03) or healthy individuals (p<0.001). The difference between the anti-HEV seroprevalence rate in AIH and RA patients did not reach the level of significance (p = 0.13), however, AIH patients were younger than individuals with RA (mean age 51 years vs. 59 years, Mann-Whitney test: p<0.001).

Anti HEV IgG-positive AIH patients were older than in anti-HEV-negative patients (mean 58 years, SD 13 years vs mean 50 years, SD 15 years, p = 0.032 Mann-Whitney test). There was no difference regarding gender distribution between anti-HEV positive versus negative AIH patients (4/16 male vs 59/192 male, p = 0.44 chi-square test), ALT levels (mean 154 U/ml, SD 347 U/ml vs mean 89 U/ml, SD 160 U/ml, p = 0.26 Mann-Whitney test) or AST levels (mean 95 U/ml, SD 157 U/ml vs mean 69 U/ml, SD 98 U/ml, p = 0.07 Mann-Whitney test).

As this study was based on the anti-HEV MP assay, we next aimed to confirm the findings by a second, independent sero-assay, the Wantai assay, which has been suggested to be more sensitive than the MP assay [16,17]. Sera of 123 AIH patients and 90 patients with chronic hepatitis B or C were investigated. Indeed, the testing with the Wantai assay confirmed that AIH patients were numerically more likely to test anti HEV positive (33%, CI 25–42) than in HBV/HCV patients (21%, CI 14–31) even though only borderline statistical significance was reached (p = 0.05).

Prevalence of HEV RNA in patients with autoimmune hepatitis

All patients with AIH, RA or HBV/HCV were also tested for HEV RNA irrespective of the presence of anti HEV antibodies. None of the RA patients or HCV/HBV-infected subjects tested HEV RNA positive. HEV RNA was detected in only one AIH patient. This was a 70 years old female patient in whom AIH had been diagnosed 5 years earlier. Immunosuppressive medication consisted of cyclosporine (125 mg/d) and prednisolone (50 mg/d). The high dose of 50 mg prednisolone had been prescribed as liver enzymes had increased despite treatment with 20 mg prednisolone per day. A liver biopsy was performed showing a lymphoplasmacytic infiltration and signs of acute inflammation and portal fibrosis (Ishak-score A3,B0,C2,D3,F3 and steatosis S1, figure 2). Immunosuppression was reduced after the HEV RNA tested positive. HEV RNA became negative after reducing the dose of prednisolone from 50 mg/d to 15 mg/d. Anti HEV IgG antibodies remained positive. Retrospective analysis of stored serum samples revealed that this patient had no detectable HEV RNA or anti HEV IgG antibodies 4 months before this episode of ALT elevation indicating that the patient had indeed acute but not chronic hepatitis E at the time of investigation.

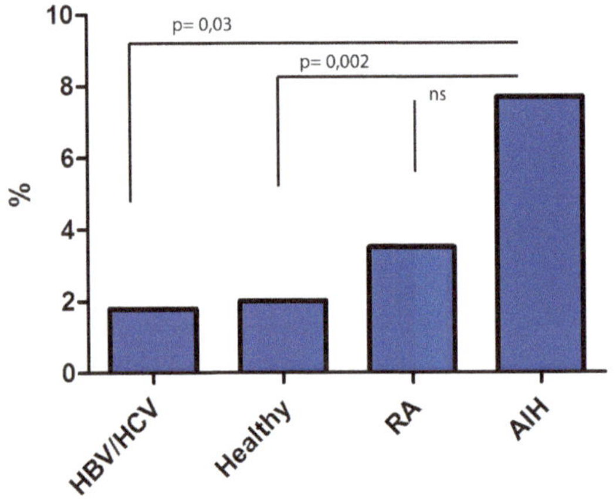

Figure 1. Seroprevalence rate of HEV specific antibodies in healthy controls, patients with chronic HBV- or HCV-infection and patients with autoimmune hepatitis.

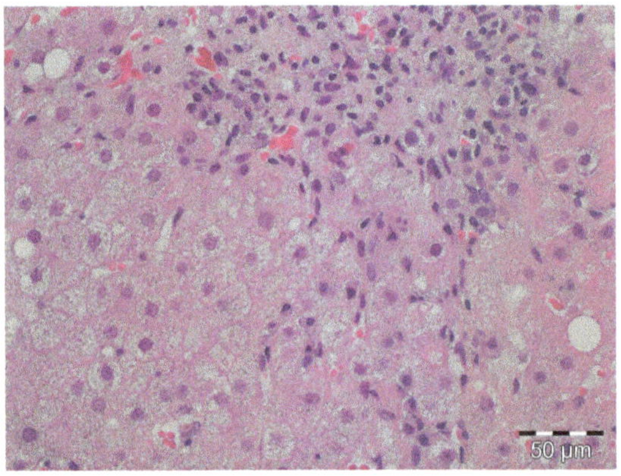

Figure 2. Histology of an autoimmune hepatitis patient with acute HEV infection. (H.E. stain, original magnification 200×).

HEV-specific T-cell responses

HEV-specific T cell responses could be studied in the anti-HEV-positive AIH patient, who tested positive for RNA and in 4 further anti-HEV positive AIH patients (figure 3). HEV-specific proliferation of CD4+ T cells was detectable in all 4 anti-HEV-positive/HEV RNA-negative AIH patients with previous HEV infection. In addition, HEV-specific CD8+ T cell responses were detectable in two of the four patients. The AIH-patient with acute hepatitis E showed a low HEV-specific T cell response in the peripheral blood when she was still viremic. However, two years after recovery, a multispecific CD4+ and CD8+ T cell response became detectable (figure 3).

Discussion

We here show that HEV antibodies may be more frequent in patients with autoimmune hepatitis than in individuals with other chronic viral liver diseases or patients with other autoimmune diseases and healthy controls. We also show that chronic hepatitis E seems not to be a major clinical problem in individuals with autoimmune hepatitis receiving standard immunosuppressive medications. However in single cases HEV infection can occur and may contribute to the severity of hepatitis.

A higher prevalence of anti HEV antibodies in patients with AIH patients has already been described previously in two smaller studies from California [18] and Sweden [19] performed in the 1990ies. Thus, our findings obtained in a larger case series seem to be in line with these earlier observations. AIH patients with anti-HEV-IgG antibodies did not show any significant differences in specific characteristic as compared to anti-HEV-negative AIH patients. In contrast to the previous studies, two cross-sectional control groups of patients another hepatic disease or with another autoimmune respectively have been studied. Of note, even though RA patients were older than patients with AIH, the anti-HEV prevalence was more than two-fold higher in AIH as compared to RA patients. Moreover, the seroprevalence rate of HBV- or HCV-infected patients was the similar to healthy individuals and more than three times lower than in AIH patients. Of note, the higher anti-HEV seroprevalence rate of AIH patients compared to

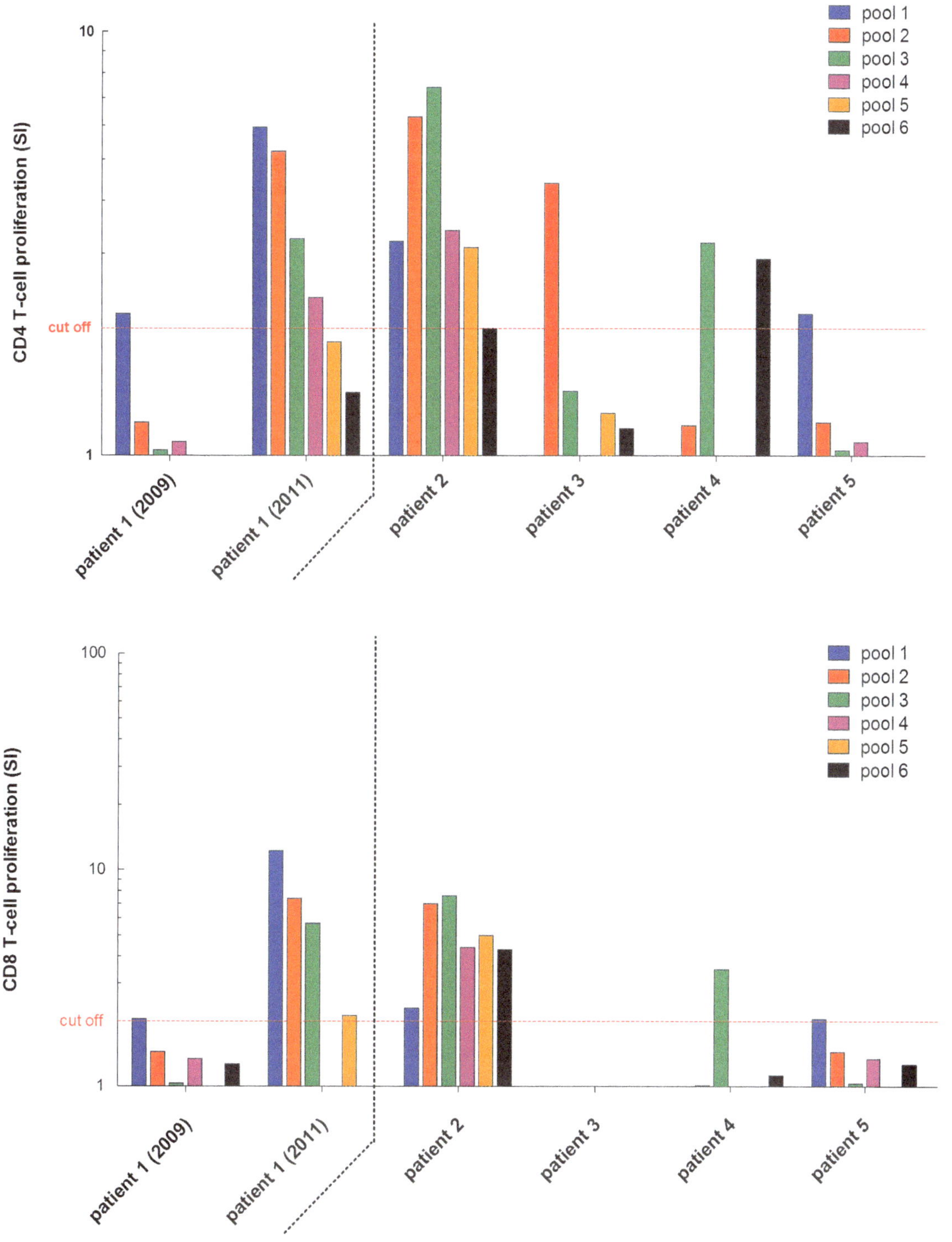

Figure 3. HEV specific T-cell responses in AIH patients (anti-HEV IgG positive).

patients with chronic viral hepatitis was confirmed by a second independent sero-assay, the Wantai assay, which has been suggested to be more sensitive and to detect much higher frequencies of anti-HEV [16,17]. Even though the "background" seroprevalence rate in chronic viral hepatitis patients was indeed almost 10-fold higher using the Wantai-assay, AIH patients were again about 1.5 fold more likely to test anti-HEV positive. Still, 95% confidence intervals overlapped in this analysis and larger cohorts would therefore need to be studied to confirm or disprove our findings.

What could be possible explanations for an increased prevalence of anti-HEV antibodies in patients with autoimmune hepatitis? One possibility might be that previous subacute HEV infections could have triggered immune events leading to the manifestation of AIH. This hypothesis would be in line with several previous studies describing an association between viral infections and subsequent development of AIH (2, 4). Specific cross-reactive humoral or T cell epitopes cross-reacting with possible auto-antigens have been described for HCV infection [20]. If these are also present during HEV infections remains to be shown. Larger studies are necessary to confirm the association between AIH and HEV-seropositivity and to get more insights into the underlying pathophyisiology.

Second, patients with autoimmune hepatitis may have distinct risk factors for acquiring HEV infections. This could include more frequent blood transfusions and medical procedures as well more frequent contacts to animals representing a potential zoonotic reservoir for HEV infection. Of note, not only pigs [21] but also several other animal species such as cats [22], shellfish [23], deer [24] or rats [25] can be carriers of HEV. Third, cross-reactive non-HEV-specific antibodies could be present in patients with AIH. The specificity of most HEV ELISA tests is not 100% but conditions determining "false-positive" results are currently unknown. Fourth, acute hepatitis E may present with histological and biochemical features of AIH and thus acute disease may be misclassified as de novo onset of AIH if HEV infection has not been excluded [26].

Persistent HEV infections have been described in organ transplant recipients receiving higher doses of immunosuppression and HIV-infected individuals with particular low CD4 counts. Studying 208 AIH patients receiving low doses of steroids alone or in combination with azathioprine, we could not identify a single case of chronic hepatitis E. This is an important clinical information suggesting that the risk to develop chronic hepatitis E should not been overestimated in patients with lower levels of immunosuppression in a non-endemic area. This finding is also well in line with our experience in patients with HIV-infection [27]. However, HEV infections can occur and thus hepatitis E should be considered in the differential diagnosis when AIH patients seem to be non-responder to immunosuppressive treatment.

Control of viral infections is believed to be mediated by both humoral and cellular immune responses. Interestingly, we detected a strong and multispecific HEV-specific T cell responses in an AIH patient who had cleared acute HEV infection previously while responses were much weaker when she was still HEV viremic. In addition, HEV-specific T cell responses were detected in three anti-HEV-positive AIH patients suggesting that these individuals had indeed contact with HEV and that unspecific cross-reactivity of the antibody assay seems to be unlikely. Future studies should investigate mechanisms potentially leading to the failure to mount an efficient adaptive cellular immune response against HEV. Overall, the findings presented in this paper are well in line with our experience in studying HEV-specific T cell responses in organ transplant recipients where both CD4+ and CD8+ T cell responses became detectable only after clearance of HEV RNA [15].

In conclusion, we show that patients with autoimmune hepatitis have a higher prevalence of anti HEV antibodies than control populations. The underlying cause for this observation remains to be determined. In addition, we did not find any evidence for an increased prevalence of chronic hepatitis E in German individuals with autoimmune hepatitis receiving standard immunosuppressive medications. However in single cases HEV infections may occur and thus hepatitis E needs to be considered in the differential diagnosis of non-response to immunosuppressive medications in AIH.

Author Contributions

Conceived and designed the experiments: SP MPM HW RR BB TW. Performed the experiments: RR BB SP SW BZ HB KR. Analyzed the data: RES RT KW JS PVS AG. Contributed reagents/materials/analysis tools: AG JS RR BB. Wrote the paper: SP HW MPM TW KR HB.

References

1. Manns MP, Strassburg CP (2001) Gastroenterology 120: 1502–17.
2. Manns MP (1993) Intervirology 35: 108–15.
3. Manns MP (1997) J Viral Hepat 4 Suppl 1: 7–10.
4. Vento S, Cainelli F (2004) Autoimmun Rev 3: 61–9.
5. Wedemeyer H, Pischke S, Manns MP (2012) Gastroenterology 142: 1388–1397 e1.
6. Rein DB, Stevens G, Theaker J, Wittenborn JS, Wiersma ST (2011) Hepatology.
7. Wedemeyer H, Rybczynska J, Pischke S, Krawczynski K (2013) Semin Liver Dis 33: 71–78.
8. Kamar N, Selves J, Mansuy JM, Ouezzani L, Peron JM, et al. (2008) N Engl J Med 358: 811–7.
9. Dalton HR, Bendall RP, Keane FE, Tedder RS, Ijaz S (2009) N Engl J Med 361: 1025–7.
10. Pischke S, Suneetha PV, Baechlein C, Barg-Hock H, Heim A, et al. (2010) Liver Transpl 16: 74–82.
11. Pischke S, Stiefel P, Franz B, Bremer B, Suneetha PV, et al. (2012) Am J Transplant 12: 3128–33.
12. Alvarez F, Berg PA, Bianchi FB, Bianchi L, Burroughs AK, et al. (1999) J Hepatol 31: 929–38.
13. Czaja AJ, Manns MP (2010), Gastroenterology 139: 58–72 e4.
14. Suneetha PV, Schlaphoff V, Wang C, Stegmann KA, Fytili P, et al. (2009) J Immunol Methods 342: 33–48.
15. Suneetha PV, Pischke S, Schlaphoff V, Grabowski J, Fytili P, et al. (2012) Hepatology 55: 695–708.
16. Wenzel JJ, Preiss J, Schemmerer M, Huber B, Jilg W (2013) J Infect Dis 207: 497–500.
17. Bendall R, Ellis V, Ijaz S, Ali R, Dalton H (2010) J Med Virol 82: 799–805.
18. Le Cann P, Tong MJ, Werneke J, Coursaget P (1997) Scand J Gastroenterol 32: 387–9.
19. Sylvan SP, Hellstrom UB, Hampl H, Kapprell HP, Troonen H (1995) Jama 273: 377–8.
20. Kammer AR, van der Burg SH, Grabscheid B, Hunziker IP, Kwappenberg KM, et al. (1999) J Exp Med 190: 169–76.
21. Goens SD, Perdue ML (2004) Anim Health Res Rev 5: 145–56.
22. Okamoto H, Takahashi M, Nishizawa T, Usui R, Kobayashi E (2004) Infection 32: 57–8.
23. Said B, Ijaz S, Kafatos G, Booth L, Thomas HL, et al. (2009) Emerg Infect Dis 15: 1738–44.
24. Tei S, Kitajima N, Ohara S, Inoue Y, Miki M, et al. (2004) J Med Virol 74: 67–70.
25. Easterbrook JD, Kaplan JB, Vanasco NB, Reeves WK, Purcell RH, et al. (2007) Epidemiol Infect 135: 1192–9.
26. Vieira CL, Baldaia C, Fatela N, Ramalho F, Cardoso C (2013) World J Hepatol 5: 152–5.
27. Pischke S, Ho H, Urbanek F, Meyer-Olsen D, Suneetha PV, et al. (2010) J Viral Hepat 17: 598–9.

23

Inverse Association between Air Pressure and Rheumatoid Arthritis Synovitis

Chikashi Terao[1]*, Motomu Hashimoto[2], Moritoshi Furu[2], Shuichiro Nakabo[3], Koichiro Ohmura[3], Ran Nakashima[3], Yoshitaka Imura[3], Naoichiro Yukawa[3], Hajime Yoshifuji[3], Fumihiko Matsuda[1], Hiromu Ito[2], Takao Fujii[2], Tsuneyo Mimori[3]

1 Center for Genomic Medicine, Kyoto University Graduate School of Medicine, Kyoto, Japan, **2** Department of the Control for Rheumatic Diseases, Kyoto University Graduate School of Medicine, Kyoto, Japan, **3** Department of Rheumatology and Clinical Immunology, Kyoto University Graduate School of Medicine, Kyoto, Japan

Abstract

Rheumatoid arthritis (RA) is a bone destructive autoimmune disease. Many patients with RA recognize fluctuations of their joint synovitis according to changes of air pressure, but the correlations between them have never been addressed in large-scale association studies. To address this point we recruited large-scale assessments of RA activity in a Japanese population, and performed an association analysis. Here, a total of 23,064 assessments of RA activity from 2,131 patients were obtained from the KURAMA (Kyoto University Rheumatoid Arthritis Management Alliance) database. Detailed correlations between air pressure and joint swelling or tenderness were analyzed separately for each of the 326 patients with more than 20 assessments to regulate intra-patient correlations. Association studies were also performed for seven consecutive days to identify the strongest correlations. Standardized multiple linear regression analysis was performed to evaluate independent influences from other meteorological factors. As a result, components of composite measures for RA disease activity revealed suggestive negative associations with air pressure. The 326 patients displayed significant negative mean correlations between air pressure and swellings or the sum of swellings and tenderness ($p = 0.00068$ and 0.00011, respectively). Among the seven consecutive days, the most significant mean negative correlations were observed for air pressure three days before evaluations of RA synovitis ($p = 1.7 \times 10^{-7}$, 0.00027, and 8.3×10^{-8}, for swellings, tenderness and the sum of them, respectively). Standardized multiple linear regression analysis revealed these associations were independent from humidity and temperature. Our findings suggest that air pressure is inversely associated with synovitis in patients with RA.

Editor: Masataka Kuwana, Keio University School of Medicine, Japan

Funding: The authors have no funding or support to report.

Competing Interests: The authors have declared that no competing interests exist.

* E-mail: a0001101@kuhp.kyoto-u.ac.jp

These authors contributed equally to this work.

Introduction

Rheumatoid arthritis (RA) is an autoimmune disorder characterized by joint synovitis and resultant joint destruction. Patients with RA present with swellings and tenderness of their joints, especially small joints such as metacarpophalangeal joints and proximal interphalangeal joints. Joint swellings and tenderness are closely related with future joint destruction [1,2] and this is why joint swellings and tenderness are included in the items for composite measures used for evaluation of RA activity [3–6]. Disease activity index (DAS) 28 is the most common composite measure in RA used for evaluation of daily RA activity and is composed of erythrocyte sedimentation rate (ESR) or C-reactive protein (CRP) as inflammatory parameters, swollen joint count (SJC) and tender joint count (TJC) for the 28 joints with or without visual analogue scale (VAS).

A large number of studies have tried to elucidate basic mechanisms of joint synovitis in RA and revealed the importance of inflammatory cytokines such as TNF-alpha and IL-6 to which biological agents were developed to target [7]. On the contrary, environmental factors which influence joint synovitis are scarcely known. Several studies with a relatively large number of subjects have reported seasonal variations of RA symptoms or joint destruction [8,9], but the relationship is still inconclusive [10–12]. Detailed meteorological differences among various seasons which cause changes in RA symptoms have not been clarified.

Through our daily medical care for patients with RA, we noticed that many patients with RA told us about the fluctuations in their joint symptoms according to changes in air pressure. In particular, many of them recognized worsening of their symptoms when the air pressure decreased such as during a typhoon in the summer. While many rheumatologists have heard of this, there have been no large-scale association studies to date addressing the relationship between air pressure and joint synovitis in RA. Previous studies addressing correlations between RA synovitis and meteorological changes included less than 100 patients with RA and the results were not consistent [10,13–18]. Previously, it was reported that a consistent microenvironment would ease joint symptoms in patients with RA [13]. While one study showed that temperature and humidity were associated with joint pain in 88 patients with RA [15], another study did not find statistically significant associations between meteorological changes and arthritic symptoms in 70 patients [16]. Another study where researchers observed 18 patients with RA for more than one year did not find significant associations and the authors concluded that this subjective belief in association by RA patients is simply an assumption that people have believed in for thousands of years [19]. However, none of the studies analyzed a large-number of joint assessments and the association is still inconclusive.

Recently, Kyoto University developed a large-scale database named "KURAMA (Kyoto University Rheumatoid Arthritis Management Alliance)" to accumulate detailed clinical information and specimen of patients with RA to uncover the basics of RA [20]. Here, we obtained 23,064 joint assessments for patients with RA from the KURAMA database and analyzed correlations between air pressure and joint synovitis in RA.

Results

Firstly, whether air pressure was correlated with daily disease activity in RA was addressed. DAS28 was selected as evaluation of RA activity for the association study. Table 1 shows the basic characteristics of the DAS28 scores and its components. The mean DAS28 score in the current patient group was 3.28, indicating low to moderate disease activity [21]. 14,999 DAS28 scores with three variables including SJC, TJC and ESR did not show a significant association with air pressure ($p = 0.18$, Table S1). Because DAS is a composite measure for assessing disease activity in RA, other RA composite measures could be associated with air pressure. Correlation analyses between air pressure and SJC, TJC, ESR, patients' VAS (pVAS) and Dr's VAS (dVAS) showed that all elements except for ESR showed suggestive or significant inverse associations with air pressure (Table S1). We also found that the sum of SJC and TJC showed a significant association with air pressure (Table S1). These results suggest that air pressure is associated with RA synovitis across different evaluations and different patients with RA. However, these analyses might be influenced by intra-patient correlations. Considering that significant associations were observed for SJC and the sum of SJC and TJC with air pressure, and that the largest number of data was available for SJC and TJC among the components of composite measures, we adopted SJC, TJC, and the sum of the two counts as best candidates showing associations with meteorological factors to obtain the maximum power for further analyses.

Secondly, correlation between air pressure and RA synovitis in each patient was analyzed to control intra-patient correlations. As the distribution of number of evaluations varied in the patients with RA, we extracted patients with more than 20 evaluations to confirm the correlations between air pressure and joint synovitis across different patients. In total, 12,061 evaluations from 326 patients were used for this analysis. The means of SJC and TJC were comparable with those in the 2,131 patients (Table 1). The overall fluctuations between SJC, TJC, or the combination of the two and air pressure are illustrated in Figure S1. Because we could not find the regular strong tendency of association between air pressure and joint synovitis through the figure, correlation coefficients between air pressure and signs of joint synovitis were calculated for each of the 326 patients. The correlation coefficients in items of synovitis demonstrated normal distributions in each item ($p \geq 0.78$, Shapiro-Wilk test, data not shown), justifying the application of t-test. The mean correlation coefficients across the 326 patients revealed significant negative correlations of air pressure with SJC and the combination of SJC with TJC (mean rho = −0.0410 and −0.0455, $p = 0.00068$ and 0.00011, respectively, Table 2). TJC showed a suggestive negative correlation (mean rho = −0.0306 and $p = 0.010$, Table 2). Figure 1 illustrates the smallest, largest and median correlation coefficients between air pressure and SJC, TJC or combination of the two among the 326 patients with RA, suggesting that negative mean correlation coefficients of RA synovitis were not brought about by patients demonstrating extreme negative correlation coefficients.

Table 1. Basic characteristics of the subjects in the current study.

Items	Overall	326 patients
Evaluation	23,064	12,061
Patient	2,131	326
Age (mean±SD)	60.7±15.0	62.4±13.6
Female ratio (%)	80.9	82.5
Stage* (mean±SD)	2.63±1.18	2.86±1.16
Class* (mean±SD)	1.92±0.70	1.94±0.70
Disease duration (year, mean±SD)	14.0±11.9	16.1±11.7
Smoking** (%)	33.6	30.8
Biologics*** (%)	19.0	46.6

*Steinbrocker's Stage and Class.
**Current smoker and ex-smoker.
***Patients who have been treated by biological agents between 2005 and 2012.
SD:standard deviation.

Thirdly, we analyzed which day showed the most significant associations between air pressure and items of joint synovitis, because it was likely that air pressure affected RA joint synovitis by an indirect mechanism taking several days. The air pressure data of six consecutive days before the date of evaluation was obtained and the same analyses using the same data set of the 326 patients were performed to evaluate associations with items of joint synovitis. As a result, the mean correlation coefficients of SJC, TJC, and the sum of SJC and TJC showed a "U-pattern" in the consecutive days (Figure 2A). The strongest associations were found three days before the joint evaluations for the three items ($p = 1.7 \times 10^{-7}$, 0.00027, and 8.3×10^{-8}, for SJC, TJC, and the sum of SJC and TJC, respectively, Figure 2A and 2B). These results strengthened correlations between air pressure and joint synovitis in RA.

Finally, whether these correlations were mainly brought about by other meteorological factors or not was addressed. Data of daily mean temperatures and humidity were obtained from the same period as air pressure. Multiple standardized linear regression analyses were performed to assess independent correlations between joint synovitis and air pressure. As a result, air pressure showed significant associations with joint synovitis in the 21,940 evaluations which were independent from temperature and humidity (beta≤ -0.0765 and $p \leq 0.0031$, Table 3). The analyses suggested that humidity also negatively influenced RA joint synovitis (Table 3). When multiple standardized linear regression analyses were performed for air pressure three days before the evaluations in each of the 326 patients with more than 20 evaluations of the 28 joints, mean coefficients of air pressure showed significant negative associations with joint synovitis ($p = 0.00023$, 0.036 and 0.0015, for SJC, TJC and the sum of SJC and TJC, respectively, Table 4). The inverse association between humidity and air pressure was also observed in this analysis ($p = 0.0019$, 0.016 and 0.0023, for SJC, TJC and the sum of SJC and TJC, respectively, data not shown).

Table 2. Mean correlation coefficients between joint synovitis and air pressure in the 326 patients.

Synovitis	Mean±SD(median)	Mean ρ±SD	P*
SJC	2.07±1.99 (1)	−0.0410±0.210	0.00068
TJC	2.08±2.19 (1)	−0.0306±0.212	0.010
SJC+TJC	4.15±3.70 (2)	−0.0455±0.207	0.00011

*p-values for Student's t-test. SD:standard deviation.

Discussion

Because environmental effects on RA synovitis are not well established, analysis with convincing results would be beneficial to manage patients with RA properly. This is the first study to address the correlations between air pressure and joint synovitis in RA with a large number of RA patients, and the first to detect significant associations between them. Our results indicate that low air pressure is associated with worsening of joint synovitis. This matches the complaints from RA patients, that they feel worsening of RA synovitis when typhoons come in the summer. Since SJC is an objective element and TJC is a subjective element of patients with RA, significant associations of air pressure with the two cannot be explained by subjective feelings of patients. Previous studies addressing correlations between meteorological effects and joint synovitis did not give consistent results [10,13–19]. The limited number of subjects (not more than 88 patients with RA) is assumed to have caused this inconsistency. In addition, although we found significant associations, the small mean correlation coefficients (ρ: −0.04~) made the previous studies difficult to detect these small effects. Because RA patients at Kyoto University Hospital frequently told us of the fluctuations in their symptoms in accordance with air pressure, among all the various meteorological

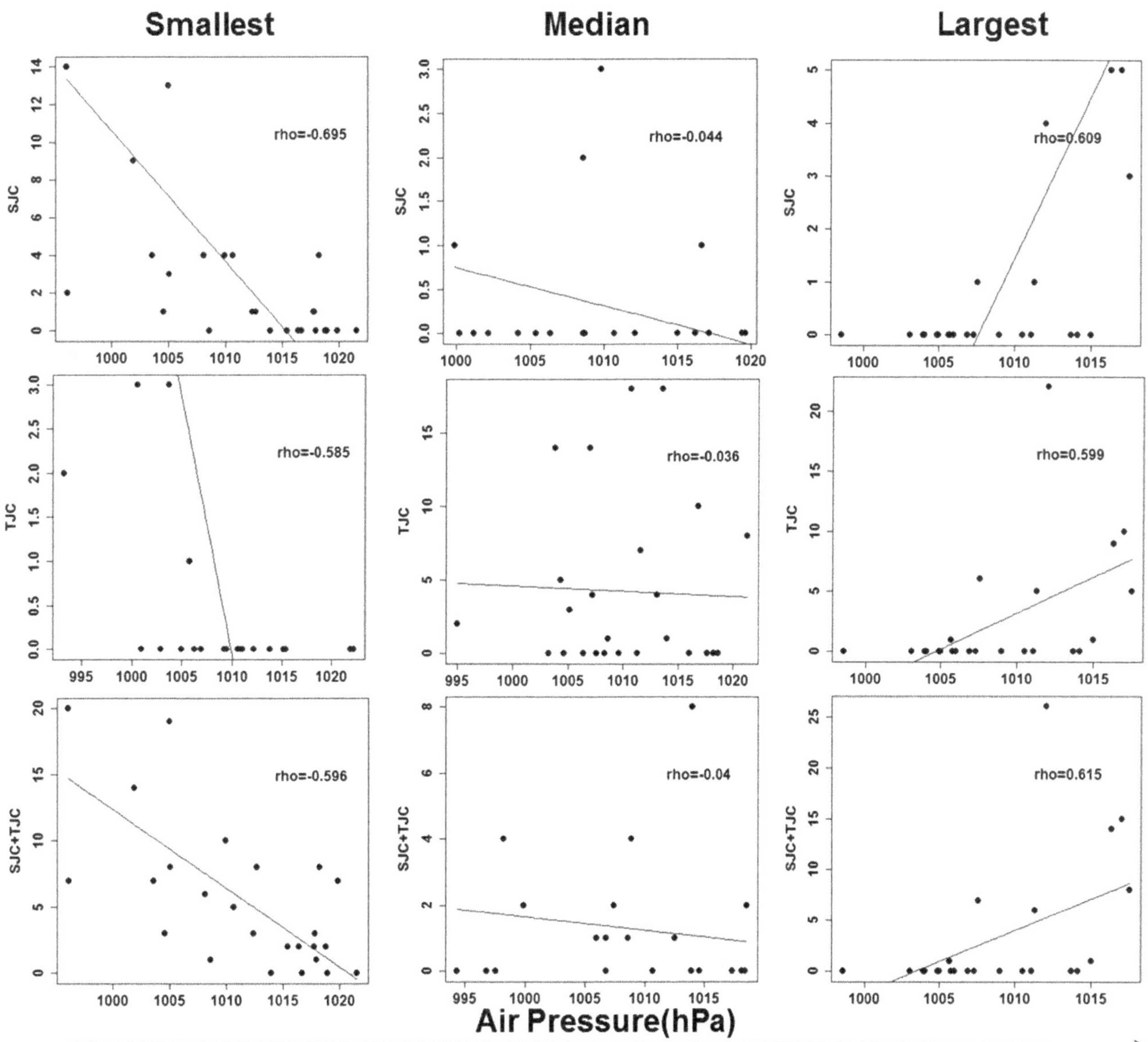

Figure 1. Correlations between joint synovitis and air pressure in RA patients. Correlation plots in patients demonstrating the smallest, median and largest correlation coefficients between joint synovitis and air pressure are illustrated in the left, middle and right panels, respectively.

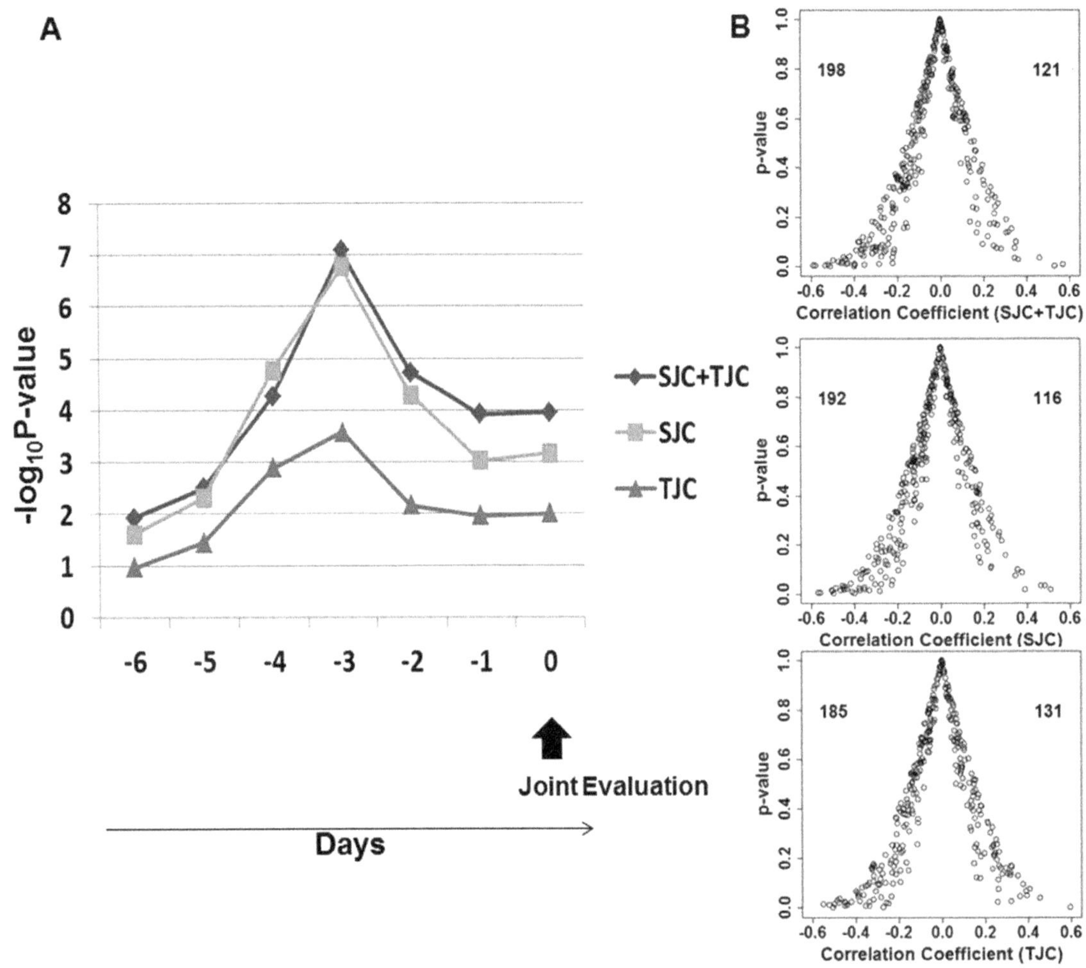

Figure 2. The strongest associations between joint synovitis and air pressure three days before joint evaluations. The 326 patients with more than 20 evaluations were analyzed. A)Associations between air pressure and joint synovitis for the seven consecutive days. Y axis indicates $-\log_{10}$P-value of Student's t-test. X axis indicates days before joint evaluations. B)Volcano plots for distribution of RA patients demonstrating positive or negative associations between joint synovitis and air pressure three days before joint evaluations. X and Y axes indicate Spearman's correlation coefficient and P-value, respectively. Numbers in the panels indicate RA patients showing positive or negative correlation coefficients. Because a part of the patients showed consistent TJC or SJC across all evaluations, the sum of the two numbers in each panel does not make 326.

factors we focused on air pressure. Another reason we only focused on air pressure was to avoid type I statistical error by performing multiple association studies.

Our data set revealed low to moderate disease activity of RA on average, which reflects the appropriateness of the treatment the patients were receiving at Kyoto Unvesity Hospital. Considering large variation of the synovitis data and large number of joint evaluations, the current data should be enough to detect correlations.

The first analysis addressing correlation between air pressure and DAS28 did not result in a significant association. However, it should be noted that all of the elements of composite measures showed the same negative direction of association with air pressure. These results may suggest common associations between

Table 3. Results of multiple standardized linear regression analysis between air pressure and joint synvoitis.

Synovitis	-	Air pressure (hPa)		Temperature (°C)		Humidity (%)	
	Mean±SD(median)	**1009.34±6.42 (1009.25)**		**16.10±8.77 (16.45)**		**63.83±9.75 (64)**	
	-	**Beta**	**P**	**Beta**	**P**	**Beta**	**P**
SJC	1.96±3.06 (1)	−0.0765	0.0031	−0.0419	0.097	−0.0996	2.8×10^{-6}
TJC	2.12±3.70 (1)	−0.105	0.00082	−0.0535	0.079	−0.0976	0.00015
SJC+TJC	4.08±5.87 (2)	−0.181	0.00027	−0.0954	0.049	−0.197	1.4×10^{-6}

Table 4. Standardized multiple linear regression analysis for air pressure 3 days before evaluations and synovitis among the 326 patients.

Synovitis	Mean±SD(median)	mean Beta±SD	P*
SJC	2.07±1.99 (1)	−0.126±0.0425	0.00023
TJC	2.08±2.19 (1)	−0.0893±0.0339	0.036
SJC+TJC	4.15±3.70 (2)	−0.215±0.0672	0.0015

*p-values for Student's t-test. SD:standard deviation.

air pressure and RA joint synovitis instead of limited association between air pressure and a specific element of RA joint synovitis. At the same time, these results may suggest that composite measures composed of multiple elements showing weak association with air pressure are not sensitive enough to detect the influence of air pressure. In addition, because many medical doctors evaluate synovitis of many patients with RA, variations among doctors in each element would be amplified in the composite measure and result in difficulty to detect significant correlations. Considering the strong association between air pressure and sum of SJC and TJC, the fine direction of association between different elements and air pressure should partly overlap but partly differ. PVAS showed the lowest mean correlation coefficient among items of composite measures. This matches our observation that many of the RA patients feel correlation between their symptoms and air pressure. Although the number of data for pVAS is limited, 81 patients with more than 15 data for pVAS revealed a suggestive inverse correlation with air pressure (mean rho = −0.0469, data not shown). Accumulation of more data for each element would detect a significant association between each element and air pressure and a fine direction of association with air pressure in each element.

Because the number of joint assessments differed among patients and it was likely that analyses using all assessments would be influenced by the specific patients with large number of joint assessments, we performed the analyses focusing on the 326 patients with more than 20 assessments to avoid intra-patient correlations. We hypothesized that correlations between air pressure and joint synovitis should be largely different among patients but a large number of patients would result in a significant deviation. We calculated a correlation coefficient in each patient separately. The results supported our hypothesis and showed a significant deviation of the mean correlation coefficient from the null hypothesis. Figure 1 presenting patients with median correlations along with Table S2 indicated that overall distributions of correlations between air pressure and joint synovitis shifted to negative correlations. Considering the size of correlation coefficients, although RA patients show a negative correlation in average between air pressure and joint synovitis, the correlation greatly vary among patients and the correlation should not be generalized.

We found the strongest associations between air pressure and signs of synovitis three days before evaluations. This may indicate that slow mechanisms underlie the correlations or that joint synovitis is prone to unknown factors which reflect past air pressure.

When we classified patients into subgroups based on positivity of disease duration, smoking, Stage, Class and usage of biological agents during the observation period, we did not find significant difference among RA subsets (data not shown). The analysis of confounding factors revealed that the association of air pressure with joint synovitis was not derived from humidity and temperature, which were selected since air pressure, humidity and temperature are representatives of meteorological factors. Although both humidity and temperature showed correlations with air pressure (rho:0.19 and 0.58, between air pressure and humidity or temperature, respectively), their correlations could not explain the association between air pressure and RA synovitis. The analysis also revealed that humidity showed a negative association with joint synovitis that is independent from temperature and air pressure. A previous study reported that a combination of increase in humidity and decrease in air pressure were associated with worsening of joint pain [14]. Their findings matched our results for air pressure, but the association of humidity was opposite to ours. Thus, the association between humidity and joint synovitis is inconclusive and further studies are required. It is notable that mean temperature was not associated with joint synovitis in a multiple standardized linear regression analysis. As increase or decrease of blood flow due to temperature is supposed to influence signs of synovitis in RA, the lack of the association may be explained by rapid influence of finely conditioned temperature in hospitals.

It is difficult to assume the basic mechanisms underlying the correlation between joint synovitis and air pressure. One possible explanation is that air pressure directly presses joint structures in patients with RA. Low air pressure results in reduced outside pressure of joints which allow joints to be swollen more easily. Enlarged space of joints would allow more inflammatory cells to enter joint space and produce inflammatory cytokines. Another explanation is involvement of autonomic nerves to regulate threshold of pain. A Japanese group reported that both decreased air pressure and temperature led to worsening of joint pain in an animal model [22,23]. The group also showed that these correlations in the animal model were mediated by sympathetic nerve, whose excitement and increase of circulating noradrenaline were brought about by decrease of air pressure [24,25]. As the current study did not reveal a strong association between joint tenderness and air pressure, involvement of sympathetic nerve with pain cannot fully explain the current results. Variations of B-cell activity due to meteorological changes could be another possibility. Our previous study reported seasonal variation of IgG in rheumatic diseases [26]. Analysis incorporating altitude of residence for each patient, whose information is not available in the current study, would give a clue for the mechanism underlying the association.

We could not conclude whether air pressure directly influences RA synovitis or if it is just a confounding factor of yet-to-be-determined factors with direct effects on RA synovitis. However, our analysis supports the patients' subjective feelings of relationship between air pressure and joint synovitis. Another study addressing correlations between air pressure and joint synvoitis estimated by imaging including ultrasound seems necessary. Further experiments and analyses between air pressure and joint symptoms in humans would clarify the detailed mechanisms. It will be interesting to determine the characteristics of patients who are susceptible to change of air pressure.

Materials and Methods

Ethical statements

The analyses in the current study were performed under policy of data analysis of the KURAMA database approved by Kyoto University Hospital Ethical Committee [20]. Written informed consent to enroll in the database described below was obtained from most of the patients, but for some patients the information regarding the construction of this database was disclosed instead of obtaining written informed consent. Participants who were informed regarding the construction of the database (instead of obtaining written informed consent) were allowed to withdraw from the study if desired. All data were de-identified and analyzed anonymously. This study was designed in accordance with the Helsinki Declaration.

Data of joint synovotis in patients with RA

A total of 23,064 evaluations of disease activity from 2,131 patients with RA were obtained with the corresponding dates of evaluations from the KURAMA database. The evaluation data contained some or all of the SJC, TJC in the 28 joints, ESR, pVAS and dVAS as well as DAS 28 as a composite measure for RA disease activity. The sum of SJC and TJC was also calculated for each evaluation. 326 patients with more than 20 evaluations of disease activity were extracted for further analysis.

Data of air pressure and other meteorological factors

Data of daily mean air pressure in Kyoto from 2005 to 2012 was obtained from the homepage of Japan Meteological Agency (http://www.jma.go.jp/jma/index.html). Data of daily mean temperature and humidity in Kyoto were also obtained in the same manner.

Statistical analysis

Correlations between mean air pressure on the day of joint evaluation and DAS28, SJC, TJC, ESR, pVAS, dVAS or sum of SJC and TJC were estimated by Spearman's correlation coefficients, using 23,064 evaluations of joint synovitis or evaluations in each of the 326 patients. The mean Spearman's correlation coefficients among the 326 patients with RA were estimated by Student's t-test under the null hypothesis that the mean was zero. Normality of distribution of correlation coefficients in the 326 patients was analyzed by Shapiro-Wilk test. A daily mean air pressure of the six days before the day of joint evaluation was also analyzed for correlations with signs of joint synovitis across the 326 patients with RA. To analyze independent effects of air pressure on joint synovitis from humidity and temperature, multiple standardized linear regression analysis was performed for 23,064 evaluations and each of the 326 patients with more than 20 evaluations. Mean beta values in the multiple standardized linear regression analysis among the 326 patients were assessed by Student's t-test under the null hypothsis that the mean beta values were zero. P-values less than 0.0071 were regarded as significant based on Bonferroni's correction. Data analysis was performed by R software (http://www.r-project.org/) or SPSS (ver 18).

Supporting Information

Figure S1 Fluctuations of air pressure and joint synovitis in the 326 patients. Fluctuations of each item are illustrated between 2005 and 2012. The three figures of SJC, TJC and combination of SJC and TJC are composed of 326 lines presenting fluctuations in the 326 patients.

Table S1 Correlation coefficients of RA joint synovitis in association with air pressure across different evaluations.

Table S2 Detailed information of the 326 RA patients.

Acknowledgments

We would like to thank Mr. Wataru Yamamoto at Kurashiki Sweet Hospital for his excellent support to establish and maintain the KURAMA database.

Author Contributions

Conceived and designed the experiments: CT MH FM HI TF TM. Analyzed the data: CT. Contributed reagents/materials/analysis tools: CT MH MF SN KO RN YI NY HY HI TF TM. Wrote the paper: CT MH.

References

1. Drossaers-Bakker KW, de Buck M, van Zeben D, Zwinderman AH, Breedveld FC, et al. (1999) Long-term course and outcome of functional capacity in rheumatoid arthritis: the effect of disease activity and radiologic damage over time. Arthritis and Rheumatism 42: 1854–1860.
2. Smolen JS, Van Der Heijde DM, St Clair EW, Emery P, Bathon JM, et al. (2006) Predictors of joint damage in patients with early rheumatoid arthritis treated with high-dose methotrexate with or without concomitant infliximab: results from the ASPIRE trial. Arthritis and Rheumatism 54: 702–710.
3. van der Heijde DM, van 't Hof MA, van Riel PL, Theunisse LA, Lubberts EW, et al. (1990) Judging disease activity in clinical practice in rheumatoid arthritis: first step in the development of a disease activity score. Annals of the Rheumatic Diseases 49: 916–920.
4. van der Heijde DM, van't Hof MA, van Riel PL, van Leeuwen MA, van Rijswijk MH, et al. (1992) Validity of single variables and composite indices for measuring disease activity in rheumatoid arthritis. Annals of the Rheumatic Diseases 51: 177–181.
5. Smolen JS, Breedveld FC, Schiff MH, Kalden JR, Emery P, et al. (2003) A simplified disease activity index for rheumatoid arthritis for use in clinical practice. Rheumatology 42: 244–257.
6. Aletaha D, Smolen JS (2007) The Simplified Disease Activity Index (SDAI) and Clinical Disease Activity Index (CDAI) to monitor patients in standard clinical care. Best Pract Res Clin Rheumatol 21: 663–675.
7. Furst DE, Keystone EC, Braun J, Breedveld FC, Burmester GR, et al. (2012) Updated consensus statement on biological agents for the treatment of rheumatic diseases, 2011. Ann Rheum Dis 71 Suppl 2: i2–45.
8. Iikuni N, Nakajima A, Inoue E, Tanaka E, Okamoto H, et al. (2007) What's in season for rheumatoid arthritis patients? Seasonal fluctuations in disease activity. Rheumatology (Oxford) 46: 846–848.
9. Mouterde G, Lukas C, Logeart I, Flipo RM, Rincheval N, et al. (2011) Predictors of radiographic progression in the ESPOIR cohort: the season of first symptoms may influence the short-term outcome in early arthritis. Ann Rheum Dis 70: 1251–1256.
10. Patberg WR, Rasker JJ (2004) Weather effects in rheumatoid arthritis: from controversy to consensus. A review. J Rheumatol 31: 1327–1334.
11. Hawley DJ, Wolfe F (1994) Effect of light and season on pain and depression in subjects with rheumatic disorders. Pain 59: 227–234.
12. de Rooy DP, Andersson ML, Knevel R, Huizinga TW, Svensson B, et al. (2012) Does the season at symptom onset influence the long-term severity of radiographic joint destruction in rheumatoid arthritis? Ann Rheum Dis 71: 2055–2056.
13. Edstrom G, Lundin G, Wramner T (1948) Investigations into the Effect of Hot, Dry Microclimate on Peripheral Circulation, etc., in Arthritic Patients. Ann Rheum Dis 7: 76–82.
14. Hollander JL (1963) Environment and musculoskeletal diseases. Arch Environ Health 6: 527–536.
15. Patberg WR, Nienhuis RL, Veringa F (1985) Relation between meteorological factors and pain in rheumatoid arthritis in a marine climate. J Rheumatol 12: 711–715.
16. Sibley JT (1985) Weather and arthritis symptoms. J Rheumatol 12: 707–710.
17. Gorin AA, Smyth JM, Weisberg JN, Affleck G, Tennen H, et al. (1999) Rheumatoid arthritis patients show weather sensitivity in daily life, but the relationship is not clinically significant. Pain 81: 173–177.
18. Strusberg I, Mendelberg RC, Serra HA, Strusberg AM (2002) Influence of weather conditions on rheumatic pain. J Rheumatol 29: 335–338.
19. Redelmeier DA, Tversky A (1996) On the belief that arthritis pain is related to the weather. Proc Natl Acad Sci U S A 93: 2895–2896.
20. Terao C, Hashimoto M, Yamamoto K, Murakami K, Ohmura K, et al. (2013) Three groups in the 28 joints for rheumatoid arthritis synovitis–analysis using more than 17,000 assessments in the KURAMA database. PLoS One 8: e59341.
21. van Riel PL, van Gestel AM (2000) Clinical outcome measures in rheumatoid arthritis. Ann Rheum Dis 59 Suppl 1: i28–31.

22. Sato J, Morimae H, Seino Y, Kobayashi T, Suzuki N, et al. (1999) Lowering barometric pressure aggravates mechanical allodynia and hyperalgesia in a rat model of neuropathic pain. Neurosci Lett 266: 21–24.
23. Sato J, Aoyama M, Yamazaki M, Okumura S, Takahashi K, et al. (2004) Artificially produced meteorological changes aggravate pain in adjuvant-induced arthritic rats. Neurosci Lett 354: 46–49.
24. Jin Y, Sato J, Yamazaki M, Omura S, Funakubo M, et al. (2008) Changes in cardiovascular parameters and plasma norepinephrine level in rats after chronic constriction injury on the sciatic nerve. Pain 135: 221–231.
25. Sato J, Morimae H, Takanari K, Seino Y, Okada T, et al. (2000) Effects of lowering ambient temperature on pain-related behaviors in a rat model of neuropathic pain. Exp Brain Res 133: 442–449.
26. Terao C, Ohmura K, Yamamoto K, Yukawa N, Kawabata D, et al. (2012) Serum IgG levels demonstrate seasonal change in connective tissue diseases: a large-scale, 4-year analysis in Japanese. Mod Rheumatol 22: 426–430.

Risk of Rheumatoid Arthritis in Patients with Type 2 Diabetes: A Nationwide Population-Based Case-Control Study

Ming-Chi Lu[1,2]⁹, Shih-Tang Yan[3]⁹, Wen-Yao Yin[2,4], Malcolm Koo[5,6]*, Ning-Sheng Lai[1,2]*

1 Division of Allergy, Immunology and Rheumatology, Dalin Tzu Chi Hospital, Buddhist Tzu Chi Medical Foundation, Chiayi, Taiwan, **2** School of Medicine, Tzu Chi University, Hualien, Taiwan, **3** Division of Endocrinology and Metabolism, Dalin Tzu Chi Hospital, Buddhist Tzu Chi Medical Foundation, Chiayi, Taiwan, **4** Division of General Surgery, Dalin Tzu Chi Hospital, Buddhist Tzu Chi Medical Foundation, Chiayi, Taiwan, **5** Department of Medical Research, Dalin Tzu Chi Hospital, Buddhist Tzu Chi Medical Foundation, Chiayi, Taiwan, **6** Dalla Lana School of Public Health, University of Toronto, Ontario, Canada

Abstract

Objective: Type 2 diabetes is associated with chronic, low-grade inflammation and could potentially trigger the progression of other, more prominent inflammatory diseases such as rheumatoid arthritis (RA). Therefore, we aimed to investigate the risk of incident RA in Taiwanese patients with type 2 diabetes using a population-based health claims database.

Methods: This nationwide, population-based, case-control study used administrative data to identify 1,416 patients with RA (age ≥20 years) as cases and 7,080 controls that were frequency-matched for sex, 10-year age group, and year of catastrophic illness certificate application date (index year). All subjects were retrospectively traced back, up to 13 years prior to the index year, for their first diagnosis of type 2 diabetes. Logistic regression analysis was conducted to quantify the association between incident RA and type 2 diabetes.

Results: The odds of developing RA were significantly higher in female (odds ratio [OR] 1.46, 95% confidence interval [95% CI] 1.24–1.72) but not in male (OR 1.00, 95% CI 0.72–1.37) patients who had previously diagnosed with type 2 diabetes. Subgroup analysis indicated that the odds of developing RA were more prominent in younger females (20 to 44 years of age) with type 2 diabetes. In addition, the odds of developing RA in female patients with type 2 diabetes were higher in those with a shorter time interval between the diagnosis of type 2 diabetes and RA.

Conclusions: This large nationwide, population-based, case-control study showed an elevated risk of RA in female Taiwanese patients with type 2 diabetes. Our findings were consistent with the hypothesis that chronic low-grade inflammation in type 2 diabetes may elicit the development of RA in genetically susceptible individuals.

Editor: Massimo Pietropaolo, University of Michigan Medical School, United States of America

Funding: These authors have no support or funding to report.

Competing Interests: The authors have declared that no competing interests exist.

* Email: m.koo@utoronto.ca (MK); tzuchilai@gmail.com (NSL)

⁹ These authors contributed equally to this work.

Introduction

The prevalence of type 2 diabetes has rapidly increased in many Asian populations, including the Taiwanese, thought to be the result of a combination of a sedentary lifestyle and unhealthy dietary habits. In Taiwan, the crude incidence of type 2 diabetes was 8 per 1,000 with a prevalence of 8.3% in 2007 [1]. Type 2 diabetes is characterized by pancreatic β cell dysfunction and insulin resistance. Obesity can trigger chronic low-grade inflammation and the resulting inflammatory mediators are detrimental to β cell function [2,3]. Modulating inflammatory reactions in patients with type 2 diabetes with the use of salsalate has been shown to improve glycemic control [6], strongly suggesting that inflammatory pathways are involved in the metabolic abnormalities of type 2 diabetes.

Rheumatoid arthritis (RA) is a chronic and disabling disease characterized by persistent synovitis, systemic inflammation, and the presence of autoantibodies [7]. The annual incidence of RA in Taiwan was 15.8 cases per 100,000 population with a female to male ratio of 4 to 1 [8]. Inflammatory mediators such as C-reactive protein (CRP), interleukin (IL)-6, and tumor necrosis factor (TNF)-α are frequently elevated in patients with type 2 diabetes [4,5] as well as in the sera of patients many years before the clinical onset of RA [9], suggesting a critical role in the immunopathogenesis of this disease. This observation also suggests that low-grade inflammation should have already existed in patients with RA during the preclinical phase. In addition, smoking causes chronic lung inflammation and could subsequently lead to the production of autoantibodies, resulting in the development of RA among genetically susceptible individuals [10]. Therefore, it is plausible that chronic low-grade inflammation observed in patients with type 2 diabetes could also contribute to the development of RA in these patients. Several studies show the risk of diabetes is higher in patients with RA, but less is known about RA risk in established type 2 diabetes [11,12]. Therefore, the aim of this case-control study was to explore the risk of incident RA in patients with type 2 diabetes using a nationwide health claims database. To our knowledge, this is the first study to investigate the risk of incident RA among patients with type 2 diabetes using nationwide, population-based data.

Materials and Methods

Data sources and study subjects

This study used a nationwide, population-based, case-control study design based on the data available from the National Health Insurance Research Database (NHIRD) in Taiwan [13].

The study protocol was reviewed and approved by the institutional review board of the Dalin Tzu Chi Hospital, Buddhist Tzu Chi Medical Foundation, Taiwan (No. 10004021). Since the NHIRD datafiles contain only de-identified secondary data, the need for informed consent from individual subjects was waived.

Using the 1997–2010 catastrophic illness datafile, a part of the NHIRD, cases were defined as new and successful applicants for the certificate of catastrophic illness with RA (International Classification of Diseases, ninth revision, clinical modification, ICD9-CM code 714.0). In Taiwan, patients with RA can apply for catastrophic illness certificates from the Bureau of National Health Insurance to become exempt from copayments for healthcare costs related to RA. The certificate is issued to patients only after their medical records, laboratory data, and imaging results have been reviewed by at least two rheumatologists. Because RA and type 2 diabetes occur primarily in adults, patients under 20 years of age were excluded from the study. The index date was defined as the date of first application of catastrophic illness certificate in the cases. A total of 1,416 patients with RA were included in the analyses.

The controls were selected from a random sample of the ambulatory care datafile of the 2000 Longitudinal Health Insurance Database (LHID2000) within the same inclusion period (January 1, 1997 to December 31, 2010) as the cases. The LHID2000 contained the claim data and registration files of both ambulatory and inpatient care expenditures for one million individuals randomly sampled from the 2000 Registry for Beneficiaries of the NHIRD. Any individual who was once a beneficiary of the National Health Insurance program during the period of 1996 to 2000 would be included in the registry. There are approximately 23,720,000 individuals in this registry, which represents more than 99% of the population in Taiwan. The National Health Research Institute confirmed that there were no significant differences in the age and sex between the LHID2000 and all beneficiaries.

Individuals identified as cases were excluded from the selection. Five controls per case were selected based on frequency matching for sex, 10-year age interval, and index year. Therefore, a total of 7,080 controls were included in the statistical analyses. The index year was defined as the same year of the index date of the matched case. The index date for each of the control subjects was assigned by using the date of a randomly selected ambulatory visit for a given index year.

Both the cases and controls were linked to the LHID2000 to obtain their ambulatory care visit data from 1997 to 2010. Patients were identified as having type 2 diabetes if they had at least three instances of ambulatory claims with a diagnosis of A-code A181 or ICD9-CM code 250.xx, except type 1 diabetes (ICD9-CM code 250.x1 or 250.x3). Patients with type 1 diabetes were excluded from this study because the disease is associated with an increased risk of several autoimmune diseases [14]. In addition, patients diagnosed with type 2 diabetes after the index date were excluded from the analyses. Therefore, only incident RA occurring after a diagnosis of type 2 diabetes were included in the final analyses.

Statistical analysis

Sex and age groups between cases and controls were compared with Chi-square test and t-test, as appropriate. Logistic regression was used to determine the odds ratio (OR) and 95% confidence interval (95% CI) of the risk of RA development with type 2 diabetes. A two-tailed P value of <0.05 was considered statistically significant. All statistical analyses were conducted using IBM SPSS Statistics software package, version 21.0 (IBM Corp, Armonk, NY, USA).

Results

We identified 1,416 patients newly diagnosed with RA with a certificate of catastrophic illness as cases, and 7,080 non-RA controls frequency-matched for sex, 10-year age interval, and index year. Table 1 shows the distribution of age and time interval between the first diagnosis of type 2 diabetes and index date in the cases and controls, stratified by sex. The mean age was 53.9 years for cases and the female to male ratio was 3.4:1. Since we frequency matched the cases and controls, there were no significant differences in their age distribution, with or without stratification by sex. However, there were significantly more patients with a longer time interval between the first diagnosis of type 2 diabetes and the index date among controls than among the cases ($P=0.003$); this difference was observed in females ($P=0.024$) but not in males ($P=0.118$).

Overall, the prevalence of type 2 diabetes was higher among RA cases (19.6%) compared with controls (15.4%) (Table 2). The odds of developing RA were significantly higher among patients who had previously diagnosed with type 2 diabetes (OR 1.34, 95% CI 1.16–1.55). When the data were analyzed after separating by sex, only female patients showed a significant association between RA and type 2 diabetes (OR 1.46, 95% CI 1.24–1.72). Therefore, we only included females in the subsequent analyses with stratification by age group (Table 3) and the time interval between the first diagnosis of type 2 diabetes and the index date (Table 4).

Subgroup analyses with stratification by age group indicated that the odds of developing RA in patients with type 2 diabetes were highest (OR 3.59, 95% CI 1.99–6.49) for the youngest age group of 20 to 44 years. The magnitude of the association was statistically significant but smaller in the two older age groups. Furthermore, stratification by the time interval between the first diagnosis of type 2 diabetes and the index date in female patients showed an increased odds of developing RA within a shorter time interval. The association was strongest with an interval of <4 years (OR 2.30, 95% CI 1.64–3.22) compared to those with an interval of 4 to <7 years (OR 1.60, 95% CI 1.13–2.26) or an interval of 7 to 11 years (OR 1.40, 95% CI 1.02–1.92). No significant associations were observed in patients with an interval of ≥11 years (OR 0.98, 95% CI 0.71–1.34).

Discussion

Previous studies based on healthcare utilization data have reported an increased risk of type 2 diabetes in patients with RA [11,12]. In contrast, our study showed that female patients with type 2 diabetes were associated with a significantly increased risk

Table 1. Characteristics of patients with rheumatoid arthritis and frequency-matched controls (N = 8,496).

Variable	Total			Males			Females		
	n (%)		*P* value	n (%)		*P* value	n (%)		*P* value
	Cases	Controls		Cases	Controls		Cases	Controls	
	1,416 (16.7)	**7,080 (83.3)**		**320 (16.7)**	**1,600 (83.3)**		**1,096 (16.7)**	**5,480 (83.3)**	
Age (years)			>0.999			>0.999			>0.999
20–29	68 (4.8)	340 (4.8)		13 (4.1)	65 (4.1)		55 (5.0)	275 (5.0)	
30–39	161 (11.4)	805 (11.4)		22 (6.9)	110 (6.9)		139 (12.7)	695 (12.7)	
40–49	310 (21.9)	1,550 (21.9)		72 (22.5)	360 (22.5)		238 (21.7)	1,190 (21.7)	
50–59	398 (28.1)	1,990 (28.1)		85 (26.6)	425 (26.6)		313 (28.6)	1,565 (28.6)	
60–69	267 (18.9)	1,335 (18.9)		53 (16.6)	265 (16.6)		214 (19.5)	1,070 (19.5)	
70–79	166 (11.7)	830 (11.7)		60 (18.8)	300 (18.8)		106 (9.7)	530 (9.7)	
80–89	42 (3.0)	210 (3.0)		14 (4.4)	70 (4.4)		28 (2.6)	140 (2.6)	
90–99	4 (0.3)	20 (0.3)		1 (0.3)	5 (0.3)		3 (0.3)	15 (0.3)	
mean (SD)	53.9 (14.1)	53.7 (14.5)	0.749	56.7 (14.4)	56.4 (15.0)	0.765	53.1 (13.9)	53.0 (14.2)	0.842
Interval between T2D diagnosis and index date (years)			0.003			0.118			0.024
<4	72 (25.9)	196 (17.9)		16 (29.6)	51 (18.8)		56 (25.0)	145 (17.6)	
4–<7	66 (23.7)	235 (21.5)		15 (27.8)	64 (23.6)		51 (22.8)	171 (20.8)	
7–<11	76 (27.3)	308 (28.2)		14 (25.9)	74 (27.3)		62 (27.7)	234 (28.5)	
≥11	64 (23.0)	354 (32.4)		9 (16.7)	82 (30.3)		55 (24.6)	272 (33.1)	

% are column percentages except in the header rows where they are row percentages.
T2D, type 2 diabetes.

Table 2. Association between type 2 diabetes and incident rheumatoid arthritis in male and female patients (N = 8,496).

	Total, n (row %) 8,496 (100)		Sex, n (row %)			
			Male		Female	
			1,920 (22.6)		6,576 (77.4)	
	Cases	Controls	Cases	Controls	Cases	Controls
	1,416 (16.7)	7,080 (83.3)	320 (16.7)	1,600 (83.3)	1,096 (16.7)	5,480 (83.3)
T2D, n (column %)	278 (19.6)	1,093 (15.4)	54 (16.9)	271 (16.9)	224 (20.4)	822 (15.0)
Odds ratio (95% CI)	1.34 (1.16–1.55)	1.00	1.00 (0.72–1.37)	1.00	1.46 (1.24–1.72)	1.00
P value	<0.001		0.978		<0.001	

T2D, type 2 diabetes; 95% CI, 95% confidence interval.

for incident RA. The increased risk of type 2 diabetes in patients with RA was proposed to be due to the long-term use of steroids during RA treatment [15]. Nevertheless, a Canadian study using a population-based health insurance database demonstrated a similar risk of incident type 2 diabetes in patients with RA, with or without adjusting for the use of oral or topical glucocorticoids [12]. Conversely, decreased insulin sensitivity was reported in patients with RA upon long-term exposure to steroids [16]. Thus, the role of long-term steroid use among patients with RA in the development of type 2 diabetes still requires further investigation. Furthermore, lifestyle changes after diagnosis of RA [17] might also contribute to an increase in the risk of developing type 2 diabetes. One health insurance database study performed in the United Kingdom concluded that the observed association between patients with RA and incident type 2 diabetes could substantially explained by obesity and lifestyle factors [18].

Our findings also showed that the risks between type 2 diabetes and incident RA were more prominent in younger female patients and in those with a shorter interval between the diagnosis of type 2 diabetes and RA. In the youngest age group of 20 to 44 years, the risk of developing RA was 3.6 times higher in patients with type 2 diabetes compared with patients without type 2 diabetes. Since both RA and type 2 diabetes are primarily chronic diseases of an older population, a strong positive association in young female patients is of concern. It is possible that these patients are genetically susceptible for developing autoimmune diseases, which tends to manifest early in life [19].

Furthermore, the association between type 2 diabetes and incident RA was found to be strongest for patients with the shortest time interval (<4 years) between the diagnosis of type 2 diabetes and the index date. Conversely, patients whose RA appeared 11 years or more after the diagnosis of type 2 diabetes were not significantly associated with the presence of type 2 diabetes. The proximity in the timing between when these two conditions occurred is consistent with the notion that type 2 diabetes and RA are related.

The possible link between type 2 diabetes and incident RA could be explained by the inflammatory responses associated with both conditions. Serum levels of IL-6 and levels of CRP are significantly elevated in patients with RA [20]. Regarding type 2 diabetes, a meta-analysis of ten prospective studies with a total of 19,709 participants revealed a significant dose-response association of IL-6 levels with risk of type 2 diabetes (relative risk, [RR] 1.31, 95% CI 1.17–1.46). This same study, based on the results from 22 cohorts of 40,735 participants, also found that elevated CRP levels were significantly associated with increased risk of type 2 diabetes (RR 1.26, 95% CI 1.16–1.37) [21]. Furthermore, in patients with inflammatory polyarthritis, insulin resistance was closely associated with the presence of rheumatoid factor (RF) and anti-citrullinated protein antibody (ACPA) [22]. These findings suggest an important role for chronic systemic inflammation in the pathogenesis of both RA and type 2 diabetes.

The use of disease-modifying antirheumatic drugs (DMRADs) such as hydroxychloroquine or tumor necrosis factor inhibitor for lowering the inflammatory response in patients with RA has been

Table 3. Association between type 2 diabetes and incident rheumatoid arthritis in female patients, stratified by age group (N = 6,576).

	Age group (years), n (row %)					
	20–44		45–64		≥65	
	1,836 (27.9)		3,282 (49.9)		1,458 (22.2)	
	Cases	Controls	Cases	Controls	Cases	Controls
	295 (16.1)	1,541 (83.9)	573 (17.5)	2,709 (82.5)	228 (15.6)	1,230 (84.4)
T2D, n (column %)	19 (6.4)	29 (1.9)	120 (20.9)	426 (15.7)	85 (37.3)	367 (29.8)
Odds ratio (95% CI)	3.59 (1.99–6.49)	1.00	1.42 (1.13–1.78)	1.00	1.40 (1.04–1.88)	1.00
P value	<0.001		0.002		0.026	

T2D, type 2 diabetes; 95% CI, 95% confidence interval.

Table 4. Association between type 2 diabetes and incident rheumatoid arthritis in female patients, stratified by the time interval between the first diagnosis of type 2 diabetes and the index date (N = 6,576).

	Time interval between the first diagnosis of type 2 diabetes mellitus and the index date (years), n (row %)							
	<4		4–<7		7–<11		≥11	
	1,763 (26.8)		1,501 (22.8)		1,594 (24.2)		1,718 (26.1)	
	Cases	Controls	Cases	Controls	Cases	Controls	Cases	Controls
	281 (15.9)	1,482 (84.1)	252 (16.8)	1,249 (83.2)	269 (16.9)	1,325 (83.1)	294 (17.1)	1,424 (82.9)
T2D, n (column %)	56 (19.9)	145 (9.8)	51 (20.2)	171 (13.7)	62 (23.0)	234 (17.7)	55 (18.7)	272 (19.1)
Odds ratio (95% CI)	2.30 (1.64–3.22)	1.00	1.60 (1.13–2.26)	1.00	1.40 (1.02–1.92)	1.00	0.98 (0.71–1.34)	1.00
P value	<0.001		0.008		0.039		0.876	

T2D, type 2 diabetes; 95% CI, 95% confidence interval.

shown to reduce the risk of developing diabetes [23,24]. Altogether, these findings suggest that the pathogenesis of type 2 diabetes and RA could be linked by a similar chronic inflammatory response profile. Nevertheless, it should be noted that there is currently no evidence demonstrating that both conditions have shared genetic mechanisms [25].

The data used in this study were based on health claims records and thus could minimize the presence of recall bias as a result of collecting exposure information prior to disease onset in typical case-control studies. Still, there were several drawbacks in our study. First, due to the lack of detailed clinical data in the NHIRD, no information in regards to radiographic reports, biochemical and serological data (such as inflammatory markers, ACPA, and RF), or lifestyle factors such as smoking was available. Although smoking is an important risk factor for RA [26], the prevalence of female smokers is under 5%, and even lower (1.8%) among older women in Taiwan [27]. Thus, the increased risk of RA in female patients with type 2 diabetes should not be affected by smoking. On the other hand, prevalence of smoking was high (45.7%) in males and could confound the association between type 2 diabetes and RA, possibly leading to a lack of association between the two diseases in male patients. Since both the humoral and cell-mediated immune responses are more active in females, it is plausible that the disease expression is related to sexual dimorphism in the immune response [28]. This might also explain a significant association was only found in females, not male patients as well.

Second, although mobility and physical activity could be adversely affected by joint symptoms in individuals many years prior to the definitive diagnosis of RA [29], which in turn can increase the risk of type 2 diabetes, the joint symptoms before the clinical onset of RA are generally mild [30]. Therefore, the effect of immobility and physical inactivity on the development of type 2 diabetes should be minimal.

Third, it is possible that the association between RA and type 2 diabetes might be partially explained by the confounding effect of obesity. Nevertheless, although obesity is a well-established risk factor for type 2 diabetes [31], previous research on the association between body mass index and RA generated inconsistent results. Early studies had indicated a moderate increase in the risk of RA with obesity [32] but newer studies generally reported that obesity was not a predisposing factor for RA [33]. In addition, a comparison study using nationally representative survey data indicated that the prevalence of obesity was lower in Taiwan (7.2%) compared with the United States (33.7%) and England (32.1%) [34]. Furthermore, no significant differences in waist circumference were found between 86 Taiwanese patients with RA and 172 age- and sex-matched population controls [35]. Therefore, it might be premature to attribute the significant association between type 2 diabetes and incident RA to the confounding effect of obesity without further investigation.

In conclusion, this large nationwide, population-based, case-control study suggested that female patients with type 2 diabetes had an increased risk of developing RA. Although our findings are consistent with the hypothesis that chronic inflammation seen in patients with type 2 diabetes could contribute to the development of RA, further investigation with adjustments for possible confounders is needed before conclusions can be drawn. Nevertheless, given the high and increasing prevalence of type 2 diabetes in Taiwanese and other Asian populations, it is important to understand the effects of type 2 diabetes on the development of RA, particularly in young females.

Acknowledgments

This study is based in part on data from the National Health Insurance Research Database provided by the National Health Insurance Administration, Ministry of Health and Welfare and managed by the National Health Research Institutes. The interpretation and conclusions contained herein do not represent those of the National Health Insurance Administration, Ministry of Health and Welfare or the National Health Research Institutes.

Author Contributions

Conceived and designed the experiments: MCL STY WYY NSL. Performed the experiments: MCL MK. Analyzed the data: MCL MK. Contributed reagents/materials/analysis tools: MCL STY WYY NSL. Wrote the paper: MCL MK.

References

1. Lin CC, Li CI, Hsiao CY, Liu CS, Yang SY, et al. (2013) Time trend analysis of the prevalence and incidence of diagnosed type 2 diabetes among adults in Taiwan from 2000 to 2007: a population-based study. BMC Public Health 13: 318.
2. Cefalu WT (2009) Inflammation, insulin resistance, and type 2 diabetes: back to the future? Diabetes 58: 307–308.
3. Kolb H, Mandrup-Poulsen T (2005) An immune origin of type 2 diabetes? Diabetologia 48: 1038–1050.
4. Aroor AR, McKarns S, Demarco VG, Jia G, Sowers JR (2013) Maladaptive immune and inflammatory pathways lead to cardiovascular insulin resistance. Metabolism 62: 1543–1552.
5. Goldberg RB (2009) Cytokine and cytokine-like inflammation markers, endothelial dysfunction, and imbalanced coagulation in development of diabetes and its complications. J Clin Endocrinol Metab 94: 3171–3182.
6. Goldfine AB, Fonseca V, Jablonski KA, Chen YD, Tipton L, et al. (2013) Salicylate (salsalate) in patients with type 2 diabetes: a randomized trial. Ann Intern Med 159: 1–12.
7. Scott DL, Wolfe F, Huizinga TW (2010) Rheumatoid arthritis. Lancet 376: 1094–1108.
8. Kuo CF, Luo SF, See LC, Chou IJ, Chang HC, et al. (2013) Rheumatoid arthritis prevalence, incidence, and mortality rates: a nationwide population study in Taiwan. Rheumatol Int 33: 355–360.
9. van Steenbergen HW, Huizinga TW, van der Helm-van Mil AH (2013) The preclinical phase of rheumatoid arthritis: what is acknowledged and what needs to be assessed? Arthritis Rheum 65: 2219–2232.
10. Baka Z, Buzás E, Nagy G (2009) Rheumatoid arthritis and smoking: putting the pieces together. Arthritis Res Ther 11: 238.
11. Su CC, Chen I, Young FN, Lian I (2013) Risk of diabetes in patients with rheumatoid arthritis: a 12-year retrospective cohort study. J Rheumatol 40: 1513–1518.
12. Solomon DH, Love TJ, Canning C, Schneeweiss S (2010) Risk of diabetes among patients with rheumatoid arthritis, psoriatic arthritis and psoriasis. Ann Rheum Dis 69: 2114–2117.
13. National Health Research Institute (2013) National Health Insurance Research Database, Taiwan. Available: http://nhird.nhri.org.tw/en/index.htm. Accessed 2014 May 23.
14. Hemminki K, Li X, Sundquist J, Sundquist K (2009) Familial association between type 1 diabetes and other autoimmune and related diseases. Diabetologia 52: 1820–1828.
15. Caldwell JR, Furst DE (1991) The efficacy and safety of low-dose corticosteroids for rheumatoid arthritis. Semin Arthritis Rheum 21: 1–11.
16. Dessein PH, Joffe BI, Stanwix AE, Christian BF, Veller M (2004) Glucocorticoids and insulin sensitivity in rheumatoid arthritis. J Rheumatol 31: 867–874.
17. Mancuso CA, Rincon M, Sayles W, Paget SA (2007) Comparison of energy expenditure from lifestyle physical activities between patients with rheumatoid arthritis and healthy controls. Arthritis Rheum 57: 672–678.
18. Dubreuil M, Rho YH, Man A, Zhu Y, Zhang Y, et al. (2013) Diabetes incidence in psoriatic arthritis, psoriasis and rheumatoid arthritis: a UK population-based cohort study. Rheumatology 53: 346–352.
19. Kim EJ, Lee J, Ryu YS, Kim JM, Jeong YG, et al. (2013) Shared epitope and radiologic progression are less prominent in elderly onset RA than young onset RA. Rheumatol Int 33: 2135–2140.
20. Chung SJ, Kwon YJ, Park MC, Park YB, Lee SK (2011) The correlation between increased serum concentrations of interleukin-6 family cytokines and disease activity in rheumatoid arthritis patients. Yonsei Med J 52: 113–120.
21. Wang X, Bao W, Liu J, Ouyang YY, Wang D, et al. (2013) Inflammatory markers and risk of type 2 diabetes: a systematic review and meta-analysis. Diabetes Care 36: 166–175.
22. Mirjafari H, Farragher TM, Verstappen SM, Yates A, Bunn D, et al. (2011) Seropositivity is associated with insulin resistance in patients with early inflammatory polyarthritis: results from the Norfolk Arthritis Register (NOAR): an observational study. Arthritis Res Ther 13: R159.
23. Solomon DH, Massarotti E, Garg R, Liu J, Canning C, et al. (2011) Association between disease-modifying antirheumatic drugs and diabetes risk in patients with rheumatoid arthritis and psoriasis. JAMA 305: 2525–2531.
24. Wasko MC, Hubert HB, Lingala VB, Elliott JR, Luggen ME, et al. (2007) Hydroxychloroquine and risk of diabetes in patients with rheumatoid arthritis. JAMA 298: 187–193.
25. Wellcome Trust Case Control Consortium (2007) Genome-wide association study of 14,000 cases of seven common diseases and 3,000 shared controls. Nature 447: 661–678.
26. Stolt P, Bengtsson C, Nordmark B, Lindblad S, Lundberg I, et al. (2003) Quantification of the influence of cigarette smoking on rheumatoid arthritis: results from a population based case-control study, using incident cases. Ann Rheum Dis 62: 835–841.
27. Tsai YW, Tsai TI, Yang CL, Kuo KN (2008) Gender differences in smoking behaviors in an Asian population. J Womens Health 17: 971–978.
28. Bouman A, Heineman MJ, Faas MM (2005) Sex hormones and the immune response in humans. Hum Reprod Update 11: 411–423.
29. Lai NS, Tsai TY, Li CY, Koo M, Yu CL, et al. (2014) Increased frequency and costs of ambulatory medical care utilization prior to the diagnosis of rheumatoid arthritis: A national population-based study. Arthritis Care Res (Hoboken) 66: 371–378.
30. van de Sande MG, de Hair MJ, van der Leij C, Klarenbeek PL, Bos WH, et al. (2011) Different stages of rheumatoid arthritis: features of the synovium in the preclinical phase. Ann Rheum Dis 70: 772–777.
31. Abdullah A, Peeters A, de Courten M, Stoelwinder J (2010) The magnitude of association between overweight and obesity and the risk of diabetes: a meta-analysis of prospective cohort studies. Diabetes Res Clin Pract 89: 309–319.
32. Voigt LF, Koepsell TD, Nelson JL, Dugowson CE, Daling JR (1994) Smoking, obesity, alcohol consumption, and the risk of rheumatoid arthritis. Epidemiology 5: 525–532.
33. Rodriguez LA, Tolosa LB, Ruigomez A, Johansson S, Wallander MA (2009) Rheumatoid arthritis in UK primary care: incidence and prior morbidity. Scand J Rheumatol 38: 173–177.
34. Vasunilashorn S, Kim JK, Crimmins EM (2013) International differences in the links between obesity and physiological dysregulation: the United States, England, and Taiwan. J Obes 2013: 618056.
35. Chen MF, Chen YM, Chen DY, Lan JL (2010) Metabolic syndrome in patients with rheumatoid arthritis: association of lifestyle with anthropometric measurements. Formosan J Rheumatol 24: 64–71.

25

Association of Cross-Reactive Antibodies Targeting Peptidyl-Arginine Deiminase 3 and 4 with Rheumatoid Arthritis-Associated Interstitial Lung Disease

Jon T. Giles[1]*, Erika Darrah[2], Sonye Danoff[3], Cheilonda Johnson[3], Felipe Andrade[2], Antony Rosen[2], Joan M. Bathon[1]

1 Division of Rheumatology, Columbia University, College of Physicians and Surgeons, New York, New York, United States of America, **2** Division of Rheumatology, Johns Hopkins University, Baltimore, Maryland, United States of America, **3** Division of Pulmonary and Critical Care Medicine, Johns Hopkins University, Baltimore, Maryland, United States of America

Abstract

Background: A subset of rheumatoid arthritis (RA) patients have detectable antibodies directed against the peptidyl-arginine deiminase (PAD) enzyme isoforms 3 and 4. Anti-PAD3/4 cross-reactive antibodies (anti-PAD3/4XR) have been shown to lower the calcium threshold required for PAD4 activation, an effect potentially relevant to the pathogenesis of RA-associated interstitial lung disease (ILD).

Methods: RA patients underwent multi-detector computed tomography (MDCT) of the chest with interpretation by a pulmonary radiologist for ILD features. A semi-quantitative ILD Score (range 0–32) was calculated. Concurrent serum samples were assessed for antibodies against PAD by immunoprecipitation with radiolabeled PAD3 and PAD4.

Results: Among the 176 RA patients studied, any ILD was observed in 58 (33%) and anti-PAD3/4XR was detected in 19 (11%). The frequency of any ILD among those with anti-PAD3/4XR was 68% vs. 29% among those with no anti-PAD (crude OR = 5.39; p = 0.002) and vs. 27% among those with anti-PAD4 that was not cross-reactive with PAD3 (crude OR = 5.74; p = 0.001). Both associations were stronger after adjustment for relevant confounders (adjusted ORs = 7.22 and 6.61, respectively; both p-values < 0.01). Among ever smokers with anti-PAD3/4XR, the adjusted frequency of any ILD was 93% vs. 17% for never smokers without the antibody (adjusted OR = 61.4; p = 0.001, p-value for the interaction of smoking with anti-PAD3/4XR < 0.05).

Conclusions: The prevalence and extent of ILD was markedly higher among RA patients with anti-PAD3/4 cross-reactive antibodies, even after accounting for relevant confounders, particularly among ever smokers. These findings may suggest etiopathologic mechanisms of RA-ILD, and their clinical utility for predicting ILD warrants additional study.

Editor: Masataka Kuwana, Keio University School of Medicine, Japan

Funding: This work was supported by National Institutes of Health (NIH) National Institute of Arthritis and Musculoskeletal and Skin Diseases (NIAMS) AR050026-01 (JMB), grant support from the Stabler Family Foundation, the Mackley Fund from Sibley Memorial Hospital, and NIH grant P30 AR053503 (AR, ED, FA), and awards from the American College of Rheumatology Research and Education Foundation Within-Our-Reach Campaign (SKD, JTG). Additional support was provided by the Johns Hopkins Bayview Medical Center General Clinical Research Center (Grant Number M01RR02719). The funders had no role in the study design, data collection and analysis, decision to publish, or preparation of the manuscript.

Competing Interests: The authors have the following interests. Antony Rosen, Erika Darrah, Felipe Andrade and Jon T. Giles are authors on a provisional patent application entitled "Human autoantibodies specific for PAD3 which are crossreactive with PAD4 and their use in the diagnosis and treatment of rheumatoid arthritis" (P12072-01) that was filed with the United States Patent and Trademark Office. There are no restrictions on sharing of study material and/or data related to the patent application. This does not alter the authors' adherence to all the PLOS ONE policies on sharing data and materials, as detailed online in the guide for authors.

* E-mail: jtg2122@columbia.edu

Introduction

Clinically significant interstitial lung disease (ILD) is observed in 8–15% of individuals with rheumatoid arthritis (RA) and is a major source of morbidity and mortality [1–4]. Prognosis after the development of symptomatic RA-ILD is poor, with life expectancy averaging only 2.6 years [1]. Progressive decline in lung function, supplemental oxygen requirement, physical disability, secondary pulmonary hypertension with right heart failure, and need for lung transplantation are severe consequences [4,5]. Subclinical RA-ILD is even more common, with radiographic ILD, as assessed using computed tomography (CT), observed in up to 50% of RA patients [6–8]. Although limited by the lack of clinical trials, there are, to date, no pharmacotherapies proven to be effective in altering the natural history of RA-ILD once symptoms have developed [9], and robust biomarkers for predicting those at risk for RA-ILD are lacking.

The pathogenesis of RA-ILD is poorly understood. One mechanistic possibility involves the presence and consequences of pulmonary citrullinated proteins. Citrullination is the posttranslational modification of arginine residues to citrulline catalyzed by the peptidyl-arginine deiminase (PAD) enzymes [10]. Citrullination results in a net loss of charge and a more hydrophobic protein, with implications for protein folding and tertiary structure [11,12]. Citrullinated proteins are present in lung tissue of patients with RA-ILD [13], idiopathic pulmonary fibrosis (IPF), and even broncho-alveolar lavage fluid from heavy smokers [14]. Repertoire expansion of antibodies against citrullinated protein antigens (ACPA) is associated with RA susceptibility [15], articular damage [16], and the presence and extent of radiographic RA-ILD [7], suggesting that citrullination of lung proteins and/or pathogenic ACPA may contribute to the pathogenesis of RA-ILD, perhaps via interfering with the normal functioning of targeted proteins or via pathologic antigen/antibody interactions.

PAD function is dependent on calcium, with maximal PAD function requiring 5–10 mM concentrations. This threshold is difficult to achieve *in vivo* and perhaps serves as a physiologic regulator of citrullination. Recently, we reported the discovery of an antibody targeting an epitope common to both PADs 3 and 4 that was highly specific for RA and was strongly associated with progression of radiographic erosions [17]. Adding purified IgG from patients with PAD3/4 cross-reactive antibodies (anti-PAD3/4XR) to PAD4 resulted in increased *in vitro* histone citrullination at physiologic concentrations of calcium, an effect not observed with the addition of anti-PAD4 that was not cross-reactive with PAD3. Accordingly, we hypothesized that RA patients with anti-PAD3/4XR would demonstrate a greater prevalence and extent of RA comorbidities in which tissue citrullination and/or pathogenic ACPA may play an etiopathologic role, such as RA-ILD.

Methods

Study Participants

Participants were enrolled in ESCAPE RA (Evaluation of Subclinical Cardiovascular disease And Predictors of Events in Rheumatoid Arthritis), a prospective cohort study investigating subclinical cardiovascular disease in RA described previously [18,19]. Participants met 1987 RA classification criteria [20], had RA≥6 months from diagnosis, and were 45–84 years of age without known prior pre-specified cardiovascular events. All patients provided written informed consent prior to enrollment, and the study and consent procedures were approved by the Institutional Review Board (IRB) of the Johns Hopkins Hospital. Ongoing analyses were approved by the Columbia University Medical Center IRB. Enrollment occurred between October 2004 and May 2006.

Outcomes

Pulmonary outcomes. As described previously [18], cardiac multi-detector row CT (MDCT) scans were obtained using standard methods [21] with 3 mm thickness on a Toshiba Aquilion 64 scanner. With cardiac MDCT, only lung parenchyma from the level of the carina to the lung bases was included. The validity of cardiac MDCT for pulmonary parenchymal disease has been evaluated, with correlation>90% compared to high-resolution CT [22]. Scans were assessable in 176 of the 195 enrolled participants (91%) by an expert pulmonary radiologist using a previously described standardized method [23] and blinded to clinical characteristics. Characteristics of the subgroup with assessable scans did not differ from those of the full cohort (data not shown). An ILD score (ILDS) was calculated based on the presence and extent of ILD features [i.e. ground glass opacification (GGO), reticulation (R), honeycombing (HC), and traction bronchiectasis (TB)] using a semi-quantitative scale (0 = none, 1 = 1–25%, 2 = 26–50%, 3 = 51–75%, 4 = 76–100%) with a maximum total score possible of 32. Intra-observer concordance for detecting no ILD was 90%, and 100% for ILDS≥3. Pulmonary function testing (PFT), consisting of spirometry and assessment of carbon monoxide diffusing capacity (DLCo), was performed according to American Thoracic Society guidelines [24] at the second study visit, occurring a mean ± standard deviation of 21±3 months post-baseline. Any restriction and impaired diffusion were both defined as≤79% of predicted for forced vital capacity (FVC) and DLCo, respectively.

Measurement of circulating anti-PAD3/4XR. Antibodies against PADs 3 and 4 were assessed as previously described [17]. Briefly, patient serum was added to [^{35}S] Methionine labeled *in vitro* transcribed and translated PAD3 or PAD4. Radiolabeled immune complexes were incubated with Protein A beads and subsequently washed and boiled in SDS sample buffer. Radiography was used to visualize immunoprecipitated proteins separated by gel electrophoresis. Proteins were quantified using densitometry and levels normalized a standard sample with the high titer anti-PAD3/4XR antibodies. Seropositivity was defined at ≥ 0.01 of the normalized value, as none of the non-RA control samples (from healthy controls and patients with psoriatic arthritis) had levels above this cutpoint [17].

Other measures. Demographics, current and past smoking, and medical and RA disease history were assessed by patient self-report. Forty-four joints were examined for swelling and tenderness by a single trained assessor and RA disease activity calculated using the Disease Activity Score for 28 joints with CRP (DAS28-CRP) [25]. The Stanford Health Assessment Questionnaire (HAQ) [26] was used to assess disability. Current and past use of glucocorticoids, biologic and non-biologic disease modifying anti-rheumatic drugs (DMARDs) was queried by detailed examiner-administered questionnaires. Radiographs of the hands and feet were scored using the van der Heijde modification of the Sharp method (SHS) [27] by a single experienced reader blinded to patient characteristics.

Other laboratory assessments. C-reactive protein (CRP) was measured by nephelometry (Dade Behring Inc., Deerfield, IL). RF was assessed by ELISA, with seropositivity defined at or above a level of 40 units. Serum samples obtained concurrently with CT scanning were assessed for anti-CCP (CCP2) using a commercial kit. The presence of shared epitope alleles in exon 2 of HLA-DRB1 was determined as previously described [19].

Statistical Methods

After exploring the distributions of all variables, group-wise differences in normally distributed continuous variables were compared using t-tests, in non-normally distributed continuous variables using the Kruskal-Wallis test, and in categorical variables using the chi-square goodness-of-fit or Fisher's exact test, as appropriate. The associations of PAD antibody status with dichotomous pulmonary outcomes were explored using ordinary logistic regression, and for continuous pulmonary outcomes with linear regression, with variables transformed to normality as required. Multivariable (MV) regression models were constructed, with potential confounders included that were associated with the primary exposure variable in univariate analyses at the $p<0.20$ significance level, to allow for residual confounding. Non-contributory covariates were excluded using the Likelihood-Ratio Test for nested models or Akaike's Information Criterion, as appropriate. Variance inflation factors were calculated to ensure that collinear covariates were not co-modeled. All calculations were performed using Intercooled Stata 12 (StataCorp, College Station, TX). A two-tailed α of 0.05 was used throughout.

Results

Among the 176 RA participants with interpretable lung CT scans, 56 (32%) had antibodies against PAD4; however, only 19 (11%) had anti-PAD3/4XR. Participant characteristics according to antibody status are summarized in Table 1. Compared with individuals negative for anti-PAD, those with anti-PAD3/4XR were slightly older and less likely to be a current smoker, with trends to significance for both. Those with anti-PAD3/4XR had a median disease duration 13 years greater than those with no anti-PAD ($p<0.001$) and were significantly more likely to be seropositive for RF or CCP2 compared with both the groups with no anti-PAD and those with anti-PAD4 not cross-reactive with PAD3, although associations with the individual autoantibodies were not as strong. As previously published [17], those with anti-PAD3/4XR had a significantly higher total SHS score compared with the other groups. Anti-PAD3/4XR was not associated with RA disease activity measures or treatments.

Anti-PAD3/4XR was Associated with CT-ILD in Unadjusted Analyses

Pulmonary outcomes according to antibody status are summarized in Table 2. Any ILD was observed in 58 participants (33%), among whom 22 (38%) demonstrated a predominant radiographic ILD pattern of GGO and 36 (62%) demonstrated R/TB/HC. The median ILD score was 0, with a range of 0–10 units. The median emphysema score was also 0, and ranged from 0–6. Among the 158 patients with PFTs, 44 (28%) had any abnormality, with 30 (21%) demonstrating restriction or impaired diffusion. Among the 168 patients with assessment of respiratory symptoms, 69 (41%) reported any symptoms, with a median number of symptoms of 0 (range 0–4).

For univariate comparisons of pulmonary outcomes according to antibody status, the prevalence of any ILD was more than double among those with anti-PAD3/4XR compared with the group with no anti-PAD and the group with anti-PAD4 that did not cross-react with PAD3 (both comparisons $p<0.05$). The prevalence of both GGO and R/TB/HC was also higher among those with anti-PAD3/4XR compared with the other antibody groups. However, anti-PAD3/4XR was not associated with PFT abnormalities, nor the presence or number of respiratory symptoms.

RA Characteristics were Associated with Radiographic ILD

The associations of participant characteristics with the presence of any ILD features on CT (i.e. an ILD score>0) are summarized

Table 1. Patient Characteristics According to PAD3/4 Cross-Reactive Antibody Status.

Characteristic	Total (n = 176)	No anti-PAD (n = 120)	Anti-PAD4 only (n = 37)	Anti-PAD3/4XR (n = 19)	p-value*
Age, years	59±9	59±8	58±9	62±7	0.093
Male, n (%)	71 (40)	43 (36)	21 (57)	8 (42)	0.60
White, n (%)	152 (86)	101 (84)	35 (95)	16 (84)	0.99
Any college, n (%)	133 (76)	86 (72)	31 (84)	16 (84)	0.25
Ever smoking, n (%)	105 (60)	80 (67)	16 (43)	10 (53)	0.23
Current smoking, n (%)	20 (11)	19 (16)	2 (5)	0 (0)	0.075
Reported lung disease (n = 168), n (%)	27 (16)	22 (19)	4 (12)	1 (6)	0.30
RA duration, years	8 (4–17)	7 (4–12)	15 (7–23)	20 (11–28)	<0.001
RF or CCP2 seropositivity, n (%)	137 (78)	87 (73)	33 (89)	18 (95)	0.043
RF seropositivity, n (%)	114 (65)	73 (61)	26 (70)	15 (79)	0.20
CCP2 seropositivity, n (%)	122 (70)	76 (64)	31 (84)	15 (79)	0.30
Any shared epitope alleles, n (%)	122 (70)	79 (67)	30 (81)	14 (74)	0.79
DAS28-CRP	3.7 (2.9–4.4)	3.6 (2.9–4.3)	3.5 (2.8–4.5)	3.8 (3.3–4.3)	0.68
CRP, mg/L	2.4 (1.1–7.7)	2.1 (1.0–7.1)	3.5 (1.5–9.5)	2.0 (1.6–5.4)	0.65
IL-6, pg/mL	3.7 (1.8–7.8)	3.6 (1.7–8.1)	3.9 (1.8–6.3)	3.7 (2.4–9.0)	0.24
Total SHS	8 (1–37)	5 (0–19)	12 (2–43)	56 (14–132)	<0.001
Pain (100 mm VAS)	21 (9–41)	21 (8–40)	23 (10–41)	20 (5–47)	0.71
HAQ-DI (0–3)	0.63 (0.12–1.25)	0.63 (0.12–1.25)	0.75 (0.12–1.25)	0.75 (0–1.88)	0.73
Current prednisone, n (%)	67 (38)	45 (38)	13 (35)	9 (47)	0.41
Current non-biologic DMARDs, n (%)	150 (86)	100 (84)	34 (92)	16 (84)	0.99
Methotrexate, n (%)	114 (65)	79 (66)	22 (59)	13 (68)	0.83
Leflunomide, n (%)	19 (11)	11 (9)	5 (14)	3 (16)	0.41
Current biologic DMARDs, n (%)	81 (46)	55 (46)	17 (46)	10 (53)	0.63
TNF inhibitors, n (%)	78 (45)	52 (44)	17 (46)	10 (53)	0.62
Number of failed DMARDs	1 (0–2)	1 (0–2)	1 (0–3)	2 (0–2)	0.75

Values are mean ± standard deviation or median (interquartile range) unless otherwise noted.
*p-values are for the comparison of the no anti-PAD vs. anti-PAD3/4XR groups.
PAD = peptidyl-arginine deiminase; anti-PAD3/4XR = anti-PAD3/4 Cross-Reactive antibodies; RA = rheumatoid arthritis; RF = rheumatoid factor; CCP2 = 2nd generation anti-cyclic citrullinated peptide antibody; DAS = disease activity score; CRP = C-reactive protein; IL = interleukin; SHS = Total modified Sharp-van der Heijde Score; HAQ = Health Assessment Questionnaire Disability Index; TNF = tumor necrosis factor; DMARD = disease modifying anti-rheumatic drug.

Table 2. Pulmonary Outcomes According to PAD3/4 Cross-Reactive Antibody Status.

Characteristic	Total (n = 176)	No anti-PAD (n = 120)	Anti-PAD4 only (n = 37)	Anti-PAD3/4XR (n = 19)	p-value*
Any ILD, n (%)	58 (33)	35 (29)	10 (27)	13 (68)	0.001
Any GGO, n (%)	22 (13)	11 (10)	6 (16)	5 (28)	0.047
Any R/TB/HC, n (%)	36 (22)	21 (19)	8 (22)	7 (39)	0.045
ILD Score, units (0–32)	0 (0–2; range 0–10)	0 (0–2; range 0–6)	0 (0–2; range 0–10)	2 (0–2; range 0–10)	0.020
Emphysema score, units (0–32)	0 (0–0; range 0–6)	0 (0–0; range 0–6)	0 (0–0; range 0–4)	0 (0–0; range 0–2)	0.77
Any PFT Abnormality (n = 158), n (%)	44 (28)	33 (29)	9 (29)	2 (13)	0.23
Any PFT Restriction or Impaired Diffusion, n (%)	30 (21)	21 (22)	8 (27)	1 (8)	0.46
Any respiratory symptoms (n = 168), n (%)	69 (41)	47 (40)	13 (38)	9 (53)	0.43
Number of respiratory symptoms	0 (0–1; range 0–4)	0 (0–1; range 0–4)	0 (0–2; range 0–4)	1 (0–1; range 0–3)	0.55

Values are median (interquartile range) unless otherwise noted.
*p-values are for the comparison of the no anti-PAD vs. anti-PAD3/4XR groups.
PAD = peptidyl-arginine deiminase; anti-PAD3/4XR = anti-PAD3/4 Cross-Reactive antibodies; RA = rheumatoid arthritis; ILD = interstitial lung disease; GGO = ground glass opacification; R/TB/HC = reticulation/traction bronchiectasis/honeycombing; PFT = pulmonary function testing; Impaired Diff = impaired diffusion.

in Table 3. Those with any ILD features on CT tended to be older than those without ILD and were more likely to be male (both with trends to significance). Any ILD was strongly associated with both current and past smoking, but not with reported lung disease. Those with any ILD were significantly more likely to be seropositive for RF or CCP2 and had a higher median circulating IL-6 level. Trends to significance were noted for higher total SHS and HAQ among those with vs. without ILD. Those with ILD were also significantly more likely to be treated with prednisone and current biologics, most of which were TNF inhibitors. ILD was not associated with methotrexate or leflunomide use, or the number of failed DMARDs. As expected, those with ILD were significantly more likely to have PFT restriction or impaired diffusion and report respiratory symptoms compared with those without ILD.

Anti-PAD3/4XR Remained Associated with Any ILD After Adjustment

Crude and adjusted associations of anti-PAD3/4XR with pulmonary outcomes are summarized in Figure 1. After adjusting for characteristics associated with either anti-PAD3/4XR or any ILD, anti-PAD3/4XR remained significantly associated with any-ILD compared with those with no anti-PAD or those with anti-PAD4 that did not cross-react with PAD3 (adjusted OR = 7.22 for the comparison of anti-PAD3/4XR vs. no anti-PAD; p = 0.001).

The Combination of Anti-PAD3/4XR with Smoking was Highly Associated with Any ILD Features

The individual and combined associations of anti-PAD3/4XR and ever smoking with any ILD are depicted in Figure 2. Before adjustment, only 16% of participants who were anti-PAD3/4XR negative and had never smoked had any ILD features on CT. The prevalence of any ILD was higher among those with either characteristic, and the magnitude of the association was similar for never smokers with anti-PAD3/4XR vs. ever smokers without the antibody. However, 90% of ever smokers seropositive for anti-PAD3/4XR demonstrated any features of ILD. The prevalence remained significantly higher for this group compared with the other groups after adjustment, resulting in an adjusted OR of 61.4 for the comparison of any ILD for ever smokers with anti-PAD3/4XR compared with never smokers without the antibody (p = 0.001).

Adjusted Associations of PAD3/4XR with Other Pulmonary Outcomes

Associations of anti-PAD3/4XR with other pulmonary outcomes are summarized in Table 4. Both GGO and R/TB/HC were significantly higher among RA patients with anti-PAD3/4XR compared to those negative for the antibody in unadjusted analyses. However, only the predominant pattern of GGO was significantly associated after MV adjustment. Additionally after MV adjustment, anti-PAD3/4XR was associated with a higher ILD Score when considered as a continuous variable. However, anti-PAD3/4XR was not associated with any abnormalities on PFTs or the presence or number of reported respiratory symptoms in either crude or adjusted analyses.

Discussion

In this first investigation of the relationship between the recently discovered RA-specific auto-antibody, anti-PAD3/4XR, and radiographic ILD, we detected a robust association for both the presence and extent of RA-ILD among patients with anti-PAD3/4XR compared with patients with no anti-PAD antibodies and even among those with anti-PAD4 antibodies that did not cross-react with PAD3. The associations were not diminished in magnitude under various relevant MV adjustment scenarios. Notably, the combination of anti-PAD3/4XR with a history of smoking was particularly robust in its association with RA-ILD, with a synergistic interaction suggested.

The etiopathology of RA-ILD is poorly understood. Adding to the complexity is heterogeneity in ILD histopathology and the high prevalence of asymptomatic disease [6]. However, in the setting of clinical symptoms the disease can be a severe and frequently lethal consequence of RA [1,4]. Citrullination of lung proteins may contribute to the pathogenesis of RA-ILD. Fibroblast and lymphocyte migration through the pulmonary extracellular matrix to areas of damage, as well as cellular differentiation and activation, are dependent on interactions between matrix and cell surface proteins that are highly regulated [28–30]. Citrullination of key matrix proteins, therefore, could result in aberrant cellular migration, differentiation, and activation resulting in abnormal

Table 3. Patient Characteristics According to the Presence of CT-ILD Features.

Characteristic	No ILD (n = 118)	Any ILD (n = 58)	p-value
Age, years	58±8	61±9	0.071
Male, n (%)	43 (36)	29 (50)	0.085
White, n (%)	101 (86)	51 (88)	0.67
Any college, n (%)	87 (74)	46 (79)	0.42
Ever smoking, n (%)	62 (53)	44 (76)	0.003
Current smoking, n (%)	7 (6)	14 (24)	<0.001
Reported lung disease (n = 168), n (%)	19 (17)	8 (14)	0.66
RA duration, years	8 (4–16)	8 (5–19)	0.22
RF or CCP2 seropositivity, n (%)	86 (73)	52 (90)	0.011
RF seropositivity, n (%)	71 (60)	43 (75)	0.047
CCP2 seropositivity, n (%)	73 (62)	49 (86)	0.001
Any shared epitope alleles, n (%)	80 (68)	43 (75)	0.34
DAS28-CRP	3.5 (2.8–4.3)	3.8 (3.2–4.5)	0.12
CRP, mg/L	2.3 (1.0–7.2)	3.5 (1.2–9.3)	0.58
IL-6, pg/mL	3.0 (1.6–7.0)	4.5 (2.3–9.5)	0.029
Total SHS	6 (0–26)	12 (2–55)	0.074
Pain (100 mm VAS)	19 (10–40)	24 (8–47)	0.52
HAQ-DI (0–3)	0.62 (0.12–1.25)	0.75 (0.25–1.50)	0.083
Current prednisone, n (%)	37 (31)	30 (52)	0.009
Current non-biologic DMARDs, n (%)	103 (88)	47 (81)	0.21
Methotrexate, n (%)	81 (69)	33 (57)	0.13
Leflunomide, n (%)	11 (9)	8 (14)	0.37
Current biologic DMARDs, n (%)	48 (41)	34 (59)	0.028
TNF inhibitors, n (%)	46 (39)	33 (57)	0.028
Number of failed DMARDs	1 (0–2)	1 (0–2)	0.80
Any PFT Abnormality (n = 158), n (%)	22 (21)	22 (43)	0.003
Any PFT Restriction or Impaired Diffusion, n (%)	12 (13)	18 (41)	<0.001
Any respiratory symptoms (n = 168), n (%)	40 (36)	29 (52)	0.046
Number of respiratory symptoms	0 (0–1)	1 (0–2)	0.017

Values are mean ± standard deviation or median (interquartile range) unless otherwise noted.
RA = rheumatoid arthritis; RF = rheumatoid factor; CCP2 = 2nd generation anti-cyclic citrullinated peptide antibody; DAS = disease activity score; CRP = C-reactive protein; IL = interleukin; SHS = Total modified Sharp-van der Heijde Score; HAQ = Health Assessment Questionnaire Disability Index; TNF = tumor necrosis factor; DMARD = disease modifying anti-rheumatic drug; ILD = interstitial lung disease; PFT = pulmonary function testing; Impaired Diff = impaired diffusion.

tissue repair, ectopic fibrosis, and dysregulated inflammation. For example, attachment and spreading of fibroblasts was impaired on plates coated with citrullinated fibronectin compared with non-citrullinated fibronectin [31]. This mechanism may not be exclusive to RA, as the presence of citrullinated proteins has been detected in the tissue targets of several autoimmune conditions, including the lungs of non-RA patients with ILD [13,14]. An additional possibility is that citrullinated proteins in the lung are targets for ACPA, an interaction that may drive ILD. This possibility is supported by recent evidence for the presence of ACPA in the sputum of RA patients [32]. However, at present, any speculative mechanistic links between citrullinated proteins in the lung, ACPA generation and pathogenesis, and ILD remain to be elucidated.

While citrullination of lung proteins may contribute to the pathogenesis of ILD, physiologic barriers limiting PAD activity may have evolved to regulate such pathologic citrullination. For one, the calcium threshold for PAD catalytic activity generally exceeds levels attainable extra-cellularly. *In vitro* experiments typically use 5–10 mM calcium concentrations for maximal PAD activity, whereas *in vivo* extra-cellular levels typically do not exceed 1.5 mM [33]. Recently [17], we showed that anti-PAD3/4XR antibodies increased the sensitivity of PAD4 to calcium allowing efficient citrullination in the context of physiologic calcium concentrations. From the same report, anti-PAD3/4XR reacted with PAD4 at a key calcium binding site that is also involved in protein-protein interactions, suggesting that the antibody may create a permissive environment for calcium activated catalysis. Therefore, the analyses presented here provide a circumstantial link between a disease manifestation in which aberrant citrullination may play a pathogenic role (i.e. ILD) and the mechanism by which citrullination may be facilitated (i.e. anti-PAD3/4XR).

Smoking is a well-established risk factor for both RA [34] and ILD [35], and, as confirmed among the cohort reported here, RA patients with a history of smoking were more likely to have radiographic ILD. Additionally, compared with non-smokers, smokers had higher levels of PAD2 in the bronchial mucosa, but

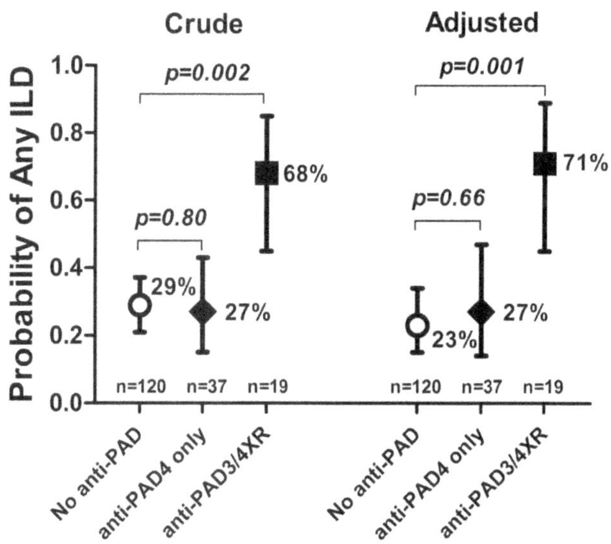

Figure 1. The Presence of anti-PAD3/4 Cross-reactive Antibodies was Associated with Radiographic RA-ILD. The cohort was grouped based on the presence of anti-PAD3/4XR antibodies (closed square), anti-PAD4 antibodies that did not cross-react with PAD3 (closed diamond), or neither reactivity (open circle). The prevalence of any ILD was more than double among those with anti-PAD3/4XR compared with those with anti-PAD4 alone or those with neither reactivity in both crude (left) and adjusted (right) analyses. Average probabilities and 95% confidence intervals are depicted. Associations adjusted for age, gender, current and past smoking, rheumatoid factor and CCP2 seropositivity, DAS28, current use of biologics and prednisone, RA duration, and total Sharp-van der Heijde Score.

no difference in the amount of protein citrullination in the same tissue [14]. In our study, the combined effect of smoking plus anti-PAD3/4XR was greater than the sum of the individual effects of either characteristic in isolation, suggesting a possible synergistic interaction. In this setting, PAD up-regulation conferred by smoking combined with the enhanced catalytic activity of PAD4 conferred by anti-PAD3/4XR could provide the stimulus for the enhanced pathogenic effect observed. Based on this circumstantial evidence, testing of this speculative mechanistic hypothesis is warranted.

The study has notable strengths and limitations. Among the strengths, scans were interpreted by the same pulmonary radiologist with decades of ILD experience, and ILD features correlated with both PFT abnormalities and respiratory symptoms. Among the limitations, cardiac MDCT differs from high-resolution CT (HRCT) in slice thickness and the lung apices were not imaged. However, while we may have missed additional ILD features exclusive to the apices (uncommon for RA-ILD), our findings are internally consistent since the same techniques were used for all patients. Owing to the characteristics of the cohort, our findings may only be generalizable to RA patients >45 years of age without prior cardiovascular events, and, notably, there were few patients with severe RA-ILD included. Additionally, the primary comparisons were cross-sectional, limiting any ability to establish temporality in the associations. Additional longitudinal work is underway exploring the temporal relationship between emergence of anti-PAD3/4XR over the time-course of RA and incident RA-ILD.

In summary, anti-PAD3/4XR seropositivity was detected in a subset of RA patients with longer standing, seropositive, destructive disease. Independent of these features, the presence of anti-PAD3/4XR remained highly associated with the presence and extent of ILD, assessed by CT scanning. Interestingly, the

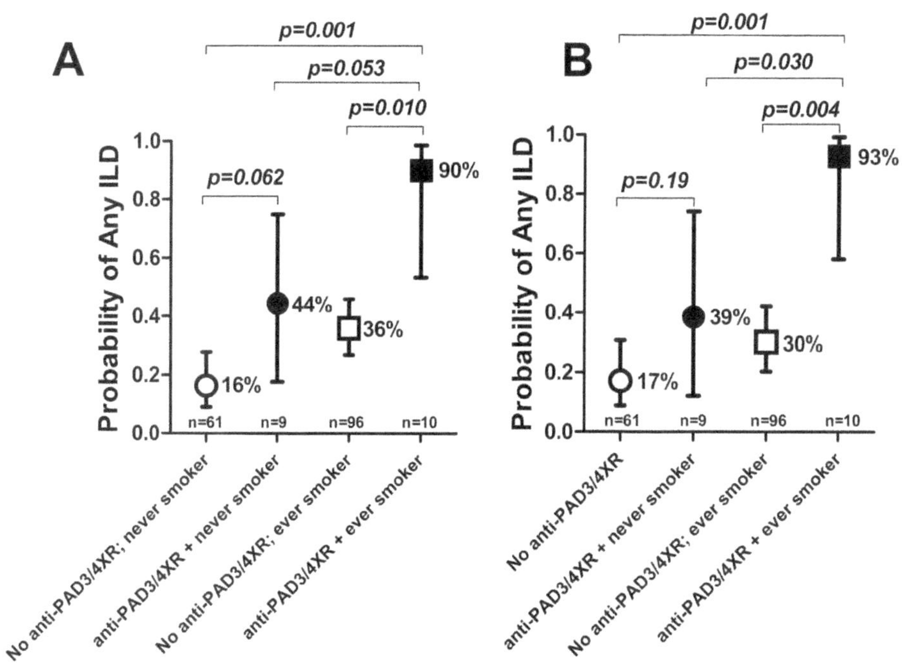

Figure 2. The Combined Effects of anti-PAD3/4 Cross-reactive Antibodies and Smoking Were Robust Indicators of Radiographic RA-ILD. The cohort was grouped based on the presence of anti-PAD3/4XR (closed markers) and history of ever smoking (i.e. current or former smokers). The association of anti-PAD3/4XR with ILD was stronger among ever smokers compared to never smokers in both crude (Panel A) and adjusted (Panel B) analyses. Average probabilities and 95% confidence intervals are depicted. Panel B associations adjusted for age, gender, rheumatoid factor and CCP2 seropositivity, DAS28, current use of methotrexate and prednisone, RA duration, and total Sharp-van der Heijde Score.

Table 4. Crude and Adjusted Associations of PAD3/4 Cross-Reactive Antibodies with Pulmonary Outcomes in RA.

Outcome	Crude		Adjusted*		Adjusted**	
	β	p-value	β	p-value	β	p-value
Any ILD†	5.39	0.001	4.37	0.011	7.22	0.001
Any GGO†	2.99	0.042	3.93	0.034	3.50	0.043
Any R/TB/HC†	2.63	0.046	1.13	0.85	2.10	0.22
Any PFT Abnormality†	0.51	0.30	0.37	0.15	0.45	0.25
Any PFT Restriction or Impaired Diffusion†	0.48	0.36	0.40	0.26	0.59	0.52
Any respiratory symptoms†	1.81	0.22	1.74	0.29	2.15	0.17
Square root ILD Score	0.61	0.004	0.52	0.022	0.61	0.002

*Adjusted for age, RA duration, RF, CCP2, IL-6, SHS.
**Adjusted for age, gender, RF, CCP2, RA duration, DAS28, prednisone use, biologic DMARD use, current and past smoking, and SHS.
†β coefficients are Odds Ratios.
ILD = interstitial lung disease; GGO = ground glass opacification; R/TB/HC = reticulation/traction bronchiectasis/honeycombing; PFT = pulmonary function testing; Impaired Diff = impaired diffusion; RA = rheumatoid arthritis; RF = rheumatoid factor; CCP2 = 2nd generation anti-cyclic citrullinated peptide antibody; DAS = disease activity score; CRP = C-reactive protein; IL = interleukin; SHS = Total modified Sharp-van der Heijde Score; DMARD = disease modifying anti-rheumatic drug.

combination of smoking history with anti-PAD3/4 antibody status was associated with a frequency of ILD to a greater extent than expected from the mere addition of their separate effects, suggesting a synergistic interaction. With additional investigation, these novel findings have potential implications for both understanding the mechanisms underlying the pathogenesis of RA-ILD and for predicting which RA patients are at risk for developing this potentially life-threatening RA extra-articular manifestation.

Acknowledgments

We would like to thank the Johns Hopkins Bayview Medical Center General Clinical Research Center and staff, the field center of the Baltimore MESA cohort, and the MESA Coordinating Center at the University of Washington, Seattle. Dr. Stanley Seigelman interpreted all of the CT scans for ILD.

We are indebted to the dedication and hard work of the ESCAPE RA Staff: Marilyn Towns, Michelle Jones, Patricia Jones, Marissa Hildebrandt, Shawn Franckowiak, and Brandy Miles and to the participants of the ESCAPE RA study who graciously agreed to take part in this research.

Drs. Uzma Haque, Clifton Bingham III, Carol Ziminski, Jill Ratain, Ira Fine, Joyce Kopicky-Burd, David McGinnis, Andrea Marx, Howard Hauptman, Achini Perera, Peter Holt, Alan Matsumoto, Megan Clowse, Gordon Lam and others generously recommended their patients for this study.

Author Contributions

Conceived and designed the experiments: JTG ED SD CJ FA AR JMB. Performed the experiments: ED FA AR. Analyzed the data: JTG. Contributed reagents/materials/analysis tools: ED FA AR JTG. Wrote the paper: JTG ED SD CJ FA AR JMB.

References

1. Bongartz T, Nannini C, Medina-Velasquez YF, Achenbach SJ, Crowson CS, et al. (2010) Incidence and mortality of interstitial lung disease in rheumatoid arthritis: a population-based study. Arthritis and Rheumatism 62: 1583–1591.
2. Koduri G, Norton S, Young A, Cox N, Davies P, et al. (2010) Interstitial lung disease has a poor prognosis in rheumatoid arthritis: results from an inception cohort. Rheumatology (Oxford) 49: 1483–1489.
3. Young A, Koduri G, Batley M, Kulinskaya E, Gough A, et al. (2007) Mortality in rheumatoid arthritis. Increased in the early course of disease, in ischaemic heart disease and in pulmonary fibrosis. Rheumatology (Oxford) 46: 350–357.
4. Olson AL, Swigris JJ, Sprunger DB, Fischer A, Fernandez-Perez ER, et al. (2011) Rheumatoid arthritis-interstitial lung disease-associated mortality. American journal of respiratory and critical care medicine 183: 372–378.
5. Solomon JJ, Ryu JH, Tazelaar HD, Myers JL, Tuder R, et al. (2013) Fibrosing interstitial pneumonia predicts survival in patients with rheumatoid arthritis-associated interstitial lung disease (RA-ILD). Respir Med 107: 1247–1252.
6. Dawson JK, Fewins HE, Desmond J, Lynch MP, Graham DR (2001) Fibrosing alveolitis in patients with rheumatoid arthritis as assessed by high resolution computed tomography, chest radiography, and pulmonary function tests. Thorax 56: 622–627.
7. Giles JT, Danoff SK, Sokolove J, Wagner CA, Winchester R, et al. (2013) Association of fine specificity and repertoire expansion of anticitrullinated peptide antibodies with rheumatoid arthritis associated interstitial lung disease. Ann Rheum Dis doi:10.1136.
8. McDonagh J, Greaves M, Wright AR, Heycock C, Owen JP, et al. (1994) High resolution computed tomography of the lungs in patients with rheumatoid arthritis and interstitial lung disease. Br J Rheumatol 33: 118–122.
9. Vij R, Strek ME (2013) Diagnosis and treatment of connective tissue disease-associated interstitial lung disease. Chest 143: 814–824.
10. Vossenaar ER, Zendman AJ, van Venrooij WJ, Pruijn GJ (2003) PAD, a growing family of citrullinating enzymes: genes, features and involvement in disease. BioEssays: news and reviews in molecular, cellular and developmental biology 25: 1106–1118.
11. Ordonez A, Martinez-Martinez I, Corrales FJ, Miqueo C, Minano A, et al. (2009) Effect of citrullination on the function and conformation of antithrombin. FEBS J 276: 6763–6772.
12. Mortier A, Loos T, Gouwy M, Ronsse I, Van Damme J, et al. (2010) Posttranslational modification of the NH2-terminal region of CXCL5 by proteases or peptidylarginine Deiminases (PAD) differently affects its biological activity. J Biol Chem 285: 29750–29759.
13. Bongartz T, Cantaert T, Atkins SR, Harle P, Myers JL, et al. (2007) Citrullination in extra-articular manifestations of rheumatoid arthritis. Rheumatology (Oxford, England) 46: 70–75.
14. Makrygiannakis D, Hermansson M, Ulfgren AK, Nicholas AP, Zendman AJ, et al. (2008) Smoking increases peptidylarginine deiminase 2 enzyme expression in human lungs and increases citrullination in BAL cells. 67: 1488–1492.
15. Sokolove J, Bromberg R, Deane KD, Lahey LJ, Derber LA, et al. (2012) Autoantibody epitope spreading in the pre-clinical phase predicts progression to rheumatoid arthritis. PloS one 7: e35296.
16. van Gaalen FA, van Aken J, Huizinga TW, Schreuder GM, Breedveld FC, et al. (2004) Association between HLA class II genes and autoantibodies to cyclic citrullinated peptides (CCPs) influences the severity of rheumatoid arthritis. Arthritis and Rheumatism 50: 2113–2121.
17. Darrah E, Giles JT, Ols ML, Bull HG, Andrade F, et al. (2013) Erosive rheumatoid arthritis is associated with antibodies that activate PAD4 by increasing calcium sensitivity. Sci Transl Med 5: 186ra165.
18. Giles JT, Szklo M, Post W, Petri M, Blumenthal RS, et al. (2009) Coronary arterial calcification in rheumatoid arthritis: comparison to the multi-ethnic study of atherosclerosis. Arthritis research & therapy 11: R36.
19. Kobayashi H, Giles JT, Polak JF, Blumenthal RS, Leffell MS, et al. (2010) Increased prevalence of carotid artery atherosclerosis in rheumatoid arthritis is artery-specific. The Journal of rheumatology 37: 730–739.
20. Arnett FC, Edworthy SM, Bloch DA, McShane DJ, Fries JF, et al. (1988) The American Rheumatism Association 1987 revised criteria for the classification of rheumatoid arthritis. Arthritis and Rheumatism 31: 315–324.

21. Carr JJ, Nelson JC, Wong ND, McNitt-Gray M, Arad Y, et al. (2005) Calcified coronary artery plaque measurement with cardiac CT in population-based studies: standardized protocol of Multi-Ethnic Study of Atherosclerosis (MESA) and Coronary Artery Risk Development in Young Adults (CARDIA) study. Radiology 234: 35–43.
22. Hoffman EA, Jiang R, Baumhauer H, Brooks MA, Carr JJ, et al. (2009) Reproducibility and validity of lung density measures from cardiac CT Scans–The Multi-Ethnic Study of Atherosclerosis (MESA) Lung Study. Academic Radiology 16: 689–699.
23. Goldin JG, Lynch DA, Strollo DC, Suh RD, Schraufnagel DE, et al. (2008) High-resolution CT scan findings in patients with symptomatic scleroderma-related interstitial lung disease. Chest 134: 358–367.
24. Miller MR, Crapo R, Hankinson J, Brusasco V, Burgos F, et al. (2005) General considerations for lung function testing. The European respiratory journal: official journal of the European Society for Clinical Respiratory Physiology 26: 153–161.
25. Prevoo ML, van 't Hof MA, Kuper HH, van Leeuwen MA, van de Putte LB, et al. (1995) Modified disease activity scores that include twenty-eight-joint counts. Development and validation in a prospective longitudinal study of patients with rheumatoid arthritis. Arthritis and Rheumatism 38: 44–48.
26. Wolfe F, Kleinheksel SM, Cathey MA, Hawley DJ, Spitz PW, et al. (1988) The clinical value of the Stanford Health Assessment Questionnaire Functional Disability Index in patients with rheumatoid arthritis. The Journal of rheumatology 15: 1480–1488.
27. van der Heijde D (2000) How to read radiographs according to the Sharp/van der Heijde method. The Journal of rheumatology 27: 261–263.
28. Felsenfeld DP, Choquet D, Sheetz MP (1996) Ligand binding regulates the directed movement of beta1 integrins on fibroblasts. Nature 383: 438–440.
29. Sheetz MP, Felsenfeld DP, Galbraith CG (1998) Cell migration: regulation of force on extracellular-matrix-integrin complexes. Trends Cell Biol 8: 51–54.
30. Luzina IG, Todd NW, Nacu N, Lockatell V, Choi J, et al. (2009) Regulation of pulmonary inflammation and fibrosis through expression of integrins alphaV-beta3 and alphaVbeta5 on pulmonary T lymphocytes. Arthritis Rheum 60: 1530–1539.
31. Shelef MA, Bennin DA, Mosher DF, Huttenlocher A (2012) Citrullination of fibronectin modulates synovial fibroblast behavior. Arthritis Res Ther 14: R240.
32. Willis VC, Demoruelle MK, Derber LA, Chartier-Logan CJ, Parish MC, et al. (2013) Sputum autoantibodies in patients with established rheumatoid arthritis and subjects at risk of future clinically apparent disease. Arthritis Rheum 65: 2545–2554.
33. Robertson WG, Marshall RW (1981) Ionized calcium in body fluids. Crit Rev Clin Lab Sci 15: 85–125.
34. Kallberg H, Ding B, Padyukov L, Bengtsson C, Ronnelid J, et al. (2011) Smoking is a major preventable risk factor for rheumatoid arthritis: estimations of risks after various exposures to cigarette smoke. Annals of the Rheumatic Diseases 70: 508–511.
35. Baumgartner KB, Samet JM, Coultas DB, Stidley CA, Hunt WC, et al. (2000) Occupational and environmental risk factors for idiopathic pulmonary fibrosis: a multicenter case-control study. Collaborating Centers. American Journal of Epidemiology 152: 307–315.

Antibodies Specific for Carbamylated Proteins Precede the Onset of Clinical Symptoms in Mice with Collagen Induced Arthritis

Jeroen N. Stoop[1*], Bi-Sheng Liu[1], Jing Shi[1], Diahann T. S. L. Jansen[1], Martin Hegen[2], Tom W. J. Huizinga[1], Leendert A. Trouw[1], René E. M. Toes[1]

1 Department of Rheumatology, Leiden University Medical Center, Leiden, The Netherlands, 2 Immunoscience Research Unit, Pfizer Worldwide Research and Development, Cambridge, Massachusetts, United States of America

Abstract

Objective: The immune response to post-translationally modified antigens is a key characteristic of rheumatoid arthritis. Carbamylation is such a posttranslational modification. Recently, we demonstrated that autoantibodies recognizing carbamylated proteins are present in sera of rheumatoid arthritis. The molecular mechanisms underlying the break of tolerance and hence the induction of anti-CarP antibody responses are unknown as well as their appearance in mouse models for systemic arthritis. Therefore we analyzed their appearance in the mouse collagen-induced arthritis model.

Methods: collagen induced arthritis was induced by immunization with type II collagen in complete Freund's adjuvant. Arthritis severity was monitored by clinical scoring and anti-CarP antibody levels were determined by ELISA.

Results: Anti-CarP antibodies were detectable in mice with collagen induced arthritis. We did not detect ACPA in mice with collagen induced arthritis. The specificity of the antibodies for carbamylated proteins was confirmed by inhibition assays and immunoblotting. Injection with complete Freund's adjuvant without type II collagen could also induce anti-CarP antibodies, however, in mice with arthritis, the anti-CarP antibody response was stronger and developed more rapidly. The onset of collagen induced arthritis was preceded by an increase of anti-CarP IgG2a levels in the serum.

Conclusion: In mice with collagen induced arthritis we did not observe an immune response against citrullinated antigens, but we did observe an immune response against carbamylated antigens. This anti-CarP response already appeared before disease onset, indicating that collagen induced arthritis can be used as an in vivo model to study anti-CarP antibodies. Our data also indicate that the tolerance to carbamylated proteins, in contrast to the response to citrullinated proteins, is easily broken and that arthritis boosts the immune response against these proteins. The anti-CarP response in mice with CIA can be used as a model for immune responses to post-translationally modified proteins.

Editor: Oliver Frey, University Hospital Jena, Germany

Funding: This work was supported by the IMI JU funded project BeTheCure, contract no 115142-2, the Dutch Arthritis Foundation, The Netherlands Organization for Scientific Research and Pfizer. Leendert Trouw receives a fellowship from Janssen biologics BV. Martin Hegen (who is an employee of Pfizer) has been involved in the design of the study and in the preparation of the manuscript in a scientific collaboration. The funders had no role in study design, data collection and analysis, decision to publish, or preparation of the manuscript.

Competing Interests: Although the authors have received funding from Pfizer and Janssen biologics BV, this does not alter adherence to PLOS ONE policies on sharing data and materials. The fact that Martin Hegen is an employee of Pfizer, does not alter adherence to PLOS ONE policies on sharing data and materials.

* Email: J.N.Stoop@lumc.nl

These authors contributed equally to this work.

Introduction

Rheumatoid arthritis (RA) is a disease characterized by a chronic inflammation of synovial joints, causing cartilage resorption and bone destruction [1]. RA affects approximately 0.5–1% of the adult population [2]. The immune response to post-translational modification of proteins is believed to play a role in the pathogenesis of RA. It is unclear how the breaking of tolerance to such modified proteins occurs. Citrullination is such a posttranslational modification. During this reaction an arginine is converted into citrulline by peptidyl arginine deiminase enzymes. This enzymatic reaction results in the generation of citrullinated antigens that are recognized by anti-citrullinated protein antibodies (ACPA; as reviewed in [3]). ACPA are diagnostic markers for rheumatoid arthritis [4] and are thought to play a role in disease pathogenesis. ACPA can activate cells and complement in vitro [5,6]. There is discussion in the literature on whether ACPA can be detected in mice with CIA. Although some groups did detect ACPA in mice with CIA [7,8], other groups could not [9]. Furthermore, conflicting results have been published on whether ACPA can modify disease in mice [7,10].

Carbamylation is a different type of post-translational modification of proteins, in which isocyanic acid reacts with the amine group of an amino acid. Carbamylation will mostly result in the conversion of lysine into homocitrulline. However, under specific conditions, other amino acids, such as arginine and cysteine and the n-terminus of a protein can also react with cyanate (as reviewed in [11]). Unlike citrullination, which is enzymatically mediated, carbamylation is a chemical reaction involving cyanate which is present in the body in equilibrium with urea. During inflammation, myeloperoxidase, which converts thiocyanate to cyanate, is released from neutrophils. This myeloperoxidase release can lead to a local increase in cyanate levels enabling further carbamylation to occur [12,13]. A schematic picture of the carbamylation of a lysine is depicted in Figure 1A.

There is evidence for a role for carbamylation in arthritis. Recently, we identified antibodies against carbamylated proteins (anti-CarP) in the serum of RA patients and showed that the presence of these antibodies is predictive of worse disease progression in ACPA negative patients [14]. We have also shown that Anti-CarP antibodies are present in arthralgia patients and that their presence predicts the development of RA, independent of the patient's ACPA status, indicating that anti-CarP might also be useful as a biomarker for seronegative RA [15]. In mice it has been reported that intra-articular injection of a citrullinated fillagrin peptide can lead to local arthritis when the animals have previously been vaccinated with a carbamylated peptide [16].

Mouse models are frequently used tools to study the break of tolerance towards self-antigens as well as the disease pathogenesis such as occurring in arthritis. The aim of this study was to gain

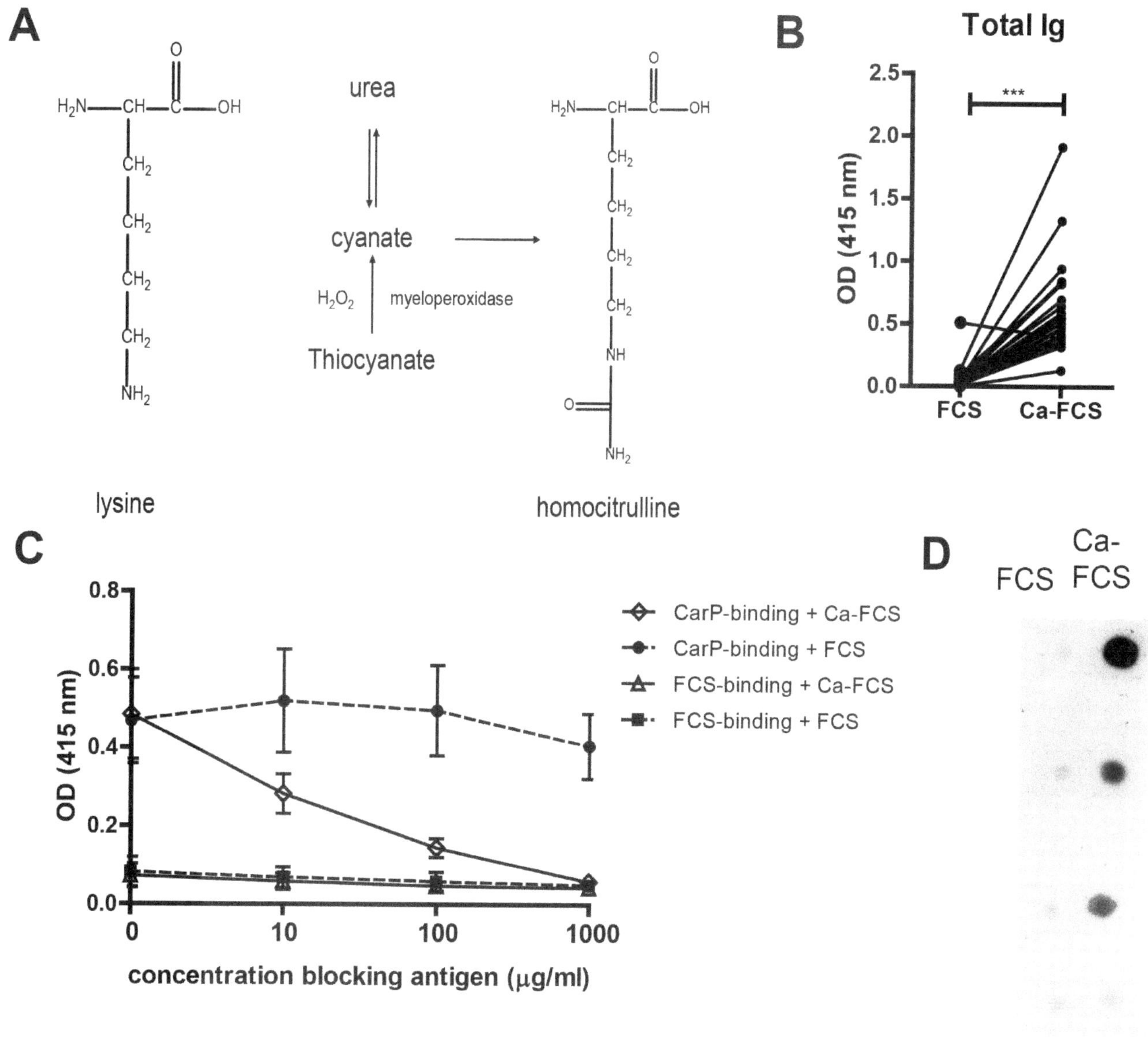

Figure 1. Anti-CarP antibodies can be detected in mice. (**A**) Schematic picture of the carbamylation process. (**B**) DBA/1J mice were immunized with CII in CFA. The antibody binding to FCS and Carbamylated-FCS (Ca-FCS) was determined by ELISA. The OD value for Ca-FCS binding and FCS binding of each sample are connected with a line. Statistical analysis was performed using a Wilcoxon paired test (n = 29). (**C**) Sera from anti-CarP positive mice were pre-incubated with different concentrations of Ca-FCS and FCS. The Ig binding to FCS and Ca-FCS was determined by ELISA (n = 4). (**D**) C57Bl/6 mice were immunized with CII in CFA. Equal amounts of Ca-FCS and FCS were blotted on a membrane. The presence of antibodies reactive to the Ca-FCS or FCS on the blots was analyzed by incubating the blots with sera from the immunized mice. A representative example of 2 independent experiments is depicted.

insight into the requirements for the emergence of anti-CarP antibody responses and to determine whether anti-CarP antibodies are also present in mice with collagen induced arthritis (CIA), the most frequently used animal model of arthritis. Here, we show for the first time that anti-CarP antibodies can be detected in mice with systemic arthritis and that the appearance of anti-CarP antibodies in the serum precedes the onset of arthritis.

Materials and Methods

Animals and arthritis induction

All animal experiments were performed conform national guidelines and the study protocol was approved by the Ethical Committee for Animal Experimentation (Dier Experimentele Commissie; DEC) of Leiden University. DBA/1J mice were obtained from our own breeding colony (originally obtained from Charles River). C57Bl/6 mice were purchased from Charles River. CIA was induced in 8–10 week old mice by injection at the tail base with 100 µg of CII emulsified in complete Freunds adjuvant (CFA). On day 21 the mice received a subcutaneous boost with 100 µg of CII in incomplete Freunds adjuvant (IFA; Sigma-Aldrich). For DBA/1J mice bovine CII (Chondrex) and CFA containing 0.5 mg/ml of *M.tuberculosis* (Difco) were used and for C57Bl/6 mice chicken CII (Chondrex) and CFA containing 2.5 mg/ml of *M.tuberculosis* (Chondrex) were used. For the CFA only immunizations PBS was used instead of CII. Arthritis severity was monitored as described earlier using a clinical score with a maximum of 15 per paw [17]. For the kinetics experiments, mice were bled before immunization, on day 7, 14, 21, 28, 35, 49 after immunization and at the end of follow up. Blood was centrifuged and serum was harvested and stored at −80°C until use.

Carbamylation and citrullination of FCS

For generating carbamylated Fetal Calf Serum (Ca-FCS) or ovalbumin (OVA; Sigma), FCS or OVA was diluted in water to a protein concentration of 4 mg/ml. The diluted FCS or OVA was incubated for 12 hours at 37°C with 1 M potassium cyanate (Sigma-Aldrich). After incubation the sample was extensively dialyzed against water (as described before [14]). Citrullinated FCS (Ci-FCS) was generated by incubation of 10 mg FCS in a volume of 1 ml containing 0.1 M Tris-HCl pH 7.6, 10 mM $CaCl_2$, and 40 U PAD4 (Sigma) for 24 hours at 37°C.

Detection of Anti-CarP antibodies ACPA by ELISA

Non-modified FCS, citrullinated-FCS (Cit-FCS) and Ca-FCS were coated overnight at a concentration of 10 µg/ml (diluted in pH 9.6 0.1 M carbonate-bicarbonate buffer) on Nunc Maxisorp plates (Thermo Scientific). The plates were washed with PBS/0.05% Tween (Sigma) and subsequently blocked for 6 hours at 4°C with 100 µl of PBS/1% BSA (Sigma). After washing, the wells were incubated with 50 µl serum 1/50 diluted in PBS/1% BSA/0.05% Tween. The ELISA plates were incubated overnight on ice. Total Ig, IgG1, and IgG2a were detected using HRP-conjugated rabbit anti-mouse Ig antibody (Dako), HRP-conjugated goat anti-mouse IgG2a, HRP-conjugated goat anti-mouse IgG2c, HRP-conjugated goat anti-mouse IgG1 (all from Southern Biotec) or HRP-conjugated rabbit anti-human IgG (Dako). HRP enzyme activity was visualized using ABTS. As a standard, serial dilutions of a pooled serum sample from mice with CIA were used.

Detection of Anti-CarP antibodies by immunoblotting

Equal amounts of FCS and Ca-FCS were loaded onto Hybond-C Extra membranes (Amersham). Blots were blocked for 1 hour with PBS/3% milk powder (ELK)/0.05% Tween for 1 hour at room temperature. The blots were washed six times with PBS/0.05% Tween. Serum from immunized C57Bl/6 mice was diluted 1:200 with PBS/3% ELK/0.05% Tween. The blots were incubated with diluted serum for 1 hour at room temperature. After six washes with PBS/0.05% Tween, blots were incubated with HRP-labeled goat anti-mouse IgG2c diluted in PBS/3% ELK/0.05% Tween for 1 hour at room temperature. Next, blots were washed and bound antibodies were visualized using enhanced chemiluminescence (Amersham).

Statistical analysis

All statistical testing was performed using Prism 5 (GraphPad Software). Outliers were determined using the Grubbs' test and excluded from the data analysis. Different groups of mice were compared using a Mann-Whitney U test. When multiple groups were compared a Kruskal-Wallis test was used followed by a Dunn's Multiple comparison test. Anti-CarP antibody levels over time were compared by calculating the area under the curve for each mouse, followed by a Mann-Whitney U test.

Results

Anti-Carp antibodies can be detected in mice

To detect anti-CarP antibodies, we developed an ELISA similar to the human anti-CarP antibody ELISA described previously [14]. Since we did not know whether mouse serum contained anti-CarP antibodies and which carbamylated proteins these antibodies would recognize, we opted to use a pool of different carbamylated antigens. It was important that this pool of antigens did not contain the antigen that was used for immunization, because this would make it difficult to determine the difference in antibody levels against the carbamylated and the non-carbamylated form of the protein. For these reasons, FCS was carbamylated (Ca-FCS) and used to coat the ELISA plates. Non-modified FCS was always included as a control to determine how much of the signal detected in the Ca-FCS coated well was specific to carbamylated proteins. As shown in figure 1B, serum from mice with CIA contains immunoglobulin's (Ig) that bind to Ca-FCS but not to non-modified FCS, indicating, for the first time, the presence of antibodies that specifically recognize carbamylated proteins in mice with CIA.

To further confirm the specificity of binding of these antibodies, we pre-incubated mouse serum containing anti-CarP antibodies with different concentrations of Ca-FCS and non-modified FCS. Following pre-incubation of the serum we performed an anti-CarP antibody ELISA. Pre-incubation with increasing concentrations of Ca-FCS blocked binding to Ca-FCS in a dose dependent manner, while pre-incubation of the sera with FCS did not affect the Ca-FCS binding (Figure 1C).

To further confirm the specificity of the antibodies using a different assay, we next tested the specificity of the antibodies by immunoblotting. Equal amounts of Ca-FCS and non-modified FCS were blotted on a nitrocellulose membrane. The presence of reactive antibodies in mouse sera was analyzed by incubating these blots with sera of four different immunized mice. On three out of four blots substrate developed on the location where Ca-FCS was blotted, but not on the location where FCS was blotted, indicating that serum from three out of four mice harbored antibodies specific for Ca-FCS (Figure 1D). The dot blot results were further reproduced with sera from an independent immunization experiment (data not shown). All tested serum samples that were positive in ELISA were also positive in these immunoblotting experiments. Together, these data indicate that anti-CarP antibodies are present in mice with CIA, and that their

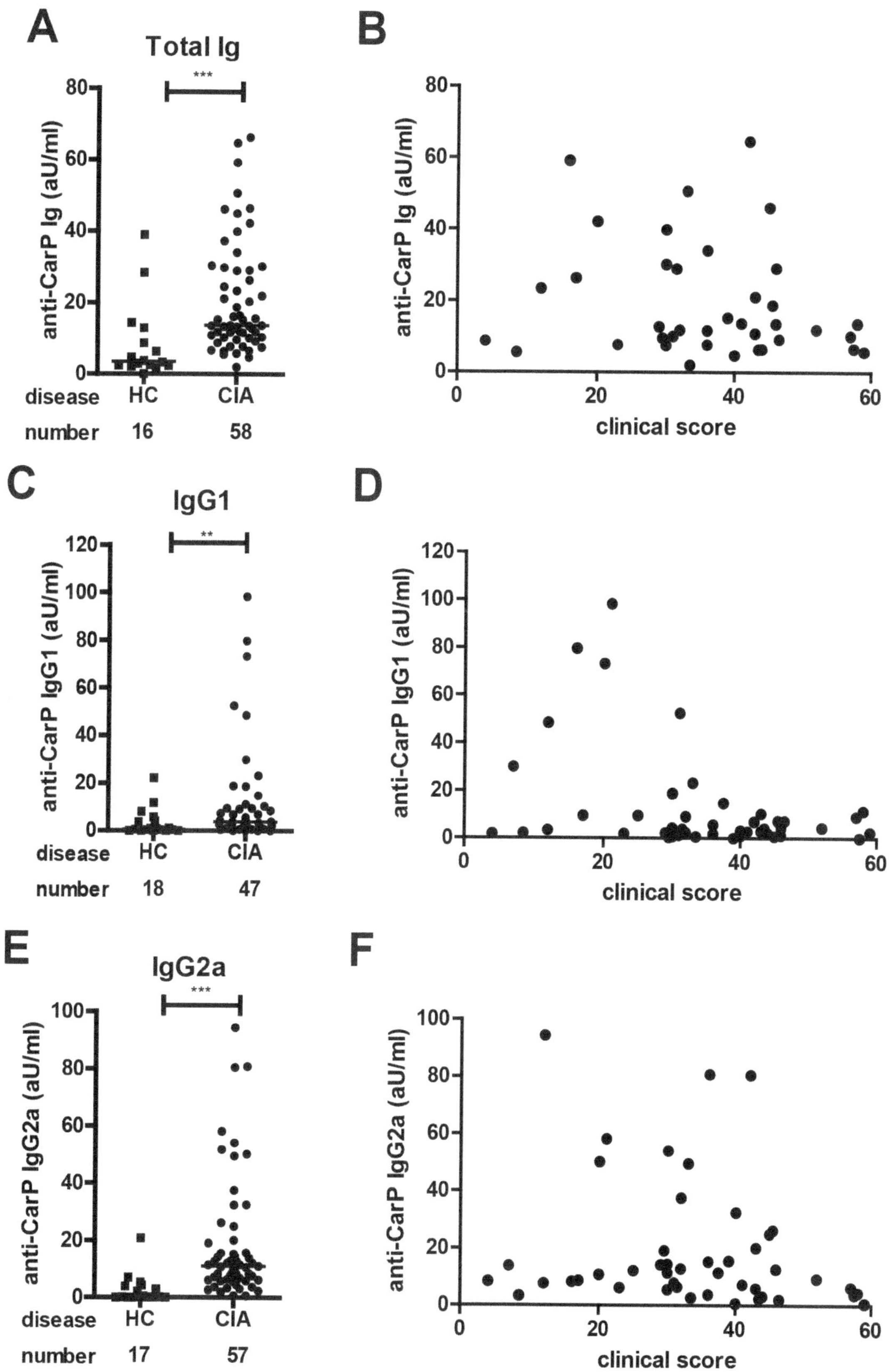

Figure 2. Mice with CIA harbor anti-CarP antibodies. CIA was induced in DBA/1J mice. After 70–90 days, serum of naïve non-immunized mice (HC; squares) and mice with CIA (dots) was harvested and anti-CarP levels were determined by ELISA. Arbitrary units were calculated using a standard curve of pooled serum from mice with CIA. The number indicates the number of mice per group. (**A**) Total Ig levels (**B**) Total Ig levels plotted against the clinical score (**C**) IgG1 levels (**D**) IgG1 levels plotted against the clinical score (**E**) IgG2a levels (**F**) IgG2a levels plotted against the clinical score. The

data is pooled data from 4 independent experiments. Every symbol represents one mouse and the bar indicates the median. Statistical analysis was performed using a Mann-Whitney test (** p<0.01, *** p<0.001).

appearance does not require immunization with specific carbamylated antigens.

Different isotypes of anti-CarP antibodies, but no ACPA, can be detected in mice with CIA

To determine whether the presence of anti-CarP antibodies in mice is related to arthritis, we compared anti-CarP antibody levels in the sera of mice with CIA and healthy non-immunized mice. Anti-CarP total Ig, IgG1 and IgG2a could be detected in mice with CIA, but not in non-immunized mice (Figure 2).

We did not detect any antibodies that recognized citrullinated FCS in sera from healthy non-immunized mice or mice with CIA, indicating that there are no ACPA present in these sera (Figure 3). ACPA positive RA serum samples were used as a positive control in the ACPA ELISA. A validation experiment demonstrating the effectiveness of this method for detecting ACPA in CCP+ patient samples is depicted in Figure S1. These results are important as they indicate that mouse B cells discriminate between proteins containing homocitrulline and citrulline and they demonstrate it is unlikely that the reactivity towards carbamylated proteins we detect is caused by cross reactivity of ACPA.

Taken together, these results show that mice with CIA have different isotypes of anti-CarP antibodies, which we could not detect in healthy mice. Furthermore, the occurrence of isotype switching indicates a role for T cell help in the anti-CarP antibody response.

The development of antibodies specific for carbamylated protein precedes disease onset in CIA

After establishing that anti-CarP antibodies are present in CIA, we next investigated whether there was a relation between anti-CarP antibody levels and disease. We first studied the kinetics of the development of the anti-CarP antibody response. CIA was induced in DBA/1J mice and the mice were bled at different time points to monitor the development of the anti-CarP antibody response over time. From day 14 after immunization onwards, anti-CarP antibodies could be detected in the sera. The anti-CarP antibody levels increased until day 21 after immunization after which the anti-CarP antibody levels stabilized (Figure 4A). We observed an increase in serum anti-CarP antibodies before the onset of clinical symptoms (Figure 4B). We did not find a correlation between anti-CarP levels and the clinical score (Figure 2).

CII-specific IgG2a antibodies are important in the pathogenesis of CIA and their levels correlate with disease severity. Therefore, we compared CII-specific IgG2a levels with anti-CarP antibody levels. We did not find a correlation between the two antibody responses (data not shown). Together, these data indicate that the onset of clinical symptoms in CIA is preceded by an increase in serum anti-CarP antibody levels.

Anti-CarP antibodies can be present independent of CIA

Because the incidence of CIA is >95% in DBA/1J mice, it is not feasible to determine whether development of anti-CarP antibody responses is specific for mice with arthritis/mice that will develop arthritis after immunization with CII in CFA. The CIA incidence is lower in C57Bl/6 mice. To study whether anti-CarP antibodies are specific for mice with CIA upon vaccination with CII in CFA, we next induced CIA in C57Bl/6 mice. In 2 independent experiments, anti-CarP IgG2c antibody levels could be detected in a proportion of the immunized C57Bl/6 mice; however their presence did not correlate with disease induction. Some immunized mice that did not develop CIA did also harbor anti-CarP antibodies. Similar to what we showed for DBA/1J mice (Figure 2), not all mice that developed CIA had detectable levels of anti-CarP antibodies indicating that the presence of anti-CarP antibodies in the circulation is not required for disease induction (Figure S2). Similar to what was observed for DBA/1J

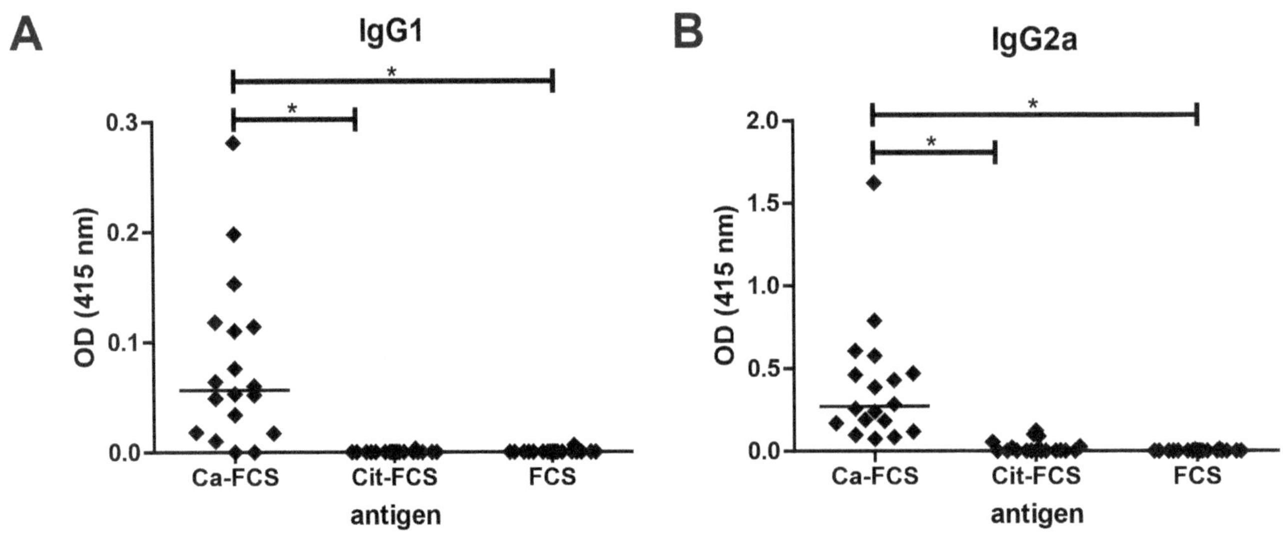

Figure 3. Anti-citrullinated protein antibodies (ACPA) could not be detected in mice with CIA. CIA was induced in DBA/1J mice. After 70–90 days, serum was harvested and anti-CarP and ACPA levels were determined by ELISA. Every symbol represents an individual mice and the line indicates the median. (**A**) IgG1 levels. (**B**) IgG2a levels. Statistical analysis was performed using a kruskall-wallis test followed by a Dunn's Multiple comparison test (* p<0.05).

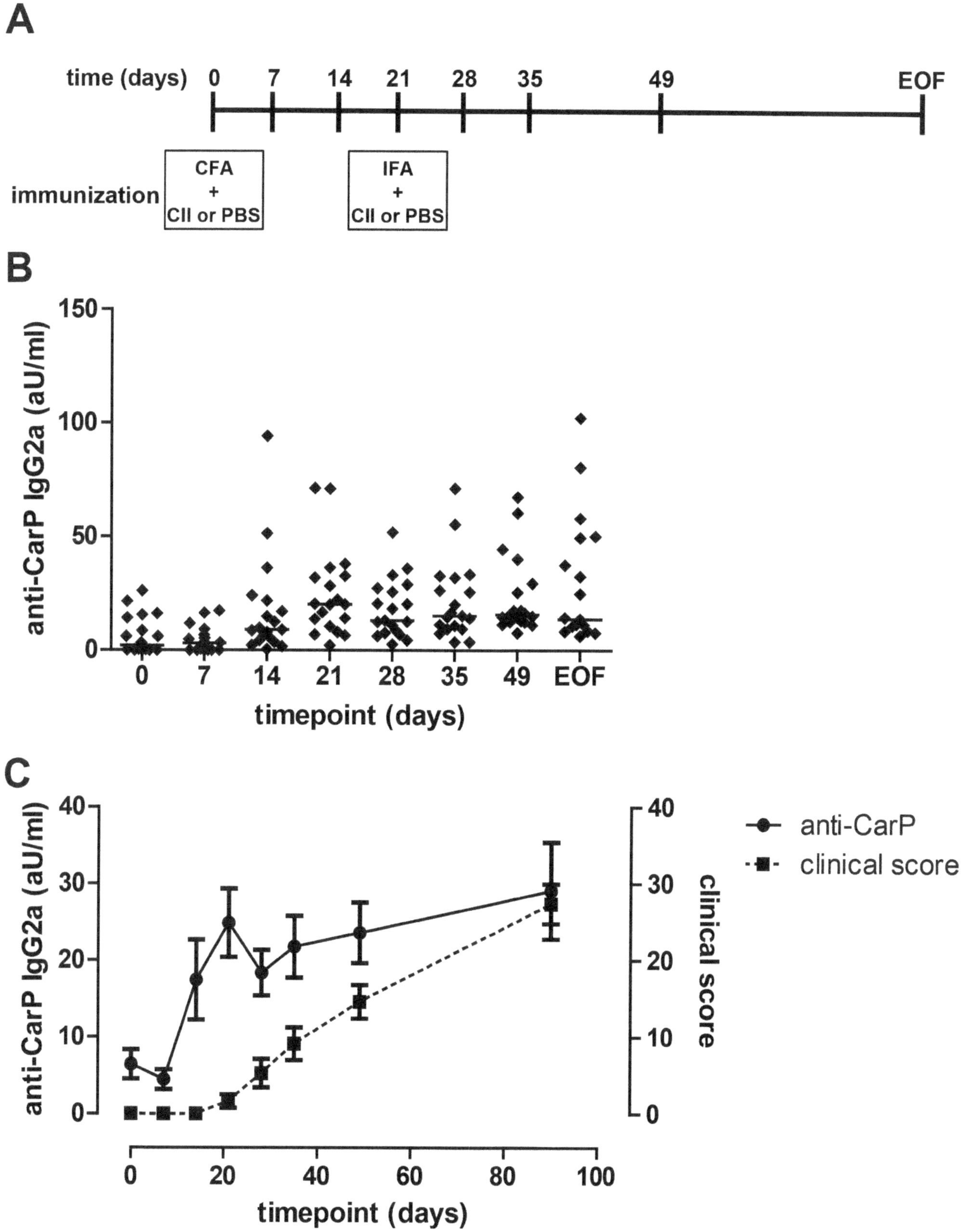

Figure 4. Kinetics of the anti-CarP response during CIA. (**A**) CIA was induced in DBA/1J mice (n = 19). The mice were immunized at day 0 and boosted at day 21. Blood was harvested from the mice at the indicated time points and serum was stored at −80. The anti-CarP antibody levels were determined in all serum samples simultaneously by ELISA at the end of the experiment. The data shown are the pooled data from 2 independent experiments that showed a similar trend. (**B**) Anti-CarP IgG2a levels were determined by ELISA. Arbitrary units were calculated using a standard curve

of pooled serum from mice with CIA. Every symbol represents one individual mouse and the line indicates the median. **(C)** Anti-CarP IgG2a antibody levels are plotted on the left Y axes and indicated by the dots with the solid line. The clinical score is plotted on the right Y-axis and indicated by the squares and the dashed line. The error bars indicate the SEM.

mice, we did not find a correlation between disease severity and clinical score (data not shown).

As we observed the presence of anti-CarP antibodies also in mice that did not develop arthritis and since immunization with CFA causes local inflammation, combined with the notion that inflammation can induce carbamylation [12,13], we hypothesized that immunization of mice with CFA without an additional antigen can be sufficient for the induction of anti-CarP antibodies. To study this notion we determined anti-CarP antibody levels in DBA/1J mice that were immunized with CFA only (followed by a boost with IFA). We detected high levels of anti-CarP in three of these nine mice. Nonetheless, the anti-CarP antibody levels in mice with CIA increased earlier as compared to the CFA immunized mice. Over the course of the first 50 days after immunization the mice with CIA displayed significantly higher levels of anti-CarP as compared to CFA only immunized mice (Figure 5). Altogether these data indicate that immunization with CFA can lead to the induction of anti-CarP antibodies, however, the kinetics are different and magnitude of response is lower as compared to mice with CIA. More importantly, these data indicate that the induction of anti-CarP antibody responses is not directly related to arthritis or vaccination with specific carbamylated antigens, but instead, suggest that an inflammatory trigger can also lead to a break of B cell tolerance to carbamylated proteins.

Discussion

A cornerstone of modern biomedical research is the use of mouse models to explore basic pathophysiological mechanisms. A key characteristic of one of the most common autoimmune diseases, rheumatoid arthritis, is the occurrence of antibody systems against post-translationally modified proteins. We now show that the mechanisms behind breaking of tolerance against post-translationally modified proteins, and in particular anti-Carp antibodies, can be studied in an animal model of arthritis. CIA is a mouse model of arthritis that shares several characteristics with RA and which is frequently used to study potential therapeutic strategies for RA [18,19]. Antibodies play a key role in the disease pathogenesis of CIA [20]. Because of the importance of antibodies in CIA, this model is an interesting tool to further study anti-CarP antibody responses. In this study we show for the first time that, like in patients with RA, anti-CarP antibodies can also be detected in a proportion of the mice with CIA, however anti-CarP positivity does not necessarily correlate with arthritis, as we also detect the presence of anti-CarP antibodies in mice without arthritis.

In a previous study it has been reported that anti-CarP antibodies could be present in mice after immunization with CFA and a specific carbamylated peptide [16], but we now demonstrate that anti-CarP antibodies are readily detectable when mice are immunized with an emulsion of CFA and non-modified proteins (eg. the commercially available CII which is used for CIA induction). We show that immunization with CFA alone (without CII) can induce anti-CarP antibodies as well. Although we cannot exclude the possibility that CFA contains some proteins that are, at least partially carbamylated, our data indicate that there is no need to immunize with extensively carbamylated proteins or carbamylated peptides to breach B cell tolerance leading to the emergence of anti-CarP antibody responses. We consider it likely that anti-CarP-Immune responses can occur resulting from inflammatory conditions induced by for example infection, as it is conceivable that such conditions lead to the carbamylation of pathogen-derived proteins or self-proteins.

We have detected different anti-CarP isotypes and subclasses. For most B cell responses T cell help, in the form of cytokines and CD40-CD40L ligation, is required for isotype switching to occur [21]. Therefore, the fact that isotype switching occurs indicates a role for T cell help in the anti-CarP antibody response.

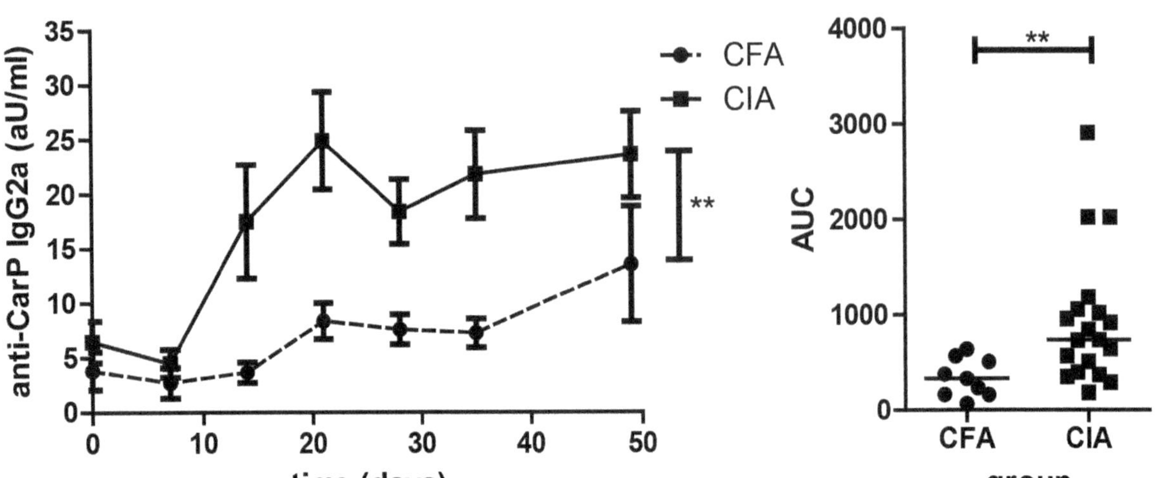

Figure 5. Anti-CarP can be detected in CFA immunized mice. DBA/1J were immunized with CII (CIA; (n = 19)) or PBS in CFA followed by a booster with CII or PBS in IFA (CFA; n = 9). Anti-CarP IgG2a levels were determined by ELISA. The data shown are the pooled data from 2 independent experiments that showed a similar trend. CFA +PBS immunized mice are depicted as circles and CIA mice are depicted as squares. The error bars indicate the SEM. In the right panel the area under curve is depicted. Every symbol represents one individual mouse and the line indicates the median. Statistical analysis was performed by comparing the area under the curve followed by a Mann-Whitney test (** $p<0.01$).

It was recently shown that ELISA can give false positive results when determining ACPA levels in mouse serum and it was suggested that immunoblotting represents a more reliable technique [10]. To exclude the possibility that we obtained false positive results in the anti-CarP antibody ELISA, we also verified the specificity of the antibodies by dot blot. In these assay's we only detected binding to Ca-FCS and not to FCS confirming the results obtained by ELISA. Since the immunoblotting assays and the ELISA gave similar results, we used ELISA for all the other experiments because it is a more high-throughput method and it allows for more reliable quantification. To further show the specificity of the anti-CarP antibodies we performed inhibition assays. Pre-incubation of the sera from mice with CIA with increasing concentrations of Ca-FCS could block Ca-FCS binding in the ELISA, while pre-incubation with non-modified FCS had no effect. The increased binding of sera to Ca-FCS cannot be explained by differences in the amount of protein that was coated on the ELISA plate. Experiments with Ca-OVA and non-modified OVA revealed that carbamylated proteins are not binding better to ELISA plates (data not shown).

Although citrullinated FCS can readily be used to demonstrate the presence of ACPA in human anti-CCP positive sera (Figure S1) we could not demonstrate the presence of ACPA in the context of the study presented. Mice with CIA can have citrullinated antigens in their inflamed tissue [9], however, no ACPA could be detected in mice with CIA indicating that the B cell tolerance to citrullinated antigens was not broken in our experiments. Nonetheless, we detected the presence of anti-CarP antibodies in most arthritic mice analyzed indicating that B cell tolerance to carbamylated antigens is broken more easily as compared to the B cell tolerance to citrullinated antigens. Whether carbamylated proteins are present in arthritic tissue will have to be addressed in future studies.

The appearance of anti-CarP antibodies in the serum before disease onset is similar to what we have found in patients [22]. Anti-CarP antibodies can be detected in serum of arthralgia patients before the onset of RA [15]. The observations that a large part of the mice with CIA harbor anti-CarP antibodies, that these antibodies precede the onset of clinical disease and that anti-CarP antibodies can be found in non-arthritic mice, nicely recapitulates the current findings in humans.

We did not find a correlation between anti-CarP levels and clinical score in our mice. However, this could be explained by the fact that the clinical score predominantly monitors the level of inflammation. Furthermore, in RA patient samples we did also not detect a correlation with the inflammation, but only with radiographic damage [14]. This issue can potentially be addressed in future studies using micro-CT imaging.

The onset of the anti-CarP antibody response during CIA is more or less similar to what has been reported for the onset of the anti-CII antibody response, since both antibodies can already be detected 2 weeks after immunization [23]. However, while anti-CII antibody levels still increase after 21 days [23], the anti-CarP antibody levels did not. Together, these findings indicate that the kinetics of the anti-CarP response are different from the anti-CII response.

Not all mice that develop CIA had detectable levels of anti-CarP antibodies in their serum, indicating that unlike CII-specific antibodies, anti-CarP antibodies are not required for disease induction. We could also detect anti-CarP antibodies in serum of immunized C57Bl/6 mice that did not develop CIA and in DBA/1J mice that were immunized with CFA (without CII). Similar observations have been made for anti-CII antibodies in C57Bl/6 mice, where after immunization all mice had anti-CII antibodies, however not all mice developed arthritis [24]. Since anti-CII antibodies are considered to be pathogenic, but can be present in non-arthritic immunized mice, the presence of anti-CarP antibodies in non-arthritic mice does not exclude the possibility that anti-CarP antibodies can play a role in disease pathogenesis as well. The potential pathogenicity of anti-CarP antibodies will have to be addressed in future studies with e.g. anti-CarP monoclonal antibodies in a similar fashion as has been described before for ACPA [7,10].

In conclusion our results indicate that immunization with CFA can lead to a break in tolerance to carbamylated antigens, resulting in the induction of a specific antibody response and that this anti-CarP antibody response is stronger in mice with arthritis compared to immunized control mice. The presence of anti-CarP antibodies in CIA indicates that the CIA model could function as an in vivo model to study anti-CarP responses.

Supporting Information

Figure S1 Citrullinated-FCS can be used to detect anti-CCP in human sera. Human sera was divided in 2 groups based on the anti-CCP status. The anti-Cit-FCS Ig levels were determined by ELISA. Every symbol represents 1 serum sample and the line indicates the median.

Figure S2 Anti-CarP antibody levels in C57Bl/6 mice. CIA was induced in C57Bl/6 mice in two independent experiments. After 70–90 days, serum of naïve non-immunized mice (squares) and immunized mice that did not develop CIA (dots) and immunized mice that developed CIA (diamonds) was harvested and anti-CarP levels were determined by ELISA. The left panel shows the first experiment and the right panel shows the second experiment.

Author Contributions

Conceived and designed the experiments: JNS BSL DTSLJ JS LAT REMT. Performed the experiments: JNS BSL DTSLJ JS. Analyzed the data: JNS BSL DTSLJ JS MH TWJH LAT REMT. Wrote the paper: JNS MH TWJH LAT REMT.

References

1. Firestein GS (2003) Evolving concepts of rheumatoid arthritis. Nature 423: 356–361.
2. Silman AJ, Pearson JE (2002) Epidemiology and genetics of rheumatoid arthritis. Arthritis Res 4 Suppl 3: S265–272.
3. Klareskog L, Ronnelid J, Lundberg K, Padyukov L, Alfredsson L (2008) Immunity to citrullinated proteins in rheumatoid arthritis. Annu Rev Immunol 26: 651–675.
4. Aletaha D, Neogi T, Silman AJ, Funovits J, Felson DT, et al. (2010) 2010 rheumatoid arthritis classification criteria: an American College of Rheumatology/European League Against Rheumatism collaborative initiative. Ann Rheum Dis 69: 1580–1588.
5. Clavel C, Nogueira L, Laurent L, Iobagiu C, Vincent C, et al. (2008) Induction of macrophage secretion of tumor necrosis factor alpha through Fcgamma receptor IIa engagement by rheumatoid arthritis-specific autoantibodies to citrullinated proteins complexed with fibrinogen. Arthritis Rheum 58: 678–688.
6. Trouw LA, Haisma EM, Levarht EW, van der Woude D, Ioan-Facsinay A, et al. (2009) Anti-cyclic citrullinated peptide antibodies from rheumatoid arthritis patients activate complement via both the classical and alternative pathways. Arthritis Rheum 60: 1923–1931.
7. Kuhn KA, Kulik L, Tomooka B, Braschler KJ, Arend WP, et al. (2006) Antibodies against citrullinated proteins enhance tissue injury in experimental autoimmune arthritis. J Clin Invest 116: 961–973.

8. Uysal H, Bockermann R, Nandakumar KS, Sehnert B, Bajtner E, et al. (2009) Structure and pathogenicity of antibodies specific for citrullinated collagen type II in experimental arthritis. J Exp Med 206: 449–462.
9. Vossenaar ER, Nijenhuis S, Helsen MM, van der Heijden A, Senshu T, et al. (2003) Citrullination of synovial proteins in murine models of rheumatoid arthritis. Arthritis Rheum 48: 2489–2500.
10. Cantaert T, Teitsma C, Tak PP, Baeten D (2013) Presence and role of anti-citrullinated protein antibodies in experimental arthritis models. Arthritis Rheum 65: 939–948.
11. Shi J, van Veelen PA, Mahler M, Janssen GM, Drijfhout JW, et al. (2014) Carbamylation and antibodies against carbamylated proteins in autoimmunity and other pathologies. Autoimmun Rev 13: 225–230.
12. Sirpal S (2009) Myeloperoxidase-mediated lipoprotein carbamylation as a mechanistic pathway for atherosclerotic vascular disease. Clin Sci (Lond) 116: 681–695.
13. Wang Z, Nicholls SJ, Rodriguez ER, Kummu O, Horkko S, et al. (2007) Protein carbamylation links inflammation, smoking, uremia and atherogenesis. Nat Med 13: 1176–1184.
14. Shi J, Knevel R, Suwannalai P, van der Linden MP, Janssen GM, et al. (2011) Autoantibodies recognizing carbamylated proteins are present in sera of patients with rheumatoid arthritis and predict joint damage. Proc Natl Acad Sci U S A 108: 17372–17377.
15. Shi J, van de Stadt LA, Levarht EW, Huizinga TW, Toes RE, et al. (2013) Anti-carbamylated protein antibodies are present in arthralgia patients and predict the development of rheumatoid arthritis. Arthritis Rheum 65: 911–915.
16. Mydel P, Wang Z, Brisslert M, Hellvard A, Dahlberg LE, et al. (2010) Carbamylation-dependent activation of T cells: a novel mechanism in the pathogenesis of autoimmune arthritis. J Immunol 184: 6882–6890.
17. van Duivenvoorde LM, Han WG, Bakker AM, Louis-Plence P, Charbonnier LM, et al. (2007) Immunomodulatory dendritic cells inhibit Th1 responses and arthritis via different mechanisms. J Immunol 179: 1506–1515.
18. Bevaart L, Vervoordeldonk MJ, Tak PP (2010) Evaluation of therapeutic targets in animal models of arthritis: how does it relate to rheumatoid arthritis? Arthritis Rheum 62: 2192–2205.
19. Kollias G, Papadaki P, Apparailly F, Vervoordeldonk MJ, Holmdahl R, et al. (2011) Animal models for arthritis: innovative tools for prevention and treatment. Ann Rheum Dis 70: 1357–1362.
20. Burkhardt H, Koller T, Engstrom A, Nandakumar KS, Turnay J, et al. (2002) Epitope-specific recognition of type II collagen by rheumatoid arthritis antibodies is shared with recognition by antibodies that are arthritogenic in collagen-induced arthritis in the mouse. Arthritis Rheum 46: 2339–2348.
21. Weinstein JS, Hernandez SG, Craft J (2012) T cells that promote B-Cell maturation in systemic autoimmunity. Immunol Rev 247: 160–171.
22. Shi J, van de Stadt LA, Levarht EW, Huizinga TW, Hamann D, et al. (2013) Anti-carbamylated protein (anti-CarP) antibodies precede the onset of rheumatoid arthritis. Ann Rheum Dis.
23. Terato K, Hasty KA, Cremer MA, Stuart JM, Townes AS, et al. (1985) Collagen-induced arthritis in mice. Localization of an arthritogenic determinant to a fragment of the type II collagen molecule. J Exp Med 162: 637–646.
24. Backlund J, Li C, Jansson E, Carlsen S, Merky P, et al. (2013) C57BL/6 mice need MHC class II Aq to develop collagen-induced arthritis dependent on autoreactive T cells. Ann Rheum Dis 72: 1225–1232.

Permissions

All chapters in this book were first published in PLOS ONE, by The Public Library of Science; hereby published with permission under the Creative Commons Attribution License or equivalent. Every chapter published in this book has been scrutinized by our experts. Their significance has been extensively debated. The topics covered herein carry significant findings which will fuel the growth of the discipline. They may even be implemented as practical applications or may be referred to as a beginning point for another development.

The contributors of this book come from diverse backgrounds, making this book a truly international effort. This book will bring forth new frontiers with its revolutionizing research information and detailed analysis of the nascent developments around the world.

We would like to thank all the contributing authors for lending their expertise to make the book truly unique. They have played a crucial role in the development of this book. Without their invaluable contributions this book wouldn't have been possible. They have made vital efforts to compile up to date information on the varied aspects of this subject to make this book a valuable addition to the collection of many professionals and students.

This book was conceptualized with the vision of imparting up-to-date information and advanced data in this field. To ensure the same, a matchless editorial board was set up. Every individual on the board went through rigorous rounds of assessment to prove their worth. After which they invested a large part of their time researching and compiling the most relevant data for our readers.

The editorial board has been involved in producing this book since its inception. They have spent rigorous hours researching and exploring the diverse topics which have resulted in the successful publishing of this book. They have passed on their knowledge of decades through this book. To expedite this challenging task, the publisher supported the team at every step. A small team of assistant editors was also appointed to further simplify the editing procedure and attain best results for the readers.

Apart from the editorial board, the designing team has also invested a significant amount of their time in understanding the subject and creating the most relevant covers. They scrutinized every image to scout for the most suitable representation of the subject and create an appropriate cover for the book.

The publishing team has been an ardent support to the editorial, designing and production team. Their endless efforts to recruit the best for this project, has resulted in the accomplishment of this book. They are a veteran in the field of academics and their pool of knowledge is as vast as their experience in printing. Their expertise and guidance has proved useful at every step. Their uncompromising quality standards have made this book an exceptional effort. Their encouragement from time to time has been an inspiration for everyone.

The publisher and the editorial board hope that this book will prove to be a valuable piece of knowledge for researchers, students, practitioners and scholars across the globe.

List of Contributors

Lucie Brosseau, Gino De Angelis, Laurianne Loew, Christine Smith, Judy King and Stéphane Poitras
School of Rehabilitation Sciences, Faculty of Health Sciences, University of Ottawa, Ottawa, Ontario, Canada

Prinon Rahman
Department of Community Health and Epidemiology, Dalhousie University, Halifax, Nova Scotia, Canada

Karine Toupin-April
Centre for Global Health, Institute of Population Health, Ottawa, Ontario, Canada

Gail Paterson
The Arthritis Society, Ottawa, Ontario, Canada

Lynn Casimiro
School of Rehabilitation Sciences, Faculty of Health Sciences, University of Ottawa, Ottawa, Ontario, Canada
Department of Academic Affairs, Montfort Hospital, Ottawa, Ontario, Canada

Sabrina Cavallo
École de Santé Publique, Université de Montré al, Montré al, Quebec, Canada

Jessica Mc Ewan
University of Ottawa Library, Ottawa, Ontario, Canada

Takashi Matsuo, Masato Mori, Koichiro Ohmura and Tsuneyo Mimori
Department of Rheumatology and Clinical Immunology, Graduate School of Medicine, Kyoto University, Kyoto, Japan

Motomu Hashimoto and Moritoshi Furu
Department of the Control for Rheumatic Diseases, Graduate School of Medicine, Kyoto University, Kyoto, Japan

Takao Fujii
Department of the Control for Rheumatic Diseases, Graduate School of Medicine, Kyoto University, Kyoto, Japan
Department of Rheumatology and Clinical Immunology, Graduate School of Medicine, Kyoto University, Kyoto, Japan

Hiroshi Kawabata
Department of Hematology and Oncology, Graduate School of Medicine, Kyoto University, Kyoto, Japan

Masahide Hamaguchi
Department of Experimental Immunology, Immunology Frontier Research Center, Osaka University, Osaka, Japan

Hiromu Ito
Department of the Control for Rheumatic Diseases, Graduate School of Medicine, Kyoto University, Kyoto, Japan
Department of Orthopedic Surgery, Graduate School of Medicine, Kyoto University, Kyoto, Japan

Chikashi Terao
Center for Genomic Medicine, Graduate School of Medicine, Kyoto University, Kyoto, Japan

Keiichi Yamamoto
Division of Clinical and Epidemiological Database, Department of Information Governance, National Cerebral and Cardiovascular Center, Osaka, Japan

Wataru Yamamoto
Department of the Control for Rheumatic Diseases, Graduate School of Medicine, Kyoto University, Kyoto, Japan
Department of Health Information Management, Kurashiki Sweet Hospital, Kurashiki, Japan

Rossella Menghini, Manfredi Tesauro, Arianna Marino, Valentina Rovella, Giuseppe Rodia and Nicola di Daniele
Department of System Medicine, University of Tor Vergata, Rome, Italy

Umberto Campia
Division of Cardiology, MedStar Heart Institute, Washington, DC, United States of America

Francesca Schinzari and Carmine Cardillo
Department of Internal Medicine, Catholic University Medical School, Rome, Italy

Barbara Tolusso, Angelo Zoli and Gianfranco Ferraccioli
Department of Rheumatology, Catholic University Medical School, Rome, Italy

Massimo Federici
Department of System Medicine, University of Tor Vergata, Rome, Italy
Center for Atherosclerosis, Policlinico Tor Vergata, Rome, Italy

Yang Song, Su-li Wang and Liang-Jing Lu
Department of Rheumatology, Ren Ji Hospital, School of Medicine, Shanghai Jiao Tong University, Shanghai, China,

Li-an Zhu, Lin Leng and Richard Bucala
Department of Medicine, Section of Rheumatology, Yale University School of Medicine, New Haven, Connecticut, United States of America

Fanlei Hu, Yingni Li, Li Zheng, Lianjie Shi, Hongjiang Liu, Xuewu Zhang, Huaqun Zhu, Sumei Tang, Lei Zhu, Liling Xu, Yuqin Yang and Zhanguo Li
Department of Rheumatology and Immunology, Peking University People's Hospital, Beijing, China

Shomi Oka, Hiroshi Furukawa Akiko Komiya, Naoshi Fukui and Shigeto Tohma
Clinical Research Center for Allergy and Rheumatology, Sagamihara Hospital, National Hospital Organization, Sagamihara, Japan

Aya Kawasaki and Naoyuki Tsuchiya
Molecular and Genetic Epidemiology Laboratory, Faculty of Medicine, University of Tsukuba, Tsukuba, Japan

Kota Shimada
Department of Rheumatology, Sagamihara Hospital, National Hospital Organization, Sagamihara, Japan
Department of Rheumatology, Tokyo Metropolitan Tama Medical Center, Fuchu, Japan

Shoji Sugii
Department of Rheumatology, Tokyo Metropolitan Tama Medical Center, Fuchu, Japan

Atsushi Hashimoto
Department of Rheumatology, Sagamihara Hospital, National Hospital Organization, Sagamihara, Japan

Satoshi Ito
Department of Rheumatology, Niigata Rheumatic Center, Shibata, Japan

Tadashi Nakamura
Department of Rheumatology, Kumamoto Shinto General Hospital, Kumamoto, Japan

Koichiro Saisho
Department of Orthopedics/Rheumatology, Miyakonojo Hospital, National Hospital Organization, Miyakonojo, Japan

Shouhei Nagaoka
Department of Rheumatology, Yokohama Minami Kyosai Hospital, Yokohama, Japan

Masao Katayama
Department of Internal Medicine, Nagoya Medical Center, National Hospital Organization, Nagoya, Japan

Shinichiro Tsunoda and Hajime Sano
Division of Rheumatology, Department of Internal Medicine, Hyogo College of Medicine, Nishinomiya, Japan

Kiyoshi Migita
Clinical Research Center, Nagasaki Medical Center, National Hospital Organization, Omura, Japan

Akiko Suda
Department of Rheumatology, Yokohama Minami Kyosai Hospital, Yokohama, Japan
Center for Rheumatic Diseases, Yokohama City University Medical Center, Yokohama, Japan

Christen Lykkegaard Andersen
Department of Hematology, Roskilde University Hospital, Roskilde, Denmark
The Research Unit for General Practice and Section of General Practice, Department of Public Health, University of Copenhagen, Copenhagen, Denmark

Hanne Lindegaard and Peter Junker
Department of Rheumatology, Odense University Hospital, Odense, Denmark

Hanne Vestergaard
Department of Hematology, Odense University Hospital, Odense, Denmark

Volkert Dirk Siersma and Niels de Fine Olivarius
The Research Unit for General Practice and Section of General Practice, Department of Public Health, University of Copenhagen, Copenhagen, Denmark

Hans Carl Hasselbalch
Department of Hematology, Roskilde University Hospital, Roskilde, Denmark

Ole Weis Bjerrum
Department of Hematology, Copenhagen University Hospital, Copenhagen, Denmark

Christian Lood, Helena Tydén, Gunnar Sturfelt, Andreas Jönsen and Anders A. Bengtsson
Department of Clinical Sciences Lund, Section of Rheumatology, Lund University and Skåne University Hospital, Lund, Sweden

Ulla Vogel
National Research Centre for the Working Environment, Copenhagen, Denmark

Birgitta Gullstrand and Lennart Truedsson
Department of Laboratory Medicine Lund, Section of Microbiology, Immunology and Glycobiology, Lund University, Lund, Sweden

Jacob Sode
Clinical Biochemistry, Immunology & Genetics, Statens Serum Institut, Copenhagen, Denmark
Department of Rheumatology, Frederiksberg Hospital, Frederiksberg, Denmark
Institute of Regional Health Research, University of Southern Denmark, Odense, Denmark

Steffen Bank
Department of Medicine, Viborg Regional Hospital, Viborg, Denmark
Biomedicine, University of Aarhus, Aarhus, Denmark

Paal Skytt Andersen
Department of Microbiology and Infection Control, Statens Serum Institut, Copenhagen, Denmark

Marianne Kragh Thomsen
Department of Clinical Microbiology, Aarhus University Hospital, Aarhus, Denmark

Merete Lund Hetland
The DANBIO Registry, Copenhagen Center for Arthritis Research, Center for Rheumatology and Spine Diseases, Glostrup Hospital, Glostrup, Denmark
Department of Clinical Medicine, Faculty of Health and Medical Sciences, University of Copenhagen, Copenhagen, Denmark

Henning Locht
Department of Rheumatology, Frederiksberg Hospital, Frederiksberg, Denmark

Niels H. H. Heegaard
Clinical Biochemistry, Immunology & Genetics, Statens Serum Institut, Copenhagen, Denmark,

Vibeke Andersen
Institute of Regional Health Research, University of Southern Denmark, Odense, Denmark
Department of Medicine, Viborg Regional Hospital, Viborg, Denmark
Organ Center, Hospital of Southern Jutland, Aabenraa, Denmark
OPEN (Odense Patient data Explorative Network), Odense University Hospital, Odense, Denmark

Manuel J. Del Rey, Regina Faré, Alicia Usategui, Abel Suárez-Fueyo and JoséL. Pablos
Servicio de Reumatología, Instituto de Investigación Hospital 12 de Octubre (i+12), Madrid, Spain

Elena Izquierdo and José L. Rodríguez-Fernández
Centro de Investigaciones Biológicas, Consejo Superior de Investigaciones Científicas, Madrid, Spain

Juan D. Cañete
Unitat d'Artritis, Servei de Reumatologia, Hospital Clínic de Barcelona and Institut d'Investigacions Biomédiques August Pí I Sunyer, Barcelona, Spain

Samuel A. Curran, David F. Lappin, Colin A. Murray and Marcello P. Riggio
Dental School, University of Glasgow, Glasgow, United Kingdom

Ivana Hollan
Hospital for Rheumatic Diseases, Lillehammer, Norway, and Feiring Heart Clinic, Feiring, Norway

Clett Erridge
Department of Cardiovascular Sciences, University of Leicester, Glenfield General Hospital, Leicester, United Kingdom

Gunnar Sturfelt
Department of Rheumatology, Lund University Hospital, Lund, Sweden

Knut Mikkelsen
Hospital for Rheumatic Diseases, Lillehammer, Norway

Oystein T. Førre
Department of Rheumatology, Oslo University Hospital, Rikshospitalet, Oslo, Norway

Sven M. Almdahl
Department of Surgery, University Hospital of North Norway, Tromsø, Norway

Magne K. Fagerhol
Department of Immunology and Transfusion Medicine, Ullevaal University Hospital, Oslo, Norway

Carl S. Goodyear
Institute of Infection Immunity and Inflammation, University of Glasgow, Glasgow, United Kingdom

Vesa-Petteri Kouri
Department of Medicine, Institute of Clinical Medicine, University of Helsinki, Helsinki, Finland
Department of Anatomy, Institute of Biomedicine, University of Helsinki, Helsinki, Finland

Juri Olkkonen and Emilia Kaivosoja
Department of Medicine, Institute of Clinical Medicine, University of Helsinki, Helsinki, Finland

Mari Ainola
Department of Medicine, Institute of Clinical Medicine, University of Helsinki, Helsinki, Finland
Department of Medicine/invärtes medicin, Helsinki University Central Hospital, Helsinki, Finland

Juuso Juhila
Research Program of Molecular Neurology and Department of Medical Genetics, Haartman Institute, University of Helsinki, Helsinki, Finland

Iiris Hovatta
Research Program of Molecular Neurology and Department of Medical Genetics, Haartman Institute, University of Helsinki, Helsinki, Finland
Department of Mental Health and Substance Abuse Services, National Institute for Health and Welfare, Helsinki, Finland

YrjöT. Konttinen
Department of Medicine, Institute of Clinical Medicine, University of Helsinki, Helsinki, Finland
Department of Medicine/invärtes medicin, Helsinki University Central Hospital, Helsinki, Finland
ORTON Orthopedic Hospital of the ORTON Foundation, Helsinki, Finland
COXA Hospital for Joint Replacement, Tampere, Finland

Jami Mandelin
Department of Medicine, Institute of Clinical Medicine, University of Helsinki, Helsinki, Finland
Department of Medicine/invärtes medicin, Helsinki University Central Hospital, Helsinki, Finland
ORTON Orthopedic Hospital of the ORTON Foundation, Helsinki, Finland

Adriá Aterido, Sara Marsal, Gabriela Ávila and Antonio Juliá
Rheumatology Research Group, Vall d'Hebron Hospital Research Institute, Barcelona, Spain

Carlos Palacio
Department of Hematology, Hospital Universitari Vall d'Hebron, Barcelona, Spain

Liseth Siemons and Peter M. ten Klooster
Arthritis Center Twente, Department of Psychology, Health & Technology, University of Twente, Enschede, the Netherlands

Harald E. Vonkeman and Mart A. F. J. van de Laar
Arthritis Center Twente, Department of Psychology, Health & Technology, University of Twente, Enschede, the Netherlands
Arthritis Center Twente, Department of Rheumatology, Medisch Spectrum Twente, Enschede, the Netherlands

Cees A. W. Glas
Department of Research Methodology, Measurement and Data Analysis, University of Twente,
Enschede, the Netherlands

Neville Gully , Richard Bright , Victor Marino , Ceilidh Marchant and Mark Bartold
Colgate Australian Clinical Dental Research, School of Dentistry, University of Adelaide, Adelaide, South Australia, Australia

Melissa Cantley and David Haynes
Discipline of Anatomy and Pathology, School of Medical Sciences, University of Adelaide, Adelaide, South Australia, Australia

Catherine Butler, Stuart Dashper and Eric Reynolds
Oral Health Collaborative Research Centre, Melbourne Dental School, The University of Melbourne, Melbourne, Victoria, Australia

Sooah Kim, Jinhua Xuan, Young Hoon Jung and Kyoung Heon Kim
Department of Biotechnology, Korea University Graduate School, Seoul, Republic of Korea

Jiwon Hwang and Hoon-Suk Cha
Samsung Medical Center, Sungkyunkwan University School of Medicine, Seoul, Republic of Korea

Anne C. Bay-Jensen, Claus Christiansen, Morten A. Karsdal, Inger Byrjalsen and Diana J. Leeming
Rheumatology, Nordic Bioscience, Herlev, Denmark

Stephanie Wichuk, Nathalie Morency and Walter P. Maksymowych
Division of Rheumatology, University of Alberta, Edmonton, Alberta, Canada

Amanda Nicholson, Elizabeth Ford, Kevin A. Davies, Helen E. Smith and Jackie Cassell
Division of Primary Care and Public Health, Brighton and Sussex Medical School, Brighton, United Kingdom

Greta Rait and Irene Petersen
Research Department of Primary Care and Population Health, University College London, London, United Kingdom

A. Rosemary Tate
Department of Informatics, University of Sussex, Brighton, United Kingdom

Qin Xiang, Lu Chen, Shengping Hou, Jing Fang, Yan Zhou, Lin Bai, Yunjia Liu and Peizeng Yang
Chongqing Key Laboratory of Ophthalmology and Chongqing Eye Institute; The First Affiliated Hospital of Chongqing Medical University, Chongqing, P. R. China

Aize Kijlstra
University Eye Clinic Maastricht, Maastricht, The Netherlands

Paula B. Donate, Thais A. Fornari and Claudia Macedo
Molecular Immunogenetics Group, Department of Genetics, Faculty of Medicine of Ribeirão Preto, University of São Paulo, Ribeirão Preto, Brazil

Fernando Q. Cunha, Thiago M. Cunha and Daniele C. B. Nascimento
Inflammation and Pain Group, Department of Pharmacology, Faculty of Medicine of Ribeirão Preto, Ribeirão Preto, Brazil

Elza T. Sakamoto-Hojo
Department of Biology, Faculty of Philosophy, Sciences and Letters of Ribeirão Preto, Ribeirão Preto, Brazil

Eduardo A. Donadi
Division of Clinical Immunology, Department of Medicine, Faculty of Medicine of Ribeirão Preto, Ribeirão Preto, Brazil

Geraldo A. Passos
Molecular Immunogenetics Group, Department of Genetics, Faculty of Medicine of Ribeirão Preto, University of São Paulo, Ribeirão Preto, Brazil
Disciplines of Genetics and Molecular Biology, Department of Morphology, Faculty of Dentistry of Ribeirão Preto, Ribeirão Preto, Brazil

Carmen Martínez
Departamento de Biología Celular, Facultad de Medicina, Universidad Complutense de Madrid, Madrid, Spain

Ana M. Ortiz, Amalia Lamana, Rosario García-Vicuña and Isidoro González-Álvaro
Servicio de Reumatología, Hospital Universitario de la Princesa, Instituto de Investigación Sanitaria la Princesa, Madrid, Spain

Yasmina Juarranz, Iria V. Seoane, Javier Leceta and Rosa P. Gomariz
Departamento de Biología Celular, Facultad de Biología, Universidad Complutense de Madrid, Madrid, Spain

Jerome Schlue
Institute for Pathology, Hannover Medical School, Hannover, Germany

Sven Pischke, Anett Gisa, Pothakamuri Venkata Suneetha, Steffen Björn Wiegand, Richard Taubert, Karsten Wursthorn, Heike Bantel, Regina Raupach, Birgit Bremer, Behrend Johann Zacher, Michael Peter Manns, Kinan Rifai and Heiner Wedemeyer
Department of Gastroenterology, Hepatology and Endocrinology, Hannover Medical School, Hannover, Germany

Reinhold Ernst Schmidt and Torsten Witte
Department of Clinical Immunology, Hannover Medical School, Hannover, Germany

Chikashi Terao and Fumihiko Matsuda
Center for Genomic Medicine, Kyoto University Graduate School of Medicine, Kyoto, Japan

Motomu Hashimoto,Hiromu Ito, Takao Fujii and Moritoshi Furu
Department of the Control for Rheumatic Diseases, Kyoto University Graduate School of Medicine, Kyoto, Japan

Shuichiro Nakabo, Koichiro Ohmura, Ran Nakashima, Yoshitaka Imura, Naoichiro Yukawa, Hajime Yoshifuji and Tsuneyo Mimori
Department of Rheumatology and Clinical Immunology, Kyoto University Graduate School of Medicine, Kyoto, Japan

Ming-Chi Lu and Ning-Sheng Lai
Division of Allergy, Immunology and Rheumatology, Dalin Tzu Chi Hospital, Buddhist Tzu Chi Medical Foundation, Chiayi, Taiwan
School of Medicine, Tzu Chi University, Hualien, Taiwan

Shih-Tang Yan
Division of Endocrinology and Metabolism, Dalin Tzu Chi Hospital, Buddhist Tzu Chi Medical Foundation, Chiayi, Taiwan

Wen-Yao Yin
School of Medicine, Tzu Chi University, Hualien, Taiwan
Division of General Surgery, Dalin Tzu Chi Hospital, Buddhist Tzu Chi Medical Foundation, Chiayi, Taiwan

Malcolm Koo
Department of Medical Research, Dalin Tzu Chi Hospital, Buddhist Tzu Chi Medical Foundation, Chiayi, Taiwan
Dalla Lana School of Public Health, University of Toronto, Ontario, Canada

Jon T. Giles and Joan M. Bathon
Division of Rheumatology, Columbia University, College of Physicians and Surgeons, New York, New York, United States of America

Erika Darrah, Felipe Andrade and Antony Rosen
Division of Rheumatology, Johns Hopkins University, Baltimore, Maryland, United States of America

Sonye Danoff and Cheilonda Johnson
Division of Pulmonary and Critical Care Medicine, Johns Hopkins University, Baltimore, Maryland, United States of America

Jeroen N. Stoop, Bi-Sheng Liu, Jing Shi, Diahann T. S. L. Jansen, Tom W. J. Huizinga, Leendert A. Trouw and René E. M. Toes
Department of Rheumatology, Leiden University Medical Center, Leiden, The Netherlands

Martin Hegen
Immunoscience Research Unit, Pfizer Worldwide Research and Development, Cambridge, Massachusetts, United States of America

Index